Role of the Transcriptome in Breast Cancer Prevention

Jose Russo • Irma H. Russo

Role of the Transcriptome in Breast Cancer Prevention

Springer

Jose Russo
Breast Cancer Research Laboratory
Fox Chase Cancer Center
Philadelphia
Pennsylvania, USA

Irma H. Russo
Breast Cancer Research Laboratory
Fox Chase Cancer Center
Philadelphia
Pennsylvania, USA

ISBN 978-1-4614-4883-9 ISBN 978-1-4614-4884-6 (eBook)
DOI 10.1007/978-1-4614-4884-6
Springer New York Heidelberg Dordrecht London

Library of Congress Control Number: 2012947988

Printed on acid-free paper

Springer is part of Springer Science+Business Media (www.springer.com)

We dedicate this book to all my trainees from whom we have received more than they ever have expected to give us. Among them Jwang Ling M.D., Eugene Agnone M.D., Francisco Martinez M.D., Gloria Calaf Ph.D., Daniel R. Ciocca M.D., Lee K. Tay Ph.D., Stephen P. Ethier Ph.D., Gustavo A. Moviglia M.D., Satori Higa M.D., Megan Mills Ph.D., Gustavo Rubio Coronel M.D., Anna Sapino M.D., Fulvio Basolo M.D., Gabriella Fontanini M.D., Josiah Ochieng Ph.D., Muneesh Tewari M.D., Ph.D., Pei-Li Zhang Ph.D., Maria Elena Alvarado M.D., Anthony Magliocco M.D., Teh-Yuan Ho Ph.D., Nandita Sohi Ph.D., Chai Yu-Li M.D., Saad El-Gendy Ph.D., Judith Gordon M.D., Eric G. Thomas D.O., Roupen Yagsessian M.D., Kunle Adesina M.D., Ph.D., Ruth Padmore M.D., Ph.D., Yun-Fu Hu Ph.D., Ana Maria Salicione Ph.D., Betsy Bove Ph.D., Yajue Huang Ph.D., Ismael Dale Cotrin Silva M.D., Ph.D., Abdel-Rahman N. Zekri M.Sc., Ph.D., Xiaoshang Jiang Ph.D., Raquel Angela Silva Soares Lino Ph.D., Hasan M. Lareef M.D., Gabriela Balogh Ph.D., Fathima Sheriff M.D., Sandra Fernandez Ph.D., Johana Vanegas M.D., Raquel Moral Ph.D., Daniel Mailo Ph.D., Ricardo Lopez Ph.D., Julia Pereira Ph.D., Hilal I. Kocdor M.D., Ph.D., Mehmet A. Kocdor M.D., Sylvana Carrea de Noronha Ph.D., Samuel Ribeiro de Noronha Ph.Dc., and Yanrong Su Ph.D.

Acknowledgment

Our special acknowledgment and thanks to *Ms. Patricia A. Russo* for her insightful editorial and stylish suggestions, for her critiques and delightful moments discussing the manuscript and ideas, to *Ms. Rose Sonlin* for verifying the accuracy of the references and the search for not easy to find articles and to *Pathology Consultation Services* from Rydal, PA, that have financed the writing and editing of this book.

Contents

Chapter 1
The Epidemiology of Breast Cancer and the Basis for Prevention

1.1 Introduction

Breast cancer is a heterogeneous and complex disease resulting from the uncontrolled growth of cells that are unique and specific to the breast. The occurrence of cancer of the breast has long been known, as documented in the Edwin Smith surgical papyrus, written between 3000 and 1500 BC [1] (Table 1.1). Although nowadays breast cancer is the malignant disease most frequently diagnosed in postmenopausal Caucasian women born in Northern European countries and in America [2–4], the disease affects women of all races and nationalities. Furthermore, its incidence around the globe is increasing in countries that are industrialized [3], as well as in those that have recently become industrialized [5, 6]. The worldwide incidence of breast cancer has increased 30–40% since the 1970s, reaching a total of 1,383,500 new cases and a mortality of 458,400 cases by 2011 [2, 4, 7].

Although the definitive cause or mechanisms behind initiation of breast cancer, whose knowledge is essential for developing strategies for its prevention, have not been identified, epidemiological, clinical, and pathological studies have uncovered novel aspects regarding the complexity of this disease [8–10]. Among these, the knowledge that age at diagnosis and ethnicity are associated with a specific tumor type and tumor behavior, and that they are in turn differently influenced by a woman's age at the first pregnancy [11, 12], indicate that the global incidence of breast cancer changes over time in relation to geography, race, and changes in lifestyle, suggesting that breast cancer risk is influenced by a multiplicity of still undefined factors.

The task at hand is to identify amongst a multiplicity of still undefined factors which ones are etiologically relevant in breast cancer risk. A common denominator for the risk of developing breast cancer has been found to be a reproductive history [8, 9, 12]. Increased breast cancer incidence and mortality were associated with nulliparity as early as the 1700s, as reported by Bernardino Ramazzini, who attributed the phenomenon to the childlessness of nuns in Italian convents [13]. MacMahon et al. [8] reported that pregnancy exerted a protective effect in women whose first

J. Russo and I.H. Russo, *Role of the Transcriptome in Breast Cancer Prevention*,
DOI 10.1007/978-1-4614-4884-6_1, © Springer Science+Business Media New York 2013

Table 1.1 Landmarks in the history of breast cancer

Year	Landmark discovery or observation
3000–1500 BC	Edwin Smith surgical papyrus describes eight cases of breast cancer in women
1700	Bernardino Ramazzini attributed the high incidence of breast cancer in nuns to their childlessness
1896	Beatson demonstrated that removal of the ovaries caused regression of advanced cancer in young women
1959	Huggins et al. demonstrated in laboratory animals that chemical carcinogens induced mammary cancer in rats, and that removal of the pituitary or the ovaries reduced tumor size
1970	MacMahon et al. reported that pregnancy exerted a protective effect in women whose first child was bore from early teens to the middle 20s
1975	Soule develops the breast cancer cell line MCF-7, which was instrumental for the discovery of the ERα
1978	Russo and Russo establish the concept the mammary gland differentiation induce by full-term pregnancy is the mechanism behind the protective effect against breast cancer

child was born from the early teen years to the middle 20s relative to a risk of 100 for nulliparous women (Table 1.1). Numerous studies have confirmed these results and have additionally reported that multiple pregnancies significantly decrease the risk of developing breast cancer after 50 years of age [8, 9] (Fig. 1.1), whereas postponement of the delivery increases a woman's breast cancer risk, which reaches the same levels observed in nulliparous women when it occurs between 30 and 34 years of age, increasing even further after 35 years [8, 9] (Fig. 1.2). An understanding of the mechanisms that determine whether a pregnancy would prevent breast cancer or would increase its risk requires taking into consideration not only the age at the first pregnancy but also the age at the time of breast cancer diagnosis, which in turn influences the stage and pathological characteristics of the tumors developed [14–16] (Table 1.1).

Pregnancy itself is a complex process that only succeeds when a woman's ovaries are fully functional and secrete estrogen and progesterone, hormones that are essential for the maintenance of pregnancy. The ovaries work under the control of the hypothalamic–pituitary–gonadal (HPG) axis [17, 18], which synchronizes the ovarian secretions with those of pituitary and placental hormones for stimulating breast development in preparation for milk production [18, 19]. Primiparous women younger than 25 years old that have elevated serum levels of hCG during the first trimester of pregnancy have a 33% decrease in risk of breast cancer diagnosis after the age of 50, whereas estrogen concentrations have been positively associated with risk of breast cancer before age 40, supporting the role of this or other pregnancy hormones in the development of breast cancer [12, 20–24] (Table 1.2).

An understanding of the relationship between pregnancy and environmental influences on breast cancer risk requires the use of experimental models that have already contributed to unraveling some of the endocrinological mechanisms mediating cancer prevention when the reproductive event precedes carcinogen exposure

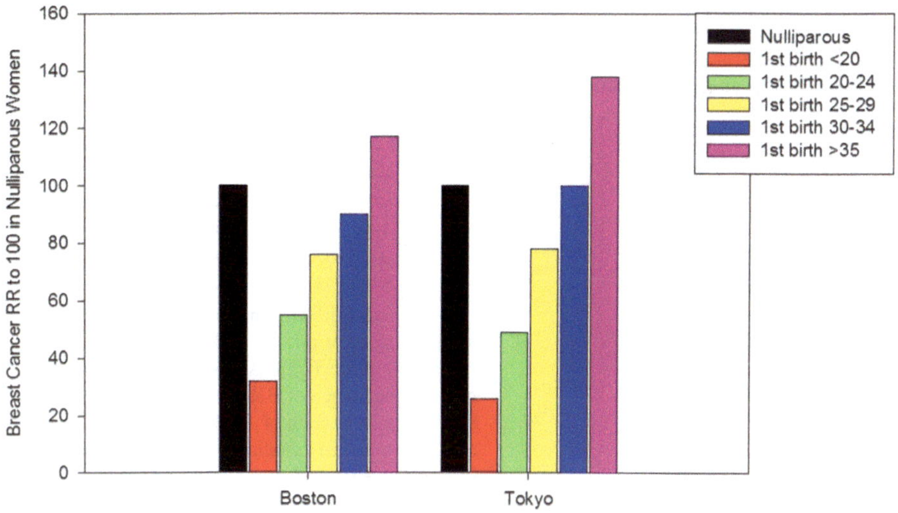

Fig. 1.1 Breast cancer relative risk (RR) by age at first pregnancy. The histogram depicts breast cancer incidence in two out seven different regions of the world (adapted from [8])

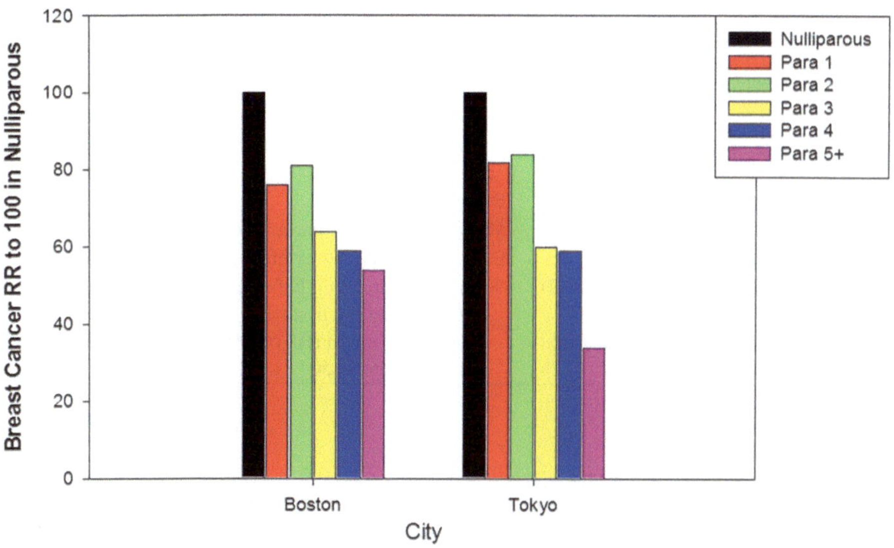

Fig. 1.2 Breast cancer relative risk (RR) by number of pregnancies. The histogram depicts breast cancer incidence in two out seven different regions of the world (adapted from [8])

[22, 25–28], or acts as a promoter of mammary cancer when it is initiated after carcinogen-induced damage has been initiated [29–31]. These models have also contributed to uncover the preventive effects of estrogen on chemically induced carcinogenesis when given alone at a moderate dose to prepubertal rats [32], or as

Table 1.2 Who is at risk in breast cancer today—a modern epidemic

Clinical relevance	Supporting data
Breast cancer as an age-related disease	Sporadic breast cancer: 95% of new cases are sporadic Diagnosed after age 50 in postmenopausal women with no family history of the disease Tend to be of low grade and predominantly estrogen receptor (ER) positive ductal carcinomas Are responsive to antiestrogen and immunotherapy
Breast cancer diagnosis before menopause	Represents ~5% of all cases Diagnosed predominantly in women with positive family history or proven inheritance of deleterious mutations in the TP53, AT, BRCA1 or BRCA2 genes. Inheritance of BRCA1/2 mutations are more frequently in women of Ashkenazi Jew or African ancestries, and in association with cancer diagnosis before age 40 The cancers developed are basal-like triple negative, characterized by absence of ER, progesterone receptor (PR), and Her2, and therefore unresponsive to endocrine or immunotherapy
Pregnancy associated breast cancer (PABC)	Diagnosed during pregnancy or within 1 or 2 years following delivery. PABC has a worse prognosis and more pronounced mortality than breast cancer diagnosed to women with no PABC The hormonal milieu of pregnancy might stimulate the progression of preexisting preneoplastic lesions
Protective effect of first full-term pregnancy from developing breast cancer after menopause	Having first child from early teens to middle 20s (early parity) Breastfeeding Multiparity in early parous women Each additional birth confers greater protection
Human chorionic gonadotropin (hCG)	Women first pregnant before age 25 with high levels of hCG during the first trimester of pregnancy have a 33% decrease in risk of breast cancer diagnosis after the age of 50

therapeutic agents when given in combination with progesterone to carcinogen-exposed rats [33]. Various natural and synthetic hormones have been reported to inhibit the progression of chemically induced mammary cancer in different strains of virgin rats [34] and in mouse models of mammary carcinogenesis [35–37]. The development of genetically engineered mice (GEM) models has greatly contributed to the understanding of gene–environmental interactions, finding that has been reported extensively in excellent publications [38–43], therefore this field will be only summarily addressed in this chapter.

The identification of the specific conditions under which the completion of one pregnancy at early age fully differentiates the breast epithelium and reduces breast cancer risk should serve as a blueprint for understanding the anatomical, physiological, endocrinological, and molecular mechanisms that need to be operational for developing rational strategies for the prevention of breast cancer in future generations. In the present chapter we will first address the strategies utilized in the rodent experimental system, secondly, we will review our knowledge on pregnancy and cancer in women, and lastly, we will address all of the other confounding factors that we need to bear in mind for understanding and solving the complex and fascinating relationships between pregnancy and cancer.

1.2 Rodent Models of Mammary Carcinogenesis

Spontaneous mammary tumors are frequently observed in long-term rodent studies [30, 44]; however, their usefulness for carcinogenicity testing is hindered by the tumors' biological characteristics, such as long latency period, variations in etiologic agents or mechanisms of tumor initiation, and pregnancy dependence in certain strains of mice [45]. The induction of hormone-dependent rat mammary tumors with chemical carcinogens, on the other hand, has become an essential model for testing the carcinogenic potential of specific chemicals, such as 3,4-benzopyrene, 3-methylcholanthrene (MCA) [46] and the polycyclic aromatic hydrocarbon (PAH) 7,12-dimethylbenz(a)anthracene (DMBA) [47], or the alkylating agent *N*-methyl-*N*-nitrosourea (MNU) [48, 49]. Chemically induced tumors developed in mice strains of low spontaneous mammary cancer incidence or in transgenic mice are adenoacanthomas or type B adenocarcinomas that are in general estrogen receptor alpha (ERα) negative [43]. However, in p53 null mice hormonal stimulation by estrogen and/or progesterone or prolactin/progesterone, markedly enhances tumorigenesis, whereas blocking estrogen signaling through ovariectomy or tamoxifen treatment greatly reduces the tumorigenic capability of the mammary epithelium, an indication that normal mammary gland and preneoplastic lesions are responsive to estrogen [43]. The majority of rat mammary tumors induced by DMBA or MNU are ductal adenocarcinomas that are ERα positive and reproduce the pathological features of the most frequent type of adenocarcinomas developed by women [50]. The characteristics of this model have opened a myriad of opportunities for dissecting the initiation, promotion, and progression steps of carcinogenesis and for translating these findings to the human situation [22, 30, 50].

1.3 Windows of Susceptibility to Carcinogenesis

The response of the mammary gland to specific carcinogenic stimuli depends upon the physiologic state of the mammary tree under the control of the endocrine system. The administration of optimal carcinogenic doses to young and sexually mature

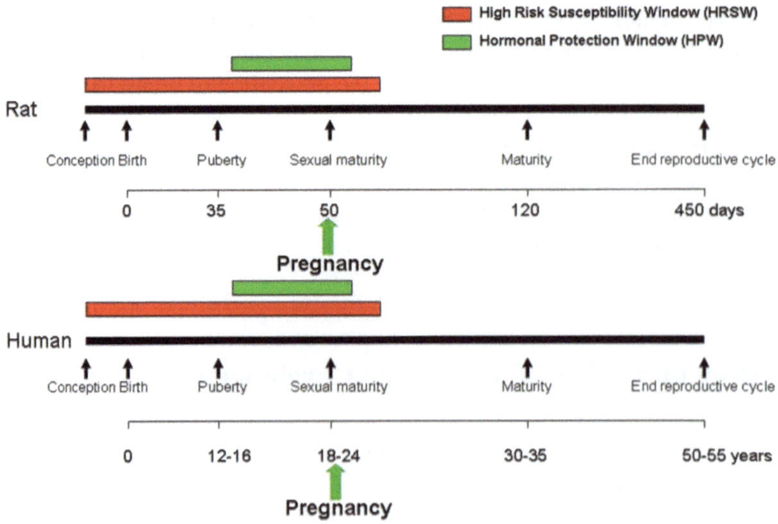

Fig. 1.3 Diagrammatic representation of mammary gland development from conception to the end of reproductive life. In both rats (*upper line*) and humans (*lower line*) the period of life that begins in uterus and persists until sexual maturity, represents a window of greater susceptibility of the mammary gland to be damaged by exogenous carcinogenic stimuli or exposure to endocrine disruptors. The differentiation of the mammary gland induced by pregnancy or the appropriate hormonal treatments needs to occur during the post-pubertal period and before the mammary epithelium has suffered any damage, representing a hormone-driven window of protection that overrides the high risk window. *HRSW* high risk susceptibility window, *red bar*; *HPW* hormonal protection window, *green bar* (from Russo IH, Russo J (2011) Pregnancy-induced changes in breast cancer risk. A review. J Mammary Gland Biol Neoplasia 16:221–233)

virgin rats induces maximal tumorigenic response [29, 30, 46–49]. This period of highest susceptibility of the mammary gland to be transformed by such stimulus represents the "high risk susceptibility window" (HRSW), which encompasses different stages of development, i.e., prenatal life, infancy, puberty, and early adulthood (Fig. 1.3). Thus, in addition to age, the tumorigenic response elicited by carcinogenic agents is modulated by the animal's endocrinological milieu prevailing at the time of exposure, as well as by endocrine and environmental influences occurring during the HRSW [51–54]. The peak of cancer incidence occurring when virgin rats reach the age of 45–55 days and have had at least two ovulatory cycles after vaginal opening [55], represents the response of numerous mammary terminal end buds (TEBs) that are predominantly composed of progenitor mammary stem cells (PMSCs). These cells have been characterized by their size, nuclear-cytoplasmic ratio and euchromatin-heterochromatin ratio, number and distribution of organelles, and proliferative activity [30, 56]. Under normal conditions, PMSCs cells are primed by ovarian hormones for expansion of the mammary parenchyma and lobular formation. Instead, when they are exposed to a carcinogen such as DMBA, the PMSCs exhibit the highest rate of carcinogen uptake and of cell proliferation [30]. Within a few days transformed PMSCs expand and form intraductal proliferations (IDPs) that

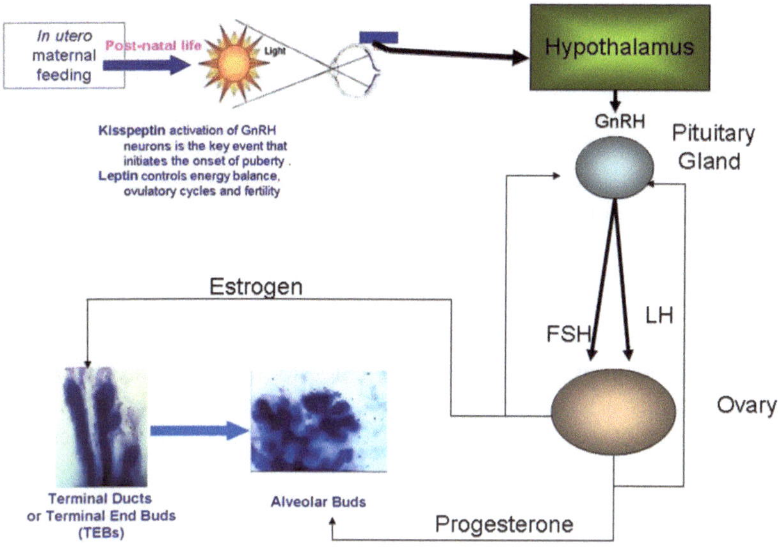

Fig. 1.4 Hypothalamic effect on gland development

progress to ductal carcinomas in situ and invasive, confirming the transition of PMSCs to mammary cancer stem cells (MCSC) under the influence of a carcinogen [56, 57]. Morphologically similar cells have been isolated from DMBA-induced mammary tumors [58]. In the mouse, the mammary gland continually undergoes postnatal developmental changes that are driven by signals from TEBs [59]. They direct ductal growth and elongation, producing a progeny of varied lineages that include luminal and myoepithelial cells under the influence of signals from the local tissue microenvironment [59].

1.4 Prevention of Mammary Cancer by Pregnancy

Under the stimulus of the first pregnancy, the mammary gland that has not been exposed to a carcinogenic insult during the early phases of the HRSW enters into a "hormonal protection window" (HPW). During this period the hormones of pregnancy will block any future damage caused by carcinogens or endocrine disruptors through the induction of mammary gland differentiation [22, 30] (Fig. 1.3). The first pregnancy is an essential step for determining the fate of the mammary gland future cancer risk. Its success depends on timely ovulation, which in turn, is the result of a sequence of neuroendocrine events (Fig. 1.4) triggered within the preoptic area (POA) and the mediobasal hypothalamus by the positive feedback of estrogen secreted by ovarian follicles and metastin (KISS-1), a natural ligand for the G protein-coupled receptor GPR54 [60, 61]. This stimulus induces the surge of gonadotropin releasing hormone (GnRH) and of luteinizing hormone (LH) for triggering ovulation. After oocyte fertilization and implantation, ovarian estrogen, progesterone, and inhibin are supplemented by rat chorionic gonadotropin and rat placental lactogen, hormones synthesized by the developing embryo and the placenta. Jointly they contribute to stimulate the mammary glands to undergo active cell proliferation and differentiation of TEBs to alveolar buds (ABs) and lobules. The contributions of the pituitary hormones prolactin (PRL) that stimulates milk production and oxytocin that enhances the secretory activity of the alveolar cells complete the functional differentiation of the mammary gland [18, 62]. Completion of pregnancy and lactation induce long-lasting structural and genomic changes in the mammary gland of different strains of rats and in mice [33]. These molecular changes ultimately result in a significant reduction in mammary cancer incidence and number of tumors per animal [25–28, 55, 56].

1.5 Prevention of Mammary Cancer by Hormones

In the absence of pregnancy, various natural and synthetic hormones have been shown to prevent the initiation of mammary cancer when they are administered to young virgin rats during the HRSW prior to the exposure to a carcinogen or an endocrine disruptor. Prepubertal administration of 10 μg 17α-estradiol to Sprague–Dawley rats significantly advances the age at vaginal opening, stimulates lobular development of the mammary gland, and reduces the incidence of DMBA-induced tumors [32]. Norethynodrel-Mestranol (NM) administered at a contraceptive and a tenfold higher dose to post-pubertal and sexually mature virgin rats result in long-lasting structural changes in the mammary gland and a dose-dependent reduction in tumor incidence [63]. Daily treatment of virgin Sprague–Dawley rats with hCG at the doses of 1, 5, 10, or 100 IU for 21 days significantly reduces adenocarcinoma incidence and number of adenocarcinomas per animal in a dose-dependent manner [22] (Fig. 1.5). Similarly, treatment with 100 IU hCG daily for 5, 10, or 15 days suffices to induce a significant degree of mammary gland differentiation and protection from cancer initiation [64] (Fig. 1.6). The reduction in cancer incidence resulting from hCG treatment is long-lasting, as demonstrated by the persistent reduction in carcinogenic response to administration of DMBA at 21, 42, or 63 days after termination of the hormonal treatment [22, 26]. In spite of the morphological regression of the mammary gland after cessation of the hormonal treatment, the analysis of mRNA reveals elevated expression of genes involved in the apoptotic pathways, which include testosterone repressed prostate message 2 (TRPM2), interleukin 1β-converting enzyme (ICE), bcl-XL, bcl-XS, p53, p21, and c-myc [65], as well as activation of tumor suppressor activity through upregulation of inhibin A and B [66, 67].

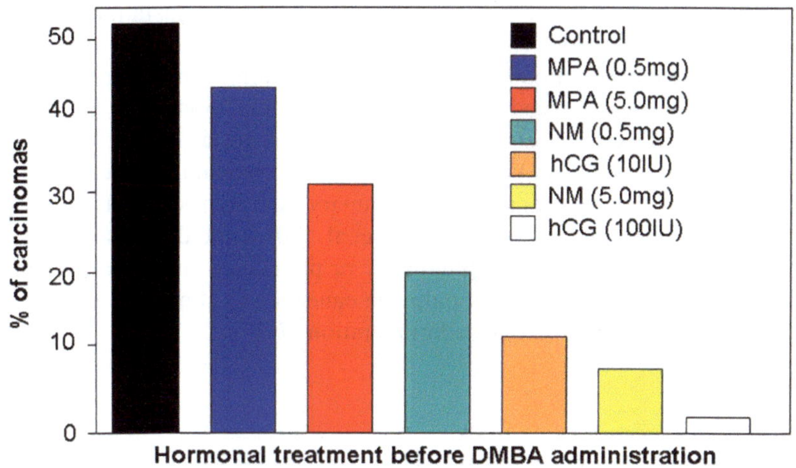

Fig. 1.5 Effect of hormonal treatment before induction of mammary cancer with dimethylbenz(a) anthracene (DMBA)

Fig. 1.6 Treatment of virgin rats with recombinant hCG prevents DMBA-induced mammary carcinogenesis

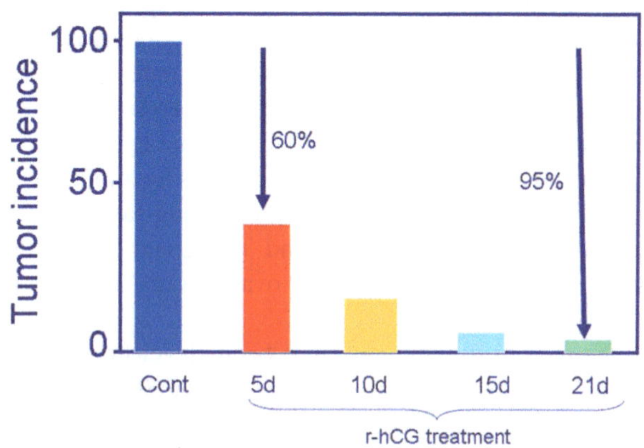

1.6 Effect of Pregnancy on Cancer Progression

It is important to take into consideration the fact that the protective effect of pregnancy or hormones acting during the HPW might be nullified if the mammary gland has been exposed to environmental carcinogens or endocrine disrupting agents before or during the early phases of the HRSW (Fig. 1.3). Pregnancy initiated 15 days after DMBA or MCA feeding [29, 68, 69] induces 100% incidence of mammary carcinomas; the tumors rapidly grow during the gestational period and are maintained by lactation. The nursing stimulus maintains the growth of DMBA-induced rat mammary carcinomas, whereas cessation of nursing causes tumor regression [68]. The enhanced growth of mammary carcinomas by pregnancy has been attributed to increased secretion of estrogen, progesterone, prolactin, placental lactogen, or relaxin [29]. Although all of these hormonal influences might be of importance in promoting the growth of mammary carcinomas, results are inconclusive, and sometimes controversial. Grubbs et al. [70] found decreased cancer incidence in MNU-treated rats after pregnancy or pregnancy and lactation, although the time of appearance of the first palpable cancers was shorter in rats becoming pregnant 10 days after carcinogen administration [70].

1.7 Effect of Hormones on Tumor Progression

The hormone dependence of breast cancer that had been established by Beatson [20] (Table 1.1) was not recognized in laboratory animals until Huggins et al. [46] demonstrated that all 3-MC treated rats exhibited a deep reduction of tumor size after hypophysectomy. Ovariectomy also reduced mammary cancer incidence by 40%; administration of daily injections of 0.1 or 0.2 μg 17β-estradiol increased mammary cancer incidence to 100%, whereas rats receiving 20 μg 17β-estradiol daily had a 70% reduction in incidence. Dihydrotestosterone treatment also decreased tumor size; whereas progesterone or diethylstilbestrol administered to ovariectomized rats increased tumor incidence and enhanced the speed of tumor growth. Blocking the action of estrogens by antiestrogens that bind to the ERα, such as tamoxifen [71] has demonstrated a long-lasting chemopreventive effect on mammary tumors both benign and malignant. Nevertheless, hormone-independent tumors continue growing after ovariectomy as well after prolonged treatment with tamoxifen [46, 71] (Table 1.3).

Numerous treatments have been developed for the extinction of chemically induced tumor in rodents. DMBA-treated Sprague–Dawley rats that begin receiving a daily injection of 100 IU hCG 20 days after carcinogen administration exhibit a significant reduction in mammary adenocarcinoma incidence and number of tumors per animals, an effect that becomes evident as early as 10 days after initiation of the hormonal treatment and persisted for 40 days after its termination [22, 25, 26] (Table 1.3). Treatment of various strains of rats with hormonal combinations, i.e., ethinyl estradiol-megestrol acetate; ethinyl estradiol-norethindrone [29, 30] or 17β-estradiol-progesterone [33] 2 weeks after NMU administration significantly inhibits tumor progression. Protection conferred by 17β-estradiol and progesterone to BALB/c mice after treatment with DMBA administration is associated with activation of p53 in response to the hormonal treatment, which is sustained to induce p21 upon carcinogen challenge [36, 40] (Table 1.3).

Table 1.3 Modulators of carcinogenic response

Biological or clinical event	Supporting data
Pregnancy after carcinogen exposure	Pregnancy initiated 15 days after DMBA or MCA feeding induces 100% incidence of mammary carcinomas [29]
	The tumors rapidly grow during the gestational period [68]
	The nursing stimulus maintains the growth of carcinogen-induced rat mammary carcinomas [69]
	Cessation of nursing causes tumor regression
Hormonal treatments after carcinogen exposure	Dihydrotestosterone—Decreases tumor size
	Progesterone or diethylstilbestrol—Administered to OVEX rats increase tumor incidence and enhance the speed of tumor growth
	Antiestrogens (Tamoxifen)—Exert a long-lasting chemopreventive effect on mammary tumors
	Ovariectomy (OVEX)—3-MC treated rats exhibit reduced mammary cancer incidence by 40% after OVEX
	17β-estradiol—Daily injections of 0.1 or 0.2 μg 17β-estradiol increase mammary cancer incidence to 100%. Daily injections of 20 μg 17β-estradiol decrease mammary cancer incidence by 70%
	Hormone-independent tumors continue growing after OVEX as well after prolonged treatment with tamoxifen
	Human chorionic gonadotropin (hCG)—Virgin Sprague–Dawley rats that receive a daily injection of 100 IU hCG starting 20 days after DMBA administration exhibit complete extinction of carcinomas in situ and significant reduction in incidence of invasive adenocarcinomas. The effect becomes evident as early as 10 days after the initiation of hormonal treatment and persists for 40 days after its termination
	17β-Estradiol-progesterone combination—Treatment of strains of rats that differ in susceptibility to carcinogens (Lewis, Wistar-Furth, Fischer 344, and Copenhagen) starting 2 weeks after NMU administration significantly inhibits tumor progression in all the strains
	Ethynyl estradiol-megesterol acetate and ethynyl estradiol-norethindrone—Administered 2 weeks after NMU treatment significantly inhibit tumor progression

(continued)

Table 1.3 (continued)

Biological or clinical event	Supporting data
Age at first pregnancy as a risk factor	Postponement of the first delivery after age 24 increases a woman's breast cancer risk
	First birth between 30 and 34 years of age is associated with a risk similar to that observed in nulliparous women
	First birth after 35 years of age increases by two third the breast cancer risk
Pregnancy associated breast cancer (PABC)	The hormonal milieu of pregnancy might stimulate the progression of preexisting preneoplastic lesions that are diagnosed during pregnancy or within 1 or 2 years following delivery
	PABC has a worse prognosis and more pronounced mortality than breast cancer diagnosed to women with no PABC
Estrogens and progestagens as carcinogens	17β-Estradiol
	Women with high levels during the first trimester of pregnancy are at increased risk of breast cancer diagnosis before 40 years of age, but decreased in women whose breast cancer was diagnosed after the age 40
	Administration to August/Copenhagen/Irish (ACI) rats induces tumors that are similar to the in situ and invasive ductal carcinomas developed by women
	In vitro it induces neoplastic transformation of the human breast epithelial cells MCF-10F, which become tumorigenic in SCID mice
	Medroxyprogesterone acetate (MPA)
	Administration to BALB/c female mice induces mammary ductal carcinomas in 80% of treated animals. The tumors are ERα and progesterone receptor positive and metastasize to lymph nodes and lung
Hormone replacement therapy (HRT) and postmenopausal breast cancer	In USA and Europe prescriptions for HRT have been linked to 25% of breast cancers (Carsten AJ (2009) S Afr Med J 99:280)
	Breast cancer incidence has decreased following the decline in the use of HRT (Renard et al (2010) Ann Oncol)
	The incidence of lobular cancer increased by 14% in association with the use of HRT (Ravdin PM (2009) Breast Dis 30:3)

1.8 Hormones as Carcinogens

The dependence of breast cancer from estrogens has been demonstrated through the induction of mammary cancer in female August/Copenhagen/Irish (ACI) rats in which administration of 17β-estradiol induces tumors that are similar to the in situ and invasive ductal carcinomas developed by women [72]. Estrogen-induced lesions are completely prevented by concomitant treatment with tamoxifen citrate (TAMc), confirming their estrogen receptor dependence [73]. The carcinogenicity of 17β-estradiol has been confirmed by in vitro experiments through the induction of neoplastic transformation of the human breast epithelial cells MCF-10F, supporting the concept that this hormone could act as an initiator of breast cancer in women [74]. The biphasic effect of estradiol on breast cancer risk is highlighted by the findings that elevated levels of estradiol in maternal serum during the first trimester of pregnancy are positively associated with risk of breast cancer before age 40, but inversely associated with risk in women whose breast cancer was diagnosed after the age 40 [19, 23]. Among the hormones used for contraception, medroxyprogesterone acetate (MPA) also has a biphasic effect when administered to rats of different ages before DMBA inoculation. MPA given for 21 days moderately increases the incidence of adenocarcinomas in 45-day-old rats, and more significantly in 75-day-old rats, whereas the same doses significantly reduced mammary cancer incidence in the 55-day-old rats, and indication that the same hormone and same dose exerts a biphasic effect that is modulated by the age of the rats at the time of initiation of treatment [75]. MPA administered to BALB/c female mice induces mammary ductal carcinomas in 80% of treated animals. The tumors are hormone-dependent ERα and progesterone receptor positive that metastasize to lymph nodes and lungs; the tumors evolve through different stages of hormone dependence that are progesterone receptor dependent [76] (Table 1.3).

1.9 When Does a Full-Term Pregnancy Reduce Breast Cancer Risk?

Pregnancy, which is the gold standard for induction of mammary gland differentiation, needs to be completed for preventing mammary cancer, as demonstrated in rats that their first pregnancy was interrupted 12 days after conception and received DMBA 21 days later [27]. Tumor incidence and number of tumors per animal in pregnancy-interrupted rats and age-matched virgin rats were similar, whereas rats that completed their pregnancy had a significantly reduced tumorigenic response. Completion of the first pregnancy results in full differentiation of the mammary gland that culminates in the secretion of milk, which persists during the length of the lactational period [18, 22]. At postweaning, the lobular structures regress and the cells that remain exhibit a marked reduction in proliferative rate, lengthening in the G_1 phase of the cell cycle, greater capabilities to repair DNA damaged by the

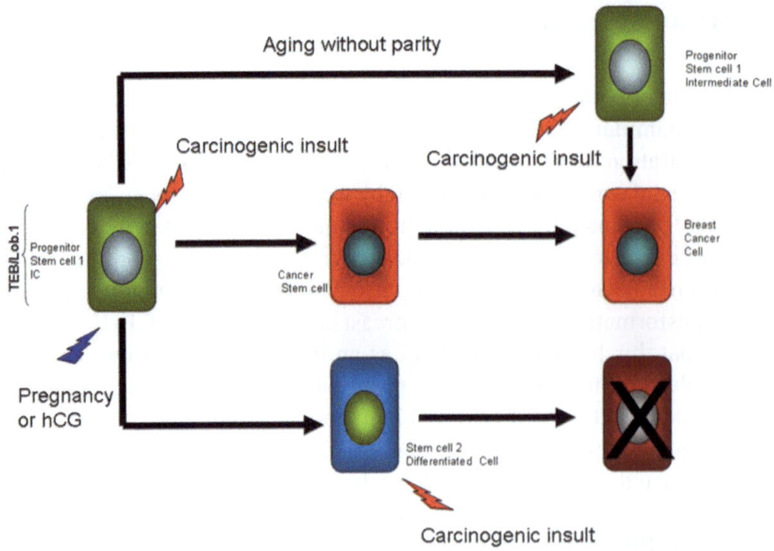

Fig. 1.7 The initially normal progenitor stem cell 1 or intermediate cell (IC) that is present in the TEB/Lob 1 and gives origin to the parenchymal tree, when affected by a carcinogen becomes the cancer stem cell (CSC) that originates breast cancer cells. With aging, in the absence of pregnancy, it remains undifferentiated; if affected by a carcinogen it would retain the capacity of becoming a CSC. Both early pregnancy or hCG treatment of virgin animals induce the differentiation of the progenitor stem cell 1 (IC) to the stem cell 2, which is resistant to be transformed by a carcinogen, although it retains the proliferative activity and capability to regenerate the complete lobular system during the next pregnancy (from Russo IH, Russo J (2011) Pregnancy-induced changes in breast cancer risk. A review. J Mammary Gland Biol Neoplasia 16:221–233)

carcinogen and lower affinity for binding DMBA to DNA [22]. These structural, functional, and molecular changes persist in the mammary gland, resulting in a significant reduction in mammary cancer incidence that is evident in various strains of rats and mice [35], in spite of histopathological differences in tumor type between these species. Blakely et al. [33] have confirmed that in four genetically distinct inbred strains of rats (Lewis, Wistar-Furth, Fischer 344, and Copenhagen) and in mice pregnancy and lactation induce similar structural and genomic changes in mammary glands studied by microarray analysis. Gene analysis identified a genomic signature that sufficed for distinguishing nulliparous from parous animals and explain the almost total refractoriness of the parous rat mammary gland to develop carcinomas after carcinogen administration [33, 77]. These observations indicate that when the development of the mammary gland has been completed by an early pregnancy, steroid hormone- or hCG treatment of virgin animals the PMSC or Stem Cell 1 has completed a first cycle of differentiation under specific hormonal influences, becoming a Stem Cell 2, which is resistant to be transformed by a carcinogen (Fig. 1.7). Although more differentiated, the Stem Cell 2 has retained the capacity to regenerate the complete lobular system required by subsequent pregnancies. This concept has been further demonstrated in transgenic WAP-driven Cre and

Rosa 26-fl-stop-fl-LacZ mice in which parity-induced mammary epithelial cells (PI-MEC) originated from differentiated cells during pregnancy, survived post lactational involution and increased their percentage with successive pregnancies [78]. PI-MEC, like the Stem Cell 2 in the parous rat mammary gland, show capacity for self-renewal and contribute to mammary outgrowth in transplantation studies. PI-MEC can function as alveolar progenitors in subsequent pregnancies, and it is thought that they would be related to differences in response to hormonal stimulation and carcinogenic agents observed between nulliparous and parous females [28, 79, 80] (Table 1.3).

The relevance of the findings that the first full-term pregnancy occurring during the HRSW but before exposure to a carcinogen prevents cancer initiation is equivalent to the well demonstrated protective effect of an early first FTP in women. A first FTP initiated approximately 2 weeks after carcinogen exposure, on the other hand, results in a high incidence of mammary cancer, a phenomenon that could explain the increased cancer risk observed in women first parous after age 30, supporting the assumption that during that lengthened HRSW the breast had been exposed to carcinogenic stimuli before pregnancy. These data emphasize the importance of discriminating whether the first pregnancy would produce protection by inducing complete differentiation of the breast activating the same mechanisms that hormonal treatments do, or would increase breast cancer risk as a consequence of genotoxic or epigenetic exposures during the HRSW (Fig. 1.3).

1.10 The Human Breast in Pregnancy and Disease

The development of the breast is a continuous process initiated by the fourth week of intrauterine life that progresses under the influence of maternal, placental, and environmental factors until birth and by diet and environmental exposures after weaning, respectively. During these periods the maturation of the HPG axis [17, 18, 81] and endogenous hormone secretions play essential roles on the development of the breast at puberty, which is driven by the initiation of ovulation and the establishment of regular menstrual cycles [82]. The architecture of the breast of normally cycling women has been widely described as composed of three main lobular structures that are classified on the basis of their degree of development into lobules type 1 (Lob 1), lobules type 2 (Lob 2), and lobules type 3 (Lob 3) [22, 83, 84] (Fig. 1.8). The breast of women that never conceived a child remains composed of Lob 1, with moderate formation of Lob 2 with successive menstrual cycles (Fig. 1.9); Lob 3 is present only occasionally during the early reproductive years. After menopause the breast further regresses, resulting in an increase in the number of Lob 1 in response to the decline in Lob 2 and Lob 3 with aging (Fig. 1.10). We postulate that the breast parenchyma of postmenopausal nulliparous women contains predominantly Stem Cells 1, which did not achieve the most differentiated stage of Stem Cell 2 due to the absence of pregnancy, therefore retaining its susceptibility to be transformed. Therefore, a carcinogenic insult or an inappropriate hormonal stimulus, such as

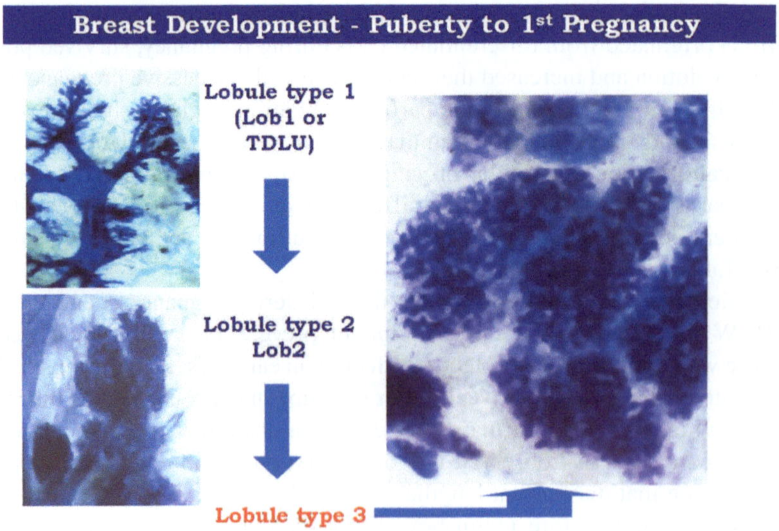

Fig. 1.8 Development of the human breast before the first pregnancy from puberty to adulthood

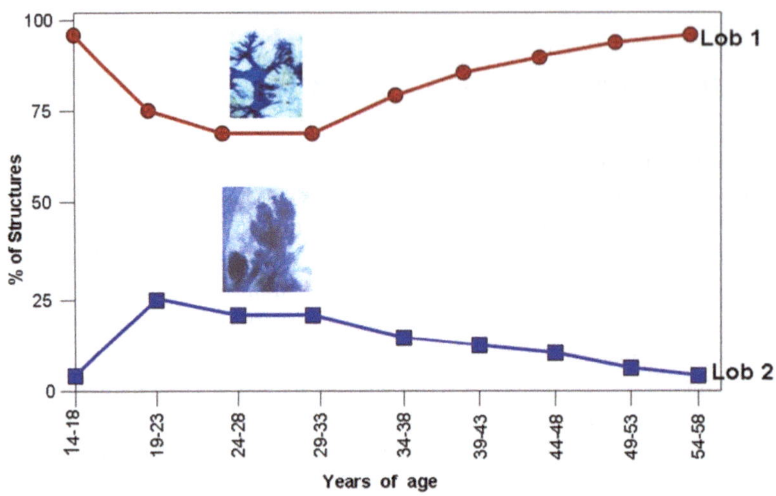

Fig. 1.9 Diagrammatic representation of the development of the breast based on the relative percentage of lobules present. From puberty to menopause, in the absence of pregnancy, lobules type 1 (Lob 1) predominate. From ages 19 to 33 a moderate reduction in the number of Lob 1 due to their progression to Lob 2 occurs in response to the hormonal stimulus of successive menstrual cycles. After menopause the number of Lob 1 increases in response to the decline in Lob 2 (from Russo IH, Russo J (2011) Pregnancy-induced changes in breast cancer risk. A review. J Mammary Gland Biol Neoplasia 16:221–233)

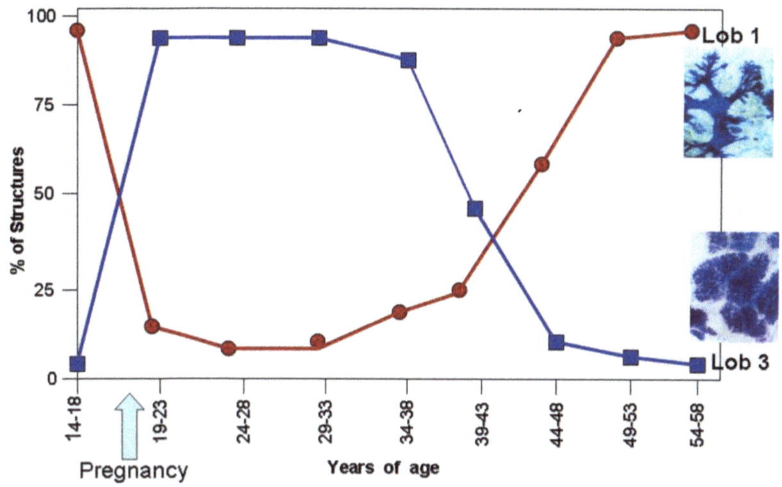

Fig. 1.10 Diagrammatic representation of the development of the breast after the first pregnancy. Lobules type 1, which predominate after 14 years of age, are rapidly replaced by Lob 2, 3, and 4 during pregnancy. Regression of Lob 4 to Lob 3 at postweaning is followed by regression of Lob 3 to Lob 1 after age 39. The increasing number of Lob 1 crosses over with Lob 3 by age 44, and continue progressively increasing after menopause (from Russo IH, Russo J (2011) Pregnancy-induced changes in breast cancer risk. A review. J Mammary Gland Biol Neoplasia 16:221–233)

hormone replacement therapy [85], would transform the Stem Cell 1 into a cancer stem cell (Fig. 1.7).

1.11 Breast Development Under the Endocrinological Influence of Pregnancy

The development of the breast from birth to puberty follows a general pattern common for all normally cycling women, with the formation of Lob 1, Lob 2, and Lob 3 [83, 84]. The progression of lobular development under the cyclic influence of ovarian hormones is rapidly accelerated during the first pregnancy, which for being successful requires the timely fertilization of an ovocyte followed by its uterine implantation. The embryo drives a process that establishes a collaboration of the newly formed placenta with the maternal environment [86]. The placenta alone elaborates a myriad of proteins, glycoproteins, steroid hormones, growth factors, tumor suppressor factors, and cytokines that control the local environment of the fetus and regulate the metabolic activities of both the mother and the fetus [87]. In addition to estrogen and progesterone, newly secreted hormones, such as human growth hormone (hGH); hCG, human placental lactogen (hPL), inhibin [88, 89] stimulate breast development and differentiation. Elevated serum levels of Metastin (KISS-1) have been detected during pregnancy [90] (Fig. 1.4), but the role of this hormone in breast development has not been identified as yet. LH, progesterone, and hCG are the main hormones driving the initial phase of growth, which is followed by the secretion of the pituitary hormone PRL that stimulates milk secretion and contributes to the development of the fully differentiated Lob 4 during the last trimester of pregnancy and lactation. After weaning Lob 4 regress to Lob 3, which persists in the breast as long as women continue cycling (Fig. 1.10). At perimenopause, the number of Lob 3 progressively decreases due to their involution to Lob 2 and Lob 1 [22].

1.12 Basis of the Protective Effect of Early Pregnancy

There exists consensus on the fact that an early pregnancy and increasing number of full-term pregnancies are associated with greater risk reduction for invasive breast cancer compared with never-pregnant women and women whose first full-term pregnancy occurred after 30 years of age [8, 9]. Data on the mechanisms mediating the protection conferred by early pregnancy or the increased risk resulting from delayed first birth in women are scant or nonexistent. These uncertainties emanate from the lack of knowledge on the cause and time of initiation of breast cancer. Epidemiological data have provided useful information on cancer causation through the identification of deleterious environmental exposures, such as radiation exposure, either accidental [91] or diagnostic and therapeutic [92]; and passive or active smoking at an early age [93]. The association of these early exposures with the development of breast cancer are an indication that the initiation of breast epithelial cell transformation took place several years before a first FTP during a window of susceptibility similar to that described in the rodent experimental model (Fig. 1.11). The hormonal milieu of pregnancy might stimulate the progression of preexisting preneoplastic lesions or small tumors that would be diagnosed during pregnancy or within 1 or 2 years following delivery as pregnancy associated breast cancer (PABC) [94], whose incidence is likely to increase because of the continuous trend towards postponement of childbearing [95, 96]. PABC diagnosed shortly after delivery has a worse prognosis and more pronounce mortality than breast cancer in women with no PABC. Unfortunately, the knowledge of the response of the breast to the hormones of pregnancy is scant and insufficient for understanding the complex interactions between pregnancy hormones required for stimulating fetal growth and breast development and those that activate differentiation pathways exerting a cancer risk reduction effect [34] (Fig. 1.11). This is a field that requires extensive investigation for clarifying these hormonal-carcinogen relationships.

Current knowledge on the development of the breast before and during pregnancy has been acquired through the study of in vivo and in vitro experimental models, autopsy material, or cancer-free breast tissues obtained from biopsies or reduction mammoplasties [22, 25, 26, 30]. Conclusions drawn through these studies had to be extrapolated to the conditions prevailing in the breast during pregnancy due to the difficulties in obtaining breast tissue specimens during the gestational

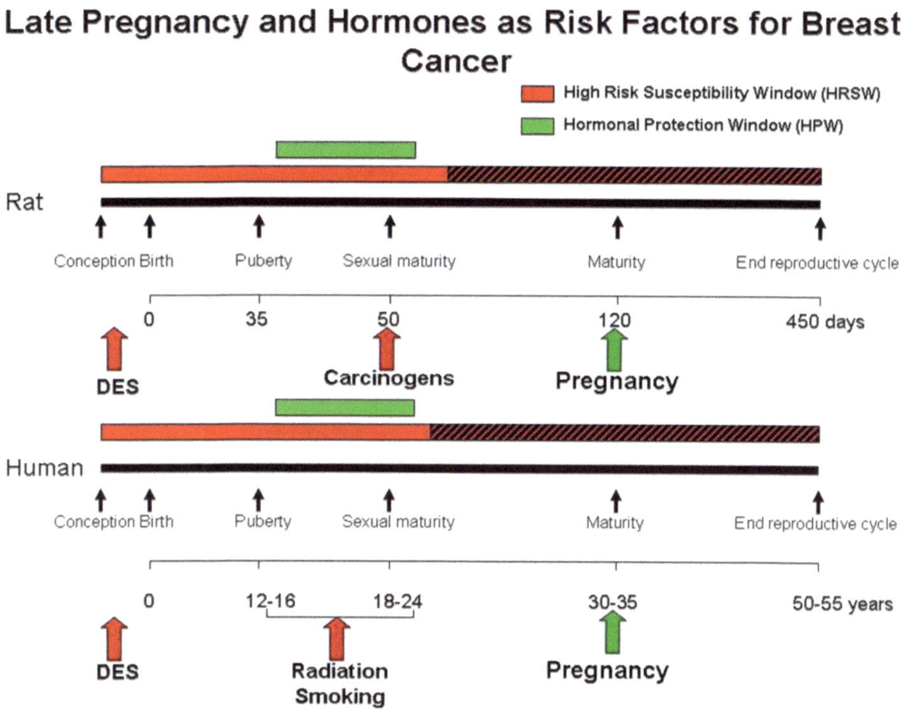

Fig. 1.11 Diagrammatic representation of mammary gland development from conception to the end of reproductive life. In both rats (*upper line*) and humans (*lower line*) as in Fig. 1.3. The hatched *red line* represents increase widening of the HRSW to hormonal factors or late pregnancy

process. In order to understand how the dramatic modifications that occur during pregnancy in the pattern of lobular development and differentiation, cell proliferation and hormone receptors influence a woman's lifetime cancer risk, it has been necessary to analyze the pattern of gene expression in the epithelium of Lob 1 in breast biopsies of parous and nulliparous postmenopausal women with a history of invasive breast cancer (cases) or benign breast disease without hyperplasia or atypia (controls). Genomic and Gene Ontology (GO) analyses revealed that the mRNA obtained from the breast of parous women free of cancer had a higher level of gene expression in processes that included proteolysis and ubiquitination, cell adhesion, response to exogenous agents, metabolism, DNA repair and replication, RNA processing, apoptosis, antiapoptosis, and chromatin modifications [97, 98]. These data indicate that parous women after menopause who had not developed breast cancer exhibit a genomic "signature" that differs from that present in the breast of parous postmenopausal women with cancer or in nulliparous women, who traditionally represent a high breast cancer risk group [97, 98] (Fig. 1.12). The importance of these findings is that they support the concept that for being protective, parity should

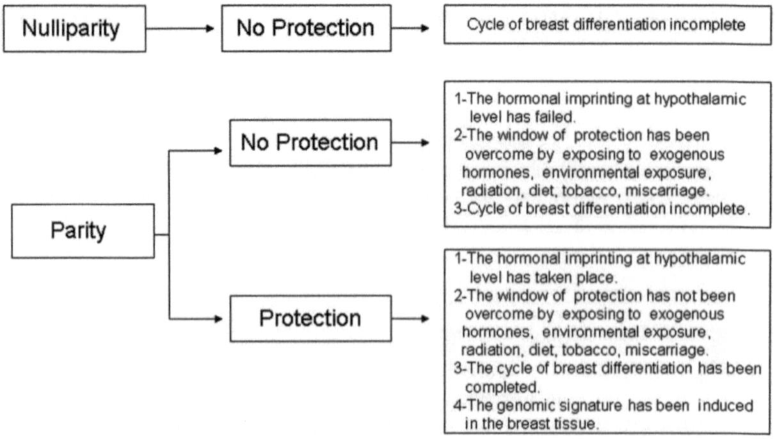

Fig. 1.12 Algorithm of breast cancer protection

occur during a specific time of breast development, which is represented by the interplay of the HRSW/HPW and that the stem progenitor cells must be programmed for differentiation before any carcinogenic insult has activated them for becoming cancer stem cells (Figs. 1.7 and 1.12). If a carcinogenic insult reaches the progenitor stem cells of the breast before the first FTP, then pregnancy, instead of being protective, might stimulate the progression of transformed cells (Fig. 1.12).

1.13 Influence of Fertility on Breast Cancer Risk

No satisfactory answer has been found to the puzzle of why women that have completed their first pregnancy before age 24 have significantly reduced risk of developing breast cancer after menopause, whereas women that become first pregnant after age 30 or that are younger than 40 years of age at the time of breast cancer diagnosis are not protected by parity. Although the exact mechanisms underlying these differences on breast cancer risk remain unclear, studies of the association of cohort fertility and breast cancer incidence have revealed that childbearing trends account at least in part for cohort variations in breast cancer incidence in the Western world. In the United States the average age of mothers at the first birth was 21.4 in 1970, increasing 3.6 years by 2006 [99]. During this period the proportion of first births to women aged 35 years and over increased nearly eight times; whereas the percentage of first time mothers under age 20 was reduced from 36 to 21%, and the number of invasive breast cancer cancers increased 2.71-fold (171%), in contrast with an increase in the female population of 1.29-fold (29%), an indication that delayed first birth played a greater role in the increased breast cancer incidence than population growth [99, 100]. These epidemiological data support our hypothesis that in order for a first FTP to be protective it should occur during specific periods of time, the HRSW/HPW interface (Figs. 1.3 and 1.12).

1.13.1 Ovarian Aging and Fertility

The understanding of the mechanisms that determine the variability in breast cancer risk in relation to age at the first full-term pregnancy requires to take into consideration not only the development and differentiation of the breast at various ages, but of the organs that control both breast development and the capabilities of women to be fertile, namely the ovary and the HPG axis [17, 18]. The fertility of a sexually mature woman is established as early as the fourth month of her fetal life, when the number of ovarian primordial follicles is set. At birth they number approximately five million; progressively decreasing to 500,000 when the girl reaches menarche [101]. Between the initiation of ovulation and up to 30 years of age, the monthly fecundity rate (MFR), i.e., the ability of a woman to become pregnant, ranges from 20 to 25% [101]. Continuous ovulation and associated follicular atresia and apoptosis further reduce the natural MFR to below 10% by age 35 and even more thereafter, resulting in either sub fertility or clinical infertility, which affects approximately 15% of women in developed countries [102]. With aging of the ovary the size of recruited follicles declines, with a concomitant reduction in the number of follicles entering maturation and of preovulatory oocytes. Under these conditions the quality of the oocytes declines, leading to lower pregnancy rates even after infertility treatments. In addition, embryo aneuploidy and miscarriage rates increase, ultimately resulting in poorer delivery rates [103] (Fig. 1.12).

1.13.2 Aging of the Hypothalamic–Pituitary–Ovarian Axis and Fertility

Although follicular depletion is a critical factor mediating both fertility and menopausal transition, the age-related decline in reproductive function is affected by changes in all levels of the HPG axis [17]. The major hormonal elements that hierarchically define this system are the hypothalamic GnRH, and the pituitary gonadotropins LH and follicle stimulating hormone (FSH) that control the synthesis and release of ovarian sex steroids and peptides. Accumulating evidence indicates that during the earliest stages of reproductive decline, changes at the level of the brain play an important role in the initiation of reproductive senescence, which is manifested as a dampened and delayed GnRH-driven proestrous LH surge [17, 103, 104]. These data emphasize the need to understand how endocrinological changes occurring in response to aging affect on the ability of the breast to respond to the hormonal effects of pregnancy or of exogenous hormones that might be used for the purposes of preventing breast cancer.

1.14 Concluding Remarks

The mechanisms described above emphasize the importance of a timely differentiation of the breast for preventing breast cancer. The fact that only full-term pregnancy occurring during a narrow window in the development of the breast would succeed in permanently inducing the molecular changes that will make the breast resistant to develop cancer imposes a heavy burden on reproductive biologists, breast specialists, endocrinologists, and molecular biologists for developing the adequate strategies for preventing breast cancer in continuously changing populations. A hope is offered by the observations that it is possible to protect the breast from cancer initiation and progression with hCG, one of the hormones produced by the human placenta. The implications of these observations are twofold: on one hand, they indicate that hCG may induce early genomic changes that control the progression of the differentiation pathway, and that these changes are permanently imprinted in the genome, regulating the long-lasting refractoriness of the breast to develop cancer. The permanence of these changes would, in turn, make them ideal surrogate markers for the evaluation of novel chemopreventive agents designed for preventing breast cancer in the future.

References

1. Breasted JH (ed) (1991) The Edwin Smith Surgical Papyrus: published in facsimile and hieroglyphic transliteration with translation and commentary in two volumes, vol 1. University of Chicago Press, Chicago
2. Clarke CA, Purdie DM, Glaser SL (2006) Population attributable risk of breast cancer in white women associated with immediately modifiable risk factors. BMC Cancer 6:170
3. Botha JL, Bray F, Sanlika R, Parkin DM (2003) Breast cancer incidence and mortality trends in 16 European countries. Eur J Cancer 39:1718–1729
4. Jemal A, Bray F, Center MM, Ferlay J, Ward E, Forman D (2011) Global cancer statistics. CA Cancer J Clin 61:69–90
5. Nagata C, Mizoue T, Tanaka K, Tsuji I, Wakai K, Inoue M et al (2006) Tobacco smoking and breast cancer risk: an evaluation based on a systematic review of epidemiological evidence among the Japanese population. Jpn J Clin Oncol 36:387–394
6. Maskarinec G, Pagano I, Chen Z, Nagata C, Gram IT (2007) Ethnic and geographic differences in mammographic density and their association with breast cancer incidence. Breast Cancer Res Treat 104:47–56
7. Althuis MD, Dozier JM, Anderson WF, Devesa SS, Brinton LA (2005) Global trends in breast cancer incidence and mortality 1973-1997. Int J Epidemiol 34:405–412
8. MacMahon B, Cole P, Lin TM, Lowe CR, Mirra AP, Ravnihar B et al (1970) Age at first birth and breast cancer risk. Bull World Health Organ 43:209–221
9. Hinkula M, Pukkala E, Kyyrönen P, Kauppila A (2001) Grand multiparity and the risk of breast cancer: population-based study in Finland. Cancer Causes Control 12:491–500
10. Ma H, Henderson KD, Sullivan-Halley J, Duan L, Marshall SF, Ursin G et al (2010) Pregnancy-related factors and the risk of breast carcinoma in situ and invasive breast cancer among postmenopausal women in the California Teachers Study cohort. Breast Cancer Res 12:R35
11. Phipps AI, Chlebowski RT, Prentice R, McTiernan A, Wactawski-Wende J, Kuller LH et al (2011) Reproductive history and oral contraceptive use in relation to risk of triple-negative breast cancer. J Natl Cancer Inst 103:1–8

12. Toniolo P, Grankvist K, Wulff M, Chen T, Johansson R, Schock H et al (2010) Human chorionic gonadotropin in pregnancy and maternal risk of breast cancer. Cancer Res 70:6779–6786
13. Mustacchi P (1961) Ramazzini and Rigoni-Stern on parity and breast cancer. Clinical impression and statistical corroboration. Arch Intern Med 108:639–642
14. Kroman N, Mouridsen HT (2003) Prognostic influence of pregnancy before, around, and after diagnosis of breast cancer. Breast 12:516–521
15. Kroman N, Melbye M, Mouridsen HT (2002) Prognostic influence of age at diagnosis in premenopausal breast cancer patients. Scand J Surg 91:305–308
16. Brinton LA, Sherman ME, Carreon JD, Anderson WF (2008) Recent trends in breast cancer among younger women in the United States. J Natl Cancer Inst 100:1643–1648
17. Downs JL, Wise PM (2009) The role of the brain in female reproductive aging. Mol Cell Endocrinol 299:32–38
18. Russo IH, Medado J, Russo J (1989) Endocrine influences on mammary gland structure and development. In: Jones TC, Mohr U, Hunt RD (eds) Integument and mammary gland of laboratory animals. Springer, Berlin, pp 252–266
19. Chen T, Lundin E, Grankvist K, Zeleniuch-Jacquotte A, Wulff M, Afanasyeva Y et al (2010) Maternal hormones during early pregnancy: a cross-sectional study. Cancer Causes Control 21:719–727
20. Beatson GT (1896) On the treatment of inoperable cases of carcinoma of the mamma: suggestions for a new method of treatment with illustrative cases. Lancet ii:104
21. Russo J, Russo IH (2006) The role of estrogen in the initiation of breast cancer. J Steroid Biochem Mol Biol 102:89–96
22. Russo J, Russo IH (eds) (2004) Molecular basis of breast cancer: prevention and treatment. Springer, Berlin
23. Lukanova A, Surcel HM, Lundin E, Kaasila M, Lakso HA, Schock H et al (2011) Circulating estrogens and progesterone during primiparous. Pregnancies and risk of maternal breast cancer. Int J Cancer 130:910–920
24. Albrektsen G, Heuch I, Thoresen S, Kvale G (2006) Clinical stage of breast cancer by parity, age at birth, and time since birth: a progressive effect of pregnancy hormones? Cancer Epidemiol Biomarkers Prev 15:65–69
25. Russo IH, Koszalka M, Gimotty PA, Russo J (1990) Protective effect of chorionic gonadotropin on DMBA-induced mammary carcinogenesis. Br J Cancer 62:243–247
26. Russo IH, Koszalka M, Russo J (1991) Comparative study of the influence of pregnancy and hormonal treatment on mammary carcinogenesis. Br J Cancer 64:481–484
27. Russo J, Russo IH (1980) Susceptibility of the mammary gland to carcinogenesis: II. Pregnancy interruption as a risk factor in tumor incidence. Am J Pathol 100:497–512
28. Russo J, Tay LK, Ciocca D, Russo IH (1983) Molecular and cellular basis of the mammary gland susceptibility to carcinogenesis. Environ Health Perspect 49:185–199
29. Welsch CW (1985) Host factors affecting the growth of carcinogen-induced rat mammary carcinomas: a review and tribute to Charles Brenton Huggins. Cancer Res 45:3415–3443
30. Russo IH, Russo J (1996) Mammary gland neoplasia in long-term rodent studies. Environ Health Perspect 104:938–967
31. McCormick GM, Moon RC (1967) Effect of nursing and litter size on growth of 7,12-dimethylbenz(a)anthracene (DMBA)-induced rat mammary tumors. Br J Cancer 21:586–591
32. Cabanes A, Wang M, Olivo S, DeAssis S, Gustafsson JA, Khan G et al (2004) Prepubertal estradiol and genistein exposures up-regulate BRCA1 mRNA and reduce mammary tumorigenesis. Carcinogenesis 25:741–748
33. Blakely CM, Stoddard AJ, Belka GK, Dugan KD, Notarfrancesco KL, Moody SE et al (2006) Hormone-induced protection against mammary tumorigenesis is conserved in multiple rat strains and identifies a core gene expression signature induced by pregnancy. Cancer Res 66:6421–6431
34. Lakshmanaswamy R, Guzman RC, Nandi S (2008) Hormonal prevention of breast cancer: significance of promotional environment. Adv Exp Med Biol 617:469–475

35. Medina D, Smith GH (1999) Chemical carcinogen-induced tumorigenesis in parous, involuted mouse mammary glands. J Natl Cancer Inst 91:967–969
36. Medina D, Kittrell FS (2003) p53 function is required for hormone-mediated protection of mouse mammary tumorigenesis. Cancer Res 63:6140–6143
37. Medina D (2007) Chemical carcinogenesis of rat and mouse mammary glands. Breast Dis 28:63–68
38. Medina D (2008) Premalignant and malignant mammary lesions induced by MMTV and chemical carcinogens. J Mammary Gland Biol Neoplasia 13:271–277
39. Shen Q, Brown PH (2005) Transgenic mouse models for the prevention of breast cancer. Mutat Res 576:93–110
40. Rajkumar L, Kittrell FS, Guzman RC, Brown PH, Nandi S, Medina D (2007) Hormone-induced protection of mammary tumorigenesis in genetically engineered mouse models. Breast Cancer Res 9:R12
41. Allred DC, Medina D (2008) The relevance of mouse models to understanding the development and progression of human breast cancer. J Mammary Gland Biol Neoplasia 13:279–288
42. Borowsky AD (2011) Choosing a mouse model: experimental biology in context—the utility and limitations of mouse models of breast cancer. Cold Spring Harb Perspect Biol 3:a009670
43. Medina D, Kittrell FS, Hill J, Shepard A, Thordarson G, Brown P (2005) Tamoxifen inhibition of estrogen receptor-alpha-negative mouse mammary tumorigenesis. Cancer Res 65:3493–3496
44. Rao GN, Piegorsch WW, Haseman JK (1987) Influence of body weight on the incidence of spontaneous tumors in rats and mice of long term studies. Am J Clin Nutr 45:252–260
45. Tarone RE, Chu KC, Ward JM (1981) Variability in the rates of some common naturally occurring tumors in Fischer 344 rats and (C57BLU6N x C3/HeN) F1 (B6C3F) mice. J Natl Cancer Inst 66:1175–1181
46. Huggins C, Briziarelli G, Sutton H (1959) Rapid induction of mammary carcinoma in the rat and the influence of hormones on the tumors. J Exp Med 709:25–42
47. Huggins C, Grand L, Fukunishi R (1964) Aromatic influences in the yields of mammary cancers following administration of 7,12-dimethylbenzanthracene. Proc Natl Acad Sci USA 57:737–742
48. Gullino PM, Pettigrew HM, Grantham FH (1975) N-nitrosomethylurea as mammary gland carcinogen in rats. J Natl Cancer Inst 54:401–414
49. Thordarson G, Lee AV, McCarty M, Van Horn K, Chu O, Chou YC et al (2001) Growth and characterization of N-methyl-N-nitrosourea-induced mammary tumors in intact and ovariectomized rats. Carcinogenesis 22:2039–2047
50. Russo J, Gusterson BA, Rogers AE, Russo IH, Wellings SR, Van Zwieten MJ (1990) Comparative study of human and rat mammary tumorigenesis. Lab Invest 62:1–32
51. Moral R, Wang R, Russo IH, Lamartiniere CA, Pereira J, Russo J (2008) Effect of prenatal exposure to the endocrine disruptor bisphenol A on mammary gland morphology and gene expression signature. J Endocrinol 196:101–112
52. Kawaguchi H, Miyoshi N, Miyamoto Y, Souda M, Umekita Y, Yasuda N et al (2009) Effects of fetal exposure to diethylstilbestrol on mammary tumorigenesis in rats. Vet Med Sci 71:1599–1608
53. Umekita Y, Souda M, Hatanaka K, Hamada T, Yoshioka T, Kawaguchi H et al (2011) Gene expression profile of terminal end buds in rat mammary glands exposed to diethylstilbestrol in neonatal period. Toxicol Lett 205:15–25
54. Goodman A, Schorge J, Greene MF (2011) The long-term effects of in utero exposures—the DES story. N Engl J Med 364:2083–2084
55. Russo IH, Russo J (2007) Primary prevention of breast cancer by hormone-induced differentiation. Recent Results Cancer Res 174:111–130
56. Russo J, Tait L, Russo IH (1983) Susceptibility of the mammary gland to carcinogenesis: III. The cell of origin of rat mammary carcinoma. Am J Pathol 113:50–66

57. Russo J, Balogh GA, Chen J, Fernandez SV, Fernbaugh R, Heulings R et al (2006) The concept of stem cell in the mammary gland and its implication in morphogenesis, cancer and prevention. Front Biosci 11:151–172
58. Bennett DC, Peachey LA, Durbin H, Rudland PS (1978) A possible mammary stem cell line. Cell 15:283–298
59. Bussard KM, Smith GH (2011) The mammary gland microenvironment directs progenitor cell fate in vivo. Int J Cell Biol. doi:10.1155/2011/451676
60. Navarro VM, Castellano JM, Fernandez-Fernandez R, Barreiro ML, Roa J, Sanchez-Criado JE et al (2004) Developmental and hormonally regulated messenger ribonucleic acid expression of KiSS-1 and its putative receptor GPR54 in rat hypothalamus and potent LH releasing activity of KiSS-1 peptide. Endocrinology 145:4565–4574
61. Kinoshita M, Tsukamura H, Adachi S, Matsui H, Uenoyama Y, Iwata K et al (2005) Involvement of central metastin in the regulation of preovulatory luteinizing hormone surge and estrous cyclicity in female rats. Endocrinology 146:4431–4436
62. Russo IH, Russo J (1998) Role of hormones in mammary cancer initiation and progression. J Mammary Gland Biol Neoplasia 3:49–61
63. Russo IH, Frederick J, Russo J (1989) Hormone prevention of mammary carcinogenesis by norethynodrel-mestranol. Breast Cancer Res Treat 14:43–56
64. Vanegas JE, Kocdor M, Pereira JS, Kocdor H, Russo J, Snider K et al (2009) Preventive effect of hCG on rat mammary carcinogenesis. AACR Annual Meeting Abstracts 2059
65. Srivastava P, Russo J, Russo IH (1997) Chorionic gonadotropin inhibits mammary carcinogenesis through activation of programmed cell death. Carcinogenesis 18:1799–1808
66. Srivastava P, Russo J, Russo IH (1999) Inhibition of rat mammary tumorigenesis by human chorionic gonadotropin is associated with increased expression of inhibin. Mol Carcinog 26:10–19
67. Russo IH, Russo J (1993) Chorionic gonadotropin: a tumoristatic and preventive agent in breast cancer. In: Teicher BA (ed) Drug resistance in oncology. Marcel Dekker, New York, pp 537–560
68. McCormick GM, Moon RC (1965) Effect of pregnancy and lactation on growth of mammary tumours induced by 7,12-dimethylbenzanthracene (DMBA). Br J Cancer 79:160–166
69. Dao TL, Sunderland H (1959) Mammary carcinogenesis by 3-methylcholanthrene: I. Hormonal aspects in tumor induction and growth. J Natl Cancer Inst 23:567–585
70. Grubbs CJ, Hill DL, McDonough KC, Peckham JC (1983) N-nitroso-N-methylurea-induced mammary carcinogenesis: effect of pregnancy on preneoplastic cells. J Natl Cancer Inst 71:625–628
71. Jordan VC (1976) Effect of tamoxifen (ICI 46,474) on the initiation and growth of DMBA-induced rat mammary carcinoma. Eur J Cancer 12:419–424
72. Weroha SJ, Li SA, Tawfik O, Li JJ (2006) Overexpression of cyclins D1 and D3 during estrogen-induced breast oncogenesis in female ACI rats. Carcinogenesis 27:491–498
73. Li SA, Weroha SJ, Tawfik O, Li JJ (2002) Prevention of solely estrogen-induced mammary tumors in female aci rats by tamoxifen: evidence for estrogen receptor mediation. J Endocrinol 175:297–305
74. Russo J, Fernandez SV, Russo PA, Fernbaugh R, Sheriff FS, Lareef HM, Garber J, Russo IH (2006) 17-Beta-estradiol induces transformation and tumorigenesis in human breast epithelial cells. FASEB J 20:1622–1634
75. Russo IH, Gimotty P, Dupuis M, Russo J (1989) Effect of medroxyprogesterone acetate on the response of the rat mammary gland to carcinogenesis. Br J Cancer 59:210–216
76. Lanari C, Lamb CA, Fabris VT, Helguero LA, Soldati R, Bottino MC et al (2009) The MPA mouse breast cancer model: evidence for a role of progesterone receptors in breast cancer. Endocr Relat Cancer 16:333–350
77. Russo J, Balogh GA, Heulings R, Mailo DA, Moral R, Russo PA et al (2006) Molecular basis of pregnancy-induced breast cancer protection. Eur J Cancer Prev 15:306–342
78. Wagner KU, Boulanger CA, Henry MD, Sgagias M, Hennighausen L, Smith GH (2002) An adjunct mammary epithelial cell population in parous females: its role in functional adaptation and tissue renewal. Development 129:1377–1386

79. Boulanger CA, Wagner KU, Smith GH (2005) Parity-induced mouse mammary epithelial cells are pluripotent, self-renewing and sensitive to TGF-beta 1 expression. Oncogene 24:552–560
80. Booth BW, Boulanger CA, Smith GH (2008) Selective segregation of DNA strands persists in long-label-retaining mammary cells during pregnancy. Breast Cancer Res 10:R90
81. Blackshaw S, Scholpp S, Placzek M, Ingraham H, Simerly R, Shimogori T (2010) Molecular pathways controlling development of thalamus and hypothalamus: from neural specification to circuit formation. J Neurosci 30:14925–14930
82. Hendriks AE, Lavens JS, Valkenburg O, Fong SL, Fauser BC, de Ridder MA et al (2011) Fertility and ovarian function in high-dose estrogen-treated tall women. J Clin Endocrinol Metab 96:1098–1105
83. Russo J, Russo IH (1987) Development of human mammary gland. In: Neville MC, Daniel C (eds) The mammary gland development, regulation and function. Plenum, New York, pp 67–93
84. Russo J, Rivera R, Russo IH (1992) Influence of age and parity on the development of the human breast. Breast Cancer Res Treat 23:211–218
85. Howell A, Evans GD (2011) Hormone replacement therapy and breast cancer. Recent Results Cancer Res 188:115–124
86. Lathi RB, Fisher SJ, Giudice LC (2006) Implantation and placental physiology in early human pregnancy: the role of the maternal decidua and the trophoblast. In: De Groot L, Jameson LJ (eds) Endocrinology. Elsevier Saunders, Philadelphia, pp 3341–3351
87. Parry S, Strauss F III (2006) Placental hormones. In: De Groot L, Jameson LJ (eds) Endocrinology. Elsevier Saunders, Philadelphia, pp 3353–3367
88. Alvarado MV, Ho T-Y, Russo J, Russo IH (1994) Human chorionic gonadotropin regulates the synthesis of inhibin in the ovary and the mammary gland of rats. Endocrine 2:1–10
89. Alvarado ME, Alvarado NE, Russo J, Russo IH (1994) Human chorionic gonadotropin inhibits proliferation and induces expression of inhibin in human breast epithelial cells *in vitro*. In Vitro 30A:4–8
90. Horikoshi Y, Matsumoto H, Takatsu Y, Ohtaki T, Kitada C, Usuki S et al (2003) Dramatic elevation of plasma metastin concentrations in human pregnancy: metastin as a novel placenta-derived hormone in humans. J Clin Endocrinol Metab 88:914–919
91. McGregor H, Land CE, Choi K, Tokuoka S, Liu PI, Wakabayashi I, Beebe GW (1977) Breast cancer incidence among atomic bomb survivors, Hiroshima and Nagaski 1950-1989. J Natl Cancer Inst 59:799–811
92. Cutuli B, Borel C, Dhermain F, Magrini SM, Wasserman TH, Bogart JA et al (2001) Breast cancer occurred after treatment for Hodgkin's disease: analysis of 133 cases. Radiother Oncol 59:247–255
93. Johnson KC, Miller AB, Collishaw NE, Palmer JR, Hammond SK, Salmon AG et al (2011) Active smoking and secondhand smoke increase breast cancer risk: the report of the Canadian Expert Panel on Tobacco Smoke and Breast Cancer Risk (2009). Tob Control 20:e2
94. Johansson AL, Andersson TM, Hsieh CC, Cnattingius S, Lambe M (2011) Increased mortality in women with breast cancer detected during pregnancy and different periods postpartum. Cancer Epidemiol Biomarkers Prev 20:1865–1872
95. Hahn RA, Moolgavkar SH (1989) Nulliparity, decade of first birth, and breast cancer in Connecticut cohorts, 1855 to 1945: an ecological study. Am J Public Health 79:1503–1507
96. Mathews TJ, Hamilton BE (2009) Delayed childbearing: more women are having their first child later in life (National Center for Health Statistics data brief No. 21). National Center for Health Statistics, Hyattsville
97. Balogh GA, Heulings R, Mailo DA, Russo PA, Sheriff F, Russo IH et al (2006) Genomic signature induced by pregnancy in the human breast. Int J Oncol 28:399–410
98. Russo J, Balogh GA, Russo IH (2008) Full-term pregnancy induces a specific genomic signature in the human breast. Cancer Epidemiol Biomarkers Prev 17:51–66
99. George K, Kamath MS (2010) Fertility and age. J Hum Reprod Sci 3:121–123

100. Homan GF, Davies M, Norman R (2007) The impact of lifestyle factors on reproductive performance in the general population and those undergoing infertility treatment. Hum Reprod Update 13:209–223
101. Gleicher N, Weghofer A, Barad DH (2011) Defining ovarian reserve to better understand ovarian aging. Reprod Biol Endocrinol 9:23
102. Danforth DR, Arbogast LK, Mroueh J, Kim MH, Kennard EA, Seifer DB et al (1998) Dimeric inhibin: a direct marker of ovarian ageing. Fertil Steril 70:119–123
103. Rance NE (2009) Menopause and the human hypothalamus: evidence for the role of kisspeptin/neurokinin B neurons in the regulation of estrogen negative feedback. Peptides 30:111–122
104. Wise PM, Smith MJ, Dubal DB, Wilson ME, Rau SW, Cashion AB et al (2002) Neuroendocrine modulation and repercussions of female reproductive aging. Recent Prog Horm Res 57:235–256

Chapter 2
An In Vivo Model of Breast Cancer Prevention

2.1 Introduction

Primary prevention is the ultimate goal for the control of breast cancer. Thus, one of the major long-standing goals of the studies conducted in the Breast Cancer Research Laboratory at the Fox Chase Cancer Center has been to develop physiological approaches that are effective for prevention of breast cancer [1–5]. Since the early 1980s, our laboratory along with other investigators have been investigating the intriguing phenomenon that pregnancy has protective effects against breast cancer in both women [6] and experimental animals, and have revealed that an early full-term pregnancy is the key physiological factor that has preventive effects on breast cancer [7–12]. It has been observed that the first full-term pregnancy at an age younger than 24 years old provides an evident protection against breast cancer [11, 13] and moreover, additional pregnancies and the prolongation of total lactation period have been shown to enhance the preventive effect even more [14–16]. The preventive effect of an early full-term pregnancy has been seen in various rodent models including out-bred Sprague–Dawley (SD) rats, inbred Lewis and Wistar-Furth rats, and inbred mice (for review see [14]). Most of these studies have revealed that the early full-term pregnancy results in a greater than 75% inhibition of the incidence of breast carcinomas [14, 17].

Pregnancy is associated with increased levels of several pregnancy-related hormones including estrogen (E) and progesterone (P), which play leading roles in orchestrating proper development and function of breast tissue [18]. In fact, pregnancy can be mimicked by the administration of E plus P, which are thought to be responsible for the diminished risk for breast cancer among women following a full-term pregnancy [18, 19]. It has been shown that a short-term administration of E plus P mimics the protective effect of parity in rats and that a treatment period as short as one-third of the gestation time is sufficient to induce protection against mammary carcinogenesis [17]. A study by Rajkumar et al. [20] has demonstrated that in nulliparous rats, a long-term protection against mammary carcinogenesis could be achieved by short-term treatments with various combinations of both natural and synthetic E and P. In addition to E and P, another key pregnancy-related hormone that is highly

J. Russo and I.H. Russo, *Role of the Transcriptome in Breast Cancer Prevention*,
DOI 10.1007/978-1-4614-4884-6_2,

secreted during pregnancy is human chorionic gonadotropin (hCG), a glycoprotein that is made by the developing embryo soon after conception and later by the syncytiotrophoblast. In 1983, our laboratory reported [21] the first finding that hCG had the protective effect on mammary carcinogenesis. Our subsequent studies ([7–9, 21, 22] and for review see [2] and references therein) have clearly demonstrated that a complete differentiation of the mammary gland conferred protection against breast cancer and that the complete differentiation of the mammary gland was attained through pregnancy and lactation. The greater differentiation of the mammary gland was manifested as permanent structural changes, consisting of the disappearance of terminal end buds (TEBs) and a diminution of the number of terminal ducts (TDs) due to their differentiation into lobules. Interestingly, we found that these events were fully mimicked through exogenous administration of hCG alone [7–9, 21, 22]. More importantly, we have shown in an experimental model [23, 24] that a short-term hCG treatment induced the molecular, cellular, pathophysiological, and morphological changes that similarly occur during pregnancy. Especially, we have revealed [3] that hCG induced specific changes in genomic signature similar to those occurring during pregnancy, which were associated with inhibition of not only the initiation and the progression of chemically induced mammary carcinomas but also the development of early lesions such as intraductal proliferations and carcinoma in situ (CIS). hCG was found to inhibit mammary tumorigenesis through both induction of differentiation and inhibition of the proliferation of human breast epithelial cells (HBEC) in vitro [25]. Consistent with our observations made in studies with animal models, a nested case-control study with a female population-based cohort [26] has revealed that women with hCG levels in the top tertile consistently had lower risks of breast cancer than women with hCG levels in the lowest tertile. All together, these observations strongly support our original notion that the elevated levels of hCG, a key placental hormone, during pregnancy confer potent protection on the long-term risk of breast cancer. These observations prompt us to continually pursue the potential applications of hCG in prevention of human breast cancer. In the present work we would like to document several aspects of our studies that will help to establish the powerful role of hCG in breast cancer prevention. We will divide our work into the following sections: (a) the differential effect of urinary hCG (u-hCG) vs. recombinant hCG (r-hCG); (b) time-dependent preventive effects of hCG on rat mammary carcinogenesis; and (c) the study of side effects of hCG in reproduction.

2.2 The Differential Effect of Urinary hCG vs. Recombinant hCG

2.2.1 Human Chorionic Gonadotropin

Up to now the main known physiological function of hCG in the female is the maintenance of the corpus luteum of pregnancy through its interaction with the ovarian lutropin-choriogonadotropin-receptor (LH-CG-R), which has been described in the human breast. This interaction activates a cascade of effects that results in increases in serum levels of estrogen and progesterone. Administration of hCG to virgin rats elicits a similar response [7, 27–31]. In addition, our studies have shown that hCG has a direct effect on the rat mammary epithelium and on HBEC in vitro [32]. hCG is currently used in the treatment of infertility and hypogonadotropic hypogonadism in males [33–36]. It has also been used for the treatment of obesity [37], and has been successfully used in Phase I/II trials in the United States for the treatment of Kaposi's sarcoma lesions in acquired immunodeficiency syndrome (AIDS) patients [38–40]. A drawback in these studies is the fact that the most common source of all commercially available hCG preparations is the urine of pregnant women, which carries numerous bioactive ovarian and placental hormone and peptide metabolites. The assessment of the specific effects of hCG, therefore, requires the use of a pure form of the hormone, such as a recombinant preparation.

Pregnancy can be considered to be the most physiological mechanism for protecting the mammary gland from malignant transformation, a conclusion supported by epidemiological data [13, 41]. The fact that hCG appears to mimic the effect of pregnancy makes the use of this protocol for cancer prevention an appealing idea that needs further exploration. Our experimental results constitute the rationale for proposing to evaluate both the therapeutic efficacy of hCG in newly diagnosed breast cancer and its potential to prevent the development of new malignancies in the patients treated with hCG for primary breast cancer. In order to identify the ultimate mechanisms responsible for pregnancy/hCG-mediated protection we compared the mammary cancer preventive and therapeutic effects of hCG obtained from the urine of pregnant women (u-hCG) with those of the pure hormone, r-hCG.

Results reported here were obtained from experimental protocols designed with two main purposes, one, to evaluate the efficacy of r-hCG in comparison with that of u-hCG and placebo in the prevention of mammary cancer by determining the potential of these hormones to inhibit the initiation of DMBA-induced rat mammary carcinomas. The second purpose was to evaluate the therapeutic efficiency of r-hCG on mammary cancer. For this objective the tumoristatic and tumoricidal efficacy of r-hCG and u-hCG on early and advanced mammary cancer was tested in intact virgin rats that had received DMBA 20 days prior to the initiation of the hormonal treatments. The effect on advanced tumor development was evaluated by starting the hormonal treatment 60 days after DMBA administration, or when tumors were already palpable.

2.2.2 Experimental Protocol

For these experiments, 450 intact virgin Sprague–Dawley rats were divided into 9 groups of 50 animals each, and randomly assigned to one of the following regimens (Fig. 2.1): Regimens 1, 2, or 3 were designed for evaluating the efficacy of r-hCG in the prevention of mammary cancer. The effect of r-hCG treatment of virgin rats on the initiation of DMBA-induced mammary carcinomas was compared with that of u-hCG, utilizing as controls age-matched placebo-treated intact virgin

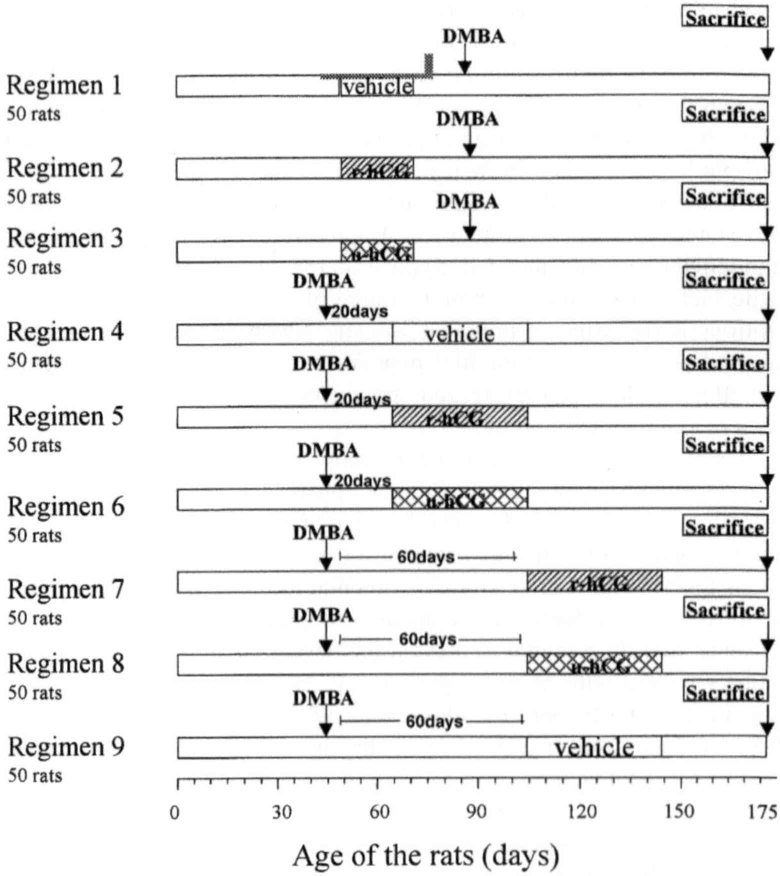

Fig. 2.1 Experimental protocol designed for testing the preventive and therapeutic efficacy of human chorionic gonadotropin (hCG) on rat mammary cancer. For these experiments, 450 intact virgin Sprague–Dawley rats were purchased from Taconic Farms (New York, NY). The animals were received when they were 40 days old. On arrival all the animals were individually and permanently numbered from 1 to 450 by ear marking with the appropriate holes and wedges. Animals from numbers 300 to 400 series were also identified by toe clipping. They were weighed, and housed three to a cage in the first 17 cages for each regimen; the last cage of each regimen housed two animals. Individual cages were sequentially numbered, and each regimen was identified by cards of different colors. The same colors were applied to all boxes containing hormones or placebo, and to syringes utilized for injecting the animals, in order to avoid errors during the injection period. The cages were placed on open racks in an environmentally controlled clean air room with a 12-h light/12-h darkness cycle. The animals were fed pellets of Purina Certified Rodent Chow 5002 and tap water ad libitum. All the procedures performed during these studies complied with the institutional and federal guidelines for the use and care of laboratory animals under protocols approved by the Institutional Animal Care and Use Committees (IACUC) of the Fox Chase Cancer: A suspension of DMBA (Sigma Chemical Co., St. Louis, MO) was prepared at a concentration of 10 mg/mL of corn oil by heating in a water bath at 95°C for 30 min. The carcinogen suspension was allowed to reach room temperature before intragastric (i.g.) instillation with a gastric cannula. Thereafter all the animals were palpated periodically for detection of tumor development and determination of tumor growth rate.

rats. Both hormones were administered at a dose of 100 IU/day for 21 days, starting when the animals were 45 days old. The 50 rats assigned to Regimen 1 received a daily intraperitoneal (i.p.) injection of 0.5 mL Ovidrel placebo for 21 days. Under Regimens 2 and 3 the same number of animals received for 21 days 100 IU/day of r-hCG (Ovidrel, Serono) or u-hCG (Steris Laboratories, Phoenix, AZ), respectively. Twenty-one days after completion of the last injection, when the animals were 87 days old, the three groups of animals were inoculated with a single intragastric (i.g.) dose of 8 mg DMBA per 100 g body weight (bw).

Regimens 4–6 were designed to test the effect of the hormonal treatments on early tumor development. All the animals received a single i.g. dose of DMBA when they were 45 days old. Twenty-one days later those animals allocated to Regimen 4 started receiving a daily i.p. injection of 0.5 mL Ovidrel placebo for 40 days. Under Regimens 5 and 6 the same number of animals received for 40 days 100 IU/day of r-hCG or u-hCG, respectively. All the animals were palpated biweekly for detection of tumor development and determination of tumor growth rate. Final tumorigenic response was evaluated 18 weeks after administration of DMBA.

Regimens 7–9 were designed to test the effect of the hormonal treatments on late tumor development. All the animals were inoculated with a single i.g. dose of 8 mg DMBA per 100 g bw when they were 45 days old. Tumorigenic response was evaluated by palpation of the right and left mammary cervical, thoracic, abdominal and inguinal areas and from ventral to dorsolateral extensions of the glands (Figs. 2.2 and 2.3). All the tumors were sequentially numbered in the order they had appeared, their location was recorded, and the rate of tumor growth was determined by measurement of tumor size with a Vernier caliper. All changes in the health status of the animals, rapid tumor growth, or skin ulceration were recorded. Those animals in which the tumors were excessively large or became ulcerated were euthanized, irrespective of the stage of the hormonal treatment, in compliance with Institutional Animal Care and Use Committees (IACUC) regulations. Those animals euthanized before initiation or before the completion of the hormonal treatments were deleted from the statistical analysis of the final tumorigenic response. Sixty days after DMBA inoculation,

Fig. 2.1 (continued) Final tumorigenic response was evaluated 18 weeks after administration of DMBA. At the end of the experiment all the animals were anesthetized with an i.p. injection of Ketamine (90 mg/kg bw)-Nembutal (40 mg/kg bw), bled through the inferior vena cava, and the serum was separated and kept frozen at –700°C. The tumors were rapidly dissected, measured in three dimensions, and serially sliced. Adjacent slices were: (1) fixed in 10% neutral buffered formalin (NBF) for histopathological and immunocytochemical analysis, (2) frozen in liquid nitrogen for estrogen receptor (ER) and progesterone receptor (PR) determinations, and (3) placed in sterile culture medium for DNA analysis by flow cytometry. Tumors that were smaller than 1 cm in diameter were fixed in 10% NBF only. In the absence of tumors the right thoracic (second and third), and the right abdominal (fourth) mammary glands were fixed in 10% NBF for histopathological evaluation of degree of gland development. The right and left ovaries of all animals were dissected, measured in three dimensions with a Vernier caliper and fixed in 10% NBF. All the internal organs were examined for evidence of metastatic nodules, adhesions, or hemorrhages. Liver, spleen, and lung changes were documented and representative fragments of tissues were fixed in 10% NBF for histopathological examination. Representative lesions were photographed

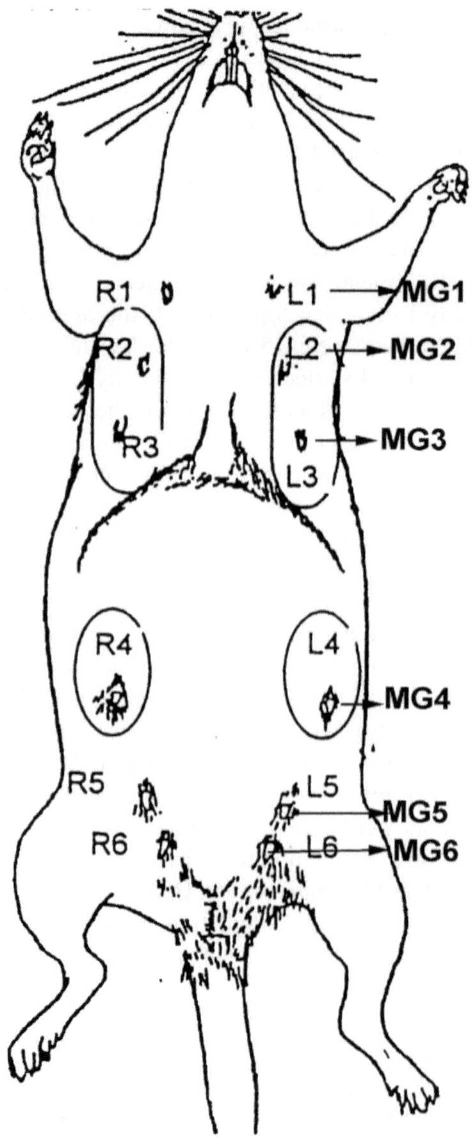

Fig. 2.2 Diagram showing the location of the mammary glands in the Sprague–Dawley rat. *MG1* mammary gland pair located in the cervical region; *MG2* and *MG3* thoracic, *MG4* abdominal; *MG5* abdomino-inguinal; and *MG6* inguino-perineal regions

Fig. 2.3 (continued) After a buffer rinse the slides were incubated for 30 min with Vectastain Elite ABC kit for mouse (Vector Laboratories, Inc., Burlingame, CA), washed in PBS buffer and incubated in peroxidase substrate solution containing hydrogen peroxide and 3,3′-diaminobenzidine-HCl (DAB) for 2 min. Sections incubated with nonimmune serum were used as negative controls. All sections were lightly counterstained with hematoxylin. Immunostaining was evaluated by examination of slides under a bright field microscope, and graded according to the intensity of the nuclear brown staining as negative (–), weak (+), moderate (++), or strong (+++), as previously described [33]. Results were expressed as the percentage of positive cells over the total number of epithelial cells counted for every specific type of lesion

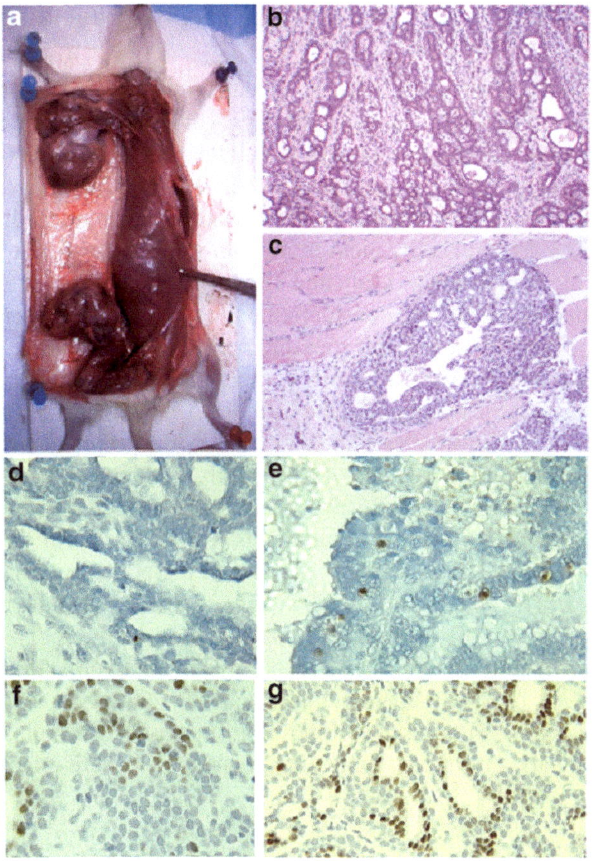

Fig. 2.3 (**a**) Gross anatomy of tumors located in thoracic mammary glands 2 and 3, and abdomino-inguinal mammary glands 4 and 5, found in animal treated with placebo (Regimen 9); (**b**) histological section of an invasive adenocarcinoma located in the cervical mammary gland of an animal treated with placebo (Regimen 4) (Hematoxylin and Eosin, ×20); (**c**) ductal CIS, found in non-tumoral breast tissue. (H&E, ×20); (**d, e**) invasive adenocarcinomas immunoreacted with ApopTag for detection of apoptotic cells, and counterstained with hematoxylin (H) (×40); (**d**) tumor in placebo-treated animal (Regimen 9); (**e**) tumor in r-hCG treated animal (Regimen 7); (**f**) Regimen 1 invasive adenocarcinoma immunoreacted with anti-estrogen receptor antibody (*brown nuclei*) and counterstained with H; (**g**) Regimen 1 invasive adenocarcinoma immunoreacted with anti-progesterone receptor antibody (*brown nuclei*) and counterstained with H; (×40). All palpable tumors, microscopic tumors, and suspicious areas exhibiting nodularity and/or discoloration that were visually identified during mammary gland dissection at necropsy were fixed in 10% neutral buffered formalin, embedded in paraffin, stained with hematoxylin-eosin, and classified according to criteria published elsewhere [14]. Mammary tumors that were fixed in formalin, dehydrated, and embedded in paraffin were cut at a thickness of 4 μm. The tissue sections were mounted on positively charged slides, deparaffinized, rehydrated, and incubated in 2% hydrogen peroxide at room temperature for 15 min for quenching endogenous peroxidase activity. The sections were sequentially incubated in two changes of Target Retrieval Solution at 98°C for 5 min each. Those slides assigned to progesterone receptor analysis (PR) were also incubated in 0.02% trypsin for 10 min. All the tissue sections were then incubated in diluted normal blocking serum for 20 min. Excess serum was blotted from the slides and the sections were incubated with either mouse monoclonal anti-estrogen receptor (ER) or anti-progesterone receptor (PR) antibodies (InnoGenex, San Ramon, CA) at a dilution of 1:400. Both antibodies were incubated in a humidity chamber at 4°C overnight, washed in buffer and the sections were incubated with rat adsorbed goat anti-mouse biotinylated secondary antibody (InnoGenex, San Ramon, CA) at room temperature for 30 min.

when the rats were 105 days old, animals allocated to Regimen 7 started receiving a daily i.p. injection of 0.5 mL r-hCG for 40 days. Under Regimens 8 and 9 the same number of animals received for 40 days 100 IU/day of u-hCG or 0.5 mL Ovidrel Placebo, respectively. Tumorigenic response was evaluated by biweekly palpation. All tumors were sequentially numbered, their location was recorded, and the rate of tumor growth was determined by measurement of tumor size with a Vernier caliper. Final tumorigenic response was evaluated 18 weeks after administration of DMBA and was evaluated by taking into consideration the following parameters: (1) Rate of tumor growth, based on sequential measurement of the two largest diameters of tumors in live animals utilizing a Vernier Caliper and expressing the results in mm, or calculating the volume by applying the formula: $V = 4/3 \times (d_1/2)(d_2/2)^2$, where V is total volume, d_1 the smallest diameter, and d_2 the largest diameter; (2) Final tumor size, based on measurement of the length, width, and height of dissected tumors with a Vernier Caliper. Results were expressed in mm. A progressively smaller tumor size in successive measurements was indicative of tumor regression. Palpable tumors that had disappeared at the time of dissection were considered to be 100% regressed. The mammary tissue in which the tumor had been originally identified was fixed in 10% NBF for histopathological analysis. This criterion was indicative of an inhibitory effect of the hormonal treatments on tumor growth; (3) Tumor necrosis in large palpable tumors, and (4) Presence of skin ulceration in live animals, indicative of rapid rate of tumor growth, more frequently found in placebo-treated animals. This condition made it mandatory to euthanize the animals.

2.2.3 *Effect of hCG in Mammary Cancer Prevention*

Regimens 1, 2, and 3. Fifty virgin rats were treated with placebo, r-hCG, or u-hCG for each one of the regimens (Fig. 2.1). The placebo or hormonal treatments were initiated when the rats were 45 days old and were administered consecutively for 21 days. Twenty-one days after the last injection, when the animals were 87 days old, they received a single i.g. dose of DMBA. One animal of Regimen 1 and one of Regimen 2 died during carcinogen administration as a consequence of acute reaction to the anesthesia; they were deleted from the study, reducing the total animal population to 49 in each one of these two regimens. All the animals appeared healthy during the injection period and thereafter throughout the length of the study, which was terminated when the animals were 175 days old.

Periodic palpation of the animals revealed that all of them were free of palpable masses before carcinogen administration. The vast majority of tumors were found at the time of autopsy and none of them were ulcerated. None of the animals were required to be euthanized before the end of the experiment. In animals treated with placebo (Regimen 1) 44 palpable masses were found in 22 of 49 animals treated (44.9%). The tumors were predominantly located in the mammary glands located in the thoracic regions, mammary gland pairs 2 (MG2) and 3 (MG3). Second in frequency were those tumors located in the MG1 and neck and ear regions (Fig. 2.2; Table 2.1). After dissection and histopathological evaluation and diagnosis of the

Table 2.1 Effect of r-hCG and u-hCG in the prevention of DMBA-induced mammary carcinogenesis

Regimen treatment	No animals	Animals with tumors/%	No. tumors/tumors per animal	Animals with carcinomas/%	No. carcinomas/carcinoma per animal	No. CIS/CIS per animal	No. benign lesions[a]/benign lesions per animal
1-Placebo	49	22/45	44/0.89	18/37	26/0.53	27/0.55	18/0.36
2-r-hCG	49	4/8	5/0.10	3/6	3/0.06	0/0.00	2/0.04
3-u-hCG	50	6/12	7/0.14	4/8	5/0.10	2/0.04	2/0.04

Statistical analysis

Regimen	Animals with tumors/%	No. tumors/tumors per animal	Animals with carcinomas/%	No. CIS/CIS per animal
1 vs. 2	$p<0.001$	$p<0.001$	$p<0.001$	$p<0.001$
1 vs. 3	$p<0.001$	$p<0.001$	$p<0.001$	$p<0.001$

[a]Benign lesions include both tumoral and non-tumoral lesions of mammary and non-mammary origin, i.e., fibromas, fibroadenomas, epidermal inclusion cyst, keratoacanthomas, lymph node and salivary gland hyperplasia, mammary cysts and duct ectasia, etc.

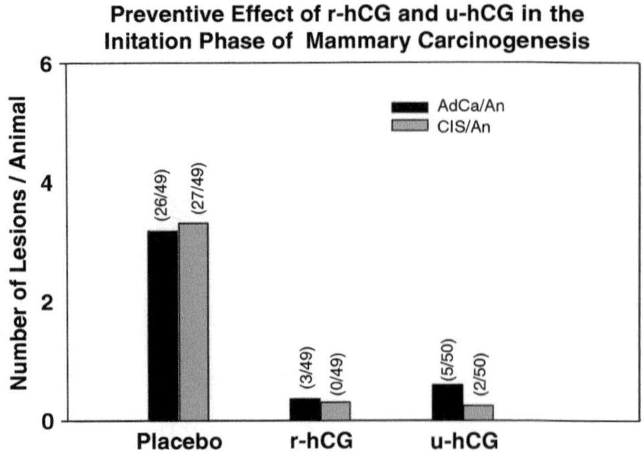

Fig. 2.4 Histogram showing in the ordinate the number of adenocarcinomas (AdCa) and carcinoma in situ (CIS) per animal. The abscissa shows the treatments received: Placebo, Regimen 1, r-hCG, Regimen 2, and u-hCG, Regimen 3, as described in Fig. 2.1. The *numbers* in *parentheses* represent the total number of lesions in the total number of animals studied

masses dissected it was found that 26 of them were invasive mammary adenocarcinomas, which were found in 18 animals (37%), representing an average of 0.53 adenocarcinomas per animal (Table 2.1). These tumors were predominantly papillary adenocarcinomas, either type I (four tumors), type II (five tumors), types II and I combined (ten tumors), and papillary carcinomas types I and II combined with cribriform pattern (seven tumors). In addition the mammary glands of the same animals contained a total of 27 in situ carcinomas, or 0.55 in situ carcinoma per animal (Table 2.1). None of these tumors exhibited necrosis or regressive changes. In four of the animals the enlarged masses represented lymph node or salivary gland hyperplasia (three enlarged lymph nodes, five enlarged salivary glands), or swollen portions of muscle, fibroadipose tissue, or mammary gland, but they were free of neoplasms.

Treatment of the animals with r-hCG (Regimen 2) significantly reduced the number of palpable tumors in all the mammary glands, neck, and ear regions. Five tumors were palpated in 4 out of 49 animals (8.1%). When the tumors were histopathologically classified, it was found that three of them were papillary adenocarcinomas, either type I, combined types I and II, and cribriform adenocarcinoma, reducing the number of animals with mammary neoplasms to three (6%) (Table 2.1; Fig. 2.4). Foci of CIS were found within invasive adenocarcinomas, but this type of lesion was not found in animals free of invasive carcinomas or bearing only benign lesions. One of the tumors detected by palpation was a benign epidermal inclusion cyst and the other an enlarged lymph node.

A total of 50 animals treated with u-hCG (Regimen 3) were evaluated at the end of the experiment. Seven tumoral masses were palpable in six of the animals (12%). Four of them were invasive papillary adenocarcinomas type I and II, and one was a papillary adenocarcinoma type I and II combined with cribriform carcinoma. These lesions and two in situ carcinomas were found in 4 out of the 50 animals (8%). The other two palpable masses were an enlarged lymph node and a benign keratoacanthoma, respectively (Table 2.1).

2.2.4 *Effect of hCG on Mammary Cancer Therapy*

2.2.4.1 Effect of r-hCG and u-hCG on Early Tumor Development

The effect of r-hCG and u-hCG was tested using Regimens 4, 5, and 6 (Fig. 2.1). Fifty virgin rats from each one of these regimens were inoculated with DMBA when they were 45 days old. One animal from Regimen 4 and one from Regimen 5 died during carcinogen administration due to acute reaction to the anesthesia. The treatment of the remaining animals with placebo, r-hCG, or u-hCG was initiated 21 days after DMBA inoculation and administered continuously for 40 days (Fig. 2.1).

Ten of the remaining 49 animals of Regimen 4 had developed at least one palpable tumor by 42 days post-DMBA administration. One animal that was severely sick died at the time of the 14th placebo injection and two animals died 12 and 14 days after the last injection, respectively. The total number of palpable tumors detected in this group was 273, which were found in 48 out of 49 animals (97.9%), averaging 5.6 tumors per animal (Table 2.2). The location of tumors was similar to that observed in animals of Regimens 1–3, although a greater percentage of tumors were found to be originating from MG2 and MG3, and lower frequencies in MG1, 4, 5, and 6, and neck-ear regions (Figs. 2.2 and 2.3). The predominant histological types were papillary adenocarcinomas type I and II (116 tumors), and combined papillary adenocarcinomas type I and II with cribriform carcinoma (68 tumors). The 87 adenocarcinomas in situ (CIS) were found in animals already bearing invasive adenocarcinomas, therefore their presence did not modify the overall tumor incidence (Table 2.2; Fig. 2.5). Among the numerous benign lesions found in this group of animals there were keratoacanthomas, epidermal inclusion cysts, intraductal papillomas, hyperplastic alveolar nodules, and mammary glands with cystic changes.

Treatment with r-hCG (Regimen 5) resulted in a reduction in the number of animals with tumors; it also reduced the total number of tumors, invasive adenocarcinomas, and carcinomas in situ (Table 2.2). The predominant types of invasive tumors were the papillary adenocarcinomas type I and II (55 tumors) and the papillary adenocarcinoma type I and II combined with cribriform carcinoma (20 tumors). Many of these tumors exhibited changes indicative of regression and differentiation, such as fibrosis, lactational charges, and necrosis, which were observed in 18 tumors. The benign lesions found consisted of keratoacanthomas, epidermal inclusion cysts, intraductal papillomas, and cystic changes; they were also reduced in number (Table 2.2).

Treatment with u-hCG (Regimen 6) also reduced the number of animals with tumors, as well as the total number of tumors, number of invasive adenocarcinomas, and carcinomas in situ (Table 2.2). The tumors found were predominantly papillary adenocarcinomas type I and II (55 tumors) and the papillary adenocarcinoma type I and II combined with cribriform carcinoma (20 tumors). Some of these tumors also exhibited fibrosis, lactational charges, and necrosis. The number of benign lesions, such as keratoacanthomas, epidermal inclusion cysts, intraductal papillomas, and cystic changes, were also reduced in number (Table 2.2).

Table 2.2 Effect of r-hCG and u-hCG on the early phase of progression of DMBA-induced mammary carcinomas

Regimen treatment	No animals	Animals with tumors/%	No. tumors/tumors per animal	Animals with carcinomas/%	No. carcinomas/carcinoma per animal	No. CIS/CIS per animal	No. benign lesions[a]/benign lesions per animal
4-Placebo	49	48/98	273/5.6	44/90	210/4.29	87/1.70	63/1.3
5-r-hCG	49	38/78	111/2.2	38/78	81/1.65	41/0.84	30/0.61
6-u-hCG	46	30/65	88/1.9	27/59	72/1.57	31/0.67	16/0.34

Statistical analysis

Regimen	Animals with tumors/%	No. tumors/tumors per animal	Animals with carcinomas/%	No. CIS/CIS per animal
4 vs. 5	$p<0.01$	$p<0.01$	$p<0.01$	$p<0.01$
4 vs. 6	$p<0.01$	$p<0.01$	$p<0.01$	$p<0.01$

[a]Benign lesions include both tumoral and non-tumoral lesions of mammary and non-mammary origin, i.e., fibromas, fibroadenomas, epidermal inclusion cyst, keratoacanthomas, lymph node and salivary gland hyperplasia, mammary cysts and duct ectasia, etc.

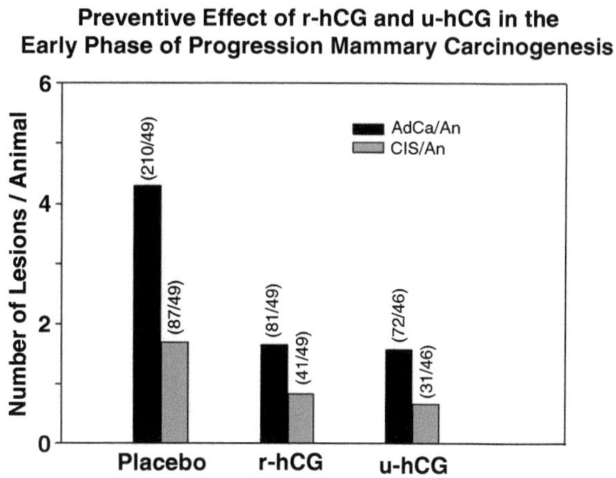

Fig. 2.5 Histogram showing in the ordinate the number of AdCa and CIS per animal in the animals treated with DMBA at the age of 45 days, and 20 days later with placebo (Regimen 4), r-hCG (Regimen 5), or u-hCG (Regimen 6). The *numbers* in *parentheses* represent the total number of lesions in the total number of animals studied

2.2.4.2 Effect of r-hCG and u-hCG on Advanced Tumor Development

The effect of r-hCG and u-hCG on advanced tumor development was tested using Regimens 7, 8, and 9 (Fig. 2.1). For these three regimens 150 animals were inoculated with DMBA when they were 45 days old. One animal from Regimen 7 died during carcinogen administration and was deleted from the study. The treatment with the hormones or placebo was initiated 60 days after DMBA administration (Fig. 1.1). At that time around 50% of the animals had already developed palpable tumors, which averaged, 1.40, 1.31, and 0.76 tumors per animal in those rats allocated to Regimens 7, 8, and 9, respectively (Table 2.3). At the end of the hormonal treatment the number of palpable tumors had increased in the three groups, although the maximal increase occurred in the placebo-treated group (Regimen 9), in which there were 119 palpable tumors, at an average of 2.90 tumors per animal. All animals that needed to be euthanized because of the rapid growth and ulceration of the tumors before completion of treatment were deleted from the final analysis of tumorigenic response. The same criterion applied to the animals treated under the three regimens, therefore 37 animals treated with r-hCG (Regimen 7), 36 treated with u-hCG (Regimen 8), and 40 animals treated with placebo (Regimen 9) were eligible for the analysis of the final tumorigenic response (Table 2.3).

Thirty-nine out of 40 animals (97.5%) in the placebo-treated group (Regimen 9) had a total of 229 tumors in a distribution similar to that described for Regimens 1–6. In addition two animals had metastatic nodules in the spleen, liver, and lungs, which were not included in the final tabulation of tumors (Table 2.4). The histopathological analysis of tumors revealed that the greatest percentage of tumors, regardless their location, was represented by invasive adenocarcinomas, papillary types I and II (129 tumors), second in frequency was the invasive adenocarcinoma papillary type I and II combined with cribriform type (34 tumors); there was a lower

Table 2.3 Effect of r-hCG and u-hCG on palpable DMBA-induced mammary tumors

	Tumorigenesis at the beginning of treatment		Tumorigenesis at the end of treatment		Tumorigenesis at the end of experiment	
Regimen treatment	No. tumors (tumor/animal)	Animal with tumor/ total no animal (%)	No. tumors (tumor/animal)	Animal with tumor/ total no animal (%)	No. tumors (tumor/animal)	Animal with tumor/ total no animal (%)
9-Placebo	36 (0.76)	20/47 (42.55)	119 (2.90)	35/40 (87.5)	229 (5.7)	39/40 (97.5)
7-r-hCG	66 (1.40)	28/47 (59.57)	79 (2.07)	28/38 (73.68)	147 (3.9)	33/37 (89.1)
8-u-hCG	63 (1.31)	27/48 (56.25)	43 (1.19)	19/36 (52.77)	122 (3.4)	32/36 (88.8)

Table 2.4 Effect of r-hCG and u-hCG on the advanced phase of progression of DMBA-induced mammary carcinomas

Regimen treatment	No animals	Animals with tumors/%	No. tumors/tumors per animal	Animals with carcinomas/%	No. carcinomas/ carcinoma per animal	No. CIS/CIS per animal	No. benign lesions[a]/ benign lesions per animal
9-Placebo	40	39/97.5	229/5.7	39/97.5	188/4.7	45/1.13	41/1.0
7-r-hCG	37	33/89.1	147/3.9	32/86.4	67/1.81	29/0.78	80/2.5
8-u-hCG	36	32/88.8	122/3.4	32/88.8	77/2.13	16/0.44	45/1.2

Statistical analysis

Regimen	Animals with tumors/%	No. tumors/tumors per animal	Animals with carcinomas/%	No. CIS/CIS per animal
9 vs. 7	$p<0.01$	$p<0.01$	$p<0.01$	$p<0.01$
9 vs. 8	$p<0.01$	$p<0.01$	$p<0.01$	$p<0.01$

[a]Benign lesions include both tumoral and non-tumoral lesions of mammary and non-mammary origin, i.e., fibromas, fibroadenomas, epidermal inclusion cyst, keratoacanthomas, lymph node and salivary gland hyperplasia, mammary cysts and duct ectasia, etc.

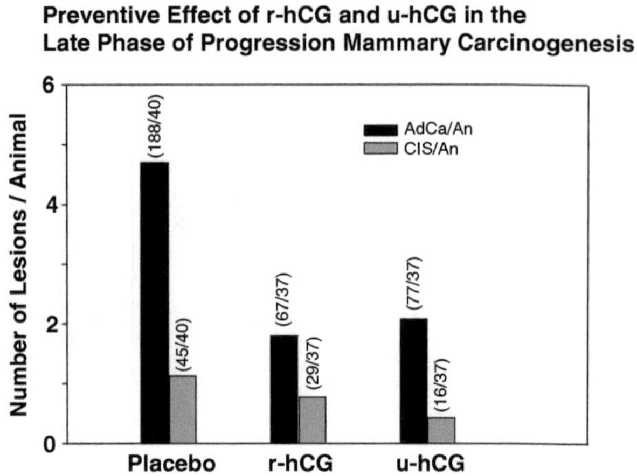

Fig. 2.6 Histogram showing in the ordinate the number of AdCa and CIS per animal in the animals treated with DMBA at the age of 45 days, and 60 days later with placebo (Regimen 9), r-hCG (Regimen 7), or u-hCG (Regimen 8). The *numbers* in *parentheses* represent the total number of lesions in the total number of animals studied

frequencies of carcinomas in situ, invasive papillary adenocarcinomas type I, and benign lesions (Table 2.4).

In the r-hCG treated group (Regimen 7), a total of 37 animals fulfilled the eligibility criteria to be included in the final analysis; 33 of them (89.1%) developed a total of 147 tumors, averaging 3.9 tumors per animal over the total number of animals at risk (Table 2.3). In two animals tumors that were palpated at the beginning of treatment had regressed completely at the time of autopsy. In this group of animals, some very large tumors consisted of an encapsulated mass of brown fluid necrotic material, with not viable tissue identifiable for additional studies, except for histopathological analysis. The histopathological analysis of tumors revealed the presence of the same tumor types found in the other regimens, namely invasive papillary adenocarcinomas type I and II, totaling 54 tumors, 10 of which exhibited necrosis, and in addition, other 30 tumors exhibited regressive and differentiation-associated changes, such as fibrosis, lactational, and cystic changes. Following in frequency among the invasive carcinomas were the papillary adenocarcinomas type I and II combined with cribriform type, 13 tumors, adenoid cystic carcinoma, 10 tumors, and papillary adenocarcinoma type I, 9 tumors. A large proportion of these lesions also exhibited fibrosis, lactational, and cystic changes. Twenty-nine carcinomas in situ, two tubular adenocarcinomas, and a variety of benign mammary lesions, which included intraductal papillomas, epidermal inclusion cysts, keratoacanthomas, hyperplastic alveolar nodules, mammary cysts, and focal areas of fibrosis were also identified in this group of animals.

Thirty-two (88.8%) out of the 36 animals of Regimen 8 that were treated with u-hCG and were eligible for the analysis of the final tumorigenic response had developed a total of 122 palpable tumors, 77 of which were invasive adenocarcinomas (Table 2.3; Fig. 2.6). The majority of them were invasive papillary adenocarcinomas type I and II, 32 tumors, pure type I, 22 tumors, and invasive papillary adenocarcinomas type I and II combined with cribriform pattern, type, 15 tumors. The number of tumors exhibiting regressive and differentiation-associated changes, such as fibrosis, lactational, and cystic changes, was markedly lower than those

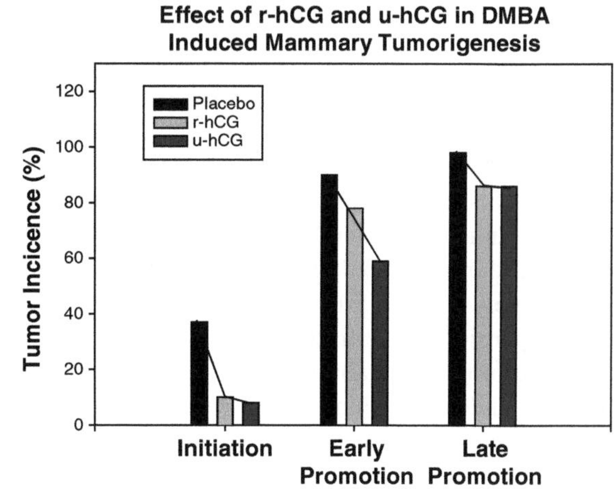

Fig. 2.7 Histogram showing in the ordinate tumor incidence in the mammary gland of virgin rats treated with placebo (Regimen 1), r-hCG (Regimen 2), or u-hCG (Regimen 3) 21 days prior to DMBA, initiation; 20 days after DMBA early promotion (Regimens 4, 5, and 6), or 60 days after DMBA administration, late promotion (Regimens 7, 8, and 9), according to the protocol shown in Fig. 2.1

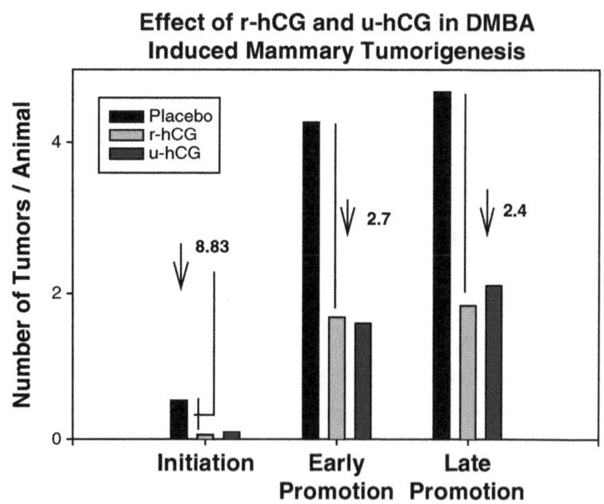

Fig. 2.8 Histogram showing in the ordinate the number of tumors per animal and in the abscissa the regimens for studying initiation (Regimens 1, 2, and 3), early promotion (Regimens 3, 4, and 5), and late promotion (Regimens 7, 8, and 9), as described in Fig. 2.1. The *arrows* and the *numbers* indicate the rate of tumor reduction as the result of treatment of the animals with r-hCG

found in animals treated with r-hCG under Regimen 7. There were six carcinomas in situ, as well as numerous benign mammary lesions, i.e., fibroadenomas, adenomas, fibromas, and intraductal papillomas. Palpable masses that were of non-mammary origin were two enlarged lymph nodes and one enlarged salivary gland.

The analysis of tumor and mammary cancer incidence as well as the number of tumors and adenocarcinomas per animal in the nine regimens studied revealed that the treatment of the virgin rats with r-hCG and u-hCG always resulted in a reduction in all parameters. The treatment with placebo initiated when the animals were 45 days old in Regimen 1 followed by carcinogen administration 20 days later, when they were 87 days old, resulted in a tumor incidence of 45%, which was significantly lower than that developed by animals treated with placebo 20 or 60 days after carcinogen administration, but that had received the carcinogen when they were 45 days old. Treatment of the animals with r-hCG and u-hCG prior to DMBA instillation further reduced the tumorigenic response (Figs. 2.7 and 2.8).

2.2.5 *Special Studies*

2.2.5.1 Cellular DNA Analysis by Flow Cytometry

Cellular DNA analysis by flow cytometry was used to evaluate cell proliferation in those tumors larger than 1 cm^3 in which there was enough tissue to serially section for histopathological and steroid receptor analyses as well. A slice of viable tumor was placed in sterile culture medium, finely minced with the help of scalpel blades, immediately fixed in 70% ethanol, and stored at −20°C until analyzed. The tumor cell suspensions were further homogenized, filtered, and the cellular DNA content was determined by staining tumor cells with the fluorescent nucleic acid dye propidium iodide (Boehringer Mannheim), that intercalates between base pairs binding to double-stranded nucleic acids. Fluorescent intensity above 600 nm was used as an indicator of cellular DNA content. The tumor cells were incubated with RNAse to degrade any double-stranded RNA that could bind propidium iodide and produce staining artifacts. The fluorescent intensity of stained cells was determined using a Becton Dickinson FACScan. The DNA content of the cells was analyzed with the Mac Cycle Software. There were no significant differences in the data collected, as depicted in Table 2.5.

2.2.5.2 Detection of Cell Cycle and Apoptotic Markers by Flow Cytometry

Mammary tumors subjected to DNA analysis by flow cytometry were also tested for their content of p53, Cyclin D1, and p21. The following fluorescein conjugated mouse monoclonal antibodies were used: Pab246, epitope mapping at amino acid residues 88–93 of mouse p53, that also recognizes rat p53, cyclin D1 (−12) epitope corresponding to amino acids 1–295, representing full length cyclin D1, specific for human, mouse and rat cyclin D1, and p21, epitope corresponding to amino acids 1–159 representing full length p21. All the antibodies were purchased from Santa Cruz Biotechnology, Inc., Santa Cruz, CA. The fluorescent intensity of stained cells was determined using a Becton Dickinson FACScan. The DNA content of the cells was analyzed with the Cell Quest Software and the data are depicted in Table 2.6. There were no significant differences detected with this method.

2.2.5.3 Immunocytochemical Detection of Inhibin

Rabbit polyclonal antibodies R-4059 and R-4072, raised in our laboratory against peptides 1-16 (YK) and [CGC] 93-104 were used in these procedures. Sections of paraffin-embedded tumors developed by animals under the nine regimen treatments were mounted on positively charged slides, deparaffinized, rehydrated, and endogenous peroxidase was quenched with 2% hydrogen peroxide. After blocking, the sections were incubated with the respective antibodies overnight, washed, and incubated

Table 2.5 Effect of r-hCG and u-hCG on the cell cycle of DMBA-induced mammary tumors

Regimen	G_1 (%)	S (%)	G_2 (%)	G_1/G_2
4	79.76±3.44	7.81±3.44	12.27±1.96	2.03±0.01
5	80.95±2.76	7.83±3.07	11.08±1.77	2.01±0.007
6	83.14±3.22	6.97±3.65	9.85±3.58	2.02±0.01
9	86.20±0.00	4.50±0.00	9.20±0.00	2.01±0.00
7	82.41±2.09	7.05±1.87	10.38±0.79	2.02±0.001
8	79.45±4.45	8.00±5.37	12.40±0.84	2.05±0.003
Statistical analysis				
Regimen	G_1	S	G_2	G_1/G_2
4 vs. 5	NS	NS	NS	NS
4 vs. 6	$p<0.07$	NS	NS	NS
9 vs. 7	NS	NS	NS	NS
9 vs. 8	NS	NS	NS	NS

Table 2.6 Effect of r-hCG and u-hCG on p53, cyclin D1, and p21 expression in DMBA-induced mammary tumors

Regimen	p53 (% of cells)	Cyclin D1 (FITC)	p21 (FITC)
4	24.56±5.93	325±142	18.38±7.62
5	24.73±6.88	196±71	17.80±8.71
6	27.06±4.02	309±106	20.96±5.41
9	42.50±0.00	276±118	18.18±7.21
7	32.58±9.96	350±116	19.15±7.34
8	35.66±12.23	288±119	17.67±2.02
Statistical analysis			
Regimen	p53	Cyclin D1	p21
4 vs. 5	NS	$p<0.05$	NS
4 vs. 6	NS	NS	NS
9 vs. 7	NS	NS	NS
9 vs. 8	NS	NS	NS

with horse anti-mouse biotinylated secondary antibody (Vector Laboratories, Inc., Burlingame, CA). Vectastain Elite ABC kit (Vector Laboratories, Inc., Burlingame, CA) was used to conjugate and 3,3′-diaminobenzidine-HCl (DAB) to reveal the immunocytochemically reacted sites. Sections incubated with pre-immune serum were used as negative controls. All sections were lightly counterstained with hematoxylin. Immunostaining was evaluated by examination of slides under a bright field microscope, and graded according to the intensity of the brown stain as negative (–), weakly (+), moderately (++), or strongly (+++) positive. Inhibin immunoreactivity was evaluated in the cytoplasm of tumor cells and in normal epithelial cells lining ducts and lobules of the non-tumoral mammary gland. The number of positively stained cells was counted, and results were expressed as a percentage and statistically analyzed in Table 2.7.

Table 2.7 Effect of r-hCG and u-hCG on inhibin expression in DMBA-induced mammary tumors

Regimen	Inhibin expression	Luminal reaction	Cytoplasmic reaction
1	+ to ++	Present	Diffuse
2	+++ to ++++	Present	Focal
3	++++	Present	Focal
4	+ to ++	Present	Diffuse
5	++++	Present	Focal
6	++++	Present	Focal
9	++	Present	Diffuse
7	++++	Present	Focal
8	++++	Present	Focal

2.2.5.4 Apoptotic Index Determination

The ApopTag in situ apoptosis detection kit from Oncor (Gaithersburg, MD) was utilized for the detection of apoptotic cells in DMBA-induced mammary carcinomas in r-hCG-, u-hCG-, or placebo-treated animals under the nine regimens under study. Paraffin-embedded tumors were sectioned at a thickness of 4 micrometers, deparaffinized and rehydrated, followed by digestion with protease K (20 g/mL) for 15 min. The sections were then placed in absolute methanol containing 0.3% H_2O_2 for 30 min to remove any endogenous peroxidase activity. Upon equilibration with reaction buffers, terminal deoxynucleotidyl transferase was added to catalyze incorporation of residues of digoxigenin-nucleotide into the new 3′-OH DNA ends generated by DNA fragmentation accompanying apoptosis. The newly incorporated digoxigenin-nucleotide complexes were detected with anti-digoxigenin antibodies utilizing standard procedures. Color was developed using 0.05% 3,3′-dimethylaminobenzene (DAB kit, Dako Corporation, Carpinteria, CA) and lightly counterstained with hematoxylin. Apoptotic response was determined by counting the number of cells containing apoptotic bodies per total number of epithelial cells that compose IDPs, in situ, and invasive carcinomas examined, and expressed as a percentage of the total. Myoepithelial cells were excluded from the count. The data are shown in Table 2.8 and Fig. 2.9.

2.2.5.5 Steroid Hormone Receptors Ligand Binding Assay

The evaluation of the content of estrogen (ER) and progesterone receptors (PR) was performed in those tumors that were large enough for performing histopathological and flow cytometric analyses (>1 cm^3) obtained from animals treated as indicated for Regimens 1–9 (Fig. 2.1). The content of ER and PR in DMBA-induced rat mammary tumors was evaluated in frozen tissues that were pulverized with a Thermovac pulverizer, homogenized, and ultracentrifuged for obtaining the cytosol fraction. The tumor cytosol fractions were incubated with increasing concentrations of

Table 2.8 Effect of r-hCG and u-hCG in the Apoptotic Index (ApopTag) and Mitotic Index of DMBA-induced mammary tumors

Regimen	Cells counted	Apoptotic cells	Apoptotic Index	Cells in mitosis	Mitotic Index
1	13,600	85	0.64+0.41	16	0.13+0.15
2	9,400	140	1.52+0.77	14	0.11+0.19
3	4,400	71	1.71+0.82	5	0.09+0.27
4	9,800	29	0.31+0.34	8	0.06+0.14
5	3,800	128	4.37+3.40	7	0.15+0.22
6	7,000	217	3.69+2.56	3	0.05+0.20
9	7,700	47	0.68+0.78	9	0.21+0.31
7	12,100	402	3.57+1.32	17	0.16+0.17
8	2,450	107	5.59+4.42	12	0.39+0.45
Statistical analysis					
Regimen			Significance		
1 vs. 2			$p<0.0003$		NS
1 vs. 3			$p<0.0001$		NS
4 vs. 5			$p<0.00006$		NS
4 vs. 6			$p<0.00001$		NS
9 vs. 7			$p<0.0000002$		NS
9 vs. 8			$p<0.0003$		NS

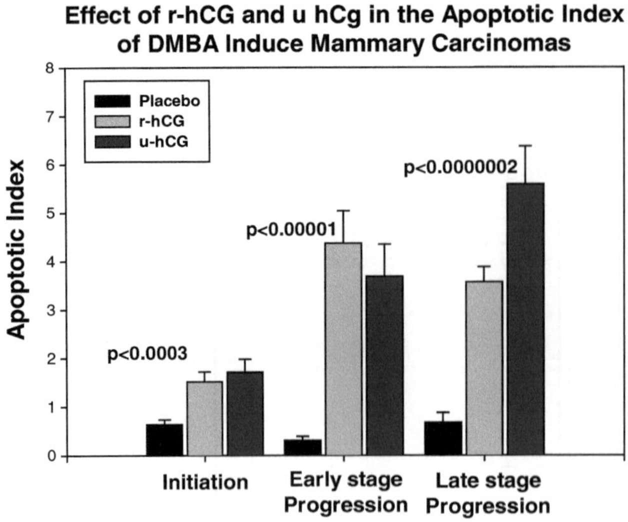

Fig. 2.9 Histogram showing in the ordinate the Apoptotic Index of adenocarcinomas and in the abscissa the regimens for studying initiation (1, 2, and 3), early promotion (3, 4, and 5), and late promotion (7, 8, and 9) of protocol described in Fig. 2.1. The significance of the difference is indicated above the *bars*

^{3}H-estradiol-17 or ^{3}H-R5020 for multipoint titration analysis using the dextran-coated charcoal method. The binding data were analyzed by the Scatchard. Lineweaver–Burk plot, which was used in the case of high receptor content. These procedures were performed according to the standards established for the assessment of estrogen receptors in human breast cancer established by the E.O.R.T.C. Breast Cancer Cooperative Group at the Antoni van Leeuwenhoek-Huis workshop in Amsterdam. The data are depicted in Table 2.9.

2.2.6 *Considerations*

Results presented here demonstrate that a 21 day treatment of young virgin rats with r-hCG (Ovidrel) prevents the initiation and inhibits the progression of DMBA-induced tumors. A 21 day treatment with Ovidrel produces a preventive effect similar to that previously demonstrated by u-hCG, even when the treatment had been terminated 21 days prior to carcinogen administration. Only 8% of Ovidrel treated animals developed tumors (the total number of tumors developed was five), whereas 44.9% of placebo-treated animals developed tumors—44 tumors in all, at an average of 0.89 tumors per animal. The group receiving u-hCG also exhibited an inhibitory effect on tumorigenesis, although the reduction was less significant than that induced by the r-hCG. The results of the present study revealed that r-hCG

Table 2.9 Effect of r-hCG and u-hCG in the expression of ER and PgR in DMBA-induced mammary tumors

Regimen	ER status	PgR status
1	15.3±7.8	31.40±5.06
2	17.3±5.4	28.18±5.12
3	16.8±7.3	28.23±2.51
4	14.7±8.1	27.25±5.54
5	15.3±6.7	50.91±27.04
6	16.0±3.9	22.57±13.47
9	17.1±4.1	36.89±18.11
7	16.5±5.7	28.57±18.18
8	15.9±8.8	32.05±14.04
Statistical analysis		
Regimen	ER status	PgR status
1 vs. 2	NS	NS
1 vs. 3	NS	NS
4 vs. 5	NS	NS
4 vs. 6	NS	NS
9 vs. 7	NS	NS
9 vs. 8	NS	NS

ER estrogen receptor; *PgR* progesterone receptor

treatment of rats previously inoculated with DMBA inhibited the development of early mammary lesions, since initiation of the hormonal treatment 20 days after carcinogen administration reduced significantly both tumor incidence and tumor burden. Both r-hCG and u-hCG exhibited similar tumor inhibitory effects. These data have a significant clinical implication, because they indicate the usefulness of the utilization of this hormonal treatment on early as well as on premalignant lesions. The lesson here is that the sooner a treatment is started the more efficient is the therapeutic effect of these hormones.

When the hormonal treatments were initiated 60 days after administration of DMBA the reduction in tumor incidence was less pronounced, but the tumor burden, expressed as the number of tumors per animal, were significantly depressed. Both r-hCG and u-hCG reduce the tumor burden significantly and reduce the growth of tumors, as evidenced by the lower number of tumors per animal after cessation of the hormonal treatments. The analysis of the final tumorigenic response demonstrated that the placebo-treated animals had 40% more tumors than those treated with either hormone. It is important to analyze the slope of the curve between the initiation (start) and finalization (stop) of the treatment shown in Fig. 2.7. Both hormones induce a decline in the slope of the curve due to the direct effect of the hormones on tumorigenesis. At the end of treatment the slope of the curve becomes steeper, but it never reaches that of the animals that had received the placebo, an indication that both hormones have an efficient therapeutic effect by reducing tumor burden by 40%. These observations suggest that r-hCG would be more efficient as a therapeutic tool when used in not only one but probably multiple cycles of treatment in order to be fully curative.

2.3 Time-Dependent Preventive Effects of Human Chorionic Gonadotropin on Rat Mammary Carcinogenesis

The present study was performed to test the hypothesis that degrees of protection by hCG against the development of breast cancer are dependent on the effective duration of hCG action at specific stages of breast development and that different duration of hCG treatment prior to carcinogen inoculation affects the degree of its protective effects [42]. The results obtained from this study indicate that even a much shorter exposure to hCG, as short as 5 days, can confer preventive effects against development of chemically induced mammary cancer in rats and that the preventive effects of hCG increased significantly with the increasing duration of its treatment. The potent inhibition of DMBA-induced mammary carcinomas in female rats by hCG treatment is reflected by significant reduction in tumor rate, the tumor load per rat, tumor size and incidence and multiplicity and significant increase in tumor latency of mammary adenocarcinomas. For this purpose we used 36 days old female virgin Sprague–Dawley rats obtained from Taconic Farm (New York, NY) that were kept for 2 weeks of acclimatization to the new environment before the beginning of the study. Four groups of 13 rats each were organized as shown in Fig. 2.10. The animals were divided into a control group and three groups that were treated with hCG for 5, 10 or 15 days, respectively. The hCG treatment was initiated when animals were 50 days old. Three weeks after the last injection five rats from each group were sacrificed and frozen samples of the left mammary glands, liver, pituitary and brain, as well as whole mounts from the right mammary glands were collected. These animals were used to record the effect of hCG in the mammary gland morphology, and to asses the direct effect on gland differentiation. The rest of the rats at age of 86 days were given a single doses of chemical carcinogen, 7,12-dimethylbenz(a)anthracene (DMBA). Every week the rats were weighed and palpated to evaluate animal's health. The tumor growth rate was determined by weekly measurement of the tumor size with a Vernier caliper to record the tumorigenic response. When a tumor was bigger than 1 cm in diameter, close monitoring was carried out to assure wellness of the animal. Four months after the DMBA administration, the animals were euthanized and the final tumorigenic responses were evaluated. In cases where the animals developed rapidly growing tumors or a tumor became ulcerated, the animals were euthanized earlier. Animals that did not develop tumors but appeared to be sick or wasted were sacrificed as soon as the diseased condition was observed [42].

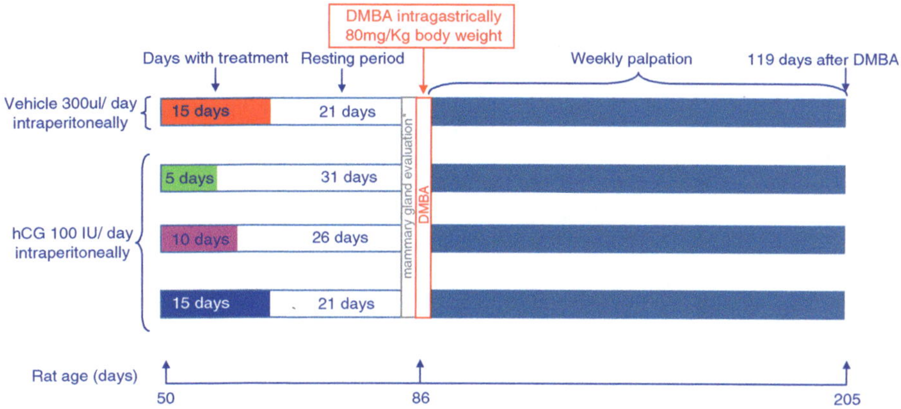

Fig. 2.10 Experimental model. At 50 days of age Sprague–Dawley rats, were treated for 0, 5, 10, or 15 days with 100 IU hCG. At 86 days of age rats were given a single dose of DMBA (80 mg/kg). Rats were followed by palpation every week, until sample collection time. The treatment was initiated when animals were 50 days old. The control group received for 15 days an intraperitoneal (i.p.) injection of bacteriostatic water (Hospira), the vehicle used for the hCG treatment; The other three groups received daily i.p. injection of 100 IU (5 μg) of r-hCG for 5-, 10- or 15-days, respectively. A constant 300 μL of r-hCG in a concentration of 16.67 μg/mL was injected intraperitoneally into each animal using an insulin syringe with a 25G 5/8 needle. The selection of this dose was based on previous work

2.3.1 *hCG Effect on Body Weight and Gland Morphology*

The average weight of the animals at the beginning of the experiment (50 days old) was between 120 and 140 g. By the time the DMBA was administrated at the age of 86 days old, their average weight was 260–280 g. At the end of the experiment (206 days old), the average weight of the animals was between 300 and 340 g. The body weight of the animals increased at the same rate in all the groups, independently of the hCG treatment (Fig. 2.11). However, the body weight among the hCG-treated groups of animals showed a trend of lower weight when compared to that of control group of animals.

Five rats from each of the group, who had received no DMBA treatment, were sacrificed 3 weeks after the last hCG injection. To determine the direct effect of hCG on mammary gland differentiation, we prepared whole mounts from the right mammary glands and stained them with toluidine blue and counted the number of terminal end buds (TEBs). The number of TEB in the control group was significantly higher than that in all the hCG-treated groups (Fig. 2.12).

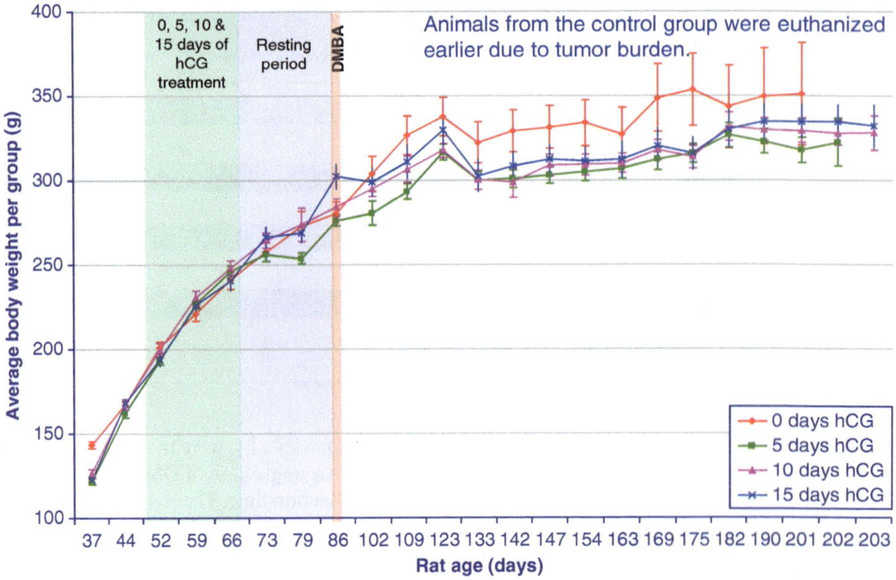

Fig. 2.11 Average weight gain

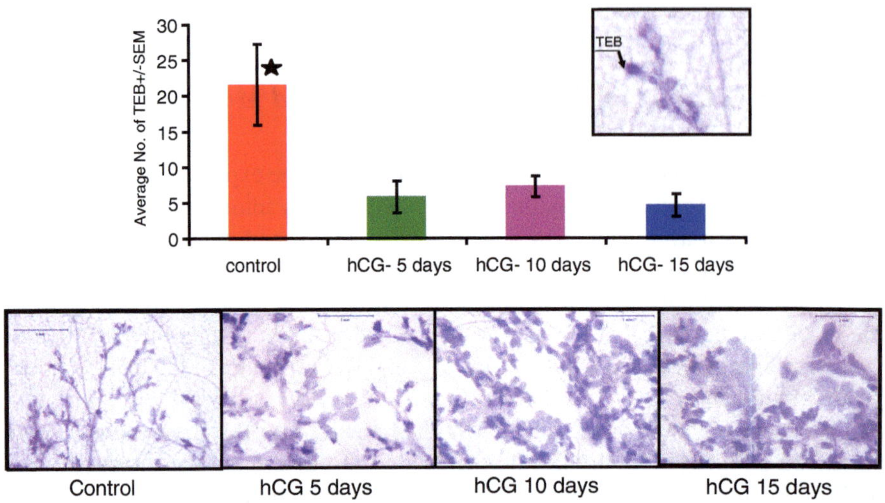

Fig. 2.12 Whole mounts were prepared from the right mammary glands as described previously [4, 13]. Briefly, the right mammary glands were first fixed in ethanol (EtOH) for 10–12 h, then defatted using acetone, rehydrated, stained using toluidine blue stain, washed with distilled water, dehydrated in graded alcohol, and stored in histoclear. Whole mounts were then mounted between glass slides using Permount

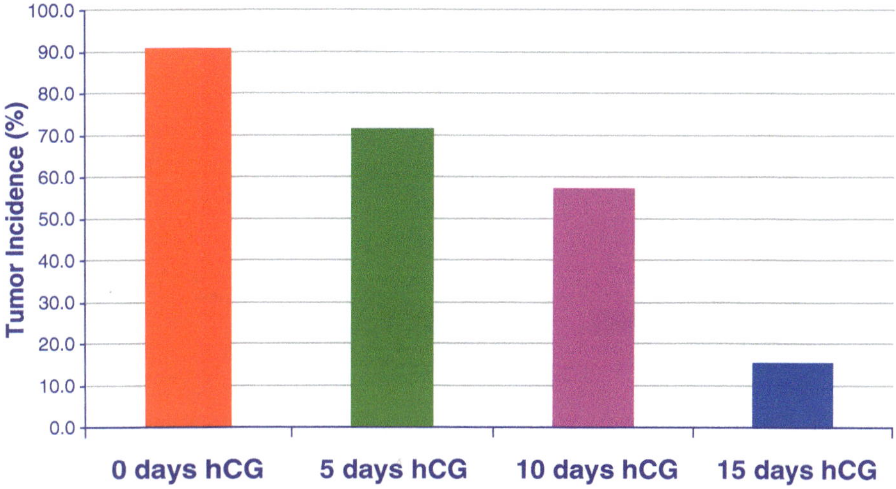

Fig. 2.13 The tumor-inducing carcinogen, 7,12-dimethylbenz(a)anthracene (DMBA) (Cat # D3254), was obtained from Sigma-Aldrich (St. Louis, MO, USA). The DMBA preparation was carried out within a glove box. All precautions for carcinogen handling were followed. The DMBA was dissolved in corn oil at a concentration of 21 mg/mL. When the animals were 86 days old, they were fasted for 24 h; under slight sedation they were administered a single intragastric (i.g.) injection of DMBA at a dose of 80 mg/kg body weight (bw). For producing muscle relaxation, the animals were sedated with 0.1 mL of ketamine/xylazine mixture at a concentration of 10 mg of xylazine per 1 mL of ketamine. For the safety of DMBA administration, the animals were housed in disposable rodent cages and moved to the carcinogen room of the LAF. The animals were kept first for 7 days at the carcinogen room and then transferred to clean cages, and moved back to the animal room and kept there until the final steps of the entire experiment. Animal euthanasia was performed when any of the following events arose: ulcerated tumor was found, the size of a tumor was found to disable the animal, and when the animal appeared to be sick or wasted. At the time points of sample collection, an intraperitoneal injection of the anesthetic agents ketamine and xylazine, prepared at a concentration of 10 mg xylazine/mL of ketamine, was administrated (90 mg/kg bw), to induce muscle relaxation and analgesia. All tumors were sequentially numbered and their location was recorded. A three and a quarter portion of each mammary gland tumor, left mammary glands 2, 3 and 4, 5, and other organs (liver, brain, and pituitary) were quickly harvested and frozen in liquid nitrogen and stored at −80°C for future studies. A piece of each mammary tumor, a piece of liver and ovary/uterus were collected and immediately fixed in 10% buffered formalin for 18–24 h. After fixation, tissues were processed overnight using the Modular Vacuum Processor I and embedded using the Leica EG1160 embedding station. Four micron sections were taken for the paraffin block of the mammary tumors and stained with H&E and examined under the light microscope. Histopathological examination followed, and all tumors were classified microscopically as benign (adenoma, cyst or fibroadenoma) or malignant lesions (CIS, adenocarcinoma) [7] by applying criteria already published [28, 29]

2.3.2 hCG Effect on Tumorigenic Response to DMBA

Several parameters related to tumorigenic responses were determined. The data for tumor frequency in the control and the hCG-treated groups are presented in Fig. 2.13. DMBA induced development of mammary tumors in 91% of the rats in

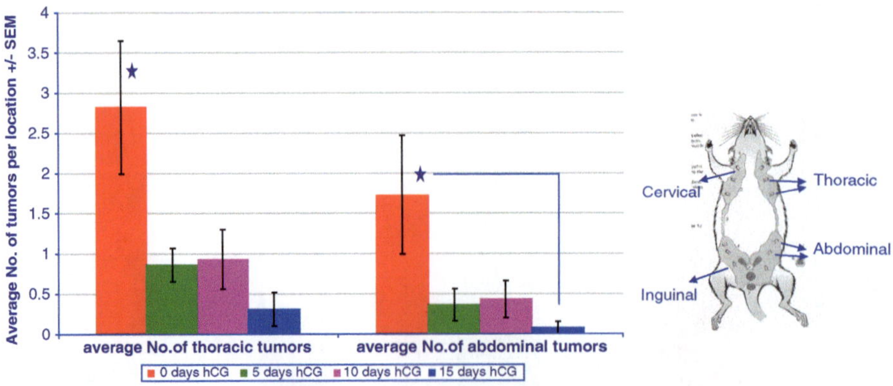

Fig. 2.14 Data from the tumorigenesis study were analyzed using the statistical programs SAS, R and SigmaStat 3.5 program. For statistical comparisons of in vivo quantifying parameters (tumor burden and tumor volume), ANOVA was used and followed by *Tukey test*. For tumor latency evaluation, *Gehan–Breslow survival analysis* was implemented and followed by *Holm–Sidak method* for multi-comparison of the differences among groups. For the comparison of tumor incidence among groups at the end of experiment, Student's *t*-test and *Chi-square test* were performed. The *p* values <0.05 were considered significant differences

the control group. Pretreatment of the animals with hCG for 5, 10, and 15 days progressively decreased the incidence of DMBA-induced mammary tumors with a statistically substantial percentage ($X^2=98.2$, df=3, $p<0.0001$). Among the hCG-treated groups, tumor frequencies were 69.2% in 5-day, 53.8% in 10-day, and 15% in 15-day groups, respectively. Furthermore, there were also statistically significant differences in tumor incidence among the hCG-treated groups. For example, tumor frequency in hCG-5 days was statistically significant different from that in hCG-10 days ($X^2=6.42$; $p=0.011$) and in hCG-15 days ($X^2=13.6$; $p<0.0001$). Cancer frequency in the 15-day hCG-treated group was remarkably lower than that in the 10-day hCG-treated group ($X^2=7.53$; $p=0.006$). The total number of thoracic tumors is statistically significantly higher in the control groups than in the hCG-treated groups (Fig. 2.14). While a total of 31 thoracic tumors were found in the control group ($n=11$), only 12, 13, and 5 thoracic tumors were found in the 5-day ($n=14$), 10-day ($n=14$) and 15-day ($n=13$) hCG-treated groups, respectively. A similar trend was also observed for the abdominal tumors. A total of 19 abdominal tumors were found in the control group ($n=11$) whereas only one abdominal tumor was found in the 15-day hCG-treated group ($n=13$).

The data of tumor multiplicity among the control and hCG-treated groups are presented in Figs. 2.15 and 2.16. The tumor load per rat in the control group was 4.5 ± 1.4 (mean ± SEM), while this number dropped to 1.2 ± 0.3, 1.4 ± 0.5 and 0.4 ± 0.2 in the 5-, 10-, and 15-day of hCG-treated groups, respectively. A *t*-test of these data indicated significant difference between the control group and the hCG-treated groups ($p<0.03$). There is a statistically significant difference between the 5- and 15-days of hCG-treated groups ($p<0.04$) (Fig. 2.16). Average number of

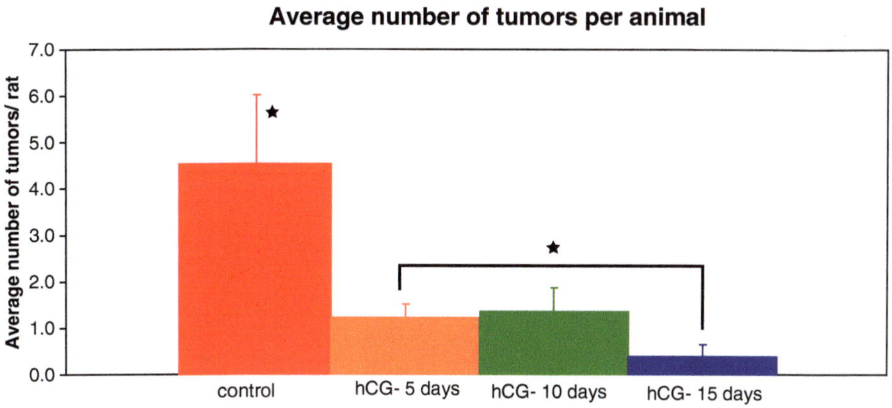

Fig. 2.15 Mean number of tumors per animal

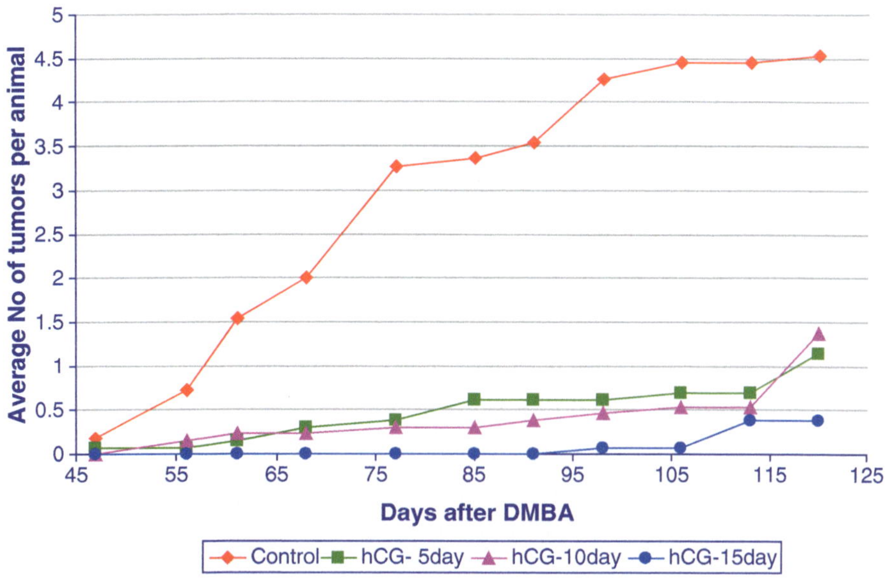

Fig. 2.16 Tumor multiplicity

tumors per rat was substantially higher in the control group in comparison with that in the hCG-treated groups (ANOVA and Tukey test, $p=0.002$). The lowest number of tumor per rat was found in the 15-day hCG-treated group; however, there was no any difference in terms of tumor quantity among treated groups. These data indicate that the 5-days of hCG treatment is as effective as 10 and 15 days of treatment in reducing tumor multiplicity.

The tumor volume was calculated using the formula: Tumor volume $= 1/2 \times ar^2 \times br$, were "$a$" is the smallest radius. The data for

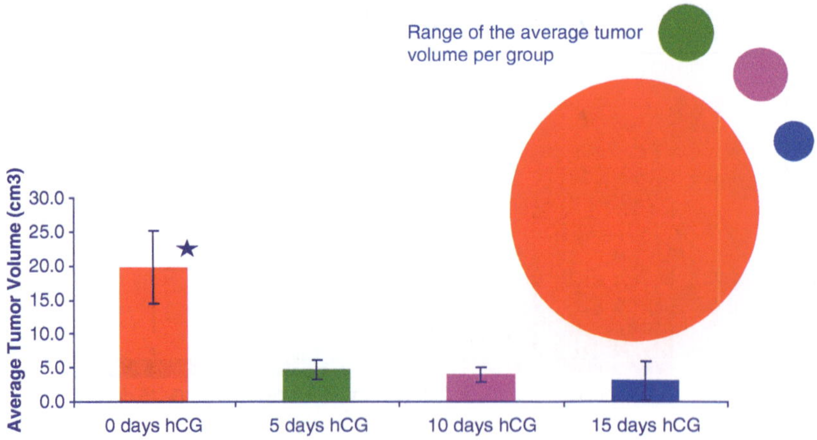

Fig. 2.17 Average tumor volume

average tumor volume among control and hCG-treated groups are presented in Fig. 2.17. It can be seen from this figure that the average tumor volume was statistically greater in the control group than in the hCG-treated groups. While the average tumor volume in the control group was 19.8 ± 1.4 cm^3 (mean ± SEM), the average tumor volumes were 1.2 ± 0.3, 1.4 ± 0.5 and 0.4 ± 0.2 cm^3 for the 5-, 10-, and 15-days groups of hCG treatment. The administration of hCG prior to the carcinogen inoculation decreased the tumor volumes dramatically (ANOVA and Tukey test; $p = <0.001$). Although the lowest tumor volumes were encountered in the hCG-15-day group, there was not a statistically significant difference among the hCG groups. Again, these data indicate that the 5-days of hCG treatment is as effective as the 10 and 15-day treatment in reducing tumor volume. Average tumor volumes were determined to be 19.7; 2.5; 2.1 and 0.46 cm^3 in control, hCG-5-day, hCG-10-day, and hCG-15-day groups respectively.

We determined the average time for tumor development among the control and hCG-treated groups after DMBA administration. The data are presented in Fig. 2.18. The average time for tumor development became progressively prolonged with increasing duration of hCG treatment (Kaplan–Meier Survival analysis: Gehan–Breslow procedure, $p = 0.019$). Average periods of tumor development were 77.9 ± 6.3 days (mean + SEM) in the control group; 87.9 ± 8 days in 5-day hCG-treated group; 92.9 ± 8.9 days in 10-day hCG-treated group and 112 ± 8.4 days in 15-day hCG-treated group. Statistically significant difference in tumor latency was found only between the control group and 15-day hCG-treated group (Holm–Sidak, $p = 0.00408$). Examination of tumor latency with The Kaplan and Meier method demonstrated that the animals treated with hCG exhibited an increased latency in development of mammary tumors. The percentage of animals with tumors decreased significantly with the increasing duration of hCG treatment. The histopathological examination on the tumor samples (Table 2.10) revealed that

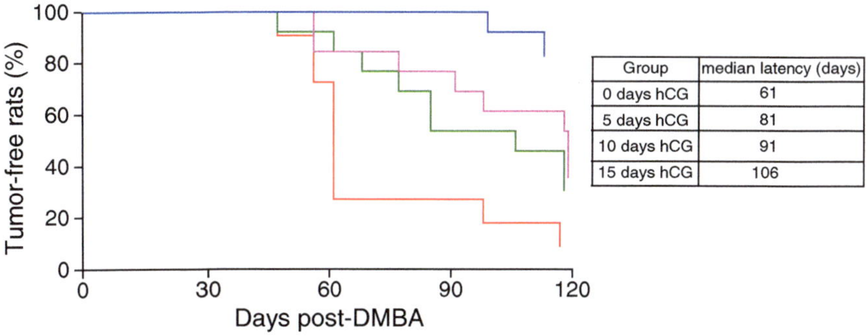

Fig. 2.18 Tumor latency (See text for details)

Table 2.10 Tumor histopathology

Group	Control	hCG-5 days	hCG-10 days	hCG-15 days
Total number of tumors	50	16	19	5
Adenocarcinomas (*n*)	49	15	19	5
Adenocarcinomas (%)	98	94	100	100
AdCa average per rat	4.5	1.2	1.4	0.4

the percentages of adenocarcinomas in all the groups ranged from 94 to 100% of the tumors.

2.3.3 Considerations on the Dose and Timing of hCG Treatment

Although the preventive effects of hCG on human breast cancer and chemically induced mammary tumor in animals have been well recognized [7–9], the data described in Sect. 2.3.2 provided additional lines of evidence that strongly support our original notion that hCG plays a pivotal role in gaining the preventive effects of an early pregnancy against breast cancer. More importantly, this study has clearly demonstrated that the duration of hCG treatment significantly affects the degree of protection of rats against the DMBA-induced development of breast cancer. Furthermore, this study indicate that while the animals who received hCG treatment still developed breast cancer, they did so much later than the animals who did not receive hCG treatment, further demonstrating the protective effects of hCG against mammary tumors. The key finding is that the preventive effects of hCG were evident as early as after 5 days of hCG treatment and were significantly enhanced as the duration of its treatment was increased and reached the maximum levels at 15 days of hCG treatment. In the present study, we examined the effects of short-term (5, 10, and 15 days) hCG treatment on inhibition of chemical carcinogen DMBA-induced development of mammary cancer in female rats. When tumor volume and

Table 2.11 Data obtained from necropsy

Group	Control	hCG-5 days	hCG-10 days	hCG-15 days
Animal per group	11	14	14	13
Animal with tumors	10	10	8	2
Total number of tumors	50	17	19	5
Toracic tumors (%)	62	71	68	80
Abdominal tumors (%)	38	29	32	20

Table 2.12 Tumorigenic response to hCG

Group	Control	hCG-5 days	hCG-10 days	hCG-15 days	*p*
Tumor multiplicity (*n*)	4.54±1.47	1.15±0.31	1.38±0.54	0.38±0.26	0.002
Tumor incidence (%)	90.9	69.2	53.8	15.4	<0.0001*
Tumor volume (cm^3)	19.76±5.37	2.48±0.88	2.11±0.88	0.46±0.44	<0.001
Tumor latency (days post-DMBA)	77.6±6.3	87.9±8	92.9±8.9	112.6±8.4	0.019[a]

*Chi-square=98.8; degree of freedom=3
[a]Gehan–Breslow survival analysis

the number of tumors per animal in the control were compared to those in three hCG-treated groups, it became obvious that all the hCG treatment regimes were effective in preventing mammary carcinogenesis. Together with this, the lowest tumor frequency was observed in the 15-day hCG-treated group and this was significantly lower than that in the 5- and 10-days hCG-treated groups. More importantly, the development period of the first tumor, i.e., tumor latency, was prolonged in 5-day hCG-treated group and significantly shifted to a later time point in the 15-day hCG-treated group. In the analysis of this parameter, the significant difference was only observed between the control and the 15-days hCG-treated groups as shown in Tables 2.10, 2.11, and 2.12. These results indicate that in order to obtain the maximum preventive effect, an optimum treatment period is necessary along with the optimum effect dose belonging to the hCG. In one of our previous studies [13], we tested the preventive effect of hCG in a 21-day period with different doses (1, 5, 10, 100 IU r-hCG in 50-day-old SD rats) before carcinogen gavage. We observed that the percentages of adenocarcinomas development, frequency and tumor burden showed a noticeable decrease as the dose increased [13]. For example, adenocarcinoma frequency was found to be 42% in 1 IU, 14% in 5 IU and 11% in 10 IU. Strikingly, no malignant tumors were encountered in 100 IU dose application. Consequently, we determined the optimum effective dose as 100 IU [43]. We also observed similar results in full-term pregnant rats before carcinogen gavage without the hCG treatment. In our previous study, we compared rats who received a 3-week hCG treatment (100 IU/day) before carcinogen gavage with rats that underwent 3 weeks of pregnancy [9]. When the carcinogen gavage was applied on the 92nd day, adenocarcinoma frequency was found to be 48% in the control group, 5.6% in the pregnancy group and 6.1% in the hCG-treated group. When the carcinogen gavage was shifted for a later time (134th day), carcinoma frequency decreased in the control group (18.5%), and a significant decrease was observed in pregnancy and hCG pretreatment groups (9.2% and 7.4% respectively). Together, these observations indicate that hCG confers potently preventive effects against chemically induced mammary tumors in a time- and dose-dependent manner, showing the pharmacological characteristics of anticancer reagents. The fact that hCG at even smaller doses and for a much short duration of its treatment confers protective effects on breast tissue reflects the effectiveness of this hormone in breast cancer prevention.

While the analysis of the molecular mechanisms underlying hCG-induced protections against mammary tumors is still under study, several mechanisms are under consideration. One of the major mechanisms by which hCG inhibits the initiation and the progression of chemically induced mammary carcinomas is its role in the induction of differentiation of the mammary gland during the first full-term pregnancy [44]. The breast tissue of normally cycling women contains three types of lobules: the undifferentiated Lobules type 1 (Lob 1), the more developed Lobules type 2 (Lob 2) and Lobules type 3 (Lob 3). The breast attains its maximum development (Lobules type 4) (Lob 4) during pregnancy and lactation. After menopause the breast regresses in both nulliparous and parous women containing only Lob 1. It has been proposed [10] that Lob 1 in the breast of nulliparous women and parous women with breast cancer never went through the process of differentiation, retaining a high concentration of epithelial cells that are targets for carcinogens and are thus susceptible to neoplastic transformation. It has been shown [13] that in the rat, the highly proliferating and undifferentiated gland of the young, virgin, intact females exhibited maximal susceptibility to neoplastic transformation. Breast cancer initiates in Lob 1, the most undifferentiated structures frequently found in the breast of young nulliparous women. We have shown [43] that a determining factor in the susceptibility of the human breast to cancer is the mammary gland architecture. The early full pregnancy stimulated mammary gland differentiation and treatment of rats with hCG mimicked pregnancy in inducing mammary gland differentiation [45]. In particular, we have demonstrated that pregnancy or hCG treatment for 21 days induces differentiation of mammary gland and shifting of stem cell 1, which is susceptible to carcinogenesis, to stem cell 2, which is refractory to carcinogenesis. Consistent with these observations, the data shown in Fig. 2.10 show that the number of TEB counted in the control-DMBA group was significantly higher compared to that of all the hCG treatments and that 5 days of hCG treatment was as effective as 10- and 15 days of hCG treatment in reduction of TEB. These results reveal a key role of hCG in induction of differentiation of mammary gland during pregnancy. Early pregnancy imprints in the breast permanent genomic changes that reduce the susceptibility of this organ to cancer. Our previous genetic signature analysis has revealed that full-term pregnancy induced specific changes in the genomic signature that are related to the control of growth and differentiation in the human breast and that hCG induced the similar genomic signature [46, 47]. The genomic signature induced by either pregnancy or hCG included activators or repressors of transcription genes, apoptosis, growth factors, cell division control, DNA repair, tumor suppressor, and cell-surface antigen genes [47].

Thus, secretion of hCG during pregnancy induces changes in genetic signature and thus, differentiation of the mammary gland, thereby making the breast tissue less susceptible to carcinogenesis.

Consistent with its role of hCG in inducing mammary gland differentiation, it has been reported [29, 48, 49] that hCG induced the expression of inhibin, a gonadal glycoprotein which is a member of the TGF superfamily of growth and differentiation factors. Inhibin regulates the production of follicle-stimulating hormone and is present in cells of the cytotrophoblast layer of human placenta at term and in primary cultures of human trophoblasts [50]. Inhibin-b subunit, considered a tumor suppressor, contributes to the process of initiation, promotion, or progression of endocrine-related cancers [51]. High levels of inhibin-a were present in the maternal serum throughout human pregnancy. Inhibin-a is derived from a placental source [52]. hCG stimulated the secretion of inhibin from cultured placental cells [50] and human breast MCF-7 cells [48]. The induction of inhibin by hCG was associated with inhibition of cell proliferation [48]. We previously observed [29] that hCG treatment induced the expression of inhibin in the cytoplasm of alveolar cells but not in ductal cells. The induction of inhibin by hCG was evident by 10-days of hCG treatment and reached maximal levels by day 15. Thereafter, the hCG-mediated induction of inhibin was detected in the stroma, which exhibited maximal expression by day 20. Once hCG treatment was terminated, the mammary gland regressed to its pretreatment condition, appearing similar both in morphology and inhibin content to that of control animals. The expression of inhibin in the mammary gland after hCG administration at the time of maximal lobuloalveolar development, and its diffusion towards the stroma during regression, suggest a critical role of inhibin as a modulator of mammary growth and differentiation. The time-course of induction of inhibin expression by hCG treatment appears to be parallel to that of hCG-induced inhibition of mammary gland tumor, indicating its role in these events. Furthermore, inhibins have been shown to regulate mammary epithelial cell differentiation through mesenchymal–epithelial interactions [53]. In these animals, inhibin-a and inhibin-b were found to be elevated in the non-tumoral mammary glands in association with lobule formation and in the tumors. Their mRNAs were also elevated in the mammary tissue, associated with increased levels of c-myc and c-jun induced by the hCG treatment. DMBA alone did not modify the expression of these genes. These findings indicate that inhibin production and gene activation are associated with both mammary gland differentiation and tumor regression.

The second mechanism by which hCG prevents the initiation and the progression of chemically induced mammary carcinomas is through its activation of programmed cell death [27, 54] and inhibition of cell proliferation [55]. Guo et al. [56] analyzed gene expression profiles of human breast cancer cells MCF-7 cells treated with hCG for 24, 48, and 96 h and identified 48 genes affected by this hormone. A cluster of genes was found to be over-expressed during the first 24 h and level off thereafter whereas other genes were maximally expressed at 96 h of treatment. These genes are involved in the regulation of cell proliferation, apoptosis, cell trafficking, and DNA. It has been shown that naturally derived hCG induced apoptosis in human breast xenografts from a mean of 5% in control to a means of 28% in hCG-treated tumors [54]. The hCG activates apoptosis likely via up-regulation of tumor suppressor factors and the modulation of apoptotic gene expression. Several tumor suppressors including p53 [57], OKL38 [58], and VHL [59] have been shown to be upregulated by hCG. The tumor suppressor p53 is extensively involved in activation of apoptosis induced by a various oxidative stresses. The expression of p53 protein was increased in hCG-pretreated mice and rats and the p53-regulated gene p21Cip1 was also increased concomitantly with p53 [25, 60]. A role of p53 in hCG-induced protection has been indicated by the study using BALB/c p53 null mammary epithelium [61]. In the mammary epithelium, the absence of *p53* gene expression abrogated the protective effect of prior pregnancy. The tumor incidence curves were superimposable in p53 null mammary epithelium treated with 7,12-dimethylbenzanthracene or pregnancy plus 7,12-dimethylbenzanthracene. These results demonstrate that p53 plays a pivotal role in hCG-induced protection. The role of p53 in hCG-induced protection has been described previously [25, 27, 32, 57]. Another tumor suppressor, OKL38, is a novel pregnancy-induced growth inhibitory gene. It has been reported [58] that the expression of OKL38 was enhanced by hCG in the rat mammary gland and ovary and that over-expression of this gene in Buffalo rat liver cells resulted in growth inhibition and cell death. Interestingly, Yao et al. [62] reported that expression of *OKL38* was enhanced by activation of p53 following DNA damage and that OKL38 induced apoptosis through localization to mitochondria and induction of cytochrome *c* release. OKL38 has been shown to be an oxidative stress response gene stimulated by oxidized phospholipids, indicating a potential role in protection against oxidative stress [63]. The VHL gene is a tumor suppressor gene encoding an E3 ubiquitin ligase that results in specific target proteins being marked for degradation. It has been shown [59] that hCG upregulated the transcript level of VHL, associated with increased expression of p53 in human granulosa lutein cells. In addition, several apoptotic genes including TRPM2, ICE, and TGF-b have been shown to be upregulated by hCG and associated with up-regulation of p53/p21Cip1in MCF-10F cells and MCF-7 [25, 45]. It is likely that p53/OKL38/VHL pathways may be involved in mediation of hCG-induced apoptosis in mammary gland. Through up-regulation of these tumor suppressors as well as other apoptotic-related genes, hCG induces programmed cell death.

Several studies [48, 55] have reported that hCG inhibited cell proliferation. The transcription factors, NF-κB, AP-1, and estrogen receptors (ERs) are involved in up-regulation of a large number of growth-related genes in breast cells. hCG treatment decreased proliferation and invasion of breast cancer MCF-7 cells by inhibiting NF-κB, and AP-1. Estrogens are potent stimuli of cell proliferation in breast epithelial cells and their proliferative effects are mediated mainly via ERa in more than 80% of all breast cancers. Pregnancy and lactation reduce estrogen levels in breast cells. Treatment of MCF-7 cells with highly purified hCG resulted in a dose- and time-dependent significant decrease in steady-state ER mRNA and protein levels as compared to controls, with the maximal decrease occurring after 4 h of culture with 10 ng/mL hCG. Furthermore, we have observed [48] that hCG, through up-regulation of inhibitin, downregulated the expression of the ERa by methylation of the CpG islands within the promoter region of this gene. It is likely that hCG inhibits estrogen-mediated breast cell proliferation by reducing the E_2/ERa-mediated signal pathways during pregnancy.

This study together with our previous studies leads us to conclude that the hormonally induced differentiation offers enormous promise for the primary prevention of breast cancer and that the ability of hCG to replicate the naturally protective effects of pregnancy against breast cancer hold significant public health value. More importantly [64], hCG enhanced the radiosensitivity of the MCF-7 breast cancer cell line, resulting in an 8–10% reduction in MCF-7 cell survival at a dose of 2 Gy, a typical dose used in conventional cancer therapy. In this regard, hCG alone and in combination with radiotherapy and/or other chemotherapies represent a new approach effective for breast cancer prevention. A clinical trial with hCG as a preventive agent against breast cancer is currently ongoing in pre-menopausal women with no previous pregnancy. Our present studies strongly point to a new hope and a great promise of breast cancer prevention.

2.4 The Study of Side Effects of hCG in Reproduction

Suppression of mammary carcinogenesis similar to pregnancy has been achieved by treatment of young virgin rats with the hCG, given daily through intraperitoneal injections for 21 days, that in the rat, is equivalent to the length of a full-term pregnancy. This treatment inhibits the development of DMBA-induced mammary carcinomas in a dose-dependent manner. hCG treatment of virgin rats affects the development of the mammary gland, mimicking the effect of pregnancy. Administration of hCG to women on day 9 of the cycle can interfere with proper folliculogenesis, ovulation and luteinisation, effects than have led researchers to propose its use as a monthly injectable contraceptive [65]. These data led us to explore the effect of hCG on the reproductive axis of the animal. In this study [66], we demonstrated that hCG administration during five estrous cycles that is around 21 days, has a contraceptive effect, and after that period pregnancy can be re-established without permanent disruption of reproductive ability and without significant side effect.

2.4.1 Experimental Evidence

To determine if the duration of hCG administration has a contraceptive effect and other side effects, including abnormalities of offspring and recovery time from the contraceptive effect, we have used 25 female Sprague–Dawley rats that were divided in five groups (Table 2.13). As a control group, the first five females were mated with one male each, in the first day of the experiment. This group received for 21 days 0.4 mL intraperitoneal injections of bacteriostatic water (Abbott Laboratories), the solvent used for the hCG injections. The other four groups received for 21 days

Table 2.13 Experimental protocol for testing the contraceptive effect of hCG

Group	21 days treatment of	Mating at
I-Control	0.400 mL of bacteriostatic water	1st day of treatment
II-hCG	0.400 mL of hCG (100 IU)	2nd day of treatment
III-hCG	0.400 mL of hCG (100 IU)	5th day of treatment
IV-hCG	0.400 mL of hCG (100 IU)	10th day of treatment
V-hCG	0.400 mL of hCG (100 IU)	15th day of treatment

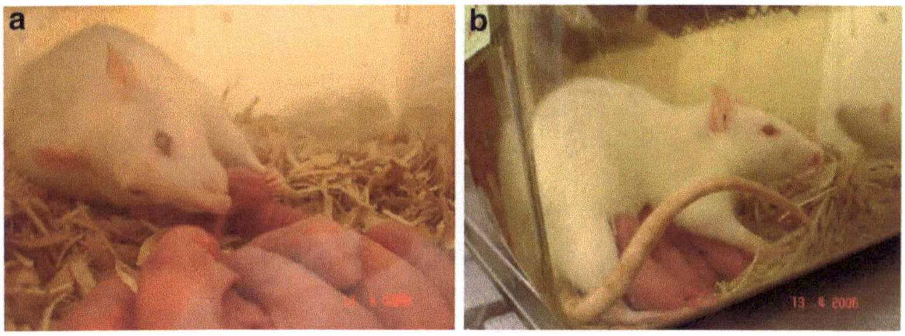

Fig. 2.19 (**a**) Rat cleaning the new born. (**b**) Rat weaning the litters

100 IU intraperitoneal injections of hCG (Ovidrel®—Serono), for 21 days with varied mating dates. Group II was mated 24 h after the first hCG injection. Groups III, IV, and V were mated 5, 10, and 15 days after the beginning of the experiment, respectively (Table 2.13). All pairs were kept together until the end of the experiment. The females were followed up to determine when they became pregnant and the length of pregnancy. When they delivered, the number of pups was recorded. The gestation period was between 20 and 23 days. During the experiment period, the rats were observed every day to follow the pregnancy and behavior. The day of the delivery was used to estimate the time when the rats got pregnant. The pups were counted and observed after birth (Fig. 2.19). After the delivery, the pups were examined for any visible abnormalities [66].

In the control group, all rats delivered between the 23rd and 27th days after mating. Therefore, we conclude that the females got pregnant approximately between the first and sixth day of mating. All control animals had between 10 and 12 pups (average = 11.2). In the treated groups, the first delivery was on the 56th day after the beginning of the hCG injections, therefore, the first treated rat became pregnant approximately on the 14th day after the end of hCG treatment. The rest of the animals became pregnant between 15 and 37 days after the end of the injections. Only 2 of 20 rats did not have any delivery until the 81st day after the end of treatment. The average number of pups of the treated group was 11.1, with no significant difference between the number of litters in the treated and control groups (Table 2.14). The pregnancies began after the end treatment and were random among the different mating dates. After the first delivery, seven treated rats became pregnant for a second time (Tables 2.13 and 2.14).

Table 2.14 Delivery data from all animals

Groups	Animal #	Delivery day	Number of pups	Sex F	Sex M	OBS	Average number of pups
Group I	1	04.13.06	11	–	–		11.2
	2	04.15.06	11	–	–		
	3	04.11.06	10	–	–		
	4	04.12.06	12	–	–		
	5	04.14.06	12	–	–		
Group II	6	05.16.06	13	4	9	Second pregnancy	11.1
	7	05.22.06	13	6	7		
	8	05.23.06	11	5	6	Second pregnancy	
	9	No delivery					
	10	05.24.06	8	4	4		
Group III	11	05.19.06	10	3	7	Second pregnancy	
	12	06.05.06	13	6	7	Second pregnancy	
	13	05.21.06	14	11	3		
	14	05.21.06	13	7	6	Second pregnancy	
	15	05.17.06	7	4	3		
Group IV	16	05.24.06	11	8	3		
	17	05.24.06	7	4	3		
	18	05.29.06	13	6	7		
	19	05.16.06	12	9	3		
	20	06.06.06	3	1	2	Second pregnancy	
Group V	21	No delivery					
	22	05.21.06	11	5	6	Large ovary	
	23	05.16.06	10	4	6	Second pregnancy	
	24	05.17.06	16	5	11		
	25	05.14.06	15	4	11		

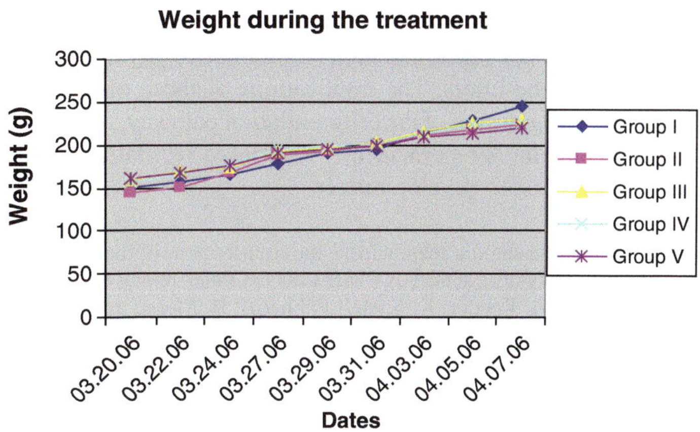

Fig. 2.20 Graph showing the average weight of different groups during the treatment

2.4.2 *Side Effect of hCG*

No visible side effects were visibly noticed in the females or in their pups. When the female rats were sacrificed, only 1 in 20 treated rats presented increased ovarian size. The weight of treated rats and control rats did not differ throughout most of the treatment. Towards the end of the experiment the control group gained more weight, which is to be expected as the control rats were by that time pregnant (Fig. 2.20). None of the rats that have received hCG during the 21 days treatment became pregnant. However, the control group, which was receiving injections of same volume of bacteriostatic water for the same period of time, and was handled in the same way, got pregnant at the beginning of the study. This experiment has shown that the hCG treatment for 21 days has a contraceptive effect in rats, and this contraceptive effect is reversible after the end of the treatment. The contraceptive effect lasted between 3 and 9 estrous cycles (15 and 37 days) after the end of the treatment. After this period, the rats recovered the ability of get pregnant and they had approximately the same number of pups as the animals who did not receive hCG.

2.5 Concluding Remarks

We have shown evidence that hCG, one of the hormones produced by the human placenta protect the mammary gland from cancer initiation and progression. This effect is induced by the natural hormone or u-hCG as well as the recombinant hormone formulation or r-hCG. The administration of this hormone for 21 days in the period of highest susceptibility of the mammary gland to carcinogenesis (50–60 days of age in the rat) produces the highest level of protection. This protection or preventive effect is also achieved by a 5 day treatment. Of practical importance is also the fact that there is not side effect in the reproductive physiology of the host or in the development of the litters. The implications of these observations indicate that hCG control the progression of the differentiation pathway, and that the changes in the mammary epithelia are permanently imprinted regulating the long-lasting refractoriness of the breast to develop cancer.

Acknowledgements We, the authors acknowledge the contributions of the many members of the Breast Cancer Research Laboratory at the Fox Chase Cancer Center among them Drs. J.E. Vanegas; M.A. Kocdor; J.S Pereira; H. Kocdor; K. Snider; F. Sheriff; R. Moral; and R. Wang, who have worked with us to generate the data described in Sects. 2.3 and 2.4 [42, 66] incorporated into this chapter and elaborated by us it into a unified concept.

References

1. Russo IH, Russo J (1993) Physiological bases of breast cancer prevention. Eur J Cancer Prev 2(suppl 3):101–111
2. Russo IH, Russo J (2000) Hormonal approach to breast cancer prevention. J Cell Biochem Suppl 34:1–6
3. Russo IH, Russo J (2007) Primary prevention of breast cancer by hormone-induced differentiation. Recent Results Cancer Res 174:111–130
4. Russo J, Russo IH (1994) Toward a physiological approach to breast cancer prevention. Cancer Epidemiol Biomarkers Prev 3:353–364
5. Russo J, Balogh G, Russo IH (2007) Breast cancer prevention. Climacteric 10(suppl 2): 47–53
6. MacMahon B, Cole P, Lin TM, Lowe CR, Mirra AP, Ravnihar B, Salber EJ, Valaoras VG, Yuasa S (1970) Age at first birth and breast cancer risk. Bull World Health Organ 43:209–221
7. Russo IH, Koszalka M, Russo J (1990) Human chorionic gonadotropin and rat mammary cancer prevention. J Natl Cancer Inst 82:1286–1289
8. Russo IH, Koszalka M, Russo J (1990) Effect of human chorionic gonadotropin on mammary gland differentiation and carcinogenesis. Carcinogenesis 11:1849–1855
9. Russo IH, Koszalka M, Russo J (1991) Comparative study of the influence of pregnancy and hormonal treatment on mammary carcinogenesis. Br J Cancer 64:481–484
10. Russo J, Romero AL, Russo IH (1994) Architectural pattern of the normal and cancerous breast under the influence of parity. Cancer Epidemiol Biomarkers Prev 3:219–224
11. Russo J, Russo IH (1980) Susceptibility of the mammary gland to carcinogenesis: II. Pregnancy interruption as a risk factor in tumor incidence. Am J Pathol 100:497–512
12. Thordarson G, Semaan S, Low C, Ochoa D, Leong H, Rajkumar L, Guzman RC, Nandi S, Talamantes F (2004) Mammary tumorigenesis in growth hormone deficient spontaneous dwarf rats; effects of hormonal treatments. Breast Cancer Res Treat 87:277–290
13. Russo J, Tay LK, Russo IH (1982) Differentiation of the mammary gland and susceptibility to carcinogenesis. Breast Cancer Res Treat 2:5–73
14. Medina D (2005) Mammary developmental fate and breast cancer risk. Endocr Relat Cancer 12:483–495
15. Vatten LJ, Romundstad PR, Trichopoulos D, Skjaerven R (2002) Pregnancy related protection against breast cancer depends on length of gestation. Br J Cancer 87:289–290
16. Yang J, Yoshizawa K, Nandi S, Tsubura A (1999) Protective effects of pregnancy and lactation against N-methyl-N-nitrosourea-induced mammary carcinomas in female Lewis rats. Carcinogenesis 20:623–628

17. Rajkumar L, Guzman RC, Yang J, Thordarson G, Talamantes F, Nandi S (2001) Short-term exposure to pregnancy levels of estrogen prevents mammary carcinogenesis. Proc Natl Acad Sci USA 98:11755–11759
18. Jerry DJ (2007) Roles for estrogen and progesterone in breast cancer prevention. Breast Cancer Res 9:102
19. Tsubura A, Uehara N, Matsuoka Y, Yoshizawa K, Yuri T (2008) Estrogen and progesterone treatment mimicking pregnancy for protection from breast cancer. In Vivo 22: 191–201
20. Rajkumar L, Guzman RC, Yang J, Thordarson G, Talamantes F, Nandi S (2004) Prevention of mammary carcinogenesis by short-term estrogen and progestin treatments. Breast Cancer Res 6:R31–R37
21. Russo J (1983) Basis of cellular autonomy in the susceptibility to carcinogenesis. Toxicol Pathol 11:149–166
22. Russo IH, Koszalka M, Gimotty PA, Russo J (1990) Protective effect of chorionic gonadotropin on DMBA-induced mammary carcinogenesis. Br J Cancer 62:243–247
23. Russo J, Mailo D, Hu YF, Balogh G, Sheriff F, Russo IH (2005) Breast differentiation and its implication in cancer prevention. Clin Cancer Res 11:931s–936s
24. Tay LK, Russo J (1985) Effect of human chorionic gonadotrophin on 7,12-dimethylbenz[a] anthracene-induced DNA binding and repair synthesis by rat mammary epithelial cells. Chem Biol Interact 55:13–21
25. Srivastava P, Russo J, Mgbonyebi OP, Russo IH (1998) Growth inhibition and activation of apoptotic gene expression by human chorionic gonadotropin in human breast epithelial cells. Anticancer Res 18:4003–4010
26. Lukanova A, Andersson R, Wulff M, Zeleniuch-Jacquotte A, Grankvist K, Dossus L, Afanasyeva Y, Johansson R, Arslan AA, Lenner P, Wadell G, Hallmans G, Toniolo P, Lundin E (2008) Human chorionic gonadotropin and alpha-fetoprotein concentrations in pregnancy and maternal risk of breast cancer: a nested case-control study. Am J Epidemiol 168:1284–1291
27. Srivastava P, Russo J, Russo IH (1997) Chorionic gonadotropin inhibits rat mammary carcinogenesis through activation of programmed cell death. Carcinogenesis 18:1799–1808
28. Alvarado ME, Alvarado NE, Russo J, Russo IH (1994) Human chorionic gonadotropin inhibits proliferation and induces expression of inhibin in human breast epithelial cells in vitro. In Vitro 30A:4–8
29. Alvarado MV, Russo J, Russo IH (1993) Immunolocalization of inhibin in the mammary gland of rats treated with hCG. J Histochem Cytochem 41:29–34
30. Russo IH, Russo J (1994) Role of hCG and inhibin in breast cancer (review). Int J Oncol 4:297–306
31. Meunier H, Rivier C, Evans R, Vale W (1988) Gonadal and extragonadal expression of inhibin a-, bA-, and bB-subunits in various tissues predicts diverse functions. Proc Natl Acad Sci USA 85:247–251
32. Srivastava P, Russo J, Estrada S, Russo IH (1996) P53 and cyclins A and D regulate the inhibition of tumor progression induced by chorionic gonadotropin. Proc Am Assoc Cancer Res 37:2a
33. Kliesch S, Behre HM, Nieschlag E (1994) High efficacy of gonadotropin or pulsatile gonadotropin-releasing hormone treatment in hypogonadotropic hypogonadal men. Eur J Endocrinol 131:347–354
34. Kauschansky A, Frydman M, Nussinovitch M, Varsano I (1995) Evaluation of human chorionic gonadotropin stimulation tests in prepubertal and early pubertal boys. Eur J Pediatr 154:890–892
35. Quenby MB, Farquharson RG (1994) Human chorionic gonadotropin supplementation in recurring pregnancy loss: a controlled trial. Fertil Steril 62:708–710
36. Chen C, Jones WR, Fern B, Forde C (1985) Monitoring embryos after in vitro fertilization using early pregnancy factor. In: Seppala M, Edwards RG (eds) In vitro fertilization and embryo transfer. Ann N Y Acad Sci 442:428

37. Bernstein L, Hanisch R, Sullivan-Halley J, Ross RK (1995) Treatment with human chorionic gonadotropin and risk of breast cancer. Cancer Epidemiol Biomarkers Prev 4:437–440
38. Gill PS, McLaughlin T, Espina BM, Tulpule A, Louie S, Lunardi-Iskandar Y, Gallo RC (1997) Phase I study of human chorionic gonadotropin given subcutaneously to patients with acquired immunodeficiency syndrome related mucocutaneous Kaposi's sarcoma. J Natl Cancer Inst 89:1797–1802
39. Gill PS, Lunardi-Iskandar Y, Louie S, Tulpule A, Zheng T, Espina BM, Besnier JM, Herman P, Levine AM, Bryant JL, Gallo RC (1996) The effect of preparations of human chorionic gonadotropin on AIDS-related Kaposi's sarcoma. N Engl J Med 335:1261–1269
40. Harris PJ (1996) Human chorionic gonadotropin hormone is antiviral. Med Hypotheses 47:71–72
41. Lambe M, Hsieh C-C, Chan H-W, Ekbom A, Trichopoulos D, Adami HO (1996) Parity, age at first and last birth, and risk of breast cancer: a population-based study in Sweden. Breast Cancer Res Treat 38:305–311
42. Vanegas JE, Kocdor MA, Pereira JS, Kocdor H, Russo J, Snider K, Sheriff F, Russo IH (2009) Preventive effect of hCG on rat mammary carcinogenesis. Proc Am Assoc Cancer Res 50:2059a
43. Russo J, Lynch H, Russo IH (2001) Mammary gland architecture as a determining factor in the susceptibility of the human breast to cancer. Breast J 7:278–291
44. Russo J, Russo IH (1995) Hormonally induced differentiation: a novel approach to breast cancer prevention. J Cell Biochem Suppl 22:58–64
45. Russo J, Wilgus G, Russo IH (1979) Susceptibility of the mammary gland to carcinogenesis: I. Differentiation of the mammary gland as determinant of tumor incidence and type of lesion. Am J Pathol 96:721–734
46. Russo J, Balogh GA, Chen J, Fernandez SV, Fernbaugh R, Heulings R, Mailo DA, Moral R, Russo PA, Sheriff F, Vanegas JE, Wang R, Russo IH (2006) The concept of stem cell in the mammary gland and its implication in morphogenesis, cancer and prevention. Front Biosci 11:151–172
47. Russo J, Balogh GA, Russo IH (2008) Full-term pregnancy induces a specific genomic signature in the human breast. Cancer Epidemiol Biomarkers Prev 17:51–66
48. Alvarado MV, Alvarado NE, Russo J, Russo IH (1994) Human chorionic gonadotropin inhibits proliferation and induces expression of inhibin in human breast epithelial cells in vitro. In Vitro Cell Dev Biol Anim 30A:4–8
49. Jiang X, Russo IH, Russo J (2002) Human chorionic gonadotropin and inhibin induce histone acetylation in human breast epithelial cells. Int J Oncol 20:77–79
50. Petraglia F, Sawchenko P, Lim AT, Rivier J, Vale W (1987) Localization, secretion, and action of inhibin in human placenta. Science 237:187–189
51. Risbridger GP, Schmitt JF, Robertson DM (2001) Activins and inhibins in endocrine and other tumors. Endocr Rev 22:836–858
52. Birdsall M, Ledger W, Groome N, Abdalla H, Muttukrishna S (1997) Inhibin A and activin A in the first trimester of human pregnancy. J Clin Endocrinol Metab 82:1557–1560
53. Robinson GW, Hennighausen L (1997) Inhibins and activins regulate mammary epithelial cell differentiation through mesenchymal-epithelial interactions. Development 124:2701–2708
54. Lopez D, Sekharam M, Coppola D, Carter WB (2008) Purified human chorionic gonadotropin induces apoptosis in breast cancer. Mol Cancer Ther 7:2837–2844
55. Rao Ch V, Li X, Manna SK, Lei ZM, Aggarwal BB (2004) Human chorionic gonadotropin decreases proliferation and invasion of breast cancer MCF-7 cells by inhibiting NF-kappaB and AP-1 activation. J Biol Chem 279:25503–25510
56. Guo S, Russo IH, Lareef MH, Russo J (2004) Effect of human chorionic gonadotropin in the gene expression profile of MCF-7 cells. Int J Oncol 24:399–407
57. Medina D (2004) Breast cancer: the protective effect of pregnancy. Clin Cancer Res 10:380S–384S
58. Ong CK, Ng CY, Leong C, Ng CP, Ong CS, Nguyen TT, Huynh H (2004) Structural characterization of three novel rat OKL38 transcripts, their tissue distributions, and their regulation by human chorionic gonadotropin. Endocrinology 145:4763–4774

59. Herr D, Keck C, Tempfer C, Pietrowski D (2004) Chorionic gonadotropin regulates the transcript level of VHL, p53, and HIF-2alpha in human granulosa lutein cells. Mol Reprod Dev 69:397–401
60. Sivaraman L, Conneely OM, Medina D, O'Malley BW (2001) p53 is a potential mediator of pregnancy and hormone-induced resistance to mammary carcinogenesis. Proc Natl Acad Sci USA 98:12379–12384
61. Medina D, Kittrell FS (2003) p53 function is required for hormone-mediated protection of mouse mammary tumorigenesis. Cancer Res 63:6140–6143
62. Yao H, Li P, Venters BJ, Zheng S, Thompson PR, Pugh BF, Wang Y (2008) Histone Arg modifications and p53 regulate the expression of OKL38, a mediator of apoptosis. J Biol Chem 283:20060–20068
63. Li R, Chen W, Yanes R, Lee S, Berliner JA (2007) OKL38 is an oxidative stress response gene stimulated by oxidized phospholipids. J Lipid Res 48:709–715
64. Pond-Tor S, Rhodes RG, Dahlberg PE, Leith JT, McMichael J, Dahlberg AE (2002) Enhancement of radiosensitivity of the MCF-7 breast cancer cell line with human chorionic gonadotropin. Breast Cancer Res Treat 72:45–51
65. Sallam HN, Sallam AN (1996) HCG as a monthly injectable contraceptive–effects of day 9 administration. Fertil Steril (Abstract Book Supplement):S58
66. Pereira J, Vanegas JV, Moral R, Russo J, Wang R, Russo IH (2009) Restoration of rodent reproductive capabilities after human gonadotropin treatment. Proc Am Assoc Cancer Res 50:2097a

Chapter 3
Comparative Effects of the Preventive Effect of Pregnancy, Steroidal Hormones, and hCG in the Transcriptomic Profile of the Rat Mammary Gland

3.1 Introduction

The response of the mammary gland to specific carcinogenic stimuli depends upon the physiologic state of the mammary tree under the control of the endocrine system. The administration of optimal carcinogenic doses to young and sexually mature virgin rats induces maximal tumorigenic response [1–6]. This period of highest susceptibility of the mammary gland to be transformed by such stimulus represents the "high risk susceptibility window" (HRSW) [7]. The peak of cancer incidence occurring when virgin rats reach the age of 45–55 days and have had at least two ovulatory cycles after vaginal opening [8] represents the response of numerous mammary terminal end buds (TEBs) that are predominantly composed of progenitor mammary stem cells (PMSCs) [2, 9]. Under the stimulus of the first pregnancy, the mammary gland that has not been exposed to a carcinogenic insult during the early phases of the HRSW enters into a "hormonal protection window" (HPW). During this period the hormones of pregnancy will block any future damage caused by carcinogens or endocrine disruptors through the induction of mammary gland differentiation [2, 10]. Completion of pregnancy induces long-lasting structural and genomic changes in the mammary gland of different strains of rats and in mice [11]. These molecular changes ultimately result in a significant reduction in mammary cancer incidence and number of tumors per animal [8, 9, 12–15]. In the absence of pregnancy, various natural and synthetic hormones have been shown to prevent the initiation of mammary cancer when they are administered to young virgin rats during the HRSW prior to the exposure to a carcinogen or an endocrine disruptor. Daily treatment of virgin Sprague–Dawley rats with hCG at the doses of 1, 5, 10, or 100 IU for 21 days significantly reduces adenocarcinoma incidence and number of adenocarcinomas per animal in a dose-dependent manner [10]. Similarly, treatment with 100 IU hCG daily for 5, 10, or 15 days suffices to induce a significant degree of mammary gland differentiation and protection from cancer initiation [16]. The reduction in cancer incidence resulting from hCG treatment is long-lasting, as demonstrated by the persistent

J. Russo and I.H. Russo, *Role of the Transcriptome in Breast Cancer Prevention*,
DOI 10.1007/978-1-4614-4884-6_3, © Springer Science+Business Media New York 2013

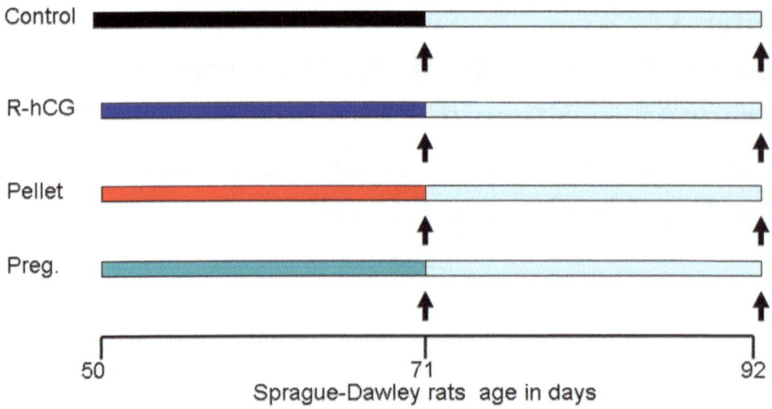

Fig. 3.1 Virgin Sprague–Dawley rats that were named as follows: Control group, received bacteriostatic water—(hCG vehicle), R-hCG (recombinant hCG 100 IU/day), Pellet (estrogen and progesterone (E+P) with a 21-day release period), and Preg (pregnancy). The r-hCG was purchased from Serono, Inc., Rockland, MA. Virgin Sprague–Dawley rats received a daily intraperitoneal (ip) injection of 100 IU suspended in 0.1 mL sterile saline. Injections started when the animals reached the age of 50 days. Injections were applied for 21 days (50 rats), which were euthanized at 21 days post-treatment, respectively. Injections were applied with 27 gauge needles, using only physical restraint while applying the injection. The estrogen-progesterone pellet implant was done in 50-day old virgin rats that were anesthetized and the subcutaneous tissue of the inter-scapular area was perforated with a needle-trocar (Innovative Research of America, FL). One pellet contains 0.72 mg pellet of 17β-estradiol (E_2) and 200 mg of progesterone (Pg). The pellets were left in place for 21 days. Hormone release was evaluated by comparing the weight of the pellets at the time of removal with their initial weight

reduction in carcinogenic response to administration of DMBA at 21, 42, or 63 days after termination of the hormonal treatment [10, 13].

It is of utmost importance to identify the molecular pathways that are responsible for the hormonally induced prevention. For this purpose we have conducted a detailed transcriptomic analysis of the resting mammary glands of Sprague–Dawley rats that have been treated for 21 days with the human chorionic gonadotropin or hCG, full term pregnancy or treatment with a pellet of estrogen and progesterone (pellet) (Fig. 3.1). The data demonstrates that the three protocols induce differentiation of the mammary gland and there are common genes that constitute the genomic signature explaining the preventive effects of these approaches. However, the transcriptomic profile induced by hCG provides a new insight in the use of this hormone as a preventive agent in human breast cancer.

3.2 Experimental Protocol

Virgin Sprague–Dawley rats that were maintained in an environmentally controlled clean air room with a 12 h light/12 h darkness cycle were distributed in four groups of 50 rats each (Fig. 3.1). All the treatments were given by intraperitoneal (ip) injection,

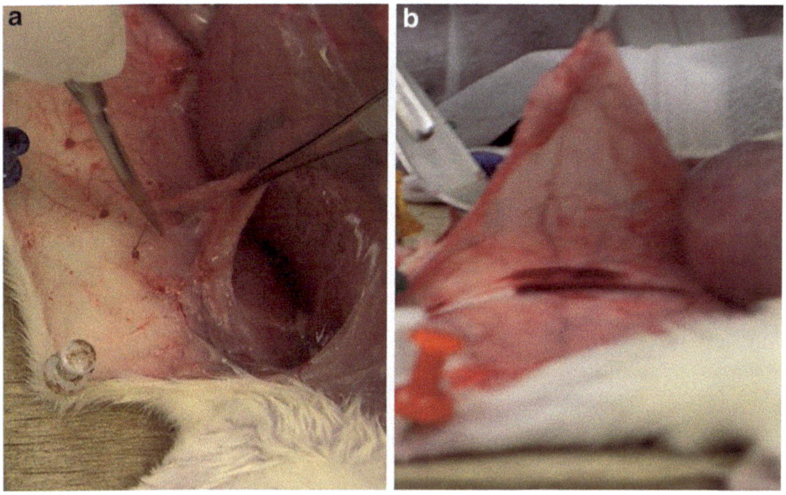

Fig. 3.2 Dissection of the thoracic (**a**) and abdominal (**b**) rat mammary gland

in a volume of 300 μL. The groups were named as follows: Control, received bacteriostatic water (hCG vehicle), hCG(r-hCG 100 IU/day), pellet (with estrogen and progesterone [E+P] as a pellet of 0.72 mg 17β estradiol [E_2] and one of 200 mg progesterone with a 21-day release period), and Preg (pregnancy). Each group received 21 consecutive days of treatment, followed by a resting period of 21 days. At the end of the resting period at age 92 days, 20 animals per group were euthanized and proceed to collect their abdominal mammary glands for histology analysis and RNA extraction. A whole mount was prepared with the right abdominal mammary gland (mg) 4, 5 and the left abdominal mammary glands were used for RNA extraction (Fig. 3.2).

3.3 Morphological Changes Induced by the Hormonal Treatment

Figure 3.3 is a schematic representation of the pathway of mammary gland differentiation from the TEBs to the formation of lobules type 1, 2, and 3. It is important to emphasize that the differentiation and branching occurring from lobules type 1 to 2 and 3 is mainly a differentiation-induced process driven by an endogenous hormonal stimulation like pregnancy or exogenous hormonal treatment like described in the protocol of Fig. 3.1.

Using the methodology described in Fig. 3.4 we have quantitated the number of structures of the rat mammary gland and expressed as the percentage of structures per mm^2 of gland; the number of TEB, Terminal ducts (TD), lob1, lob2, and lob3 at the end of the treatment and 21 days post treatment are shown in Figs. 3.5a and 3.5b respectively. The control rat mammary glands are devoid of lob2 and 3 (Fig. 3.4a–c).

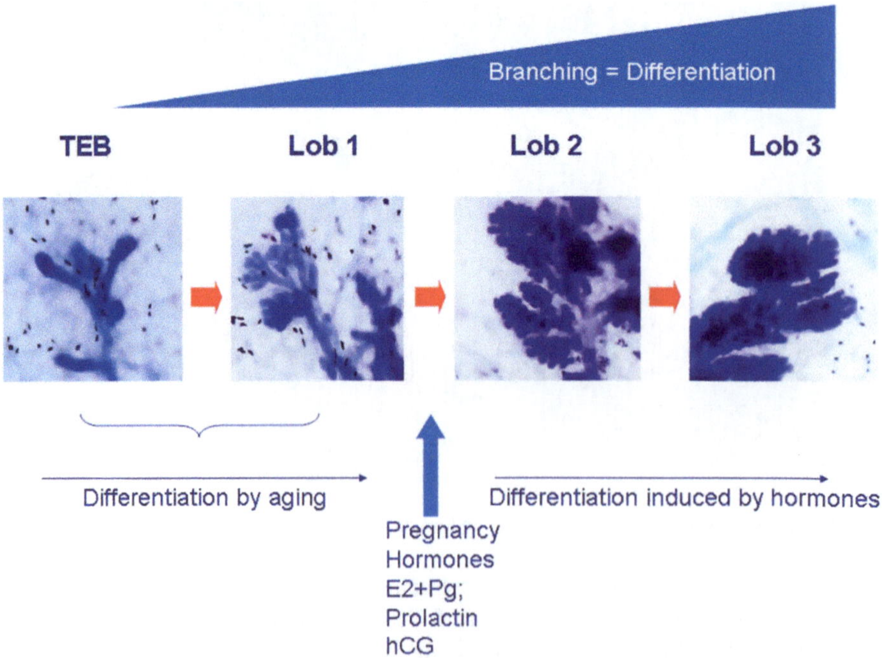

Fig. 3.3 Pathway of mammary gland differentiation from the terminal end buds (TEB) to the formation of lobules type 1, 2, and 3. Differentiation and branching occurring from lobules type 1 to 2 and 3 are mainly driven by an endogenous hormonal stimulation like pregnancy of exogenous hormonal treatment

Pregnancy and r-hCG stimulate the gland differentiation completely to lob3 at the end of treatment (Figs. 3.4d, i and 3.5a). The animals treated with the estrogen and progesterone pellet also presented profuse lobular development but there were areas of the glands that were not stimulated as shown in Fig. 3.4e–g whereas other areas were fully developed as shown in Fig. 3.4h. This is quantitated in the histogram depicted in Fig. 3.5a. After 21 days of mammary gland regression post pregnancy or post hCG treatment none of the rat mammary glands contain TEB but regression to TD lob1 and 2 is observed. The animals treated with the estrogen and progesterone pellet instead contained, in addition to TD, Lob1, 2, and 3, a great percentage of TEB as the control indicating that the mammary gland has not been completely differentiated by this treatment (Fig. 3.5b).

3.4 Transcriptomic Profile

Gene expression profiles were determined using whole genome Agilent microarrays of rat containing ~41,000 probes representing ~19,000 with unique gene symbol. We have used different FDR (False Discovery Rate) and *p*-values to determine

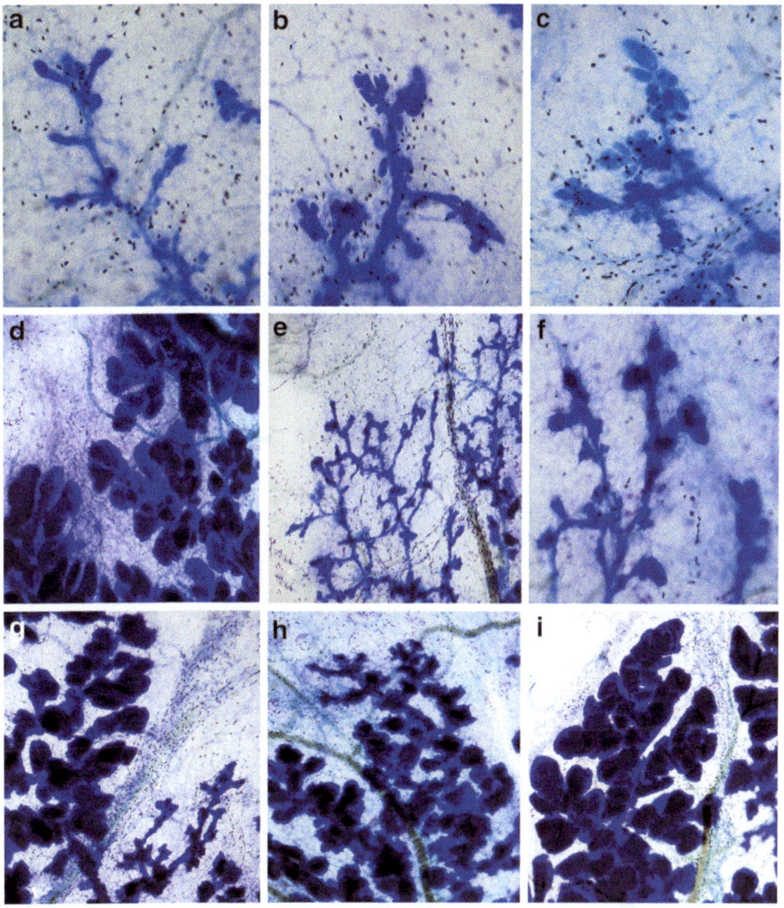

Fig. 3.4 Whole mounts of the rat mammary glands stained with toluidine blue. (**a–c**) Rat mammary gland of a virgin female control rat obtained at 72 days of ag e showing prominent TEBs (**a**), lobules type 1 (**b** and **c**) and numerous mast cells in the stroma. (**d**) Profuse formation of Lob3 in the mammary gland of an animal that received r-hCG for 21 days. (**e–h**) Mammary gland of a rat receiving the hormonal stimulation of a pellet implant showing TD and TEB (**e**, **f**) lob1 (*right*) and and lob3 (*left side*)(**g**) and only lob 3 (**h**). (**i**) Rat mammary gland with profuse lobular development (Lob 3) at the end of pregnancy

which are the most relevant genes detected using different stringency criteria in the rat mammary gland of animals treated with hCG, the pellet, and pregnancy over the control (Table 3.1). hCG treatment is the only one that induces significant genomic changes when the FDR of 5 and 10 and a fold change of 1.5 and 2 are utilized (Table 3.1). When the $p<0.001$ and twofold change are used as a cutting point (Table 3.1) we identified seven common genes that are upregulated in the mammary gland of the three groups of animals compared with the untreated ones (Table 3.2). The most relevant genes are the *Encl* (*Rattus norvegicus* ectodermal-neural cortex 1) and *Lcn2* (*Rattus norvegicus* lipocalin 2).

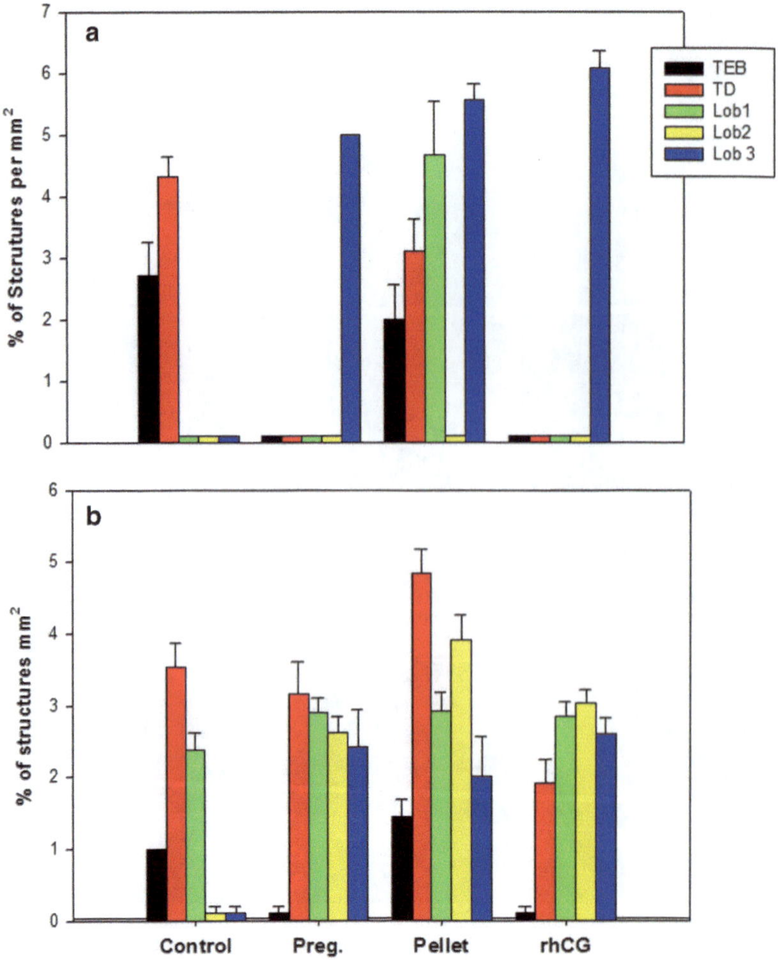

Fig. 3.5 Histogram depicting the percentage of structures per sq mm of mammary gland. (**a**) At the end of treatment. (**b**) 21 days post treatment

We ran DAVID [17] to test the function association of the three gene subsets with GO biological processes. As it is shown in Fig. 3.6 there are three GO commons to the treated animals that are associated with immune response, transport, and development. Among the genes in the GO immune response are the *Hspala* (heat shock 70 kDa protein 1A), *Kngl* (kininogen1), *Pla2g7* (phospholipase A2), group VII (platelet-activating factor [PAF] acetylhydrolase, plasma), *Lcn2* (lipocalin 2), *Cd14* (CD14 molecule), *Sectmlb* (secreted and transmembrane 1B), *Lbp* (lipopolysaccharide-binding protein), and *Cfi* (complement factor I) (Table 3.3). The GO for transport listed in Table 3.3 contains the following genes *Lcn2, LOC259246, Crhr2, Crabp2, Adfp, Scnnlg, Slc13a2*, and *Lbp*. Some of these genes overlap with the GO immune response and development. In the GO for development the most significant genes are *Hspala, Kngl, Kngl1l, Duox, Crhr2*, and *Spp1* (Table 3.3).

Table 3.1 Number of differentially expressed genes in each condition compared to the control using different cut-offs

	Number of genes			Comparisons			
Cut-offs	hCG	Pellet	Preg	hCG Pellet	hCG Preg	Pellet Preg	All
FDR 5% FC2	57	2	1	0	1	0	0
FDR 5% FC1.5	209	2	1	0	1	0	0
FDR 10% FC2	128	3	2	0	1	0	0
FDR 10% FC1.5	477	3	2	0	2	0	0
p-Value 0.001 FC2	67	35	27	8	10	12	7
p-Value 0.001 FC1.5	250	80	55	12	19	21	10
p-Value 0.01 FC2	220	112	85	33	38	50	28
p-Value 0.01 FC1.5	683	280	237	68	87	105	53

FDR false discovery rate; *FC* fold change; *Preg* pregnancy

Table 3.2 Genes found to be differentially expressed in all the three conditions ($p<0.001$ and fold change at least 2.0)

			Fold change		
Gene symbol	Systematic name	Description	hCG	Pellet	Preg
AA874941	AA874941	AA874941 UI-R-E0-ci-d-06-0-UI.s1 UI-R-E0 *Rattus norvegicus* cDNA clone UI-R-E0-ci-d-06-0-UI 3′ similar to gi [AA874941]	2.42	3.01	2.59
Cfi	NM_024157	*Rattus norvegicus* complement factor I (Cfi), mRNA [NM_024157]	7.57	6.72	6.05
Encl	NM_001003401	*Rattus norvegicus* ectodermal-neural cortex 1 (Encl), mRNA [NM_001003401]	2.08	2.26	2.01
Lcn2	NM_130741	*Rattus norvegicus* lipocalin 2 (Lcn2), mRNA [NM_130741]	3.78	4.99	4.53
Map3k6_predicted	XM_232732	PREDICTED: *Rattus norvegicus* mitogen-activated protein kinase kinase kinase 6 (predicted) (Map3k6_predicted), mRNA [XM_232732]	2.04	2.09	2.00
Thedc1	NM_022705	*Rattus norvegicus* thioesterase domain containing 1 (Thedc1), mRNA [NM_022705]	7.05	13.64	10.29
XM_234581	XM_234581	*Rattus norvegicus* similar to immunoglobulin alpha heavy chain (LOC314487), mRNA [XM_234581]	3.32	4.05	10.42

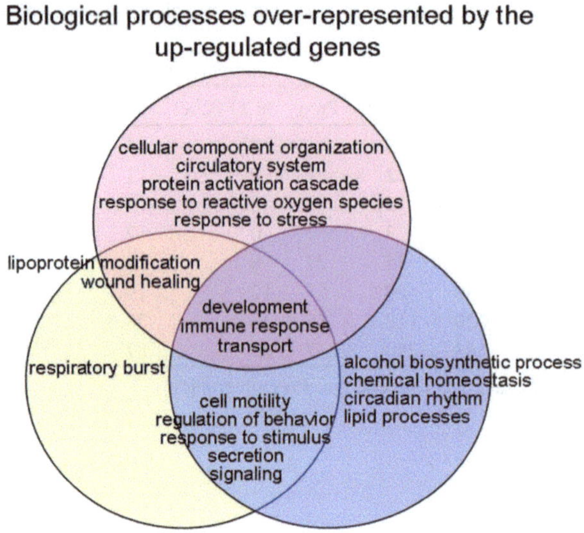

Fig. 3.6 Venn diagram depicting the biological processes of the upregulated genes in the rat mammary under three different prevention strategies. Total RNA was isolated from 15 frozen mammary glands per group using RNeasy Lipid Tissue Mini Kit (Qiagen Inc., Valencia, CA), following manufacturer's protocol and treated with DNase I. RNA concentration and quality were assessed using NanoDrop ND-1000 spectrophotometer (NanoDrop Technologies, Wilmington, DE) and Agilent 2100 Bioanalyzer capillary electrophoresis (Agilent Technologies, Palo Alto, CA), respectively. From the 15 RNA samples of each group, we obtained five different samples for hybridization by pooling the RNA of three rats. 200 ng of total RNA from five pools per group was prepared for the microarray hybridization using the Quick Amp Labeling Kit-one color (Agilent Technologies, Palo Alto, CA) following the manufacturer's protocol. Labeled cRNAs were hybridized to Whole rat genome-4X44K oligo microarrays (G4112F, Agilent Technologies). In this study we identified genes differentially expressed between the following pairwise comparisons: hCG vs. control, E2+P pellet vs. control, and pregnancy vs. control. Normalization and statistical analysis of 20 one-color arrays were conducted using limma package of Bioconductor under R environment. Background correction was performed using "normexp" method in the package to adjust the local median background estimates. The resulting data were then normalized using "quantile" method whose goal is to impose to each array the same empirical distribution of intensities. The statistical analysis of normalized log 2-ratio data was carried out by applying empirical Bayes moderated *t*-test provided in limma software. The *p*-values and the FDR using Benjamini–Hochberg method were calculated for every comparison. We set a cut-off of fold change at least 2.0 and *p*-value below 0.01 to select differentially expressed genes. For each comparison, all genes with fold change of at least 2.0 and *p*-values less than 0.01 were considered for functional analysis. The analyses were carried out independently for up- and downregulated genes. To identify the gene ontologies (GO) terms in the biological process category that were overrepresented among the differentially expressed genes, we performed conditional hypergeometric tests in the Bioconductor *GOstats* package. GO terms with *p*-values below 0.01 were considered enriched. Then, manually, equivalent GO terms were grouped together in larger classes of biological functions. The differentially expressed genes were also imported into Ingenuity Pathway Analysis (IPA version: 11904312) based on the Ingenuity Pathways Knowledge Base (IPKB), where each interaction in IPKB is supported by the underlying publications and structured functional annotation (http://www.ingenuity.com/). Statistical scores were then assigned to rank the resulting networks and pathways using Fisher's right tailed exact tests, where the significantly enriched pathways (p-value <0.01) were selected

Table 3.3 Biological processes overrepresented among the upregulated genes in all three conditions

Symbol	Name
Immune response	
hCG (GO:0002460, GO:0002682, GO:0006959, GO:0045087, GO:0006958, GO:0002449, GO:0050778, GO:0016064)	
C4bpa	Complement component 4 binding protein, alpha
Hspa1a	Heat shock 70 kDa protein 1A
Cfi	Complement factor I
Kng1	Kininogen 1
Pla2g7	Phospholipase A2, group VII (platelet-activating factor acetylhydrolase, plasma)
Lcn2	Lipocalin 2
Cd14	CD14 molecule
Pellet (GO:0006955)	
Lcn2	Lipocalin 2
Sectm1b	Secreted and transmembrane 1B
Cfi	Complement factor I
Pregnancy (GO:0045087, GO:0002687, GO:0002376, GO:0032755, GO:0002688, GO:0002232, GO:0032490)	
Lcn2	Lipocalin 2
Lbp	Lipopolysaccharide-binding protein
Cfi	Complement factor I
Pla2g7	Phospholipase A2, group VII (platelet-activating factor acetylhydrolase, plasma)
Sectm1b	Secreted and transmembrane 1B
Crhr2	Corticotropin releasing hormone receptor 2
Transport	
hCG (GO:0015891, GO:0033212, GO:0000041)	
Lcn2	Lipocalin 2
Slc39a8	Solute carrier family 39 (zinc transporter), member 8
Pellet (GO:0015833, GO:0006869, GO:0048241, GO:0015891, GO:0033212, GO:0090281)	
LOC259246	Alpha-2u globulin PGCL1
Crhr2	Corticotropin releasing hormone receptor 2
Crabp2	Cellular retinoic acid-binding protein 2
Adfp	Adipose differentiation-related protein
Lcn2	Lipocalin 2
Pregnancy (GO:0033212, GO:0090281, GO:0030001, GO:0015891, GO:0015920, GO:0033037)	
Lcn2	Lipocalin 2
Crhr2	Corticotropin releasing hormone receptor 2

(continued)

Table 3.3 (continued)

Symbol	Name
Scnn1g	Sodium channel, nonvoltage-gated 1, gamma
Slc13a2	Solute carrier family 13 (sodium-dependent dicarboxylate transporter), member 2
Lbp	Lipopolysaccharide-binding protein
Development	
hCG (GO:0035150, GO:0042335)	
Hspa1a	Heat shock 70 kDa protein 1A
Kng1	Kininogen 1
Kng1l1	Kininogen 1-like 1
Duox1	Dual oxidase 1
Pellet (GO:0048630, GO:0070584)	
Crhr2	Corticotropin releasing hormone receptor 2
LOC259246	Alpha-2u globulin PGCL1
Pregnancy (GO:0048685, GO:0070571, GO:0048670)	
Spp1	Secreted phosphoprotein 1

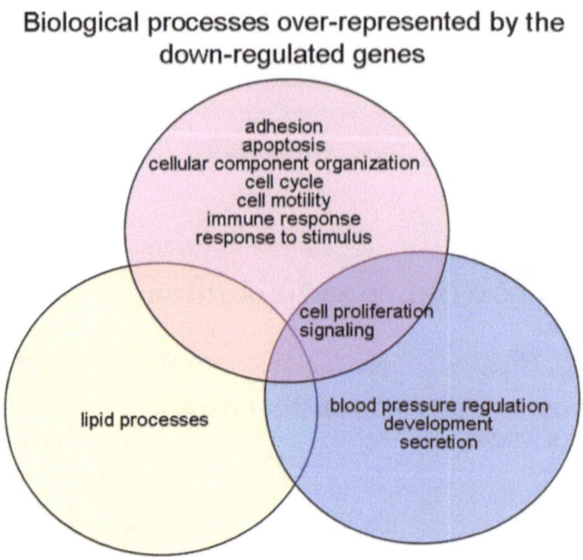

Fig. 3.7 Venn diagram depicting the biological processes of the downregulated genes in the rat mammary under three different prevention strategies

There are no common downregulated genes among the three prevention modalities (Fig. 3.7). However there are specific downregulated GO biological processes for each preventive modalities (Figs. 3.7 and 3.8) and the same apply for upregulated genes (Figs. 3.6 and 3.9). hCG induces the highest number of downregulated genes and GO biological processes including adhesion, apoptosis, cellular component

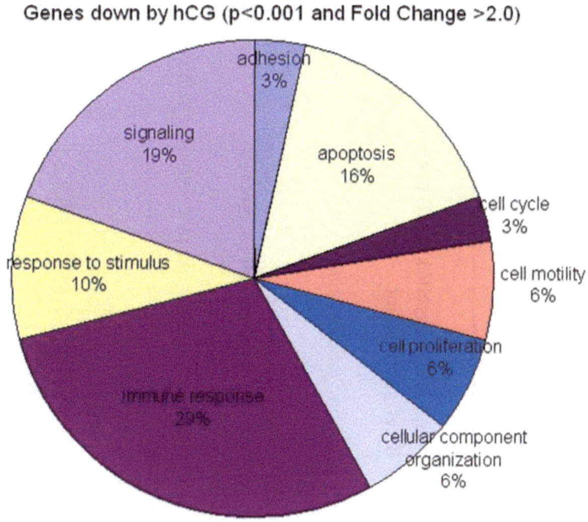

Fig. 3.8 Downregulated genes in the rat mammary under hCG treatment

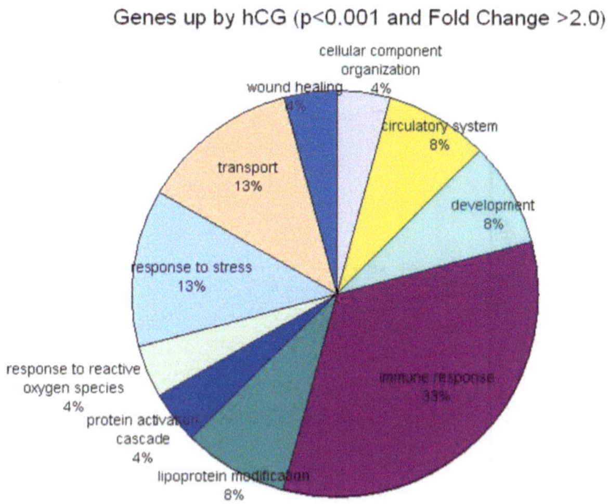

Fig. 3.9 Upregulated genes in the rat mammary under hCG treatment

organization, cell cycle, cell motility, immune response, and response to stimulus (Figs. 3.7, 3.8 and Table 3.4). The same apply to the upregulated genes with over-represented GO for cellular component organization, circulatory system, protein activation cascade, response to oxygen species, and response to stress (Figs. 3.6, 3.9 and Table 3.5).

Pregnancy only downregulates the GO biological process related to lipid metabolism (Figs. 3.7, 3.10 and Table 3.6) and upregulates the GO biological process related to respiratory burst (Figs. 3.6, 3.11 and Table 3.7). The estrogen and progesterone combination modality of prevention downregulated the GO biological

Table 3.4 Biological processes overrepresented among the genes downregulated by hCG

GOBPID	*P*-value	Odds ratio	Exp count	Count	Size	Term
GO:0006955	0	14.395	1	5	438	Immune response
GO:0043123	0	36.898	0	3	85	Positive regulation of I-kappaB kinase/NF-kappaB cascade
GO:0030890	0.001	76.125	0	2	26	Positive regulation of B-cell proliferation
GO:0045321	0.001	13.992	0	4	320	Leukocyte activation
GO:0035417	0.001	Inf	0	1	1	Negative regulation of mitotic prometaphase
GO:0035759	0.001	Inf	0	1	1	Mesangial cell-matrix adhesion
GO:2000508	0.001	Inf	0	1	1	Regulation of dendritic cell chemotaxis
GO:2000529	0.001	Inf	0	1	1	Positive regulation of myeloid dendritic cell chemotaxis
GO:0042981	0.002	7.86	1	5	768	Regulation of apoptosis
GO:0002768	0.002	33.722	0	2	56	Immune response-regulating cell surface receptor signaling pathway
GO:0010941	0.002	7.443	1	5	807	Regulation of cell death
GO:0050864	0.003	31.937	0	2	59	Regulation of B-cell activation
GO:2000353	0.003	832.545	0	1	2	Positive regulation of endothelial cell apoptosis
GO:0032946	0.004	25.6	0	2	73	Positive regulation of mononuclear cell proliferation
GO:0001768	0.004	416.227	0	1	3	Establishment of T-cell polarity
GO:0012501	0.004	6.547	1	5	906	Programmed cell death
GO:0016265	0.005	6.151	1	5	958	Death
GO:0070842	0.005	277.455	0	1	4	Aggresome assembly
GO:0048584	0.006	7.107	1	4	606	Positive regulation of response to stimulus
GO:0002684	0.007	9.709	0	3	307	Positive regulation of immune system process
GO:0035556	0.007	5.601	1	5	1,041	Intracellular signal transduction
GO:0048304	0.008	166.436	0	1	6	Positive regulation of isotype switching to IgG isotypes
GO:0050670	0.008	17.413	0	2	106	Regulation of lymphocyte proliferation
GO:0070663	0.009	16.761	0	2	110	Regulation of leukocyte proliferation
GO:0031274	0.009	138.682	0	1	7	Positive regulation of pseudopodium assembly
GO:0032862	0.009	138.682	0	1	7	Activation of Rho GTPase activity

GO:0033194	0.009	138.682	0	1	7	Response to hydroperoxide
GO:0034695	0.009	138.682	0	1	7	Response to prostaglandin E stimulus
GO:0023051	0.01	5.244	1	5	1,103	Regulation of signaling
GO:0010627	0.01	8.39	0	3	353	Regulation of intracellular protein kinase cascade
GO:0051251	0.01	15.868	0	2	116	Positive regulation of lymphocyte activation

Table 3.5 Biological processes overrepresented among the genes upregulated by hCG

GOBPID	*P*-value	Odds ratio	Exp count	Count	Size	Term
GO:0045087	0.001	12.898	0	4	178	Innate immune response
GO:0006958	0.001	63.438	0	2	18	Complement activation, classical pathway
GO:0035150	0.001	15.812	0	3	104	Regulation of tube size
GO:0002449	0.002	15.351	0	3	107	Lymphocyte-mediated immunity
GO:0002460	0.002	14.916	0	3	110	Adaptive immune response based on somatic recombination of immune receptors built from immunoglobulin superfamily domains
GO:0003018	0.002	13.989	0	3	117	Vascular process in circulatory system
GO:0006950	0.002	6.31	1	6	912	Response to stress
GO:0002682	0.002	6.506	1	5	451	Regulation of immune system process
GO:0072376	0.003	27.369	0	2	39	Protein activation cascade
GO:0070301	0.003	26.646	0	2	40	Cellular response to hydrogen peroxide
GO:0015891	0.004	481.579	0	1	2	Siderophore transport
GO:0033212	0.004	481.579	0	1	2	Iron assimilation
GO:0042335	0.004	481.579	0	1	2	Cuticle development
GO:0090084	0.004	481.579	0	1	2	Negative regulation of inclusion body assembly
GO:0042311	0.005	21.522	0	2	49	Vasodilation
GO:0006959	0.005	20.639	0	2	51	Humoral immune response
GO:0034441	0.007	240.763	0	1	3	Plasma lipoprotein particle oxidation
GO:0050778	0.007	8.697	0	3	185	Positive regulation of immune response
GO:0033554	0.007	4.89	1	5	589	Cellular response to stress
GO:0016064	0.008	16.835	0	2	62	Immunoglobulin-mediated immune response
GO:0000041	0.008	16.557	0	2	63	Transition metal ion transport
GO:0042160	0.009	160.491	0	1	4	Lipoprotein modification
GO:0009408	0.01	15.065	0	2	69	Response to heat
GO:0042060	0.01	7.663	0	3	209	Wound healing

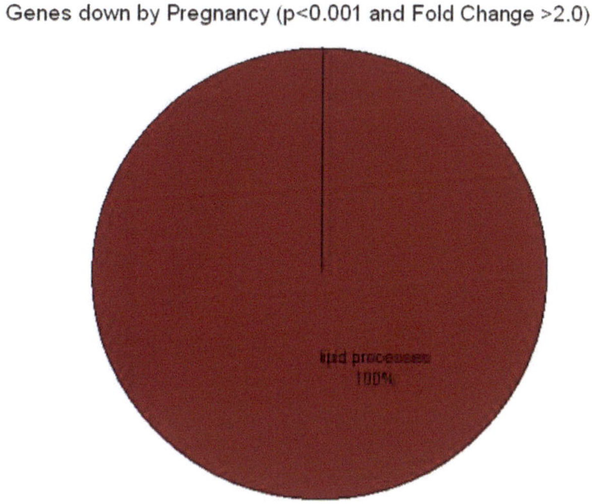

Fig. 3.10 Downregulated genes in the rat mammary after pregnancy

Table 3.6 Biological processes overrepresented among the genes downregulated by pregnancy

GOBPID	*P*-value	Odds ratio	Exp count	Count	Size	Term
GO:0019433	0.001	Inf	0	1	13	Triglyceride catabolic process
GO:0044269	0.002	Inf	0	1	15	Glycerol ether catabolic process
GO:0046461	0.002	Inf	0	1	15	Neutral lipid catabolic process
GO:0046503	0.002	Inf	0	1	19	Glycerolipid catabolic process
GO:0019432	0.003	Inf	0	1	29	Triglyceride biosynthetic process
GO:0046460	0.003	Inf	0	1	29	Neutral lipid biosynthetic process
GO:0046504	0.003	Inf	0	1	31	Glycerol ether biosynthetic process
GO:0006639	0.007	Inf	0	1	64	Acylglycerol metabolic process
GO:0045017	0.009	Inf	0	1	81	Glycerolipid biosynthetic process
GO:0018904	0.009	Inf	0	1	86	Organic ether metabolic process

processes related to blood pressure regulation, development, and secretion (Figs. 3.7, 3.12 and Table 3.8), whereas the upregulated GO processes are related to alcohol biosynthesis, chemical homeostasis, circadian rhythm, and lipid metabolism (Figs. 3.6, 3.13 and Table 3.9).

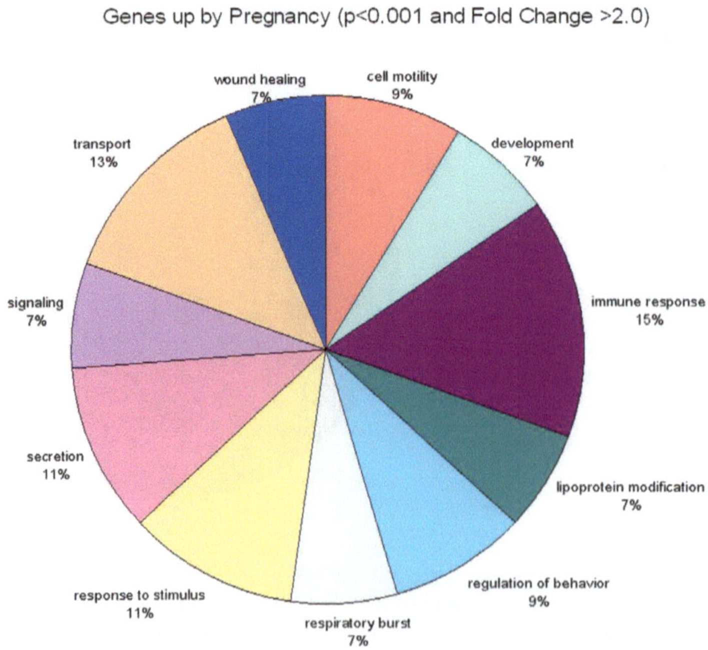

Fig. 3.11 Upregulated genes in the rat mammary gland after pregnancy

3.4.1 Functional Significance of the Common Genes Induced by the Three Preventive Modalities

As depicted in Table 3.2 and Fig. 3.14 there are few genes that are upregulated in the three preventive strategies that indicate a common mechanism for pregnancy, estrogen and progesterone and hCG treatment that could explain the preventive effect induced by these three different but not mutually exclusive effects. One of the genes is the ectodermal-neural cortex 1 or *Enc1*, which is a member of the kelch family of genes that is an actin-binding protein and plays a pivotal role in neuronal and adipocyte differentiation [18, 19]; this gene could have a role in the mammary gland differentiation induced by these three preventive modalities. *Enc1* is downregulated in neuroblastoma tumors conferring a tumor suppressor function. This gene encodes a protein that is a substrate-specific adapter of an E3 ubiquitin-protein ligase complex which mediates the ubiquitination and subsequent proteasomal degradation of target proteins [20]. Transient expression of *Enc1* reduced steady-state levels of *Nrf2* that is a transcription factor and the master regulator of a cellular defense mechanism against environmental insults. This could indicate that this gene functions as a negative regulator of *Nrf2* through suppressing Nrf2 protein translation [21]. *EncC1* has been identified as a tumor suppressor gene in melanoma [22]. The levels of *Enc1* mRNA and protein were stimulated by LH/human chorionic gonadotropin (hCG)

Table 3.7 Biological processes overrepresented among the genes upregulated by pregnancy

GOBPID	*P*-value	Odds ratio	Exp count	Count	Size	Term
GO:0035313	0	184.828	0	2	11	Wound healing, spreading of epidermal cells
GO:0050795	0	30.227	0	3	93	Regulation of behavior
GO:0032755	0.001	61.488	0	2	29	Positive regulation of interleukin-6 production
GO:0002688	0.001	50.275	0	2	35	Regulation of leukocyte chemotaxis
GO:0002232	0.001	Inf	0	1	1	Leukocyte chemotaxis involved in inflammatory response
GO:0014064	0.001	Inf	0	1	1	Positive regulation of serotonin secretion
GO:0035482	0.001	Inf	0	1	1	Gastric motility
GO:0048685	0.001	Inf	0	1	1	Negative regulation of collateral sprouting of intact axon in response to injury
GO:0060265	0.001	Inf	0	1	1	Positive regulation of respiratory burst involved in inflammatory response
GO:2000293	0.001	Inf	0	1	1	Negative regulation of defecation
GO:0045087	0.002	15.399	0	3	178	Innate immune response
GO:0002687	0.002	37.661	0	2	46	Positive regulation of leukocyte migration
GO:0050921	0.002	33.8	0	2	51	Positive regulation of chemotaxis
GO:0015891	0.003	763.083	0	1	2	Siderophore transport
GO:0015920	0.003	763.083	0	1	2	Lipopolysaccharide transport
GO:0033037	0.003	763.083	0	1	2	Polysaccharide localization
GO:0033212	0.003	763.083	0	1	2	Iron assimilation
GO:0090281	0.003	763.083	0	1	2	Negative regulation of calcium ion import
GO:2000252	0.003	763.083	0	1	2	Negative regulation of feeding behavior
GO:0030001	0.003	8.501	1	4	459	Metal ion transport
GO:0032101	0.004	11.594	0	3	234	Regulation of response to external stimulus
GO:0002376	0.004	6.407	1	5	819	Immune system process
GO:0048870	0.004	7.913	1	4	491	Cell motility
GO:0034441	0.004	381.5	0	1	3	Plasma lipoprotein particle oxidation

(continued)

Table 3.7 (continued)

GOBPID	*P*-value	Odds ratio	Exp count	Count	Size	Term
GO:0043950	0.004	381.5	0	1	3	Positive regulation of cAMP-mediated signaling
GO:0043951	0.004	381.5	0	1	3	Negative regulation of cAMP-mediated signaling
GO:0061179	0.004	381.5	0	1	3	Negative regulation of insulin secretion involved in cellular response to glucose stimulus
GO:0070571	0.004	381.5	0	1	3	Negative regulation of neuron projection regeneration
GO:0071222	0.005	23.27	0	2	73	Cellular response to lipopolysaccharide
GO:0009611	0.005	7.25	1	4	533	Response to wounding
GO:0002679	0.006	254.306	0	1	4	Respiratory burst involved in defense response
GO:0034145	0.006	254.306	0	1	4	Positive regulation of toll-like receptor 4 signaling pathway
GO:0042160	0.006	254.306	0	1	4	Lipoprotein modification
GO:0060054	0.006	254.306	0	1	4	Positive regulation of epithelial cell proliferation involved in wound healing
GO:0060326	0.006	20.632	0	2	82	Cell chemotaxis
GO:0071216	0.006	19.88	0	2	85	Cellular response to biotic stimulus
GO:0010700	0.007	190.708	0	1	5	Negative regulation of norepinephrine secretion
GO:0032277	0.007	190.708	0	1	5	Negative regulation of gonadotropin secretion
GO:0032490	0.007	190.708	0	1	5	Detection of molecule of bacterial origin
GO:0048670	0.007	190.708	0	1	5	Regulation of collateral sprouting
GO:0060263	0.007	190.708	0	1	5	Regulation of respiratory burst
GO:0071223	0.007	190.708	0	1	5	Cellular response to lipoteichoic acid
GO:0090026	0.007	190.708	0	1	5	Positive regulation of monocyte chemotaxis
GO:0048584	0.008	6.317	1	4	606	Positive regulation of response to stimulus
GO:0032811	0.008	152.55	0	1	6	Negative regulation of epinephrine secretion
GO:0034374	0.008	152.55	0	1	6	Low-density lipoprotein particle remodeling

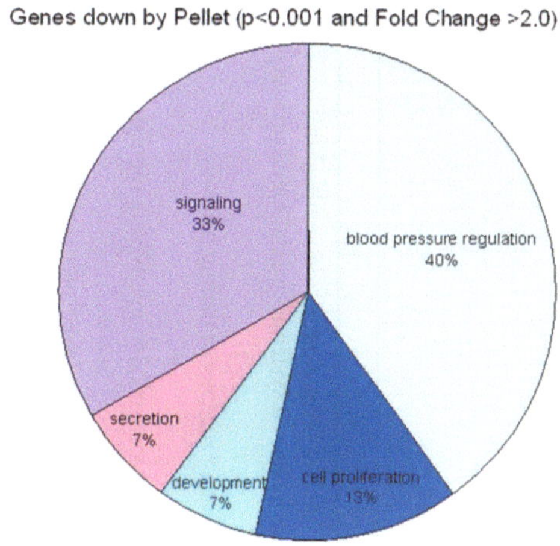

Fig. 3.12 Genes downregulated in the rat mammary gland under pellet treatment

within 3 h both in vivo and in vitro in the ovary. In situ hybridization analysis revealed that *Enc1* mRNA was localized not only in theca/interstitial cells but also in granulosa cells of preovulatory follicles but not of growing follicles in pregnant mare's serum gonadotropin/hCG-treated ovaries. LH-induced Enc1 expression was suppressed by a high dose of protein kinase C inhibitor RO 31-8220 (10 μM) but not by low doses of RO 31-8220 (0.1–1.0 μM), suggesting the involvement of atypical protein kinase C. Enc1 was detected in both nucleus and cytoplasm that was increased by LH/hCG treatment. Both biochemical and morphological analysis revealed that LH/hCG treatment increased actin polymerization within 3 h in granulosa cells. Interestingly, Enc1 physically associated with actin and treatment with cytochalasin D, an actin-depolymerizing agent, abolished this association. Confocal microscopy further demonstrated the colocalization of Enc1 with filamentous actin (F-actin). LH/hCG stimulates Enc1 expression and increases F-actin formation in granulosa cells implicating the role of Enc1 in cytoskeletal reorganization during the differentiation of granulosa cells [19]. The same mechanism could be applied to the rat mammary gland.

Among the overexpressed genes common to the effect of hCG and hormones of pregnancies (Table 3.2) is the lipocalin 2 (*Lcn2*) that is an iron-trafficking protein involved in multiple processes such as apoptosis, innate immunity, and renal development. *Lcn2* is involved in apoptosis due to interleukin-3 (IL3) deprivation: iron-loaded form increases intracellular iron concentration without promoting apoptosis, while iron-free form decreases intracellular iron levels, inducing expression of the proapoptotic protein BCL2L11/BIM, resulting in apoptosis. Whereas its function in apoptosis could be relevant to the rat mammary gland treated with the preventive agents, its role in breast cancer has been suggested to be different. For example *Lcn2* is upregulated in several epithelial cancers, including breast [23, 24] and prostate cancer, and implicated as a key mediator of breast cancer progression. The tumor cell

Table 3.8 Biological processes overrepresented among the genes downregulated by pellet

GOBPID	*P*-value	Odds ratio	Exp count	Count	Size	Term
GO:0001986	0.001	Inf	0	1	1	Negative regulation of the force of heart contraction involved in baroreceptor response to increased systemic arterial blood pressure
GO:0002158	0.001	Inf	0	1	1	Osteoclast proliferation
GO:0031547	0.001	Inf	0	1	1	Brain-derived neurotrophic factor receptor signaling pathway
GO:0046548	0.002	1145.125	0	1	2	Retinal rod cell development
GO:0001994	0.003	572.5	0	1	3	Norepinephrine-epinephrine vasoconstriction involved in regulation of systemic arterial blood pressure
GO:0071883	0.003	572.5	0	1	3	Activation of MAPK activity by adrenergic receptor signaling pathway
GO:0035625	0.004	381.625	0	1	4	Epidermal growth factor-activated receptor transactivation by G-protein coupled receptor signaling pathway
GO:0001978	0.005	286.188	0	1	5	Regulation of systemic arterial blood pressure by carotid sinus baroreceptor feedback
GO:0008217	0.005	22.477	0	2	117	Regulation of blood pressure
GO:0071875	0.006	217.952	0	1	7	Adrenergic receptor signaling pathway
GO:0033688	0.007	190.75	0	1	7	Regulation of osteoblast proliferation
GO:0001993	0.008	163.482	0	1	8	Regulation of systemic arterial blood pressure by norepinephrine-epinephrine
GO:0035810	0.008	163.482	0	1	8	Positive regulation of urine volume
GO:0030157	0.009	143.031	0	1	9	Pancreatic juice secretion
GO:0032148	0.009	143.031	0	1	9	Activation of protein kinase B activity

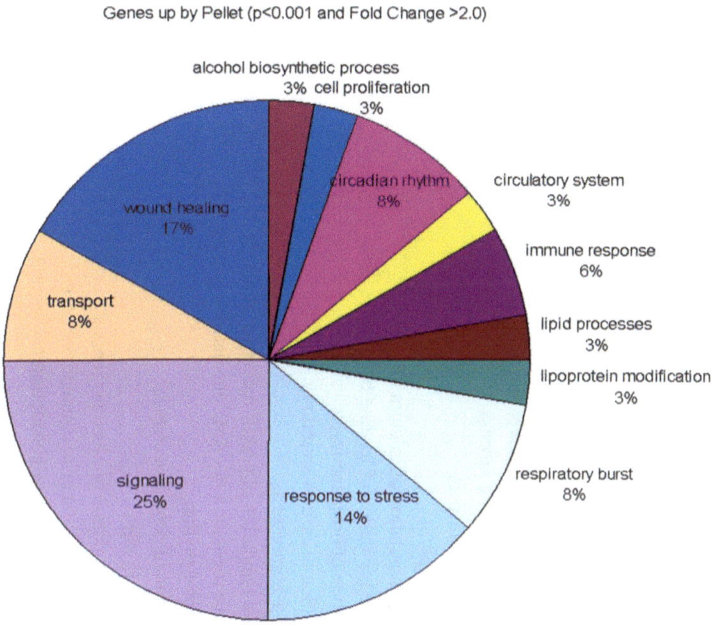

Fig. 3.13 Upregulated genes in the rat mammary gland under pellet treatment

regulates unfolded protein response (UPR) and activates *Lcn2* production in prostate cancer cells in an NF-κB-dependent manner [25]. *Lcn2* has also been associated with cell migration by controlling *NFAT1* and *NFAT5* that are acting as pro-invasive and pro-migratory transcription factors in breast carcinoma, contributing to the formation of metastases. *NFAT3* is specifically expressed in estrogen receptor alpha positive (ERA+) breast cancer cells and inhibits by itself the invasion capacity of ERA+ breast cancer cells, needing to cooperate with ERA to inhibit their migration. Conversely, *NFAT3* downregulation results in actin reorganization associated with increased migration and invasion capabilities. *NFAT3* signaling reduces migration through inhibition of Lipocalin 2 gene expression. *NFAT3/LCN2* axis critically controls motility in breast cancer [26]. In the spontaneous mammary tumor mouse model showing that MMTV-ErbB2 (V664E) mice lacking *Lcn2* had significantly delayed mammary tumor formation and metastasis with reduced matrix metalloproteinase-9 activity in the blood. LCN2 expression is upregulated by HER2/phosphoinositide 3-kinase/AKT/NF-κB pathway. Decreasing LCN2 expression significantly reduced the invasion and migration ability of HER2(+) breast cancer cells. Furthermore, injecting an anti-mouse LCN2 antibody into mice bearing established murine breast tumors resulted in significant blockage of lung metastasis. These findings indicate that LCN2 is a critical factor in enhancing breast tumor formation and progression possibly in part by stabilizing matrix metalloproteinase-9 [27]. *Lcn2* has been shown to induce the epithelial to mesenchymal transition (EMT) in breast cancer cells and to promote breast tumor invasion. Estrogen receptor alpha may

Table 3.9 Biological processes overrepresented among the genes upregulated by pellet

GOBPID	*P*-value	Odds ratio	Exp count	Count	Size	Term
GO:0061179	0	2617.429	0	2	3	Negative regulation of insulin secretion involved in cellular response to glucose stimulus
GO:0090278	0	96.667	0	2	29	Negative regulation of peptide hormone secretion
GO:0071326	0	84.157	0	2	33	Cellular response to monosaccharide stimulus
GO:0071333	0	84.157	0	2	33	Cellular response to glucose stimulus
GO:0014064	0.001	Inf	0	1	1	Positive regulation of serotonin secretion
GO:0035482	0.001	Inf	0	1	1	Gastric motility
GO:2000293	0.001	Inf	0	1	1	Negative regulation of defecation
GO:0046165	0.002	38.785	0	2	69	Alcohol biosynthetic process
GO:0015891	0.002	1145.125	0	1	2	Siderophore transport
GO:0033212	0.002	1145.125	0	1	2	Iron assimilation
GO:0090281	0.002	1145.125	0	1	2	Negative regulation of calcium ion import
GO:2000252	0.002	1145.125	0	1	2	Negative regulation of feeding behavior
GO:0010817	0.002	16.219	0	3	277	Regulation of hormone levels
GO:0050796	0.002	35.573	0	2	75	Regulation of insulin secretion
GO:0042593	0.003	31.638	0	2	84	Glucose homeostasis
GO:0043950	0.003	572.5	0	1	3	Positive regulation of cAMP-mediated signaling
GO:0043951	0.003	572.5	0	1	3	Negative regulation of cAMP-mediated signaling
GO:0045475	0.003	572.5	0	1	3	Locomotor rhythm
GO:0002791	0.003	30.511	0	2	87	Regulation of peptide secretion
GO:0007623	0.003	28.8	0	2	92	Circadian rhythm
GO:0045721	0.004	381.625	0	1	4	Negative regulation of gluconeogenesis
GO:0010700	0.005	286.188	0	1	5	Negative regulation of norepinephrine secretion
GO:0032277	0.005	286.188	0	1	5	Negative regulation of gonadotropin secretion
GO:0046883	0.005	22.88	0	2	115	Regulation of hormone secretion
GO:0009746	0.006	21.712	0	2	121	Response to hexose stimulus
GO:0032811	0.006	228.925	0	1	6	Negative regulation of epinephrine secretion
GO:0015833	0.007	20.326	0	2	129	Peptide transport

GO:0006869	0.007	19.851	0	2	132	Lipid transport
GO:0006955	0.007	10.031	0	3	438	Immune response
GO:0009743	0.008	18.683	0	2	140	Response to carbohydrate stimulus
GO:0048630	0.008	163.482	0	1	8	Skeletal muscle tissue growth
GO:0070584	0.008	163.482	0	1	8	Mitochondrion morphogenesis
GO:0055082	0.008	9.703	0	3	452	Cellular chemical homeostasis
GO:0010888	0.009	143.031	0	1	9	Negative regulation of lipid storage
GO:0048241	0.009	143.031	0	1	9	Epinephrine transport
GO:0032874	0.01	127.125	0	1	10	Positive regulation of stress-activated MAPK cascade

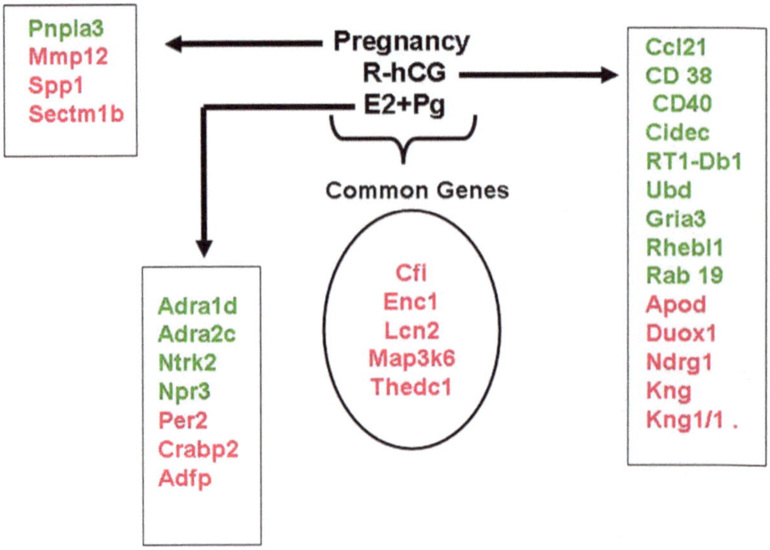

Fig. 3.14 Common genes and specific transcripts expressed in the rat mammary gland following pregnancy, r-hCG, and pellet treatment using $p<0.001$ and FC of 2.0

participate in the pathway that leads to *Lcn2*-induced EMT. Preliminary evidence also suggests that *Lcn2* may be useful as a potential noninvasive urinary biomarker of breast cancer. Elevated levels of *Lcn2* have also been reported in other human cancers. The potential roles of *Lcn2* in epithelial tumors as well as leukemia have been assumed [28, 29]. Therefore it is not clear the role of *Lcn2* in the regressed rat mammary gland after pregnancy and hormonal treatment that have shown to confer protection against DMBA induced carcinogenesis. It has been postulated [30] that the overexpression of uterocalin or lipocalin in the mammary glands of parous animals compared with virgin animals have a function that would suppress inflammation, and uterocalin was an excellent candidate for the gene that contributes to long-term protection of the mammary gland from breast cancer. The reasoning is that uterocalin stimulates apoptosis of neutrophils, but not of macrophages [31], whereas neutrophils are important in the acute phase responders, macrophages play a subsequent, but extremely important role in the inflammatory response; this role is to engulf apoptotic neutrophils and to subdue the inflammatory response [32]. Activated neutrophils, while essential for combating microbial infections, also produce numerous oxidative and carcinogenic products. Carcinogens such as DMBA must be metabolized (bioactivated) to become carcinogenic in vivo [33]. The ability of activated neutrophils to metabolize and produce active carcinogenic species has been proposed as an explanation of why epithelial cells in the breast are sensitive targets for chemical carcinogenesis despite their own limited bioactivation capacity [34]. Thus, the extent of DNA damage and mutation in a tissue increases in parallel with the average number of activated neutrophils present over time [30].

There are a group of genes that are upregulated in the hCG-treated, pregnant and pregnancy hormone treated animals that are related to the inflammatory response (Table 3.2). One of them is the complement factor I (*Cfi*) and the other is the complement factor B (*Cfb*). The *Cfi* gene encodes a serine proteinase that is essential for regulating the complement cascade and is responsible for cleaving the alpha-chains of *C4b* and *C3b* in the presence of the cofactors C4-binding protein and factor H respectively. The *Cfb* encodes complement factor B, a component of the alternative pathway of complement activation. Factor B circulates in the blood as a single chain polypeptide and is part of the alternate pathway of the complement system cleaved by factor D into two fragments: Ba and Bb. Bb, a serine protease, then combines with complement factor 3b to generate the C3 or C5 convertase. It has also been implicated in proliferation and differentiation of preactivated B lymphocytes, rapid spreading of peripheral blood monocytes, stimulation of lymphocyte blastogenesis, and lysis of erythrocytes. Ba inhibits the proliferation of preactivated B lymphocytes. Therefore it is possible that these gene products are regulating the response to inflammation in the involuted breast but their functional role is unclear.

Map3k6 or mitogen-activated protein kinase kinase kinase 6 is upregulated by the preventive treatments. This gene encodes a member of the serine/threonine protein kinase family. The encoded kinase was identified by its interaction with MAP3K5/ASK, a protein kinase, and an activator of c-Jun kinase (MAPK7/JNK) and MAPK14/p38 kinase. This kinase was found to weakly activate MAPK7, but not MAPK1/extracellular signal-regulated kinase (ERK) or MAPK14. An alternatively spliced transcript variant has been found for this gene, but its biological validity has not been determined and the biological function of *Map3k6* in the prevention properties of the pregnancy, hCG, and the steroid pellet is unknown. A gene that is also in this category is the *Thedc1* or oleoyl-ACP hydrolase also known as thioesterase domain containing 1. This gene is involved in fatty acid biosynthesis chain termination and release of the free fatty acid product is achieved by hydrolysis of the thio ester by a thioesterase I, a component of the fatty acid synthetase complex. The chain length of the released fatty acid is usually C16. However, in the mammary glands of nonruminant mammals, and in the uropygial gland of certain waterfowl there exists a second thioesterase which releases medium-chain length fatty acids (C8 to C2).

3.4.2 Functional Significance of the Biological Processes Overrepresented Among the Upregulated Genes Induced by the Three Preventive Modalities

3.4.2.1 GO for Immune Response

Among the genes that are part of the GO immune response are those already discussed above such as the *Enc1, Lcn2, and Cfi*. Another gene that is part of this GO is the corticotropin releasing hormone receptor 2 (*Crhr2*) that encoded a protein that belongs to the G-protein coupled receptor 2 family, and the subfamily of corticotropin releasing hormone receptor [35, 36]. This receptor shows high affinity for corticotropin releasing hormone (CRH), and also binds CRH-related peptides such as urocortin. CRH is synthesized in the hypothalamus, and plays an important role in coordinating the endocrine, autonomic, and behavioral responses to stress and immune challenge [37]. Corticotropin-releasing hormone (CRH) family peptides as well as their receptors have been shown to exhibit various functions in hippocampus [38]. CRH receptors activation on collapsin response mediator protein 3 (CRMP3) has shown to have an inhibitory effect on CRMP3 expression that was completely reversed by CRHR2 antagonist but not by CRHR1 antagonist. CRHR2 activation decreases CRMP3 expression in hippocampal neurons via a mechanism that is dependent on PLC/PKC signaling pathways [36]. The corticotrophin-releasing hormone (CRH) family of peptides modulates intestinal inflammation and the CRH receptor 2 suppresses postnatal angiogenesis in mice [39]. The role of *Crhr2* in the rat mammary gland is unknown.

The phospholipase A2, group VII (*Pla2g7*) is a gene that is part of the biological process controlling immune response. The protein encoded by this gene is a secreted enzyme that catalyzes the degradation of PAF to biologically inactive products. It modulates the action of PAF by hydrolyzing the sn-2 ester bond to yield the biologically inactive lyso-PAF. It has specificity for substrates with a short residue at the sn-2 position and is inactive against long-chain phospholipids. Phospholipases are a group of enzymes that hydrolyze phospholipids into fatty acids and other lipophilic molecules. PLA is subdivided into PLA1 which cleave phospholipids at the sn-1 ester bond and PLA2, which cleave at the sn-2 bond. Their most common substrate is phosphatidylcholine, which generates lysophosphatidylcholine and arachidonic acid. PLA is regulated by phosphorylation and by intracellular Ca^{2+} concentrations. Phospholipases are ubiquitously expressed and have diverse biological functions including roles in inflammation, cell growth, signaling and death, and maintenance of membrane phospholipids [40, 41]. Knockdown of *Pla2g7* resulted in downregulation of smooth muscle-specific markers in vitro and impairment of SMC differentiation in vivo, whereas enforced expression of *Pla2g7* enhanced smooth muscle cells (SMC) differentiation and increased reactive oxygen species (ROS) generation. Importantly, enforced expression of *Pla2g7* significantly increased the binding of serum response factor to SMC differentiation gene promoters, resulting in SMC differentiation, which was abolished by free radical scavenger and flavoprotein inhibitor of NADPH oxidase but not hydrogen peroxide inhibitor. Nuclear factor erythroid 2-related factor 3 (*Nrf3*) regulates *Pla2g7* gene expression through direct binding to the promoter regions of *Pla2g7* gene. *Pla2g7* plays a crucial physiological role in SMC differentiation from stem cells, and the fine interactions between *Nrf3* and *Pla2g7* are essential for SMC differentiation from stem cells [40]. Whereas we do not know if this effect is also important in the differentiation of the rat mammary gland post pregnancy and hormonal treatment it's a plausible explanation. There are also reports pointing *Pla2g7* as a cancer-selective biomarker in 50% of prostate cancers and associates with aggressive disease. The alterations induced by *Pla2g7* silencing highlighted the potential of *Pla2g7* inhibition as an anti-proliferative, pro-apoptotic and anti-migratorial therapeutic approach in prostate cancer. Moreover, the anti-proliferative effect of *Pla2g7* silencing was potentiated by lipid-lowering statins in prostate cancer cells [41]. The role of *Pla2g7* gene in atherosclerosis remains controversial [42], whereas in glioblastoma it is associated with survival [43]. *Pla2g7* is highly expressed in prostate cancer and functional studies using RNA interference indicated that it is essential for cell growth and survival. Clinical validation confirmed high *PLA2G7* expression, especially in ERG oncogene-positive prostate cancers, and its silencing sensitized ERG-positive prostate cancer cells to oxidative stress [44].

Kininogen 1 (*Kng1*) is upregulated in the rat mammary glands treated with hCG or hormones related to pregnancy. This gene uses alternative splicing to generate two different proteins—high molecular weight kininogen (HMWK) and low molecular weight kininogen (LMWK). HMWK is essential for blood coagulation and assembly of the kallikrein-kinin system. Also, bradykinin, a peptide causing numerous physiological effects, is released from HMWK. In contrast to HMWK, LMWK is not involved in blood coagulation. Three transcript variants encoding different isoforms have been found for this gene [45, 46]. The functional role of these molecules in mammary gland differentiation and its potential marker of prevention warrant further investigation.

The lipopolysaccharide-binding protein (*Lbp*) is upregulated in the rat mammary gland. The protein encoded by this gene is involved in the acute-phase immunologic response to Gram-negative bacterial infections. Gram-negative bacteria contain a glycolipid, lipopolysaccharide (LPS) on their outer cell wall. Together with bactericidal permeability-increasing protein (BPI), the encoded protein binds LPS and interacts with the CD14 receptor, probably playing a role in regulating LPS-dependent monocyte responses. Studies in mice suggest that the encoded protein is necessary for the rapid acute-phase response to LPS but not for the clearance of LPS from circulation. This protein is part of a family of structurally and functionally related proteins, including BPI, plasma cholesteryl ester transfer protein (CETP), and phospholipid transfer protein (PLTP). Finally, this gene is found on chromosome 20, immediately downstream of the BPI gene and binds to the lipid A moiety of bacterial LPSs, a glycolipid present in the outer membrane of all Gram-negative bacteria. The LBP/LPS complex seems to interact with the CD14 receptor that is also upregulated in the rat mammary glands of treated animals (Table 3.2) and may play a pivotal role in inflammation and innate immunity through its ability to accelerate the "reverse LPS transport" pathway [47]. It has been suggested that lipocalin gene expression is regulated in vivo by LPS. Lipocalin expression is also stimulated in cultured cells by LPS and polyIC [48, 49]. Both LPS and polyIC act through toll-like receptors for which NF-κB is the primary downstream transcription factor [50, 51].

The complement system plays a pivotal protective role in the innate immune response to many pathogens [52, 53] and they are upregulated in the rat mammary gland of treated animals (Table 3.3). *C4bpa* is also upregulated in the cow mammary gland infected with coliform bacteria that are the most common etiologic agents in severe mastitis [54]. Patients suffering from primary Sjögren's syndrome (pSS) display low levels of complement components C3 and/or C4 which is associated with increased risk of non-Hodgkin's lymphoma. C4b-binding protein (C4BP) is a major fluid-phase complement inhibitor which can influence C4 and C3 levels. Plasma levels of C4BP were analyzed in pSS patients ($n=86$) and in controls ($n=68$) by ELISA. C4BP levels from 49 patients were correlated to disease activity markers and autoantibody profiles. Total C4BP plasma levels were significantly higher in pSS patients compared with controls. C4BP levels correlated to the acute phase response, to levels of C4 and C3 as well as to the CD4+/CD8+ T-cell ratio. C4BP levels were inversely related to IgG levels, extent of autoantibody production and global disease activity. C3dg levels, a marker of complement activation, displayed a negative correlation to C4 levels but interestingly not to C4BP levels. C4BP levels are increased in patients suffering from pSS proportional to their acute phase response. However, in the most active cases, with the most widespread autoantibody production, C4BP levels were decreased in parallel with levels of C3 and C4 and CD4+ T cells, suggesting that disturbed complement regulation may contribute to pathogenicity in pSS [55]. The specific role of the complement pathway in the prevention of breast cancer is unknown.

The *Hspa1a* or heat shock 70 kDa protein 1A is upregulated in the rat mammary glands of treated rats. The *Hspa1a* is an intronless gene that encodes a 70 kDa heat shock protein which is a member of the heat shock protein 70 family. In conjunction with other heat shock proteins, this protein stabilizes existing proteins against aggregation and mediates the folding of newly translated proteins in the cytosol and in organelles [56, 57]. It is also involved in the ubiquitin-proteasome pathway through interaction with the AU-rich element RNA-binding protein 1. The gene is located in the major histocompatibility complex class III region, in a cluster with two closely related genes which encode similar proteins. In cooperation with other chaperones, Hsp70s stabilize preexistent proteins against aggregation and mediate the folding of newly translated polypeptides in the cytosol as well as within organelles [58]. These chaperones participate in all these processes through their ability to recognize nonnative conformations of other proteins [59]. They bind extended peptide segments with a net hydrophobic character exposed by polypeptides during translation and membrane translocation, or following stress-induced damage [60, 61]. In case of rotavirus A, infection serves as a post-attachment receptor for the virus to facilitate entry into the cell. HSPA2 and HSPA1 proteins are expressed in a cell-type-specific manner. The most pronounced cell-type expression pattern was found for HSPA2 protein. In the case of stratified squamous epithelia of the skin and esophagus, as well as in ciliated pseudostratified columnar epithelium lining respiratory tract, the HSPA2 positive cells were located in the basal layer. In the colon, small intestine and bronchus epithelia HSPA2 were detected in goblet cells. In adrenal gland cortex HSPA2 expression was limited to cells of zona reticularis [56]. Overexpression of HSPA1A protected cells from heat-induced cell death, whereas overexpression of HSPA6 did not [57].

The ret proto-oncogene (*RET*) is a transmembrane receptor required for the development of neuroendocrine and urogenital cell types. Activation of RET has roles in cell growth, migration, or differentiation. Cell lines stably expressing either the RET9 or RET51 protein isoforms induces upregulation of stress response genes such as HSPA1A, HSPA1B, and HSPA1L. Other members of several HSP families and HSP70-interacting molecules that were associated with stress response protein complexes involved in protein maturation were also specifically upregulated by RET, whereas those associated with the roles of HSP70 in protein degradation were downregulated or unaffected. The major mechanism of stress response induction is activation of the heat shock transcription factor HSF1. RET expression leads to increased HSF1 activation, which correlates with increased expression of stress response genes. The data suggest that RET may be directly responsible for expression of stress response proteins and the initiation of stress response [62].

As it is depicted in Table 3.3, *Cd14* molecule or *Cd14* antigen is upregulated in the mammary gland of rats treated with preventive agents. The protein encoded by this gene is a surface antigen that is preferentially expressed on monocytes/macrophages. CD14 cooperates with other proteins to mediate the innate immune response to bacterial LPS. Alternative splicing results in multiple transcript variants encoding the same protein. CD14 cooperates with MD-2 and TLR4 to mediate the innate immune response to bacterial LPS. CD14 acts via MyD88, TIRAP, and TRAF6, leading to NF-κB activation, cytokine secretion, and the inflammatory response. CD14 upregulates cell surface molecules, including adhesion molecules [63–65]. For example dendritic cells (DCs) are key effectors in innate immunity and play critical roles in triggering adaptive immune responses. FLT3 ligand (FLT3-L) is essential for DC development from hematopoietic progenitors. In a phase I clinical trial, FLT3-L administration significantly increased the frequency and absolute number of blood DC precursors without affecting other mature cell lineages during the 6-week course of FLT3-L therapy. After 14 days of FLT3-L administration, the number of blood CD11c+DCs, plasmacytoid DCs (PDCs), and CD14+ monocytes increased by 5.3-, 2.9-, 3.8-fold, respectively, and was maintained at increased levels throughout FLT3-L therapy. FLT3-L-increased blood DCs in HCT patients were immature and had modest enhancing effects on in vitro T-cell proliferation to antigens and natural killer (NK) cell function [63]. Presence of functional immune system is critical for any attempt aimed at improving survival of breast cancer patients by strategies based on immune system manipulation. In 11 patients, the phenotype was evaluated before and during the chemotherapy by combination of doxorubicin and paclitaxel (AT). Compared with controls breast cancer patients had significantly higher relative and absolute numbers of CD3 HLA-DR+, CD3+CD69+, and CD14+CD16+, and significantly lower percentages of CD3 and CD8+CD28+ cells. After one cycle of AT, the absolute numbers of CD3, CD3+CD4+, CD3+CD8+, and CD8+CD28+ cells increased significantly. This indicated T-cell activation in breast cancer patients. Administration of AT may lead to an increase in functional T cells in peripheral blood, indicating a potential for combining chemotherapy with immunotherapy in the treatment of breast cancer patients [67]. Administration of stem cell factor (SCF) has been proven to enhance cytokine-induced mobilization of CD34+ hematopoietic progenitor cells (HPC) into the peripheral blood (PB). As far as the CD34-PB leukocyte subsets are concerned, monocytes CD14+ displayed the earliest recovery after mobilization predicting neutrophil recovery 1 day in advance

[65]. Macrophages activated by macrophage-colony stimulating factor (M-CSF) are potent immune effector cells and can mediate both in vitro cytotoxicity and antitumor effects in vivo. Nineteen patients with metastatic melanoma received a 14-day continuous intravenous infusion of 80 μg/kg/day of recombinant human M-CSF. R24 was administered daily by intravenous infusion on days 6–10 at doses of 1, 3, 10, 30, and 50 μg/m^2/day. All patients developed a monocytosis characterized by increased expression of the antigen HLA-DR and decreased expression of CD14, a phenotype reported to represent a subpopulation of monocytes active in mediating antibody-directed cellular cytotoxicity [66]. The specific functional role of CD14 and the secreted and transmembrane protein 1B or *Sectmlb* in the rat mammary glands is not clear [67].

3.4.2.2 GO for Transport

Several genes related to the cell transport biological processes are upregulated in the mammary gland of rats subjected to the three preventive modalities (Table 3.3). Among them is the *Slc39a8* or solute carrier family 39 (zinc transporter), member 8. This gene encodes a member of the SLC39 family of solute-carrier genes, which show structural characteristics of zinc transporters. The encoded protein is glycosylated and found in the plasma membrane and mitochondria, and functions in the cellular import of zinc at the onset of inflammation. It is also thought to be the primary transporter of the toxic cation cadmium, which is found in cigarette smoke. Multiple transcript variants encoding different isoforms have been found for this gene [68–70]. The Zrt/Irt-related protein 8 (ZIP8) encoded by *Slc39a8* is an important zinc transporter involved in cellular cadmium incorporation. mRNA and protein levels of ZIP8 were decreased in cadmium-resistant metallothionein-null (A7) cells, leading to a decrease in cadmium accumulation. Epigenetic silencing of the *Slc39a8* gene by DNA hypermethylation is involved in the downregulation of ZIP8 expression. A7 cells showed a higher mRNA level of DNA methyltransferase 3b than parental cells. Hypermethylation of the CpG island of the *Slc39a8* gene was detected in A7 cells. Treatment of A7 cells with 5-aza-deoxycytidine, an inhibitor of DNA methyltransferase, caused demethylation of the CpG island of the *Slc39a8* gene and enhancement of mRNA and protein levels of ZIP8. In response to the recovery of ZIP8 expression, A7 cells treated with 5-aza-deoxycytidine showed an increase in cadmium accumulation and consequently an increase in sensitivity to cadmium. These results suggest that epigenetic silencing of the *Slc39a8* gene by DNA hypermethylation plays an important role in the downregulation of ZIP8 in cadmium-resistant metallothionein-null cells [71]. In addition ZIP8 is highly expressed in T cells derived from human subjects. T-cell ZIP8 expression was markedly upregulated upon in vitro activation. T cells collected from human subjects who had received oral zinc supplementation (15 mg/day) had higher expression of the activation marker IFN-gamma upon in vitro activation, indicating a potentiating effect of zinc on T-cell activation. Similarly, in vitro zinc treatment of T cells along with activation resulted in increased IFN-gamma expression with a maximum effect at 3.1 μM. Knockdown of ZIP8 in T cells by siRNA decreased ZIP8 levels in nonactivated and activated cells and concomitantly reduced secretion of IFN-gamma and perforin, both signatures of activation. Overexpression of ZIP8 by transient transfection caused T cells to exhibit enhanced activation. Confocal microscopy established that ZIP8 is localized to the lysosome where ZIP8 abundance is increased upon activation. Loss of lysosomal labile zinc in response to activation was measured by flow cytometry using a zinc fluorophore. Zinc between 0.8 and 3.1 μM reduced CN phosphatase activity. CN was also inhibited by the CN inhibitor FK506 and ZIP8 overexpression. The results suggest that zinc at low concentrations, through inhibition of CN, sustains phosphorylation of the transcription factor CREB, yielding greater IFN-gamma expression in T cells. ZIP8, through control of zinc transport from the lysosome, may provide a secondary level of IFN-gamma regulation in T cells [72]. Zinc is essential for normal erythroid cell functions and therefore intracellular zinc homeostasis during erythroid differentiation is tightly regulated. Zinc transporters ZnT1 and Zip10 are important for zinc homeostasis in erythrocytes and respond to the dietary zinc supply [73].

The endoderm germ layer is patterned along the anterior–posterior (A–P) axis before the formation of a gut tube (embryonic day [e] 7.5–8.5 in mouse) and 8 molecular markers that are expressed in discrete domains of the gastrula stage endoderm (e7.5) suggest that a significant level of pattern exists in the endoderm before the formation of a gut tube. Three genes *Tmprss2, NM_029639*, and *Dsp* are expressed in a presumptive midgut domain overlying the node, a domain for which molecular markers have not previously been identified. Two genes, *Klf5* and *Epha2*, are expressed in posterior endoderm associated with the primitive streak. Expression of these five genes persists in the midgut and/or hindgut at e8.5, 9.5, and 10.5, suggesting that these genes are markers of these domains throughout these stages of development. Three other genes *Slc39a8, Amot*, and *Dp1l1* are expressed in the visceral endoderm at e7.5. Starting at e9.5, *Dp1l1* is expressed de novo in the liver, midgut, and hindgut. This suggests that presumptive midgut and hindgut domains are being established at the molecular level by the end of gastrulation, and emphasize the importance of endoderm patterning before the formation of the fetal gut and the role of *Slc39a8* in differentiation process [74]. Another gene related to cell transport is *Slc13a2* or solute carrier family 13 (sodium-dependent dicarboxylate transporter) member 2 (Table 3.3) that functions as cotransporter of sodium ions and dicarboxylates such as succinate and citrate. It is known that metabolically generated acid is the major physiological stimulus for increasing proximal tubule citrate reabsorption, which leads to a decrease in citrate excretion [75]; however its role in the rat mammary gland is not clear. The same apply to the *Scnn1g* or sodium channel, voltage-gated, type I, beta (Table 3.3). The voltage-gated sodium channels are heteromeric proteins that function in the generation and propagation of action potentials in muscle and neuronal cells. They are composed of one alpha and two beta subunits, where the alpha subunit provides channel activity and the beta-1 subunit modulates the kinetics of channel inactivation.

Table 3.10 Biological processes and downregulated genes in hCG group

Symbol	Name
Adhesion (GO:0035759)	
Ccl21	Chemokine (C-C motif) ligand 21
Apoptosis (GO:0012501, GO:0016265, GO:0042981, GO:0010941, GO:2000353)	
Cd40	CD40 molecule, TNF receptor superfamily member 5
Cd38	CD38 molecule
Ubd	Ubiquitin D
Ccl21	Chemokine (C-C motif) ligand 21
Cidec	Cell death-inducing DFFA-like effector c
Cell cycle (GO:0035417)	
Ubd	Ubiquitin D
Cell motility (GO:2000508, GO:2000529)	
Ccl21	Chemokine (C-C motif) ligand 21
Cell proliferation (GO:0030890, GO:0032946)	
Cd40	CD40 molecule, TNF receptor superfamily member 5
Cd38	CD38 molecule
Cellular component organization (GO:0070842, GO:0031274)	
Ubd	Ubiquitin D
Ccl21	Chemokine (C-C motif) ligand 21
Immune response (GO:0001768, GO:0002684, GO:0048304, GO:0006955, GO:0045321, GO:0050864, GO:0050670, GO:0070663, GO:0051251)	
Ccl21	Chemokine (C-C motif) ligand 21
Cd40	CD40 molecule, TNF receptor superfamily member 5
Cd38	CD38 molecule
Ubd	Ubiquitin D
RT1-Db1	RT1 class II, locus Db1
Response to stimulus (GO:0048584, GO:0033194, GO:0034695)	
Cd40	CD40 molecule, TNF receptor superfamily member 5
Cd38	CD38 molecule
Ubd	Ubiquitin D
Ccl21	Chemokine (C-C motif) ligand 21
Signaling (GO:0032862, GO:0023051, GO:0043123, GO:0002768, GO:0035556, GO:0010627)	
Ccl21	Chemokine (C-C motif) ligand 21
Cd40	CD40 molecule, TNF receptor superfamily member 5
Cd38	CD38 molecule
Ubd	Ubiquitin D
Gria3	Glutamate receptor, ionotrophic, AMPA 3
Rhebl1	Ras homolog enriched in brain like 1
Rab19	RAB19, member RAS oncogene family

3.4.3 Transcriptome Profile Induced by hCG

As it is depicted in the Tables 3.10 and 3.11 and Figs. 3.14 and 3.15 hCG induces significant number of genes that are down- and upregulated in the mammary gland comprising different GO biological processes. Among the downregulated genes by hCG are the *Ccl21, CD38, CD40, Cidec, RT1-Db1, Ubd, Gria3, Rhebl1* and *Rab19.*

Table 3.11 Biological processes and upregulated genes in hCG group

Symbol	Name
Cellular component organization (GO:0090084)	
Hspa1a	Heat shock 70 kDa protein 1A
Circulatory system (GO:0003018, GO:0042311)	
Hspa1a	Heat shock 70 kDa protein 1A
Kng1	Kininogen 1
Kng1l1	Kininogen 1-like 1
Development (GO:0035150, GO:0042335)	
Hspa1a	Heat shock 70 kDa protein 1A
Kng1	Kininogen 1
Kng1l1	Kininogen 1-like 1
Duox1	Dual oxidase 1
Immune response (GO:0002460, GO:0002682, GO:0006959, GO:0045087, GO:0006958, GO:0002449, GO:0050778, GO:0016064)	
C4bpa	Complement component 4 binding protein, alpha
Hspa1a	Heat shock 70 kDa protein 1A
Cfi	Complement factor I
Kng1	Kininogen 1
Pla2g7	Phospholipase A2, group VII (platelet-activating factor acetylhydrolase, plasma)
Lcn2	Lipocalin 2
Cd14	CD14 molecule
Lipoprotein modification (GO:0034441, GO:0042160)	
Pla2g7	Phospholipase A2, group VII (platelet-activating factor acetylhydrolase, plasma)
Protein activation cascade (GO:0072376)	
C4bpa	Complement component 4 binding protein, alpha
Cfi	Complement factor I
Response to reactive oxygen species (GO:0070301)	
Lcn2	Lipocalin 2
Duox1	Dual oxidase 1
Response to stress (GO:0006950, GO:0033554, GO:0009408)	
C4bpa	Complement component 4 binding protein, alpha
Scnn1g	Sodium channel, nonvoltage-gated 1, gamma
Kng1	Kininogen 1
Kng1l1	Kininogen 1-like 1
Mapk13	Mitogen-activated protein kinase 13
Cfi	Complement factor I
Lcn2	Lipocalin 2
Hspa1a	Heat shock 70 kDa protein 1A
Apod	Apolipoprotein D
Duox1	Dual oxidase 1
Ndrg1	N-myc downstream regulated 1
Cd14	CD14 molecule
Transport (GO:0015891, GO:0033212, GO:0000041)	
Lcn2	Lipocalin 2
Slc39a8	Solute carrier family 39 (zinc transporter), member 8
Wound healing (GO:0042060)	
Scnn1g	Sodium channel, nonvoltage-gated 1, gamma
Kng1	Kininogen 1
Apod	Apolipoprotein D

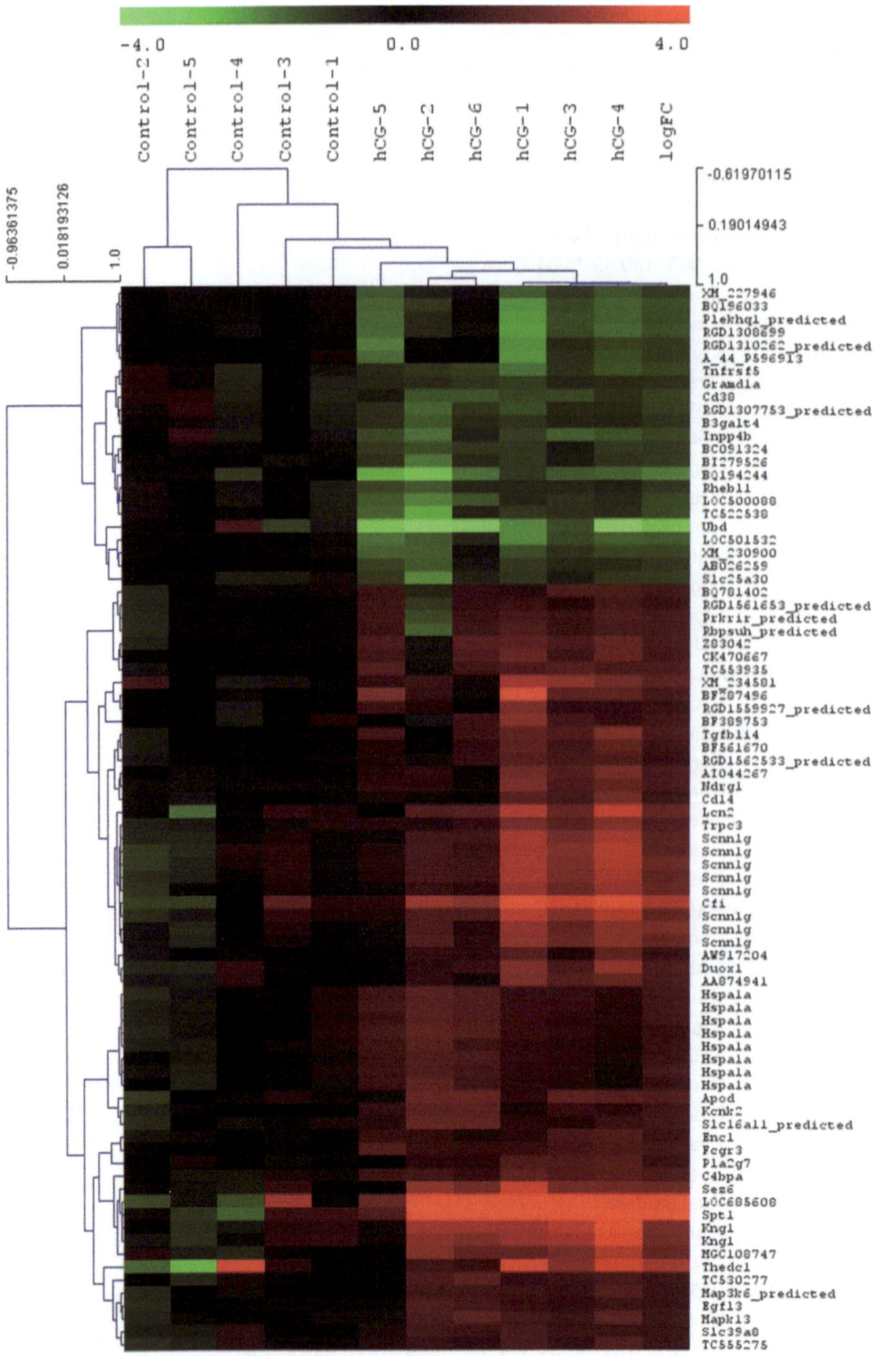

Fig. 3.15 Heat map showing the up- (*red*) and downregulated genes (*green*) of hCG-treated rat mammary glands

Ccl21-chemokine (C-C motif) ligand 21-chemokine (C-C motif) ligand 21 (previous names: small inducible cytokine subfamily A (Cys–Cys), member 21) is downregulated in the rat mammary gland in hCG treated animals. *CCL21* gene is part of several biological processes (Table 3.10) and is one of several CC cytokine genes clustered on the p-arm of chromosome 9. Cytokines are a family of secreted proteins involved in immunoregulatory and inflammatory processes. The CC cytokines are proteins characterized by two adjacent cysteines [76]. Similar to other chemokines the protein encoded by this gene inhibits hemopoiesis and stimulates chemotaxis. Therefore in the rat mammary gland it could be an anti-inflammatory protein controlling the regression of the hCG stimulated gland. This protein is chemotactic and binds to chemokine receptor CCR7 on mature dendritic cells (DCs) and distinct T- and B-cell subpopulations but not for macrophages or neutrophils [80]. The cytokine encoded by this gene may also play a role in mediating homing of lymphocytes to secondary lymphoid organs. It is a high affinity functional ligand for chemokine receptor 7 (CCR7) that is expressed on T and B lymphocytes and a known receptor for another member of the cytokine family (small inducible cytokine A19). Dendritic cells (DCs) must travel through lymphatics to carry skin antigens into lymph nodes. Activated DCs move directionally toward lymphatics, contact *Ccl21* puncta, and migrate through portals into the lumen indicating that the Ccl21-CCR7 axis plays a dual role in DC mobilization, promoting both chemotaxis and arrest of DCs on lymphatic endothelium [77]. In addition *Ccl21* recruits normal immune cells and metastasizing tumor cells to lymph nodes through activation of the G-protein coupled receptor CCR7 [76] and facilitates the migration of lung cancer by changing the concentration of intracellular Ca^{2+}. The Ccl21-CCR7 axis may play an important role in non-small cell lung cancer invasion and metastasis [78] and regulates the encounters between DC and T cells and thus is a key regulator of adaptive immune responses [79]. *Therefore the downregulation of Ccl21 in the rat mammary gland can be an important mechanism by which hCG modifies the immune response to neoplastically transformed mammary epithelial cells using this pathway as a preventive protective factor against cancer*. Supporting this concept is the finding that *Cd40* and *Cd38* are also downregulated by hCG. The CD40 molecule or TNF receptor superfamily member 5, has been found to be essential in mediating a broad variety of immune and inflammatory responses, including T-cell-dependent immunoglobulin class switching, memory B-cell development, and germinal center formation. AT-hook transcription factor *AKNA* is reported to coordinately regulate the expression of this receptor and its ligand, which may be important for homotypic cell interactions. Adaptor protein TNFR2 interacts with this receptor and serves as a mediator of the signal transduction. Abrogation of the CD40 using antibody against this protein in combination with IL2 induces regression of large mesothelioma tumors. NK cells contributed to CD40-driven systemic immunity leading to resolution of untreated distal tumors. IL-2 treatment led to increased proportions of NK cells in tumors and dLNs, and in the absence of NK cells, IL-2 lost its

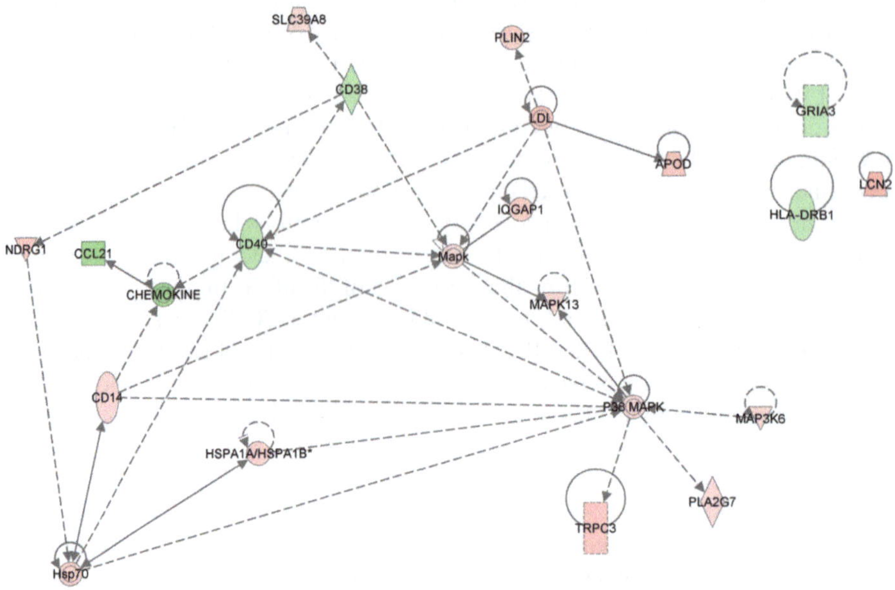

Fig. 3.16 Networking of genes depicted in the mammary glands of hCG-treated rats

therapeutic effect [80]. Abrogation of *CD40* in gastric carcinoma has shown to be mediated by upregulation of *GADD45A, C-JUN,* and *BCL-2*, and downregulation of *CYCLIN D1, CDC6, TNFR10B, c-IAP2*, and *ORC5L* pointing toward an induced apoptosis mechanism [81].

The other gene downregulated by hCG is the *Cd38* that is a novel multifunctional ectoenzyme that mediates the release of brain oxytocin [82] and widely expressed in cells and tissues especially in leukocytes [83, 84]. CD38 also functions in cell adhesion, signal transduction, and calcium signaling [85]. CD38 is a multifunctional enzyme that can not only generate cyclic adenosine diphosphate-ribose (cADPR)—a key Ca(2+)-mobilizing second messenger—by consuming NAD(+), but also hydrolyze extracellular NAD(+). Silencing of CD38 led to significantly decreased survival of the glial cells and decreased levels can lead to apoptosis of the microglial cells, as assessed by flow cytometry-based Annexin V/7-AAD assay, caspase-3 immunostaining, and Hoechst staining assays [86]. CD38 and CD40 are networking together with other hCG downregulated genes as it is depicted in Fig. 3.16. This indicate that silencing or downregulation of *Cd38, Cd40*, and *Ccl21* may drive the program cell death pathway that is one the biological process detected in the hCG treated rat mammary glands as a mechanism of cancer prevention [87, 88].

It is less clear how the downregulation of the *Cidec* that encodes a member of the cell death-inducing DNA fragmentation factor-like effector family [89] affect the preventive effect of hCG. *Cidec* plays an important role in apoptosis. The encoded protein promotes lipid droplet formation in adipocytes and may mediate adipocyte apoptosis via PI3K, and it regulates expression of each protein via Akt1/2- and JNK2-dependent pathways, respectively, in human adipocytes [90]. However it has been shown that cell death-inducing DNA fragmentation factor-alpha (DFFA)-like effector (CIDE) proteins including CIDEA, CIDEB, and CIDEC/fat-specific protein 27 (Fsp27) are associated with a reduction of lipid droplet size in white adipose tissue and increased metabolic rate. Using a glycoproteomics approach has shown that posttranslational regulation of CIDE proteins via glycosylation modulates transforming growth factor (TGF)-beta 1-dependent apoptosis. In a study using mouse embryonic fibroblasts derived from CIDEA-deficient mice revealed that 5′ AMP-activated protein kinase (AMPK) activity is regulated by CIDEA-mediated ubiquitin-dependent proteasomal degradation via a protein interaction with the AMPK beta subunit [91, 92]. Human adenovirus type 36 (Ad-36) is associated with obesity and it has been shown that Ad-36 induced lipid droplets in the cultured skeletal muscle cells and this process may be mediated by promoting Cidec/FSP27 expression [93]. The specific role of this gene in the rat mammary gland needs further investigation.

A gene that is significantly downregulated by hCG is the *Ubd* or ubiquitin D. The functional role of this gene is very broad behaving as a protein modifier that can be covalently attached to target protein and subsequently leads to their degradation by the 26S proteasome, in a NUB1L-dependent manner. *Ubd* probably functions as a survival factor regulating TNF-alpha-induced and LPS-mediated activation of the central mediator of innate immunity NF-κB by promoting TNF-alpha-mediated proteasomal degradation of ubiquitinated-I-kappa-B-alpha. The gene may be involved in dendritic cell (DC) maturation, the process by which immature dendritic cells differentiate into fully competent antigen-presenting cells that initiate T-cell responses. This gene may be involved in the formation of aggresomes when proteasome is saturated or impaired. Mediates apoptosis in a caspase-dependent manner, especially in renal epithelium and tubular cells during renal diseases such as polycystic kidney disease and Human immunodeficiency virus (HIV)-associated nephropathy. *Altogether these multiple functions probably improve the immune competence of the rat mammary gland against a carcinogenic stimulus.*

A gene that is downregulated by hCG is the *Gria3*, previously called glutamate receptor, ionotrophic or AMPA 3 that could play a role in the differentiation and in the prevention mechanism, although it does not network with the other genes modified by the hCG (Fig. 3.16). It is known that glutamate receptors are the predominant excitatory neurotransmitter receptors in the mammalian brain and are activated in a variety of normal neurophysiologic processes [94]. L-glutamate acts as an excitatory neurotransmitter at many synapses in the central nervous system. Binding of the excitatory neurotransmitter L-glutamate induces a conformation change, leading to the opening of the cation channel, and thereby converts the chemical signal to an electrical impulse. Of great interest is that *GRIA3* also may play an important role in cell proliferation, apoptosis, and cell migration of human pancreatic cancer tissues. Knock-down of Gria3 significantly reduced proliferation and migration and enhanced apoptosis. In contrast, overexpression of Gria3 significantly reduced apoptosis and enhanced both proliferation and tumor cell migration. Gria3 could be confirmed as a downstream effector of CUX1 and was expressed in pancreatic cancer tissues. In vivo, Gria3 significantly enhanced the growth of subcutaneous xenografts. Inhibitors of glutamate receptors such as GYKI52466 and SYM2206 significantly decreased survival of pancreatic cancer cells, suggesting the presence of glutamate signaling in pancreatic cancer. In conclusion, Gria3 plays a role as a mediator of tumor progression in pancreatic cancer downstream CUX1 [95] and it could *be an important modulator of the reduction of cell proliferation observed in the rat mammary gland under the effect of hCG and activation of the programmed cell death cascade* [87, 88]. This pathway also can be synergistically activated by the *Rhebl1* that also is downregulated by hCG. *Rhebl1* or Ras homolog enriched in brain like 1 belongs to the Ras family of small GTPases that regulates a wide variety of cellular functions that include cell growth, differentiation, and transformation. Rhebl1 belongs to the Rheb branch of small GTPase proteins. The cDNA sequence contains an open reading frame of 551 bp, encoding a putative protein of 183 amino acid residues. The expression pattern of Rhebl1 showed that it was ubiquitously expressed in 17 tissues. Rhebl1 gene encodes a 20.69 kDa protein, localized in cytoplasm when in HEK 293T cells strongly activated the transcriptional activities of NF-κB, while the mutant (D60K) only weakly activates NF-κB-mediated transcription. Rhebl1 is a positive regulator of NF-κB-mediated gene transcription [96, 97]. The small G protein Rheb is known to promote mammalian target of rapamycin (mTOR) signaling [98] and is a downstream target of the small GTPase-activating proteins TSC1 and TSC2 [96]. This signaling pathway is regulating cell growth, mitogenesis, and apoptosis in various cell types [99, 100]. The functional role of the *Rhebl1* downregulation in the rat mammary gland is significant since the activation of MTOR is activated in several cancers such as renal cell cancer [101] and its inhibition by rapamycin and inhibitor of mTOR has shown promise in the treatment of renal carcinoma. Similar mechanism has been implicated in the pathogenesis of lymphangioleiomyomatosis-associated angiomyolipomas [102].

Another member of the signaling pathway that is downregulated by hCG is the *Rab19* that is a small GTPase of the Rab subfamily. Northern blot analysis of the distribution of the *Rab19* mRNA in various adult mouse tissues and NIH 3T3 fibroblasts revealed that is expressed in a tissue-specific manner. Its transcript was detected at high levels in intestine, lung, and spleen, and at a lower level in kidney. In contrast, liver, brain, heart, and NIH 3T3 fibroblasts contain only very little or no detectable *Rab19* mRNA [103, 104]. The functional role of *Rab19* has been linked to golgins, long coiled-coil proteins that localize to particular Golgi subdomains via their C termini, that are regulators of vesicle sorting [105].

Table 3.11 and Figs. 3.14 and 3.15 depict the genes that are upregulated in the mammary gland only by hCG. There is a set of genes related to response to stress such as the apolipoprotein D and lipocalin 2. The *ApodD* gene encodes a component of high-density lipoprotein that has no marked similarity to other apolipoprotein sequences but has a high degree of homology to plasma retinol-binding protein and other members of the alpha 2 microglobulin protein superfamily of carrier proteins, also known as lipocalins. Apolipoprotein D is a direct transcriptional target of the p53 family member genes and its expression is specifically upregulated by either TAp73 or TAp63 but not significantly by p53 [106]. Using small interference RNA designed to target p73 abolishes induction of apoD transcription following cisplatin treatment. There is a p73/p63-binding site in the promoter of the apoD gene that is responsive to the p53 family members. The ectopic expression of TAp73 as well as the addition of recombinant human apoD to culture medium induced the osteoblastic differentiation of the human osteosarcoma cell line Saos-2, as assessed by alkaline phosphatase activity. Importantly, *ApodD* knockdown abrogated p73-mediated alkaline phosphatase induction. Moreover, TAp73-mediated apoD expression was able to induce morphological differentiation, as well as expression of neuronal markers, in the human neuroblastoma cell line SH-SY5Y [106]. These results suggest that apoD induction may mediate the activity of p73 in normal development and it is also responsible for the differentiation effect observed in the mammary gland of animals treated with hCG or pregnancy hormones. The role of apoD in differentiation seems to be well conserved because it is also found associated with bone differentiation [107], adipocyte differentiation [108, 109], and that could be a marker of cellular differentiation and growth arrest [110]. The functional role of this gene in the rat mammary gland and its role in prevention requires further investigation.

Another important gene that is also specifically upregulated by hCG treatment is the *Ndrg1*-N myc downstream regulated 1. This gene is a member of the N-myc downregulated gene family which belongs to the alpha/beta hydrolase superfamily and may have a growth inhibitory role [111, 112]. The protein encoded by this gene is a cytoplasmic protein involved in stress responses, hormone responses, cell growth, and differentiation [113]. It is necessary for p53-mediated caspase activation and apoptosis [114]. Glycoprotein transmembrane nmb (*GPNMB*) gene overexpression in prostate carcinoma cells significantly attenuated cell proliferation and invasion and exerted antitumorigenic activity in vitro and in vivo. *GPNMB* overexpression induced the gene expressions of N-myc downstream regulated gene 1 and maspin in PC-3 cells. Doxorubicin treatment or transient overexpression of p53 increased *GPNMB* expression. The enhancement of *Ndrg1* and maspin gene expressions may account for the anti-proliferative and anti-invasive function of *GPNMB* in prostate cancer cells [111]. *Ndrg1* is also linked to *Wnt*, whose signaling has pivotal roles in tumor progression and metastasis. The tumor metastasis suppressor gene *Ndrg1*, interacts with the Wnt receptor LRP6, followed by blocking of the Wnt signaling, and therefore, orchestrates a cellular network that impairs the metastatic progression of tumor cells. Importantly, restoring *Ndrg1* expression by a small molecule compound significantly suppressed the capability of otherwise highly metastatic tumor cells to thrive in circulation and distant organs in animal models. The analysis of clinical cohorts data indicates that *WNT+/NDRG−/LRP+* signature has a strong predictable value for recurrence-free survival of cancer patients [115]. The upregulation of *Ndrg1* by hCG is also mimicked by indol-3-carbinol [116]. The importance of this is that N-myc downstream regulated gene-1 participates in carcinogenesis, angiogenesis, metastases, and anticancer drug resistance. The expression pattern of N-myc downstream regulated gene-1 following treatment of the human colonic cancer cell lines HCT-116 (a well differentiated with wild-type p53 gene) and Colo-320 (poorly differentiated with mutant p53 gene), with 3,3′-diindolylmethane, a well-established proapoptotic agent product derived from indole-3-carbinol disclosed inhibition of cell viability in a dose-dependent manner, mediated through apoptosis induction. The increased expression of N-myc downstream regulated gene-1 was detected only in the poorly differentiated colon cancer cell lines Colo-320 hCG induced apoptosis may represent a regulator of N-myc downstream regulated gene-1 in the mammary gland as it has been shown poorly differentiated colonic cancer cells [116].

Metastatic tumor cells become dormant and how and why tumors recur in target organs are not well understood. Bone morphogenetic protein 7 (BMP7) secreted from bone stromal cells induces senescence in prostate cancer stem-like cells (CSCs) by activating p38 mitogen-activated protein kinase and increasing expression of the cell cycle inhibitor, p21, and the metastasis suppressor gene, *NDRG1*. This effect of BMP7 depended on BMPR2 (BMP receptor 2), and BMPR2 expression inversely correlated with recurrence and bone metastasis in prostate cancer patients. Importantly, this BMP7-induced senescence in CSCs was reversible upon withdrawal of BMP7. Furthermore, treatment of mice with BMP7 significantly suppressed the growth of CSCs in bone, whereas the withdrawal of BMP7 restarted growth of these cells. These results suggest that the BMP7-BMPR2-p38-NDRG1 axis plays a critical role in dormancy and recurrence of prostate CSCs in bone [117]. N-Myc downstream-regulated gene 1 is a ubiquitous cellular protein that is upregulated under a multitude of stress and growth-regulatory conditions including hCG (Table 3.11). Free radical nitric oxide (•NO) interaction with the chelatable iron pool (CIP) and the appearance of dinitrosyliron complexes (DNIC) are key determinants in upregulating *NDRG1* using HCC 1806 triple negative breast cancer cells [118]. *Therefore the finding that Nrdg1 is upregulated specifically by hCG (Fig. 3.14) indicates the importance of this gene in the preventive strategy of mammary cancer.*

hCG specifically upregulates the dual oxidase 1 or *Duox1* (Figs. 3.14 and 3.15). The protein encoded by DUOX1 is a glycoprotein and a member of the NADPH oxidase family. *Duox1* plays a role in thyroid hormones synthesis [119–121], in lactoperoxidase-mediated antimicrobial defense at the surface of mucosa [122], and has been found to be expressed at higher frequencies in tumor specimens [123]. Although hydrogen peroxide H_2O_2 is better known for its cytotoxic effects, it has been shown also to play a crucial role in eukaryotic signal transduction [124]. Urothelial cells produce H_2O_2 in response to a calcium signal. Using a gene-deficient mouse model has demonstrated that H_2O_2 is produced by the NADPH oxidase Duox1, which is expressed in the mouse urothelium [125]. Of interest is the role of the mammalian Numb-interacting protein 1 (Nip1) in regulation of neuronal differentiation in stem cells [126]. The highest expression of Nip1 was observed in undifferentiated neuronal stem cells and was associated with Duox1-mediated ROS production. Ectopic nip1 expression in embryonal carcinoma cells induced neuronal differentiation, and this phenotype was also linked to elevated ROS production. The neuronal differentiation in nip1-overexpressing was achieved in a retinoic acid-independent manner and was corroborated by an increase in the expression of the neuronal basic helix-loop-helix transcription factors and neural-lineage cell markers. Depletion of nip1 by short hairpin RNA led to a decrease in the expression of neuronal basic helix-loop-helix transcription factors and ROS [126]. *This indicates that in the mammary gland the overexpression of Duox 1 could be an intrinsic regulator of cell fate.* The DUOXA1/NIP1 interacting protein functions as a maturation factor for the dual oxidase 1. DUOXA1/NIP1 expression has been reported in noninvasive MCF7 cells and low expression in highly metastatic cells with impaired p53 functions linking the expression of DUOXA1 with p53. An inhibition of cell proliferation associated with upregulation of p21(Cip1/WAF1) was observed in MDA-MB-231 cells following transfection of DUOXA1. The transient DUOXA1 overexpression also inhibited expression of cell-surface integrin alphaVbeta5 and CD9, which is associated with impaired spreading ability. However, there was no difference in expression of these proteins in Duox1-depleted cells. The observed effects coincided with an increase in ROS generation. These data demonstrate that DUOXA1 transient overexpression affected the cell–cell adhesion by modulating the actin cytoskeleton, and sensitized cells to doxorubicin [127]. The overexpression of Duox 1 in the breast epithelial cells could be indicative of an oxidative antimicrobial protection as has been shown in the differentiated primary human airway epithelial cells challenged with *Pseudomonas aeruginosa* flagellin or IFN-gamma [128]. *Caenorhabditis elegans* Duox 1 seems to play also an important role in the barrier epithelium as an ancient, highly conserved innate immune defense mechanism. The airway epithelium represents a key mechanism of innate airway host defense, through enhanced production of H_2O_2, which mediates cellular signaling pathways that regulate the production of various inflammatory mediators. Production of the CXC chemokine interleukin (IL)-8/CXCL8 forms a common epithelial response to many diverse stimuli, including bacterial and viral triggers, environmental oxidants, and other biological mediators, suggesting the potential involvement of a common signaling pathway that may involve Duox1-dependent H_2O_2 production [129].

Among the protein activation cascade upregulated by hCG are the complement factor I (Cfi) and the complement factor B (Cfb), which have been discussed in the previous section.

Other genes like *Kng1* are part of multiple biological processes such as development, response to stress, and circulatory system. Kininogen 1 (*Kng1*) gene uses alternative splicing to generate two different proteins—HMWK and LMWK. HMWK is essential for blood coagulation and assembly of the kallikrein-kinin system. Also, bradykinin, a peptide causing numerous physiological effects, is released from HMWK. In contrast to HMWK, LMWK is not involved in blood coagulation. Three transcript variants encoding different isoforms have been found for this gene. Kininogens are inhibitors of thiol proteases; HMW-kininogen plays an important role in blood coagulation by helping to position optimally prekallikrein and factor XI next to factor XII; HMW-kininogen inhibits the thrombin- and plasmin-induced aggregation of thrombocytes; the active peptide bradykinin that is released from HMW-kininogen shows a variety of physiological effects: influence in smooth muscle contraction, induction of hypotension, natriuresis and diuresis, decrease in blood glucose level, it is a mediator of inflammation and causes increase in vascular permeability, stimulation of nociceptors release of other mediators of inflammation (e.g., prostaglandins), it has a cardioprotective effect (directly via bradykinin action, indirectly via endothelium-derived relaxing factor action); LMW-kininogen inhibits the aggregation of thrombocytes; LMW-kininogen is in contrast to HMW-kininogen not involved in blood clotting. In addition KNG1 is associated with adiponectin. The KNG-ADIPOQ haplotype has been strongly associated with adiponectin levels in Filipinos [45] and diabetic nephropathy [46]. The role in the rat mammary gland has not been determined.

3.4.4 Transcriptome Profile Induced by Pregnancy

The biological processes downregulated (Table 3.12) by pregnancy are slightly different from those induced by hCG. There is only one downregulated gene in the mammary gland post pregnancy the *Pnpla3* or patatin-like phospholipase domain containing 3 (Fig. 3.14). The protein encoded by this gene is a triacylglycerol lipase that mediates triacylglycerol hydrolysis in adipocytes and hepatocytes [130, 131]. The encoded protein, which appears to be membrane bound, may be involved in the balance of energy usage/storage in adipocytes. It is a multifunctional enzyme that has both triacylglycerol lipase and acylglycerol *O*-acyltransferase activities. The functional role in the mammary gland and cancer prevention needs further studies.

The upregulated genes induced by pregnancy are listed in Table 3.13 and few of them are specifically induced by pregnancy; among them are *Mmp12* (matrix metallopeptidase 12), *Spp1* (secreted phosphoprotein 1), and *Sectm1b* (secreted and transmembrane 1B) (Figs. 3.14 and 3.17). *Mmp12* encodes a protein of the matrix metalloproteinase (MMP) family that is involved in the breakdown of extracellular matrix (ECM) in normal physiological processes, such as embryonic development, reproduction, and tissue remodeling, as well as in disease processes, such as cancer and metastasis. MMPs, also called matrixins, are zinc-dependent endopeptidases that are the major proteases involved in ECM degradation. MMPs are capable of degrading a wide range of extracellular molecules and a number of bioactive molecules. Twenty-four matrixin genes have been identified in humans, which can be organized into six groups based on domain organization and substrate preference: Collagenases (MMP-1, -8, and -13), Gelatinases (MMP-2 and -9), Stromelysins (MMP-3, -10, and -11), Matrilysin (MMP-7 and -26), Membrane-type (MT)-MMPs (MMP-14, -15, -16, -17, -24, and -25), and others (MMP-12, -19, -20, -21, -23, -27, and -28). MMP activity is regulated by two major endogenous inhibitors: alpha2-macroglobulin and tissue inhibitors of metalloproteases (TIMPs). MMPs play a central role in cell proliferation, migration, differentiation, angiogenesis, apoptosis, and host defences. Deregulation of MMPs has been implicated in many diseases including arthritis, chronic ulcers, encephalomyelitis, and cancer [132–137]. The MMPs have been implicated in tumor invasion and metastasis both by

Table 3.12 Biological processes and downregulated genes in the pregnancy group

Symbol	Name
Lipid processes (GO:0046503, GO:0019432, GO:0046460, GO:0019433, GO:0044269, GO:0046461, GO:0046504, GO:0006639, GO:0045017, GO:0018904)	
Pnpla3	Patatin-like phospholipase domain containing 3

Table 3.13 Biological processes and upregulated genes in the pregnancy group

Symbol	Name
Cell motility (GO:0090026, GO:0050921, GO:0048870, GO:0060326)	
Pla2g7	Phospholipase A2, group VII (platelet-activating factor acetylhydrolase, plasma)
Lbp	Lipopolysaccharide-binding protein
Mmp12	Matrix metallopeptidase 12
Scnn1g	Sodium channel, nonvoltage-gated 1, gamma
Development (GO:0048685, GO:0070571, GO:0048670)	
Spp1	Secreted phosphoprotein 1
Immune response (GO:0045087, GO:0002687, GO:0002376, GO:0032755, GO:0002688, GO:0002232, GO:0032490)	
Lcn2	Lipocalin 2
Lbp	Lipopolysaccharide-binding protein
Cfi	Complement factor I
Pla2g7	Phospholipase A2, group VII (platelet-activating factor acetylhydrolase, plasma)
Sectm1b	Secreted and transmembrane 1B
Crhr2	Corticotropin releasing hormone receptor 2
Lipoprotein modification (GO:0034441, GO:0042160, GO:0034374)	
Pla2g7	Phospholipase A2, group VII (platelet-activating factor acetylhydrolase, plasma)
Regulation of behavior (GO:2000252, GO:0050795, GO:0035482, GO:2000293)	
Crhr2	Corticotropin releasing hormone receptor 2
Lbp	Lipopolysaccharide-binding protein
Pla2g7	Phospholipase A2, group VII (platelet-activating factor acetylhydrolase, plasma)
Respiratory burst (GO:0060265, GO:0002679, GO:0060263)	
Lbp	Lipopolysaccharide-binding protein
Response to stimulus (GO:0071223, GO:0048584, GO:0032101, GO:0071222, GO:0071216)	
Lbp	Lipopolysaccharide-binding protein
Pla2g7	Phospholipase A2, group VII (platelet-activating factor acetylhydrolase, plasma)
Crhr2	Corticotropin releasing hormone receptor 2
Cfi	Complement factor I
Spp1	Secreted phosphoprotein 1
Lcn2	Lipocalin 2
Secretion (GO:0032277, GO:0032811, GO:0014064, GO:0061179, GO:0010700)	
Crhr2	Corticotropin releasing hormone receptor 2

(continued)

Table 3.13 (continued)

Symbol	Name
Signaling (GO:0043950, GO:0043951, GO:0034145)	
Crhr2	Corticotropin releasing hormone receptor 2
Lbp	Lipopolysaccharide-binding protein
Transport (GO:0033212, GO:0090281, GO:0030001, GO:0015891, GO:0015920, GO:0033037)	
Lcn2	Lipocalin 2
Crhr2	Corticotropin releasing hormone receptor 2
Scnn1g	Sodium channel, nonvoltage-gated 1, gamma
Slc13a2	Solute carrier family 13 (sodium-dependent dicarboxylate transporter), member 2
Lbp	Lipopolysaccharide-binding protein
Wound healing (GO:0035313, GO:0009611, GO:0060054)	
Mmp12	Matrix metallopeptidase 12
Scnn1g	Sodium channel, nonvoltage-gated 1, gamma
Spp1	Secreted phosphoprotein 1
Lbp	Lipopolysaccharide-binding protein

immunohistochemical studies and from the observation that specific metalloproteinase inhibitors block tumor invasion and metastasis. Oligonucleotide primers for 13 MMPs (MMP-1, -2, -3, -7, -8, -9, -10, -11, -12, -13, -14, -15, -16) were optimized for use in RT-PCR to determine the pattern of MMP mRNA expression in 84 normal and transformed or carcinogen transformed human cell lines and strains derived from different tissues. The results demonstrated one or more cell lines which express 13 members of the MMP family. Overexpression of the H-ras oncoprotein correlates with upregulation of MMP-9 and demonstrates that overexpression of v-sis also upregulates MMP-9. A cell line immortalized following myc expression was found to upregulate MMP-7, MMP-11, and MMP-13. Inappropriate expression of several MMP mRNAs was detected in breast, prostate, bone, colon, and oral tumor-derived cell lines. Identification of at least one cell line expressing each of 13 MMPs and the observation of oncogene-induced expression of several MMPs should facilitate analysis of the transcriptional mechanisms controlling each MMP [138].

The secreted phosphoprotein 1 (*Spp1*) is significantly upregulated in the rat mammary gland. *Spp1* has been previously named osteopontin (*OPN*) or bone sialoprotein I. Spp1 binds tightly to hydroxyapatite. Spp1 appears to form an integral part of the mineralized matrix and it acts as a cytokine involved in enhancing production of interferon-gamma and interleukin-12 and reducing production of interleukin-10 and is essential in the pathway that leads to type I immunity. SPP1 has been reported significantly upregulated in ductal carcinoma in situ [139] and in higher grades of breast carcinoma. This increase in expression also correlates with enhanced expressions of several oncogenic molecules (urokinase-type plasminogen activator [uPA], matrix metalloproteinase-2/-9 [MMP-2 and -9]) and increased angiogenic potential of breast carcinoma. Silencing of *OPN* by its specific small

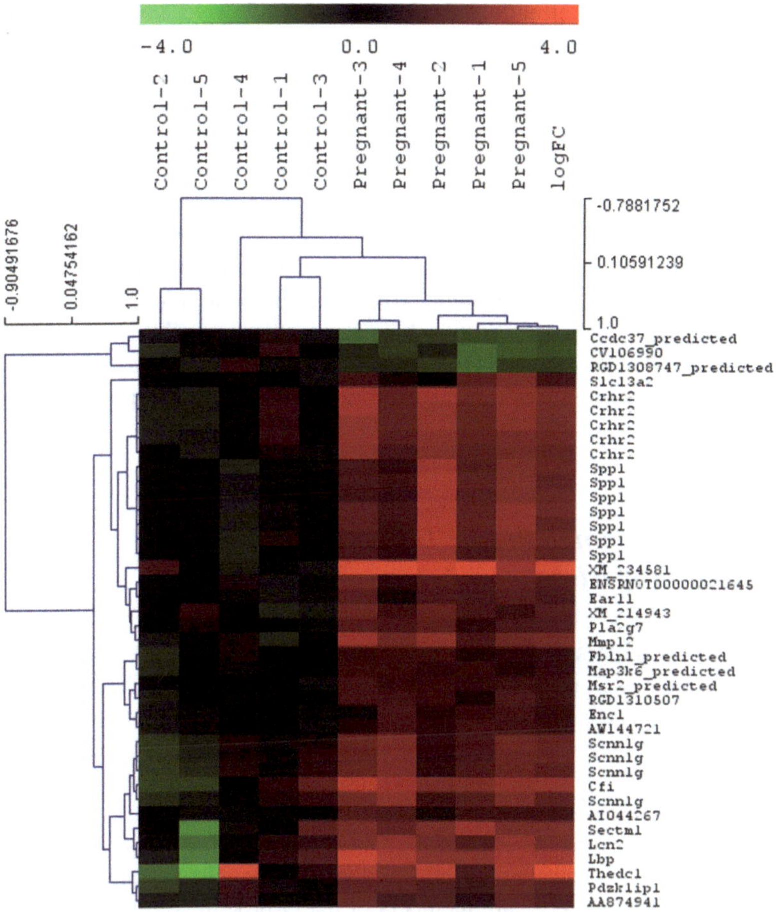

Fig. 3.17 Heat map showing the up- (*red*) and downregulated genes (*green*) of post pregnant rat mammary glands

interfering RNA (siRNA) downregulates the expressions of oncogenic molecules such as uPA, MMP-2 and -9 resulting in inhibition of in vitro cell motility and in vivo tumorigenicity in mice. $OPN^{-/-}$ mice showed slower progression of tumor growth in breast cancer model as compared to wild-type mice [140]. *OPN* has been also linked to metastatic function in lung and prostate cancers [141]. In vitro cells overexpressing *OPN* demonstrated increased anchorage-independent growth in soft agar ($p=0.001$) and increased RGD (Arg–Gly–Asp) integrin-dependent adhesion ($p=0.045$). Following mammary fat pad injection of nude mice, cells overexpressing *OPN* showed increased lymphovascular invasion, lymph node metastases, and lung micrometastases at earlier time points ($p=0.024$). Loss of the RGD region partially abrogated this effect in the lymphatics ($p=0.038$). These findings indicate that *OPN* is a key molecular player involved in lymphatic metastasis of breast cancer, potentially by affecting RGD-mediated adhesive interactions and by enhancing the establishment/persistence of tumor cells in the lymphatics [142]. *OPN* functions in tumor progression by upregulation of hyaluronan synthase 2 (HAS2) [143]. *OPN* enhances CD44s mRNA expression, increases cell surface expression of CD44 variant forms without a change in mRNA levels, and stimulates cell migration [144]. *OPN* might play a different role in the pathogenesis of endometrial cancer by complexing with CEACAM1 and could be relevant for invasive growth of such lesions [145]. Of interest is that parous mammary glands before MNU treatment showed upregulation of multiple differentiation-related genes, such as whey acidic protein (*Wap*), casein beta (*Csn2*), casein gamma (*Csng*), *Lbp*, secreted phosphoprotein 1, or *Spp1* and glycosylation-dependent cell adhesion molecule 1 (*Glycam1*) [146]. The functional role of *Spp1* or *OPN* as well as the *Sectm1b* or secreted and transmembrane 1B [67] in the normal mammary gland is unknown.

3.4.5 Transcriptome Profile Induced by Estrogen and Progesterone

The biological processes downregulated (Table 3.14) and upregulated (Table 3.15) by estrogen and progesterone are different from those induced by hCG and pregnancy. There are specific genes that are up- and downregulated by the treatment of estrogen and progesterone whose role in the prevention of mammary carcinogenesis in the rat is not known (Figs. 3.14 and 3.18). Among the downregulated genes that are specific for the estrogen and progesterone treatment are *Adra1d* (adrenergic, alpha-1D-, receptor); *Adra2c* (adrenergic, alpha-2C-, receptor); *Ntrk2* (neurotrophic tyrosine kinase, receptor, type 2); and *Npr3* (natriuretic peptide receptor C/guanylate cyclase C) (Figs. 3.14 and 3.18). *Adra1* and *Adra2c* are members of the G-protein coupled receptor superfamily [147–149]. They activate mitogenic responses and regulate growth and proliferation of many cells. Breast cancer mortality is frequently associated with metastatic disease. Metastasis models have shown adrenoceptor (AR) stimulation induces cell migration which is inhibited by adrenoceptor antagonist drugs. Adrenoceptors were not found to be independent predictors of clinical outcome. Alpha1b and α2c AR are overexpressed in basal-like breast tumors of poor prognosis. Strong β(2) adrenoceptor expression is seen in patients with a luminal (ER+) tumor phenotype and good prognosis, due to benefits derived from hormonal therapy [150]. The expression of alpha(2)-adrenoceptors was analyzed at the RNA (RT-PCR) and protein ([^{3}H]-rauwolscine binding and immunocytochemistry) levels in different human breast cell lines, and the biological activity assessed by [(3)H]-thymidine incorporation. The cancer IBH-6, IBH-7, and MCF-7 and the non-tumor HBL-100 cell-line expressed both alpha(2B)- and alpha(2C)-adrenoceptor-subtypes. A single subtype was expressed in malignant HS-578T (alpha(2A)) and MDA-MB-231 and non-tumor MCF-10A cells (alpha(2B)). All cell lines exhibited significant binding for the specific antagonist [(3) H]-rauwolscine. The alpha-, alpha(2)-, and the alpha(1)-compounds with known

Table 3.14 Biological processes and downregulated genes in the pellet group

Symbol	Name
Signaling (GO:0071875, GO:0032148, GO:0031547, GO:0071883, GO:0035625)	
Adra1d	Adrenergic, alpha-1D-, receptor
Adra2c	Adrenergic, alpha-2C-, receptor
Ntrk2	Neurotrophic tyrosine kinase, receptor, type 2
Secretion (GO:0030157)	
Npr3	Natriuretic peptide receptor C/guanylate cyclase C (atrionatriuretic peptide receptor C)
Development (GO:0046548)	
Ntrk2	Neurotrophic tyrosine kinase, receptor, type 2
Cell proliferation (GO:0002158, GO:0033688)	
Npr3	Natriuretic peptide receptor C/guanylate cyclase C (atrionatriuretic)
Blood pressure regulation (GO:0008217, GO:0001993, GO:0001986, GO:0001994, GO:0001978, GO:0035810)	
Npr3	Natriuretic peptide receptor C/guanylate cyclase C (atrionatriuretic peptide receptor C)
Adra1d	Adrenergic, alpha-1D-, receptor

affinity for alpha(2)-adrenoceptors, including epinephrine, norepinephrine, yohimbine, clonidine, rauwolscine, and prazosin, competed significantly with binding in MCF-7 cells. In addition, IBH-6, IBH-7, and MCF-7 cells showed significant staining with specific antibodies against alpha(2B)- and alpha(2C)-adrenoceptor-subtypes, when tested by immunocytochemistry. In all cell lines, the specific agonist clonidine or oxymetazoline stimulated [(3)H]-thymidine incorporation. EC(50) values were in the range of 20–50 fM for IBH-6, IBH-7, and HS-578T; 0.14 pM for MCF-7; 2–82 pM for HBL-100 and MCF-10A cells, and a biphasic behavior with a maximum value at 38.0 pM was observed for MDA-MB-231 cells. The specific alpha(2)-adrenergic antagonist rauwolscine always reversed this stimulation at 0.1 nM. Alpha(2)-adrenoceptors are expressed in human epithelial breast cell lines and activation of these receptors was associated with an enhancement of cell proliferation [151, 152].

Another gene downregulated by the estrogen and progesterone treatment is the *Npr3* or natriuretic peptide receptor C/guanylate cyclase C. This gene encodes one of three natriuretic peptide receptors. Natriuretic peptides are small peptides which regulate blood volume and pressure, pulmonary hypertension, and cardiac function as well as some metabolic and growth processes. The main physiological role of NP receptors is in homeostasis of body fluid volume. Medulloblastoma patients with *NPR3*-positive tumors exhibited a significantly diminished progression-free and overall survival irrespective of their metastatic status [153]. In acute myeloid leukemia *NPR3* is associated with high expression of insulin-like growth factor binding protein 7 (IGFBP7) that regulates the proliferation of leukemic cells and might be involved in chemotherapy resistance [154].

Among the upregulated genes (Table 3.15, and Figs. 3.14 and 3.18) that are specific for the estrogen and progesterone preventive strategy are LOC259246 (alpha-2u globulin PGCL1); *Per2* (period homolog 2 (*Drosophila*)); *Crabp2* (cellular retinoic

Table 3.15 Biological processes and upregulated genes in the pellet group

Symbol	Name
Alcohol biosynthetic process (GO:0046165)	
LOC259246	Alpha-2u globulin PGCL1
Crhr2	Corticotropin releasing hormone receptor 2
Cell motility (GO:0045475)	
LOC259246	Alpha-2u globulin PGCL1
Chemical homeostasis (GO:0042593, GO:0045721, GO:0055082)	
LOC259246	Alpha-2u globulin PGCL1
Crhr2	Corticotropin releasing hormone receptor 2
Lcn2	Lipocalin 2
Circadian rhythm (GO:0007623)	
LOC259246	Alpha-2u globulin PGCL1
Per2	Period homolog 2 (*Drosophila*)
Development (GO:0048630, GO:0070584)	
Crhr2	Corticotropin releasing hormone receptor 2
LOC259246	Alpha-2u globulin PGCL1
Immune response (GO:0006955)	
Lcn2	Lipocalin 2
Sectm1b	Secreted and transmembrane 1B
Cfi	Complement factor I
Lipid processes (GO:0010888)	
LOC259246	Alpha-2u globulin PGCL1
Regulation of behavior (GO:0035482, GO:2000293, GO:2000252)	
Crhr2	Corticotropin releasing hormone receptor 2
Response to stimulus (GO:0009746, GO:0009743, GO:0071326, GO:0071333, GO:0050796)	
LOC259246	Alpha-2u globulin PGCL1
Crhr2	Corticotropin releasing hormone receptor 2
Secretion (GO:0010817, GO:0002791, GO:0010700, GO:0061179, GO:0090278, GO:0014064, GO:0032277, GO:0046883, GO:0032811)	
LOC259246	Alpha-2u globulin PGCL1
Crabp2	Cellular retinoic acid-binding protein 2
Crhr2	Corticotropin releasing hormone receptor 2
Signaling (GO:0043950, GO:0043951, GO:0032874)	
Crhr2	Corticotropin releasing hormone receptor 2
Transport (GO:0015833, GO:0006869, GO:0048241, GO:0015891, GO:0033212, GO:0090281)	
LOC259246	Alpha-2u globulin PGCL1
Crhr2	Corticotropin releasing hormone receptor 2
Crabp2	Cellular retinoic acid-binding protein 2
Adfp	Adipose differentiation-related protein
Lcn2	Lipocalin 2

acid-binding protein 2); and *Adfp* (adipose differentiation-related protein). Of great interest is *Per2* a gene that is a member of the Period family of genes and is expressed in a circadian pattern in the suprachiasmatic nucleus, the primary circadian pacemaker in the mammalian brain. Genes in this family encode components of the circadian rhythms of locomotor activity, metabolism, and behavior. Circadian expression in the suprachiasmatic nucleus continues in constant darkness, and a shift in the light/

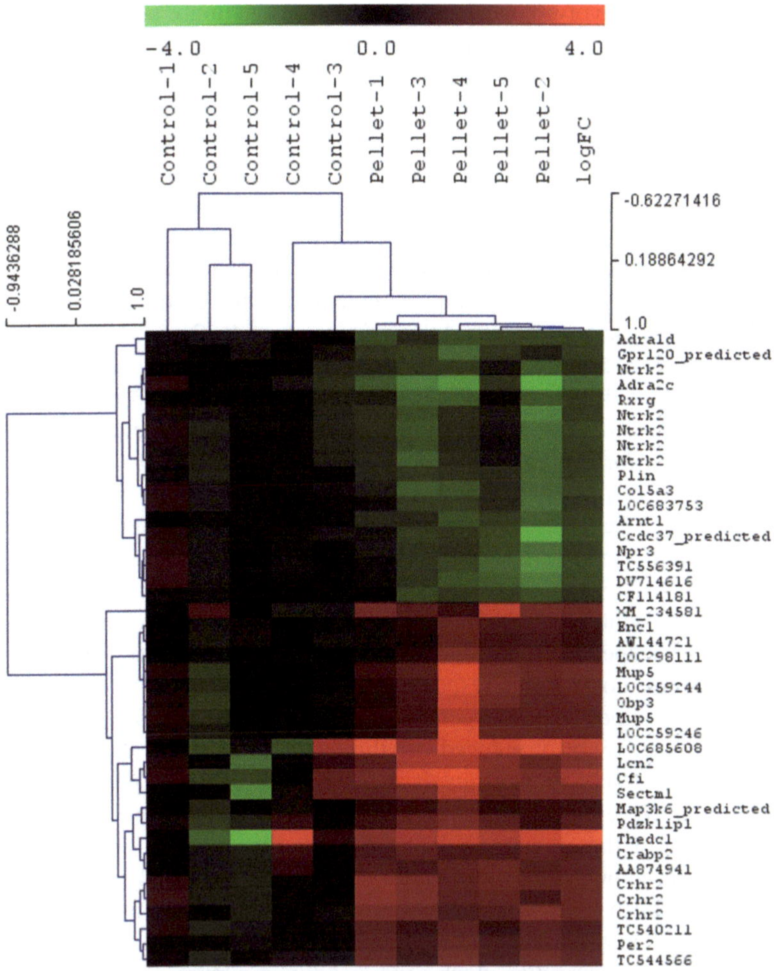

Fig. 3.18 Heat map showing the up- (*red*) and downregulated genes (*green*) of post pellet treated rat mammary glands

dark cycle evokes a proportional shift of gene expression in the suprachiasmatic nucleus. *Per2* influences clock function by interacting with other circadian regulatory proteins and transporting them to the nucleus. It negatively regulates *CLOCK*, *NPAS2-BMAL1*, and *BMAL2*-induced transactivation [155]. Genetic ablation of *mPer1* and *mPer2* function results in a complete loss of circadian rhythm control based on wheel running activity in mice. In addition, these animals also display apparent premature aging and significant increase in neoplastic and hyperplastic phenotypes. When challenged by gamma-radiation, *mPer2*-deficient mice respond by rapid hair graying, are deficient in p53-mediated apoptosis in thymocytes, and have robust tumor occurrences. The circadian clock function is very important for cell cycle, DNA damage response, and tumor suppression in vivo. Temporal expression of genes involved in cell cycle regulation and tumor suppression, such as *c-Myc*, *Cyclin D1*, *Cyclin A*, *Mdm-2*, and *Gadd45alpha*, is deregulated in *mPer2* mutant mice. In addition, genetic studies have demonstrated that many key regulators of cell cycle and growth control are also important circadian clock regulators confirming the critical role of circadian function in organism homeostasis [156]. Studies of human breast and endometrial cancers revealed that the loss and deregulation of PERIOD 1 and 2 proteins is common in the tumor cells [156]. The expression of PER1, PER2, PER3, CRY1, CRY2, CKIε, and BMAL1 has been found in several cancers [157, 158]. Methylselenocysteine reduced the incidence of *N*-nitroso-*N*-methylurea (NMU)-induced mammary carcinomas in Fischer 344 rats by 63%. Methylselenocysteine also increased the expression of *Per2* and D-binding protein (*Dbp*), providing evidence for a link between circadian rhythm and chemoprevention. NMU disrupted the expression of core circadian genes (*Per1*, *PER2*, *Cry1*, *Cry2*, and *RevErbAalpha*) and circadian-controlled genes, including melatonin receptor 1alpha (*Mtnria*), estrogen receptors (*ERalpha* and *ERbeta*), and growth-regulatory genes (*Trp53*, *p21*, *Gadd45alpha*, and *c-Myc*) in mammary glands of Fischer 344 rats. By contrast, dietary methylselenocysteine (3 ppm selenium) given for 30 days significantly enhanced the circadian expression of these genes (except for *Cry1* and *Cry2*). The largest effect was on the levels of the *Per2*, *Mtnria*, and *ERbeta* mRNAs, which showed 16.5-, 4.7-, and 9.5-fold increases in their rhythm-adjusted means, respectively, and 44.5-, 6.5-, and 9.7-fold increases in amplitude as compared with the control diet, respectively. Methylselenocysteine also shifted the peak expression times of these genes to Zeitgeber time 12 (ZT12; lights off). Methylselenocysteine also induced rhythmic expression of *Trp53*, *p21*, and *Gadd45alpha* mRNAs with peak levels at ZT12, when *c-Myc* expression was at its lowest level. However, methylselenocysteine had no significant effect on the circadian expression of these genes in liver. These results suggest that dietary methylselenocysteine counteracted the disruptive effect of NMU on circadian expression of genes essential to normal mammary cell growth and differentiation [159] and indicate that *Per2* may act as a tumor suppressor gene and preventive of mammary cancer. *PER2*, a core circadian clock gene, has tumor suppressor properties and is mutated or downregulated in human breast cancers. Using siRNA and shRNA to downregulate *Per2* expression in vitro *and* in vivo for measuring cancer cell proliferation, tumor growth rate, and several molecular pathways relevant to cancer growth and their circadian organizations, it has been shown that downregulation of functional *Per2* gene expression increases Cyclin D and Cyclin E levels and doubles in vitro breast cancer cell proliferation ($p<0.05$). Downregulation of *Per2* also accelerates in vivo tumor growth and doubles the daily amplitude of the tumor growth rhythm ($p<0.05$). *Per2* links the circadian cycle to the ERalpha signaling network; for example suppression of *Per2* levels leads to ERalpha stabilization. In turn, *Per2* itself is estrogen inducible in these cells, suggesting a feedback mechanism to attenuate stimulation by estrogen. In addition, overexpression of *Per2* in breast cancer cells leads to significant growth inhibition, loss of clonogenic ability and apoptosis. Taken together, these results further support a critical role for peripheral circadian regulation in tissue homeostasis and suggest a novel role for clock genes in estrogen receptor-positive breast cancer.

3.5 Enrichment of the Genomic Signature of Prevention

In this study we have used a gene set enrichment analysis using a cut-off value of $p<0.01$ and a fold change of 2 as indicated in Table 3.1; using this strategy we have increased the number of common genes among the three prevention modalities from 7 to 28, as depicted in Table 3.16 and Figs. 3.19 and 3.20. The identified common biological processes are depicted in Figs. 3.21 and 3.22 and in Tables 3.17 and 3.18. Among the known genes that are common and that were not detected using more stringent criteria are *Apod*, *Cldn4*, *Crb3*, *Crhr2*, *Duox1*, *Irx2*, *Kng1*, *Lbp*, *Mmp12*, *Pdzk1ip1*, *Scnn1g*, *Sectm1*, *Spp1*, *Tgfb3*, *Trim29*, and *Wap*. There are biological processes that are more representatively expressed under hCG treatment (Figs. 3.23, 3.24, and 3.25 and Tables 3.19 and 3.20), Pregnancy (Figs. 3.26, 3.27, and 3.28 and Tables 3.21 and 3.22), and pellet (Figs. 3.29, 3.30, and 3.31 and Tables 3.23 and 3.24). The number of genes per biological processes is better represented under hCG treatment (Tables 3.25 and 3.26) than for pregnancy (Tables 3.27 and 3.28) or pellet (Tables 3.29 and 3.30).

The gene enrichment procedure allows a better discrimination of the genes that are common to the three prevention modalities. For example, *Sectm1* that was only observed in the pregnancy group before using more stringent criteria now is shown among the three treatments and the same occurs for the *Apod*, *Duox1*, and *Kng1* that were only observed in the hCG treated group are now common to the three treatments. Of interest is that other genes like *Cldn4*, *Crb3*, *Crhr2*, *Irx2*, *Kng1*, *Mmp12*, *Pdzk1ip1*, *Scnn1g*, *Tgfb3*, *Trim29*, and *Wap* are now part of the signature of prevention (Fig. 3.32). Among the genes common to pregnancy and the pellet are the *Sectm1*, *Bhlhb3*, *B3galt3*, *Wfdc2*, *Cc28*, *Qscn6*, *Cldn7*, *Gzma*, *Eps812*, *St6galnac2*, *Slc55a1*, *Muc1*, *Cd24*, *Krt1-19*, and *Cfb* (Fig. 3.19). There are only two known common genes between hCG and the pellet, *Spt1* and *Trp63*. The common known genes between hCG and pregnancy are the *Pla2g7*, *Trpc3*, and *Scnn1b* (Fig. 3.19).

A gene that is commonly upregulated by the three prevention strategies is the Dual oxidase 1 or *Duox1*, which has been discussed in the previous section. The overexpression of *Duox 1* in the breast epithelial cells could be indicative of an oxidative antimicrobial protection as has been shown in the differentiated primary human airway epithelial cells challenged with *P. aeruginosa* flagellin or IFN-gamma [128]. *C. elegans* seems to play also an important role in the barrier epithelium as an ancient, highly conserved innate immune defense mechanism. The airway epithelium represents a key mechanism of innate airway host defense, through enhanced production of H_2O_2, which mediates cellular signaling pathways that regulate the production of various inflammatory mediators. Production of the CXC chemokine interleukin (IL)-8/CXCL8 forms a common epithelial response to many diverse stimuli, including bacterial and viral triggers, environmental oxidants, and other

Table 3.16 Genes found to be differentially expressed in all the three conditions ($p<0.01$ and fold chance at least 2.0)

			Fold change		
Gene symbol	Systematic name	Gene name	hCG	Pellet	Preg
TC540900	TC540900	Unknown	0.45	0.40	0.45
AA874941	AA874941	AA874941 UI-R-E0-ci-d-06-0-UI.s1 UI-R-E0 *Rattus norvegicus* cDNA clone UI-R-E0-ci-d-06-0-UI 3′ similar to gi [AA874941]	2.42	3.01	2.59
Apod	NM_012777	*Rattus norvegicus* apolipoprotein D (Apod), mRNA [NM_012777]	2.80	2.02	2.22
Cfi	NM_024157	*Rattus norvegicus* complement factor I (Cfi), mRNA [NM_024157]	7.57	6.72	6.05
Cldn4	NM_001012022	*Rattus norvegicus* claudin 4 (Cldn4), mRNA [NM_001012022]	3.57	3.70	3.84
Crb3	NM_001025661	*Rattus norvegicus* crumbs homolog 3 (*Drosophila*) (Crb3), mRNA [NM_001025661]	2.40	2.31	2.39
Crhr2	NM_022714	*Rattus norvegicus* corticotropin releasing hormone receptor 2 (Crhr2), mRNA [NM_022714]	2.99	3.78	4.84
Duox1	NM_153739	*Rattus norvegicus* dual oxidase 1 (Duox1), mRNA [NM_153739]	2.71	2.79	2.62
Enc1	NM_001003401	*Rattus norvegicus* ectodermal-neural cortex 1 (Enc1), mRNA [NM_001003401]	2.08	2.26	2.01
Irx2	NM_001039505	*Rattus norvegicus* Iroquois related homeobox 2 (*Drosophila*) (Irx2), mRNA [NM_001039505]	3.08	3.50	3.07
Kng1	NM_012696	*Rattus norvegicus* kininogen 1 (Kng1), mRNA [NM_012696]	4.42	3.14	3.69
Lbp	NM_017208	*Rattus norvegicus* lipopolysaccharide-binding protein (Lbp), mRNA [NM_017208]	3.53	4.84	6.57
Lcn2	NM_130741	*Rattus norvegicus* lipocalin 2 (Lcn2), mRNA [NM_130741]	3.78	4.99	4.53
LOC685608	XM_001065355	Predicted: *Rattus norvegicus* hypothetical protein LOC685608 (LOC685608), mRNA [XM_001065355]	25.41	8.42	4.99
Map3k6_predicted	XM_232732	Predicted: *Rattus norvegicus* mitogen-activated protein kinase kinase kinase 6 (predicted) (Map3k6_predicted), mRNA [XM_232732]	2.04	2.09	2.00
MGC108747	NM_001009628	*Rattus norvegicus* similar to alpha-1 major acute phase protein prepeptide (MGC108747), mRNA [NM_001009628]	3.64	2.65	2.70
Mmp12	NM_053963	*Rattus norvegicus* matrix metallopeptidase 12 (Mmp12), mRNA [NM_053963]	2.87	3.31	4.57
Pdzk1ip1	NM_130401	*Rattus norvegicus* PDZK1 interacting protein 1 (Pdzk1ip1), mRNA [NM_130401]	2.27	2.97	2.87
RGD1306601_predicted	XM_230527	Predicted: *Rattus norvegicus* similar to cDNA sequence BC019755 (predicted) (RGD1306601_predicted), mRNA [XM_230527]	2.76	2.78	2.71
Scnn1g	NM_017046	*Rattus norvegicus* sodium channel, nonvoltage-gated 1 gamma (Scnn1g), mRNA [NM_017046]	4.88	2.97	3.76

Sectm1	NM_199082	*Rattus norvegicus* secreted and transmembrane 1 (Sectm1), mRNA [NM_199082]	3.52	4.44	4.77
Spp1	NM_012881	*Rattus norvegicus* secreted phosphoprotein 1 (Spp1), mRNA [NM_012881]	2.46	2.85	3.98
TC523154	TC523154	Q91842 (Q91842) *Xenopus laevis* U2 snRNA gene, partial (6%) [TC523154]	2.16	2.33	2.19
Tgfb3	NM_013174	*Rattus norvegicus* transforming growth factor, beta3 (Tgfb3), mRNA [NM_013174]	2.54	2.85	3.07
Thedc1	NM_022705	*Rattus norvegicus* thioesterase domain containing 1 (Thedc1), mRNA [NM_022705]	7.05	13.64	10.29
Trim29_predicted	XM_236207	Predicted: *Rattus norvegicus* tripartite motif protein 29 (predicted) (Trim29_predicted), mRNA [XM_236207]	3.05	2.64	2.54
Wap	NM_053751	*Rattus norvegicus* whey acidic protein (Wap), mRNA [NM_053751]	17.44	17.10	14.38
XM_234581	XM_234581	*Rattus norvegicus* similar to immunoglobulin alpha heavy chain (LOC314487), mRNA [XM_234581]	3.32	4.05	10.42

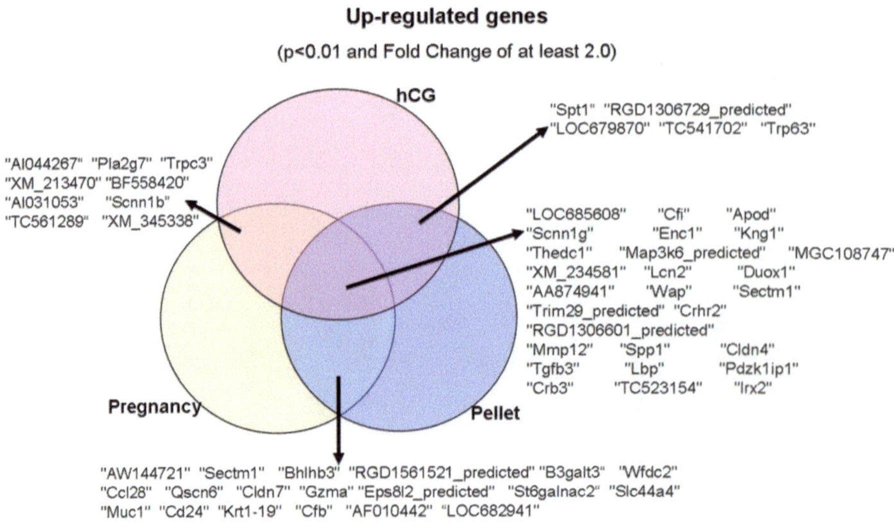

Fig. 3.19 Venn diagram depicting the biological processes of the upregulated genes in the rat mammary under three different prevention strategies using a $p<0.01$ and FC of 2.0

Fig. 3.20 Venn diagram depicting the biological processes of the downregulated genes in the rat mammary gland under three different prevention strategies using a $p<0.01$ and FC of 2.0

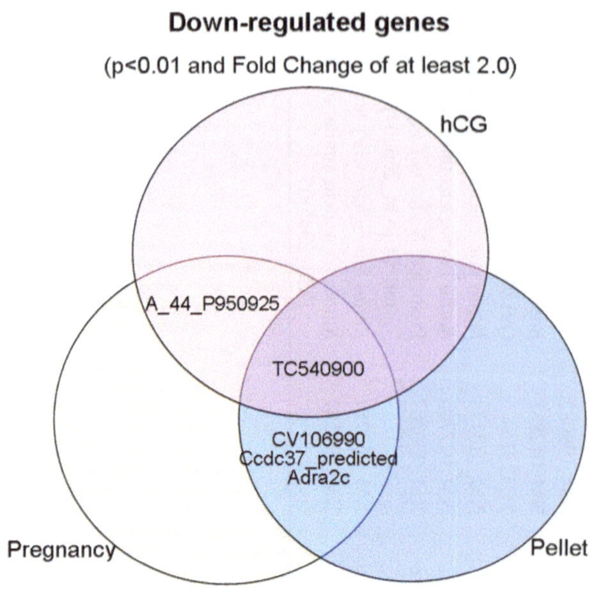

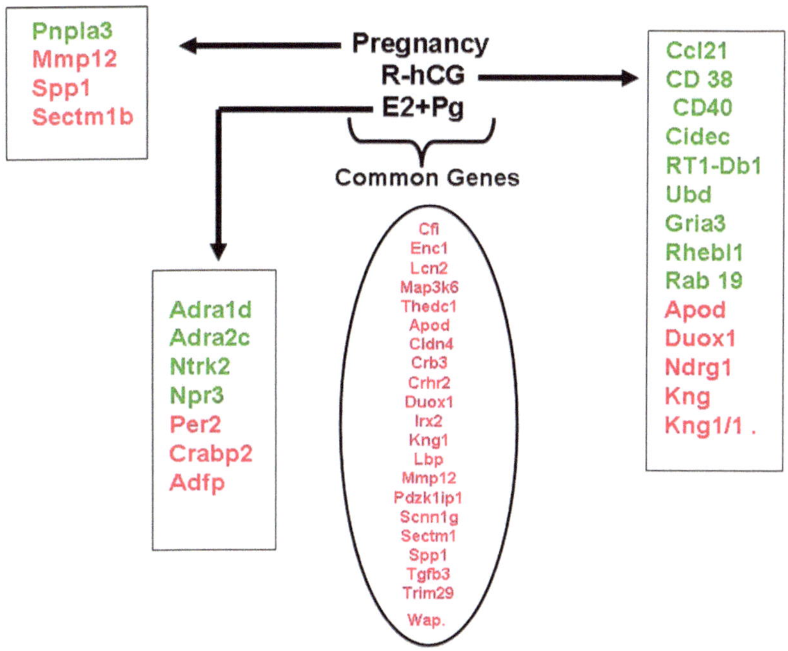

Fig. 3.21 Common genes and specific transcripts expressed in the rat mammary gland following pregnancy, hCG and pellets using a $p<0.01$ and FC of 2.0

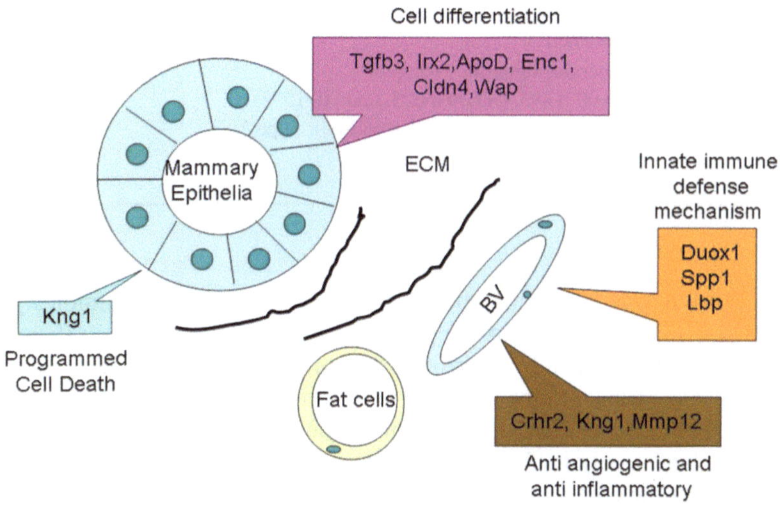

Fig. 3.22 Schematic representation of the different biological processes involved in the prevention signature

Table 3.17 Biological processes overrepresented among the downregulated genes in all three conditions

Symbol	Name
Signaling	
hCG (GO:0035556, GO:0043123, GO:0009967, GO:0023051, GO:0046425, GO:0035023, GO:0032321, GO:0010627)	
Cflar	CASP8 and FADD-like apoptosis regulator
Stk17b	Serine/threonine kinase 17b
Cd40	CD40 molecule, TNF receptor superfamily member 5
Arhgap4	Rho GTPase-activating protein 4
Prkcb	Protein kinase C, beta
Hcls1	Hematopoietic cell-specific Lyn substrate 1
Ubd	Ubiquitin D
Plcg2	Phospholipase C, gamma 2
Ccl21	Chemokine (C-C motif) ligand 21
Zap70	Zeta-chain (TCR) associated protein kinase
Rhoh	Ras homolog gene family, member H
Rhebl1	Ras homolog enriched in brain like 1
Clcf1	Cardiotrophin-like cytokine factor 1
Rac2	Ras-related C3 botulinum toxin substrate 2 (rho family, small GTP-binding protein Rac2)
Il22ra2	Interleukin 22 receptor, alpha 2
Rab19	RAB19, member RAS oncogene family
Ghrl	Ghrelin/obestatin prepropeptide
Kcnn4	Potassium intermediate/small conductance calcium-activated channel, subfamily N, member 4
Cd38	CD38 molecule
Arhgap15	Rho GTPase-activating protein 15
Gria3	Glutamate receptor, ionotrophic, AMPA 3
Pregnancy (GO:0071883, GO:0035625, GO:0032148, GO:2000273, GO:0045742, GO:0007176, GO:0061098)	
Adra2c	Adrenergic, alpha-2C-, receptor
Pellet (GO:0031547, GO:0071883, GO:0035625, GO:0071875)	
Ntrk2	Neurotrophic tyrosine kinase, receptor, type 2
Adra2c	Adrenergic, alpha-2C-, receptor
Adra1d	Adrenergic, alpha-1D-, receptor

biological mediators, suggesting the potential involvement of a common signaling pathway that may involve Duox1-dependent H_2O_2 production [160]. Therefore in the mammary gland *Duox 1* may protect the epithelial cells of exogenous stressor and may also contribute to the signature of differentiation conferred by pregnancy, hormonal treatment, and hCG. A common phenotypical pattern induced in the mammary gland by these three preventive strategies is the lobular development associated with the production of milk-like proteins that are indication of gland differentiation. One of these proteins is the whey acidic protein or *Wap*. *Wap* is the major milk protein in certain mammals and has been found in two monotremes,

Table 3.18 Biological processes overrepresented among the upregulated genes in all three conditions

Symbol	Name
Cellular metabolic process	
hCG (GO:0019546, GO:0052548, GO:0010466)	
Padi3	Peptidyl arginine deiminase, type III
Serpinb5	Serpin peptidase inhibitor, clade B (ovalbumin), member 5
Hspa1a	Heat shock 70 kDa protein 1A
Kng1	Kininogen 1
Foxq1	Forkhead box Q1
Wap	Whey acidic protein
Pregnancy (GO:0006709, GO:0032078, GO:0032074)	
Akr1c18	Aldo-keto reductase family 1, member C18
Gzma	Granzyme A
Pellet (GO:0044253, GO:0032078, GO:0032074)	
Tgfb3	Transforming growth factor, beta3
Ctgf	Connective tissue growth factor
Gzma	Granzyme A
Circulatory system	
hCG (GO:0008015)	
Gja1	Gap junction protein, alpha 1
Hspa1a	Heat shock 70 kDa protein 1A
Kng1	Kininogen 1
Kng1l1	Kininogen 1-like 1
Crhr2	Corticotropin releasing hormone receptor 2
Pregnancy (GO:0034107, GO:0034119)	
Cd24	CD24 molecule
Pellet (GO:0034107, GO:0034119)	
Cd24	CD24 molecule
Development	
hCG (GO:0031069, GO:0009888, GO:0030855, GO:0048627, GO:0048685, GO:0060529, GO:0048732, GO:0060512)	
Tp63	Tumor protein p63
Igfbp5	Insulin-like growth factor binding protein 5
Foxq1	Forkhead box Q1
Serpinb5	Serpin peptidase inhibitor, clade B (ovalbumin), member 5
Cebpb	CCAAT/enhancer-binding protein (C/EBP), beta
Gja1	Gap junction protein, alpha 1
Apod	Apolipoprotein D
Spp1	Secreted phosphoprotein 1
Tgfb3	Transforming growth factor, beta3
Crhr2	Corticotropin releasing hormone receptor 2
Bambi	BMP and activin membrane-bound inhibitor, homolog (*Xenopus laevis*)
Sdc1	Syndecan 1
Pregnancy (GO:0031103, GO:0048685, GO:0034103, GO:0042335, GO:0043932)	
Apod	Apolipoprotein D
Spp1	Secreted phosphoprotein 1

(continued)

Table 3.18 (continued)

Symbol	Name
Chl1	Cell adhesion molecule with homology to L1CAM
Cd24	CD24 molecule
Duox1	Dual oxidase 1
Tgfb3	Transforming growth factor, beta3
Pellet (GO:0048685, GO:0060529, GO:0034103, GO:0042335, GO:0043932, GO:0045617, GO:0060197, GO:0031103)	
Spp1	Secreted phosphoprotein 1
Tp63	Tumor protein p63
Cd24	CD24 molecule
Duox1	Dual oxidase 1
Tgfb3	Transforming growth factor, beta3
Apod	Apolipoprotein D
Immune response	
hCG (GO:0032755, GO:0001817, GO:0045087, GO:0006954, GO:0006958, GO:0032760, GO:0002232, GO:0060265, GO:0002252, GO:0050776)	
Lbp	Lipopolysaccharide-binding protein
Mapk13	Mitogen-activated protein kinase 13
Crhr2	Corticotropin releasing hormone receptor 2
Cebpb	CCAAT/enhancer-binding protein (C/EBP), beta
Tgfb3	Transforming growth factor, beta3
Cd14	CD14 molecule
Lcn2	Lipocalin 2
C4bpa	Complement component 4 binding protein, alpha
Cfi	Complement factor I
Kng1	Kininogen 1
Sdc1	Syndecan 1
Spp1	Secreted phosphoprotein 1
Kng1l1	Kininogen 1-like 1
Hspa1a	Heat shock 70 kDa protein 1A
Pregnancy (GO:0002682, GO:0001818, GO:0002232, GO:0032913, GO:0042103, GO:0046014, GO:0060265, GO:0032755, GO:0006954, GO:0045087, GO:0002690, GO:0006956, GO:0050778, GO:0002842)	
Kng1	Kininogen 1
Cd24	CD24 molecule
Tgfb3	Transforming growth factor, beta3
Cfb	Complement factor B
Lbp	Lipopolysaccharide-binding protein
Pla2g7	Phospholipase A2, group VII (platelet-activating factor acetylhydrolase, plasma)
Cfi	Complement factor I
Crhr2	Corticotropin releasing hormone receptor 2
Spp1	Secreted phosphoprotein 1
Kng1l1	Kininogen 1-like 1
Lcn2	Lipocalin 2

(continued)

Table 3.18 (continued)

Symbol	Name
Pellet (GO:0002237, GO:0001818, GO:0002232, GO:0032913, GO:0042103, GO:0046014, GO:0060265, GO:0032755, GO:0006954, GO:0045087, GO:0006956, GO:0002842, GO:0050778)	
Lcn2	Lipocalin 2
Cd24	CD24 molecule
Aqp2	Aquaporin 2 (collecting duct)
Cfb	Complement factor B
Lbp	Lipopolysaccharide-binding protein
Tgfb3	Transforming growth factor, beta3
Crhr2	Corticotropin releasing hormone receptor 2
Kng1	Kininogen 1
Spp1	Secreted phosphoprotein 1
Kng1l1	Kininogen 1-like 1
Cfi	Complement factor I
Localization	
hCG (GO:0051674, GO:0032879)	
Mmp12	Matrix metallopeptidase 12
Gja1	Gap junction protein, alpha 1
Scnn1b	Sodium channel, nonvoltage-gated 1, beta
Scnn1g	Sodium channel, nonvoltage-gated 1, gamma
Igfbp5	Insulin-like growth factor binding protein 5
Lbp	Lipopolysaccharide-binding protein
Pla2g7	Phospholipase A2, group VII (platelet-activating factor acetylhydrolase, plasma)
Bambi	BMP and activin membrane-bound inhibitor, homolog (*Xenopus laevis*)
Kcnk2	Potassium channel, subfamily K, member 2
Tgfb3	Transforming growth factor, beta3
Cd14	CD14 molecule
Crhr2	Corticotropin releasing hormone receptor 2
Pregnancy (GO:0033037)	
Lbp	Lipopolysaccharide-binding protein
Pellet (GO:0033037)	
Lbp	Lipopolysaccharide-binding protein
Response to stimulus	
hCG (GO:0071223, GO:0071222, GO:0071216, GO:0050909)	
Lbp	Lipopolysaccharide-binding protein
Cd14	CD14 molecule
Lcn2	Lipocalin 2
Scnn1b	Sodium channel, nonvoltage-gated 1, beta
Scnn1g	Sodium channel, nonvoltage-gated 1, gamma
Pregnancy (GO:0010033, GO:0070887, GO:0050909, GO:0050795, GO:0048545, GO:2000252, GO:0032103)	
Lcn2	Lipocalin 2
Cyp2e1	Cytochrome P450, family 2, subfamily e, polypeptide 1
Cd24	CD24 molecule
Spp1	Secreted phosphoprotein 1

(continued)

Table 3.18 (continued)

Symbol	Name
Tgfb3	Transforming growth factor, beta3
Duox1	Dual oxidase 1
Cfb	Complement factor B
Lbp	Lipopolysaccharide-binding protein
Adfp	Adipose differentiation-related protein
Cldn4	Claudin 4
Krt19	Keratin 19
Crhr2	Corticotropin releasing hormone receptor 2
Prkaa2	Protein kinase, AMP-activated, alpha 2 catalytic subunit
Pla2g7	Phospholipase A2, group VII (platelet-activating factor acetylhydrolase, plasma)
Scnn1b	Sodium channel, nonvoltage-gated 1, beta
Scnn1g	Sodium channel, nonvoltage-gated 1, gamma
Pellet (GO:0009725, GO:0043627, GO:0071280, GO:2000252, GO:0071326, GO:0071333)	
Cd24	CD24 molecule
Mfge8	Milk fat globule-EGF factor 8 protein
Spp1	Secreted phosphoprotein 1
Aqp2	Aquaporin 2 (collecting duct)
Tgfb3	Transforming growth factor, beta3
LOC259246	Alpha-2u globulin PGCL1
Cldn4	Claudin 4
Abcg2	ATP-binding cassette, subfamily G (WHITE), member 2
Krt19	Keratin 19
Ctgf	Connective tissue growth factor
Crhr2	Corticotropin releasing hormone receptor 2
Response to stress	
hCG (GO:0006950, GO:0033554)	
Mmp12	Matrix metallopeptidase 12
C4bpa	Complement component 4 binding protein, alpha
Gja1	Gap junction protein, alpha 1
Scnn1b	Sodium channel, nonvoltage-gated 1, beta
Scnn1g	Sodium channel, nonvoltage-gated 1, gamma
Kng1	Kininogen 1
Sdc1	Syndecan 1
Tgfb3	Transforming growth factor, beta3
Kng1l1	Kininogen 1-like 1
Penk	Proenkephalin
Lbp	Lipopolysaccharide-binding protein
Mapk13	Mitogen-activated protein kinase 13
Cd14	CD14 molecule
Cfi	Complement factor I
Lcn2	Lipocalin 2
Hspa1a	Heat shock 70 kDa protein 1A
Tp63	Tumor protein p63
Apod	Apolipoprotein D
Spp1	Secreted phosphoprotein 1

(continued)

Table 3.18 (continued)

Symbol	Name
Duox1	Dual oxidase 1
Ndrg1	N-myc downstream regulated 1
Crhr2	Corticotropin releasing hormone receptor 2
Pregnancy (GO:0006950)	
Mmp12	Matrix metallopeptidase 12
Lcn2	Lipocalin 2
Scnn1b	Sodium channel, nonvoltage-gated 1, beta
Scnn1g	Sodium channel, nonvoltage-gated 1, gamma
Kng1	Kininogen 1
Cd24	CD24 molecule
Apod	Apolipoprotein D
Spp1	Secreted phosphoprotein 1
Tgfb3	Transforming growth factor, beta3
Duox1	Dual oxidase 1
Kng1l1	Kininogen 1-like 1
Cfb	Complement factor B
Lbp	Lipopolysaccharide-binding protein
Crhr2	Corticotropin releasing hormone receptor 2
Prkaa2	Protein kinase, AMP-activated, alpha 2 catalytic subunit
Cfi	Complement factor I
Chl1	Cell adhesion molecule with homology to L1CAM
Pellet (GO:0006950)	
Mmp12	Matrix metallopeptidase 12
Lcn2	Lipocalin 2
Aldoc	Aldolase C, fructose-bisphosphate
Tp63	Tumor protein p63
Scnn1g	Sodium channel, nonvoltage-gated 1, gamma
Kng1	Kininogen 1
Cd24	CD24 molecule
Apod	Apolipoprotein D
Spp1	Secreted phosphoprotein 1
Aqp2	Aquaporin 2 (collecting duct)
Tgfb3	Transforming growth factor, beta3
Duox1	Dual oxidase 1
Kng1l1	Kininogen 1-like 1
Cfb	Complement factor B
Lbp	Lipopolysaccharide-binding protein
Ctgf	Connective tissue growth factor
Crhr2	Corticotropin releasing hormone receptor 2
Cfi	Complement factor I
Secretion	
hCG (GO:0014064)	
Crhr2	Corticotropin releasing hormone receptor 2
Pregnancy (GO:0014064)	
Crhr2	Corticotropin releasing hormone receptor 2
Pellet (GO:0061179, GO:0014064, GO:0090278)	

(continued)

Table 3.18 (continued)

Symbol	Name
LOC259246	Alpha-2u globulin PGCL1
Crhr2	Corticotropin releasing hormone receptor 2
Transport	
hCG (GO:0010232, GO:0035482, GO:2000293, GO:0030001)	
Gja1	Gap junction protein, alpha 1
Crhr2	Corticotropin releasing hormone receptor 2
Lcn2	Lipocalin 2
Kcnk2	Potassium channel, subfamily K, member 2
Scnn1b	Sodium channel, nonvoltage-gated 1, beta
Scnn1g	Sodium channel, nonvoltage-gated 1, gamma
Slc39a8	Solute carrier family 39 (zinc transporter), member 8
Pregnancy (GO:0032600, GO:0035482, GO:2000293, GO:0015891, GO:0015920, GO:0032594, GO:0090281)	
Cd24	CD24 molecule
Crhr2	Corticotropin releasing hormone receptor 2
Lcn2	Lipocalin 2
Lbp	Lipopolysaccharide-binding protein
Pellet (GO:0032600, GO:0035482, GO:2000293, GO:0015891, GO:0015920, GO:0032594, GO:0090281)	
Cd24	CD24 molecule
Crhr2	Corticotropin releasing hormone receptor 2
Lcn2	Lipocalin 2
Lbp	Lipopolysaccharide-binding protein
Wound healing	
hCG (GO:0042060, GO:0035313)	
Mmp12	Matrix metallopeptidase 12
Gja1	Gap junction protein, alpha 1
Scnn1b	Sodium channel, nonvoltage-gated 1, beta
Scnn1g	Sodium channel, nonvoltage-gated 1, gamma
Kng1	Kininogen 1
Sdc1	Syndecan 1
Apod	Apolipoprotein D
Tgfb3	Transforming growth factor, beta3
Pregnancy (GO:0035313, GO:0042060)	
Mmp12	Matrix metallopeptidase 12
Scnn1b	Sodium channel, nonvoltage-gated 1, beta
Scnn1g	Sodium channel, nonvoltage-gated 1, gamma
Kng1	Kininogen 1
Apod	Apolipoprotein D
Tgfb3	Transforming growth factor, beta3
Pellet (GO:0035313, GO:0042060)	
Mmp12	Matrix metallopeptidase 12
Scnn1g	Sodium channel, nonvoltage-gated 1, gamma
Kng1	Kininogen 1
Apod	Apolipoprotein D
Tgfb3	Transforming growth factor, beta3

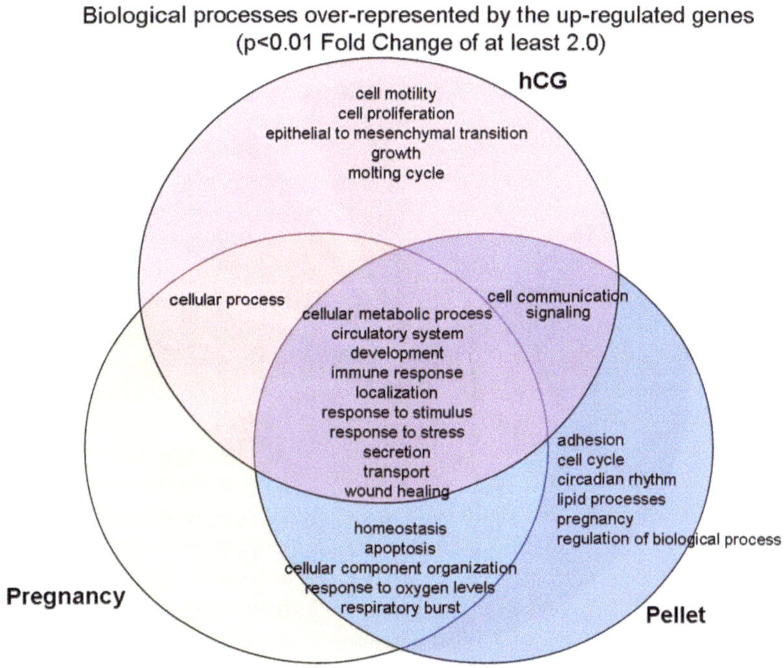

Fig. 3.23 Venn diagram depicting the biological processes of the upregulated genes in the rat mammary gland under three different prevention strategies using a $p < 0.01$ and FC of 2.0

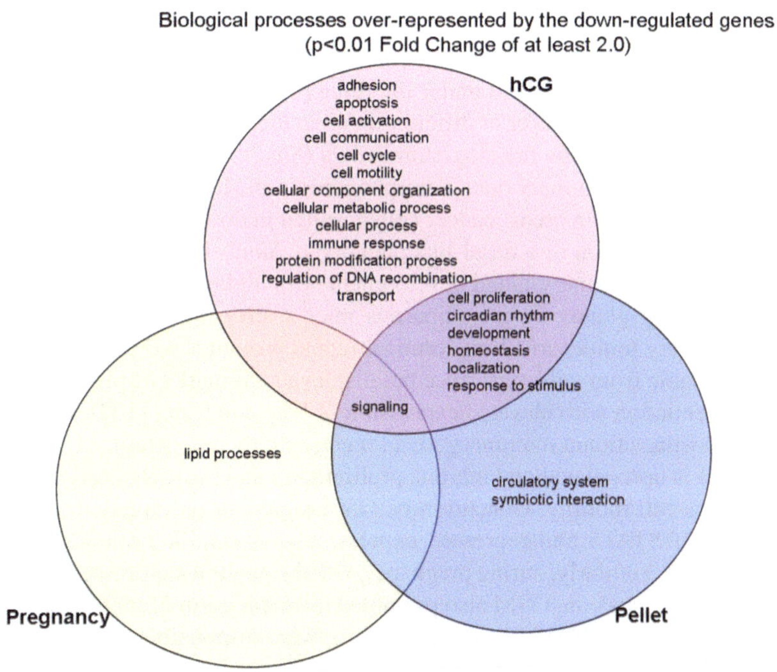

Fig. 3.24 Venn diagram depicting the biological processes of the downregulated genes in the rat mammary gland under three different prevention strategies using a $p < 0.01$ and FC of 2.0

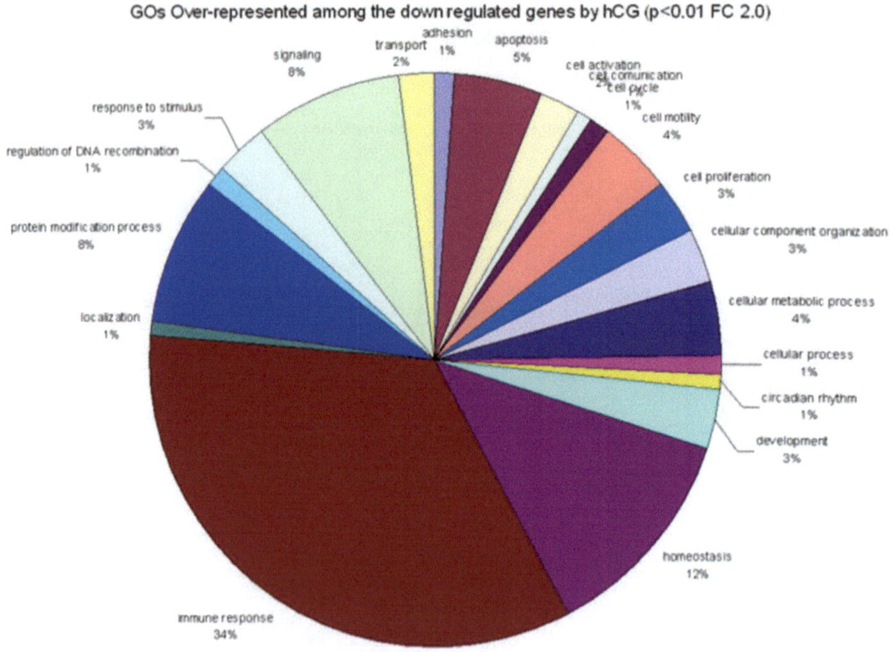

Fig. 3.25 Gene ontology of the overrepresented genes downregulated by hCG in the rat mammary gland using a $p < 0.01$ and FC of 2.0

three marsupials, rodents, rabbits, pigs, and camels. *Wap* is significantly upregulated in the rat mammary gland under the three preventive strategies tested, and it has been shown to be a marker of differentiation in diethylstilbestrol-treated women [161]. *Wap* is regulated by the singleminded 2s (*Sim2s*) transcription factor that is required for proper mammary ductal morphogenesis and luminal epithelial differentiation. Loss of *Sim2s* in breast cancer cells resulted in downregulation of epithelial markers and acquisition of a basal-like phenotype. *Sim2s* is developmentally regulated throughout mammary gland development with highest expression during lactation. Mammary glands from nulliparous mice expressing *Sim2s* driven by the mouse mammary tumor virus long terminal repeat promoter were morphologically indistinguishable from wild-type mice but displayed hallmarks of precocious lactogenic differentiation with elevated expression of Wap and Csn2 [162]. It is of interest that in postlactational mammary gland regression the oncostatin M (OSM) also named Spp1 is upregulated and inhibits proliferation and promotes cell detachment and enhances cell motility. Concurrently, OSM signaling precipitated the dephosphorylation of STAT5 and repressed expression of the milk protein genes beta-casein and Wap. Similarly, during pregnancy, OSM signaling suppressed beta-casein and *Wap* gene expression. OSM also promoted the expression of metalloproteinases MMP3, MMP12, and MMP14, which, in vitro, were responsible for OSM-specific apoptosis [163].

Table 3.19 Biological processes overrepresented among the genes downregulated by hCG ($p<0.01$ and FC 2.0)

GOBPID	*P*-value	Odds ratio	Exp count	Count	Size	Term
GO:0006955	0	8.776	3	17	438	Immune response
GO:0002429	0	27.598	0	7	53	Immune response-activating cell surface receptor signaling pathway
GO:0002684	0	8.864	2	13	307	Positive regulation of immune system process
GO:0002764	0	15.5	1	8	103	Immune response-regulating signaling pathway
GO:0002253	0	11.837	1	8	132	Activation of immune response
GO:0050670	0	12.748	1	7	106	Regulation of lymphocyte proliferation
GO:0001775	0	8.738	1	9	224	Cell activation
GO:0070663	0	12.248	1	7	110	Regulation of leukocyte proliferation
GO:0032946	0	15.886	0	6	73	Positive regulation of mononuclear cell proliferation
GO:0030890	0	31.19	0	4	26	Positive regulation of B-cell proliferation
GO:0002694	0	7.837	1	8	194	Regulation of leukocyte activation
GO:0002520	0	5.809	2	10	332	Immune system development
GO:0050852	0	26.38	0	4	30	T-cell receptor signaling pathway
GO:0046649	0	14.309	0	5	77	Lymphocyte activation
GO:0051251	0	9.63	1	6	116	Positive regulation of lymphocyte activation
GO:0030097	0	5.746	2	9	297	Hemopoiesis
GO:0006816	0	7.235	1	7	180	Calcium ion transport
GO:0035556	0	3.358	6	17	1,041	Intracellular signal transduction
GO:0050853	0	33.7	0	3	18	B-cell receptor signaling pathway
GO:0043123	0	10.858	1	5	85	Positive regulation of I-kappaB kinase/NF-kappaB cascade
GO:0050867	0	8.005	1	6	138	Positive regulation of cell activation
GO:0042098	0	10.337	1	5	89	T-cell proliferation
GO:0072511	0	6.403	1	7	202	Divalent inorganic cation transport
GO:0002312	0	25.261	0	3	23	B-cell activation involved in immune response
GO:0050864	0	12.431	0	4	59	Regulation of B-cell activation
GO:0043067	0.001	77.702	0	2	7	Regulation of programmed cell death
GO:0048584	0.001	6.244	1	6	201	Positive regulation of response to stimulus

(continued)

Table 3.19 (continued)

GOBPID	*P*-value	Odds ratio	Exp count	Count	Size	Term
GO:0009967	0.001	4.128	3	9	405	Positive regulation of signal transduction
GO:0048522	0.001	2.885	8	17	1,360	Positive regulation of cellular process
GO:0023051	0.001	2.882	7	16	1,103	Regulation of signaling
GO:0018212	0.001	7.331	1	5	123	Peptidyl-tyrosine modification
GO:0046632	0.001	16.278	0	3	34	Alpha-beta T-cell differentiation
GO:0002366	0.001	9.347	0	4	77	Leukocyte activation involved in immune response
GO:0006874	0.001	5.496	1	6	197	Cellular calcium ion homeostasis
GO:0007260	0.001	15.288	0	3	36	Tyrosine phosphorylation of STAT protein
GO:0007204	0.002	6.493	1	5	138	Elevation of cytosolic calcium ion concentration
GO:0043368	0.002	41.391	0	2	10	Positive T-cell selection
GO:0045830	0.002	41.391	0	2	10	Positive regulation of isotype switching
GO:0006464	0.002	2.603	8	17	1,296	Protein modification process
GO:0055082	0.002	3.67	3	9	452	Cellular chemical homeostasis
GO:0050801	0.002	3.661	3	9	453	Ion homeostasis
GO:0016265	0.002	2.818	6	14	958	Death
GO:0072507	0.002	5.138	1	6	210	Divalent inorganic cation homeostasis
GO:0030098	0.002	8.459	1	4	89	Lymphocyte differentiation
GO:0042981	0.002	2.948	5	12	768	Regulation of apoptosis
GO:0030183	0.003	12.294	0	3	44	B-cell differentiation
GO:0051607	0.003	12.294	0	3	44	Defense response to virus
GO:0050730	0.003	7.401	1	4	96	Regulation of peptidyl-tyrosine phosphorylation
GO:0046640	0.003	27.582	0	2	14	Regulation of alpha-beta T-cell proliferation
GO:0055065	0.004	4.465	1	6	240	Metal ion homeostasis
GO:0042325	0.004	3.203	3	9	513	Regulation of phosphorylation
GO:0001934	0.004	5.12	1	5	173	Positive regulation of protein phosphorylation
GO:0046425	0.004	10.071	0	3	53	Regulation of JAK-STAT cascade
GO:0032943	0.004	10.035	0	3	59	Mononuclear cell proliferation

GO:0030003	0.005	4.223	2	6	253	Cellular cation homeostasis
GO:0009605	0.005	2.669	5	12	840	Response to external stimulus
GO:0032879	0.005	2.647	5	12	846	Regulation of localization
GO:0060548	0.005	3.33	3	8	434	Negative regulation of cell death
GO:0051174	0.005	3.086	3	9	531	Regulation of phosphorus metabolic process
GO:0008284	0.005	3.322	3	8	435	Positive regulation of cell proliferation
GO:0030838	0.005	20.677	0	2	18	Positive regulation of actin filament polymerization
GO:0042516	0.005	20.677	0	2	18	Regulation of tyrosine phosphorylation of Stat3 protein
GO:0045687	0.005	20.677	0	2	18	Positive regulation of glial cell differentiation
GO:0060255	0.006	2.139	12	21	1,974	Regulation of macromolecule metabolic process
GO:0048873	0.006	19.459	0	2	19	Homeostasis of number of cells within a tissue
GO:0010646	0.006	2.579	5	12	866	Regulation of cell communication
GO:0002316	0.006	Inf	0	1	1	Follicular B-cell differentiation
GO:0002432	0.006	Inf	0	1	1	Granuloma formation
GO:0010037	0.006	Inf	0	1	1	Response to carbon dioxide
GO:0010764	0.006	Inf	0	1	1	Negative regulation of fibroblast migration
GO:0021747	0.006	Inf	0	1	1	Cochlear nucleus development
GO:0030322	0.006	Inf	0	1	1	Stabilization of membrane potential
GO:0032848	0.006	Inf	0	1	1	Negative regulation of cellular pH reduction
GO:0035408	0.006	Inf	0	1	1	Histone H3-T6 phosphorylation
GO:0035417	0.006	Inf	0	1	1	Negative regulation of mitotic prometaphase
GO:0035759	0.006	Inf	0	1	1	Mesangial cell-matrix adhesion
GO:0042322	0.006	Inf	0	1	1	Negative regulation of circadian sleep/wake cycle, REM sleep
GO:0043375	0.006	Inf	0	1	1	CD8-positive, alpha-beta T-cell lineage commitment
GO:0043420	0.006	Inf	0	1	1	Anthranilate metabolic process
GO:0046671	0.006	Inf	0	1	1	Negative regulation of retinal cell programmed cell death
GO:0051126	0.006	Inf	0	1	1	Negative regulation of actin nucleation
GO:2000508	0.006	Inf	0	1	1	Regulation of dendritic cell chemotaxis

(continued)

Table 3.19 (continued)

GOBPID	*P*-value	Odds ratio	Exp count	Count	Size	Term
GO:2000529	0.006	Inf	0	1	1	Positive regulation of myeloid dendritic cell chemotaxis
GO:0040012	0.006	3.959	2	6	269	Regulation of locomotion
GO:0008154	0.006	8.674	0	3	61	Actin polymerization or depolymerization
GO:0060249	0.007	5.804	1	4	121	Anatomical structure homeostasis
GO:0048871	0.007	5.657	1	4	124	Multicellular organismal homeostasis
GO:0045937	0.007	4.468	1	5	197	Positive regulation of phosphate metabolic process
GO:0002204	0.007	17.407	0	2	21	Somatic recombination of immunoglobulin genes involved in immune response
GO:0035023	0.008	8.111	0	3	65	Regulation of Rho protein signal transduction
GO:0002697	0.008	5.517	1	4	127	Regulation of immune effector process
GO:0032321	0.008	16.535	0	2	22	Positive regulation of Rho GTPase activity
GO:0010627	0.008	3.729	2	6	300	Regulation of intracellular protein kinase cascade
GO:0000018	0.009	15.745	0	2	23	Regulation of DNA recombination
GO:0043029	0.009	15.745	0	2	23	T-cell homeostasis
GO:0048002	0.009	15.745	0	2	23	Antigen processing and presentation of peptide antigen
GO:0002381	0.01	15.028	0	2	24	Immunoglobulin production involved in immunoglobulin-mediated immune response

Table 3.20 Biological processes overrepresented among the genes upregulated by hCG ($p<0.01$ and FC 2.0)

GOBPID	*P*-value	Odds ratio	Exp count	Count	Size	Term
GO:0042060	0	9.106	1	8	209	Wound healing
GO:0035313	0	77.693	0	3	11	Wound healing, spreading of epidermal cells
GO:0006950	0	4.546	4	14	951	Response to stress
GO:0031069	0	44.367	0	3	17	Hair follicle morphogenesis
GO:0071223	0	135.126	0	2	5	Cellular response to lipoteichoic acid
GO:0032755	0	23.858	0	3	29	Positive regulation of interleukin-6 production
GO:0001817	0	6.844	1	6	197	Regulation of cytokine production
GO:0048630	0.001	67.541	0	2	8	Skeletal muscle tissue growth
GO:0009888	0.001	3.583	4	11	728	Tissue development
GO:0030855	0.001	7.074	1	5	156	Epithelial cell differentiation
GO:0048518	0.002	2.59	11	20	2,049	Positive regulation of biological process
GO:0045087	0.002	6.16	1	5	178	Innate immune response
GO:0016477	0.002	3.917	2	8	462	Cell migration
GO:0022404	0.003	12.13	0	3	54	Molting cycle process
GO:0042633	0.003	11.895	0	3	55	Hair cycle
GO:0006954	0.003	4.727	1	6	280	Inflammatory response
GO:0051674	0.003	3.67	3	8	491	Localization of cell
GO:0006958	0.004	25.3	0	2	18	Complement activation, classical pathway
GO:0030512	0.004	25.3	0	2	18	Negative regulation of transforming growth factor beta receptor signaling pathway
GO:0010718	0.004	23.809	0	2	19	Positive regulation of epithelial to mesenchymal transition
GO:0009967	0.004	3.837	2	7	405	Positive regulation of signal transduction
GO:0040007	0.004	3.45	3	8	520	Growth
GO:0008283	0.005	2.855	5	11	893	Cell proliferation
GO:0032760	0.005	21.298	0	2	21	Positive regulation of tumor necrosis factor production
GO:0002232	0.005	Inf	0	1	1	Leukocyte chemotaxis involved in inflammatory response
GO:0007499	0.005	Inf	0	1	1	Ectoderm and mesoderm interaction

(continued)

Table 3.20 (continued)

GOBPID	*P*-value	Odds ratio	Exp count	Count	Size	Term
GO:0010232	0.005	Inf	0	1	1	Vascular transport
GO:0014064	0.005	Inf	0	1	1	Positive regulation of serotonin secretion
GO:0019546	0.005	Inf	0	1	1	Arginine deiminase pathway
GO:0035482	0.005	Inf	0	1	1	Gastric motility
GO:0048627	0.005	Inf	0	1	1	Myoblast development
GO:0048685	0.005	Inf	0	1	1	Negative regulation of collateral sprouting of intact axon in response to injury
GO:0060265	0.005	Inf	0	1	1	Positive regulation of respiratory burst involved in inflammatory response
GO:0060529	0.005	Inf	0	1	1	Squamous basal epithelial stem cell differentiation involved in prostate gland acinus development
GO:2000293	0.005	Inf	0	1	1	Negative regulation of defecation
GO:0048732	0.005	4.91	1	5	221	Gland development
GO:0002252	0.005	4.886	1	5	222	Immune effector process
GO:0050678	0.005	6.194	1	4	139	Regulation of epithelial cell proliferation
GO:0060512	0.006	19.266	0	2	23	Prostate gland morphogenesis
GO:0071222	0.006	8.819	0	3	73	Cellular response to lipopolysaccharide
GO:0052548	0.006	5.884	1	4	146	Regulation of endopeptidase activity
GO:0008015	0.008	4.388	1	5	246	Blood circulation
GO:0030001	0.008	3.358	2	7	459	Metal ion transport
GO:0006928	0.009	3.067	3	8	580	Cellular component movement
GO:0050776	0.009	4.296	1	5	251	Regulation of immune response
GO:0040011	0.009	3.033	3	8	586	Locomotion
GO:0071216	0.009	7.518	0	3	85	Cellular response to biotic stimulus
GO:0032879	0.009	2.679	4	10	846	Regulation of localization
GO:0033554	0.009	3.016	3	8	589	Cellular response to stress
GO:0050909	0.01	14.974	0	2	29	Sensory perception of taste
GO:0010466	0.01	7.427	0	3	86	Negative regulation of peptidase activity

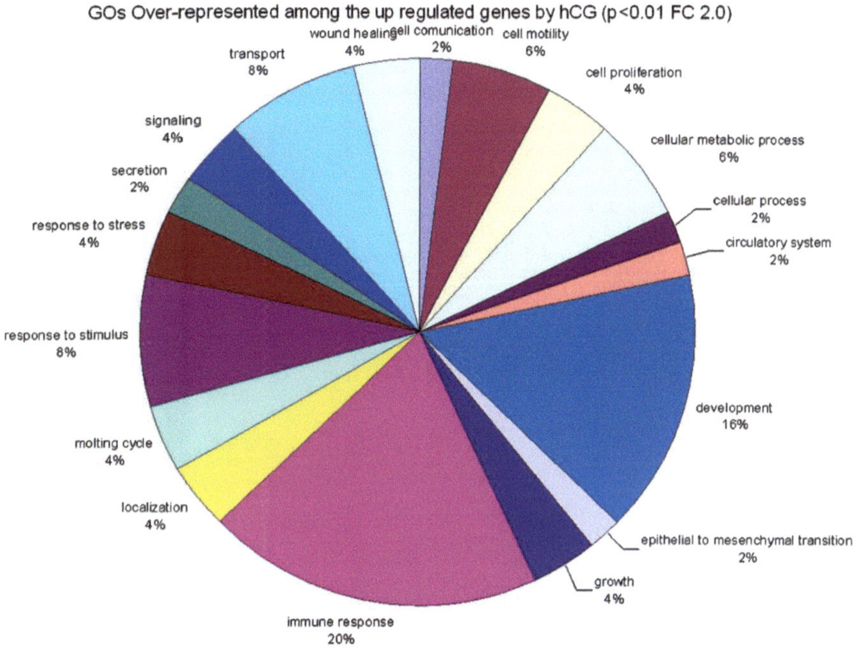

Fig. 3.26 Gene ontology of the overrepresented genes upregulated by hCG in the rat mammary gland using a $p<0.01$ and FC of 2.0

A gene that is overexpressed in the rat mammary glands of rats subjected to the three prevention modalities is the *Tgfb3* or transforming growth factor beta3 that encodes a member of the TGF-beta family of proteins. The encoded protein is secreted and is involved in embryogenesis and cell differentiation. The transforming growth factor-beta family of polypeptides (TGF-beta1, TGF-beta2, and TGF-beta3) is involved in the regulation of cellular processes, including cell division, differentiation, motility, adhesion, and death [164–169]. TGF-beta signals by binding the TGF-beta type II receptor (TGF-betaRII) which transphosphorylates and activates the type I receptor (TGF-betaRI). Activated TGF-betaRI then phosphorylates a subset of SMAD proteins, Smad2 and Smad3, which translocate to the nucleus where they form transcription complexes with DNA binding factors and co-activators/co-repressors. TGF-beta functions as a tumor suppressor by inhibiting the cell cycle in the G1 phase. Administration of TGF-beta is able to protect against mammary tumor development in transgenic mouse models in vivo [167, 168, 170–172]. TGF-beta3 may play a protective role against tumorigenesis in a range of tissues including the skin, breast, oral, and gastric mucosa [173]. During rodent mammary gland involution there is a dramatic increase in the expression of the Tgfb3 [174]. Persistent pregnancy-induced changes in mammary gene expression that are tightly associated with protection against tumorigenesis in multiple inbred rat strains have implicated alterations in transforming growth factor-beta signaling. IGF-I treatment of parous

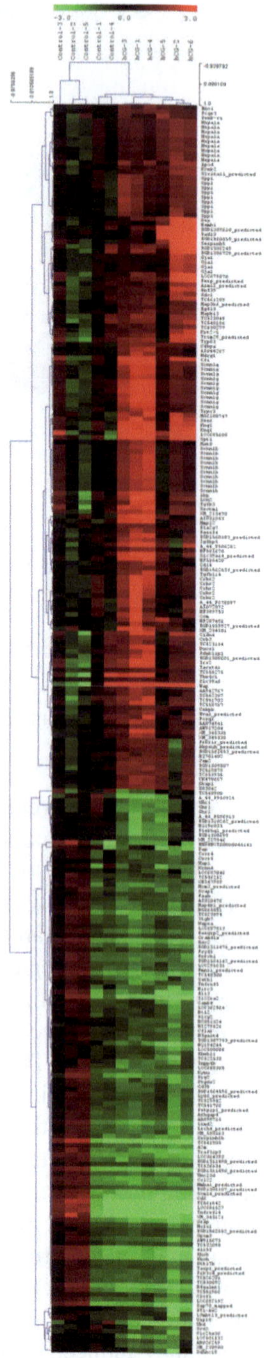

Fig. 3.27 Heat map showing the up- (*red*) and downregulated genes (*green*) of hCG treated rat mammary glands using a $p < 0.01$ and FC of 2.0

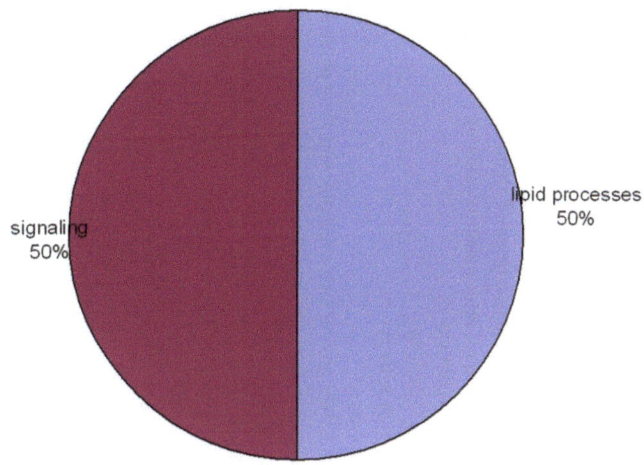

Fig. 3.28 Gene Ontology of overrepresented genes downregulated in the mammary gland of rats after pregnancy using a $p<0.01$ and FC of 2.0

rats increased mammary tumor incidence to 83%, as compared with 16% in parous rats treated with 17β-estradiol plus progesterone only. Tumor incidence and average number of tumors per animal did not differ between IGF-I-treated parous rats and age-matched virgin rats. Thordarson et al. [166] demonstrated that at the time of *N*-methyl-*N*-nitrosourea exposure, DNA content was lowest but the alpha-lactalbumin concentration was highest in the mammary glands of untreated parous rats in comparison with age-matched virgin and IGF-I-treated parous rats [166]. The protein levels of estrogen receptor-alpha in the mammary gland were significantly higher in the age-matched virgin animals than in untreated parous and IGF-I-treated parous rats. Phosphorylation (activation) of the extracellular signal-regulated kinase-1/2 (ERK1/2) and expression of the progesterone receptor were both increased in IGF-I-treated parous rats, as compared with those in untreated parous and age-matched virgin rats. Expressions of cyclin D1 and tgfb3 in the mammary gland were lower in the age-matched virgin rats than in the untreated parous and IGF-I-treated parous rats [166]. All this indicate that tgfb3 is a common pathway in cancer prevention induced by the three different treatment modalities (Figs. 3.32 and 3.33).

The iroquois homeobox 2 (*Irx2*) is upregulated by hCG and pregnancy hormones in the rat mammary gland. The Iroquois (Irx) genes encode homeoproteins conserved during evolution. Vertebrate genomes contain six Irx genes organized in two clusters, IrxA (which harbors Irx1, Irx2, and Irx4) and IrxB (which harbors Irx3, Irx5, and Irx6). The five Irx genes display largely overlapping expression patterns and contribute to neural patterning. All Irx genes are required for proper

Table 3.21 Biological processes overrepresented among the genes downregulated by pregnancy ($p < 0.01$ and FC 2.0)

GOBPID	*P*-value	Odds ratio	Exp count	Count	Size	Term
GO:0071883	0.001	4583.5	0	1	3	Activation of MAPK activity by adrenergic receptor signaling pathway
GO:0035625	0.001	3055.333	0	1	4	Epidermal growth factor-activated receptor transactivation by G-protein coupled receptor signaling pathway
GO:0032148	0.002	1145.125	0	1	9	Activation of protein kinase B activity
GO:2000273	0.002	915.9	0	1	11	Positive regulation of receptor activity
GO:0019433	0.003	763.083	0	1	13	Triglyceride catabolic process
GO:0045742	0.003	704.308	0	1	14	Positive regulation of epidermal growth factor receptor signaling pathway
GO:0007176	0.003	653.929	0	1	15	Regulation of epidermal growth factor-activated receptor activity
GO:0044269	0.003	653.929	0	1	15	Glycerol ether catabolic process
GO:0046461	0.003	653.929	0	1	15	Neutral lipid catabolic process
GO:0061098	0.004	538.353	0	1	18	Positive regulation of protein tyrosine kinase activity
GO:0046503	0.004	508.389	0	1	19	Glycerolipid catabolic process
GO:0019432	0.006	326.464	0	1	29	Triglyceride biosynthetic process
GO:0046460	0.006	326.464	0	1	29	Neutral lipid biosynthetic process
GO:0046504	0.007	304.633	0	1	31	Glycerol ether biosynthetic process

Table 3.22 Biological processes overrepresented among the genes upregulated by pregnancy ($p<0.01$ and FC 2.0)

GOBPID	*P*-value	Odds ratio	Exp count	Count	Size	Term
GO:0035313	0	92.463	0	3	11	Wound healing, spreading of epidermal cells
GO:0006950	0	3.692	7	17	1,540	Response to stress
GO:0042060	0	7.761	1	6	209	Wound healing
GO:0031103	0	25.448	0	3	32	Axon regeneration
GO:0045730	0.001	43.636	0	2	13	Respiratory burst
GO:0010033	0.002	2.951	6	13	1,294	Response to organic substance
GO:0002682	0.003	4.15	2	7	451	Regulation of immune system process
GO:0001818	0.003	11.487	0	3	67	Negative regulation of cytokine production
GO:0006921	0.004	23.976	0	2	22	Cellular component disassembly involved in apoptosis
GO:0002232	0.004	Inf	0	1	1	Leukocyte chemotaxis involved in inflammatory response
GO:0006709	0.004	Inf	0	1	1	Progesterone catabolic process
GO:0014064	0.004	Inf	0	1	1	Positive regulation of serotonin secretion
GO:0032078	0.004	Inf	0	1	1	Negative regulation of endodeoxyribonuclease activity
GO:0032600	0.004	Inf	0	1	1	Chemokine receptor transport out of membrane raft
GO:0032913	0.004	Inf	0	1	1	Negative regulation of transforming growth factor beta3 production
GO:0034107	0.004	Inf	0	1	1	Negative regulation of erythrocyte clearance
GO:0034119	0.004	Inf	0	1	1	Negative regulation of erythrocyte aggregation
GO:0035482	0.004	Inf	0	1	1	Gastric motility
GO:0042103	0.004	Inf	0	1	1	Positive regulation of T-cell homeostatic proliferation
GO:0046014	0.004	Inf	0	1	1	Negative regulation of T-cell homeostatic proliferation
GO:0048685	0.004	Inf	0	1	1	Negative regulation of collateral sprouting of intact axon in response to injury
GO:0060265	0.004	Inf	0	1	1	Positive regulation of respiratory burst involved in inflammatory response
GO:2000293	0.004	Inf	0	1	1	Negative regulation of defecation
GO:0070887	0.007	3.044	4	9	804	Cellular response to chemical stimulus
GO:0032755	0.007	17.747	0	2	29	Positive regulation of interleukin-6 production
GO:0034103	0.007	17.747	0	2	29	Regulation of tissue remodeling

(continued)

Table 3.22 (continued)

GOBPID	*P*-value	Odds ratio	Exp count	Count	Size	Term
GO:0050909	0.007	17.747	0	2	29	Sensory perception of taste
GO:0006954	0.007	4.601	1	5	280	Inflammatory response
GO:0045087	0.007	5.72	1	4	178	Innate immune response
GO:0050795	0.008	8.145	0	3	93	Regulation of behavior
GO:0002690	0.008	16.519	0	2	31	Positive regulation of leukocyte chemotaxis
GO:0006956	0.008	16.519	0	2	31	Complement activation
GO:0051704	0.008	3.401	2	7	543	Multi-organism process
GO:0031346	0.008	7.88	0	3	96	Positive regulation of cell projection organization
GO:0050778	0.008	5.494	1	4	185	Positive regulation of immune response
GO:0048545	0.008	3.792	2	6	412	Response to steroid hormone stimulus
GO:0002842	0.009	234.103	0	1	2	Positive regulation of T-cell-mediated immune response to tumor cell
GO:0006922	0.009	234.103	0	1	2	Cleavage of lamin
GO:0015891	0.009	234.103	0	1	2	Siderophore transport
GO:0015920	0.009	234.103	0	1	2	Lipopolysaccharide transport
GO:0032074	0.009	234.103	0	1	2	Negative regulation of nuclease activity
GO:0032594	0.009	234.103	0	1	2	Protein transport within lipid bilayer
GO:0033037	0.009	234.103	0	1	2	Polysaccharide localization
GO:0033212	0.009	234.103	0	1	2	Iron assimilation
GO:0042335	0.009	234.103	0	1	2	Cuticle development
GO:0043932	0.009	234.103	0	1	2	Ossification involved in bone remodeling
GO:0070483	0.009	234.103	0	1	2	Detection of hypoxia
GO:0090281	0.009	234.103	0	1	2	Negative regulation of calcium ion import
GO:2000252	0.009	234.103	0	1	2	Negative regulation of feeding behavior
GO:0032103	0.01	7.474	0	3	101	Positive regulation of response to external stimulus

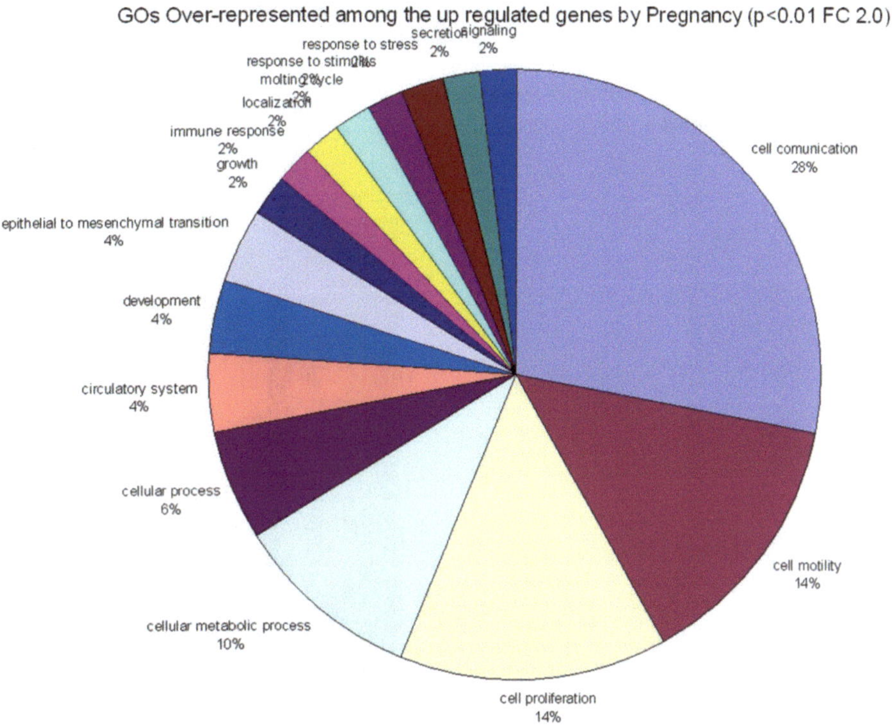

Fig. 3.29 Gene ontology of the overrepresented genes upregulated by pregnancy in the rat mammary gland using a $p<0.01$ and FC of 2.0

formation of posterior forebrain, midbrain, hindbrain and, to a lesser extent, spinal cord [175–177]. IRX2 methylated in 85–100% of the squamous cell carcinomas [178] and is overexpressed in 3D prostate cultures [179]. CpG islands in the HOXA cluster and other homeobox (Irx2, DLX2, NKX2-2) genes were significantly more methylated in Luminal A tumors [180]. Irx2a is expressed in the developing retina and that knockdown of irx2a results in a retinal phenotype strikingly similar to that of irx1a morphants. The expression of irx2a in retina ganglion cells was shown to be irx1a- and ath5-dependent suggesting that irx1a and ath5 are transcriptional regulators of irx2a. Furthermore, irx2a expression could rescue impaired propagation of shh waves in irx1a morphants. Together, these observations suggest that Irx2 functions downstream of irx1a to control shh expression in the retina. There is a transcriptional cascade of ath5-irx1a-irx2a in the regulation of hedgehog waves during vertebrate retinal development [181]. Comparative studies in *Xenopus* and mouse have identified Irx1, Irx2, and Irx3 as an evolutionary conserved subset of Irx genes, whose expression represents the earliest manifestation of intermediate compartment patterning in the developing vertebrate nephron discovered to date. Intermediate tubule progenitors will give rise to epithelia of Henle's loop in mammals. Loss-of-function studies

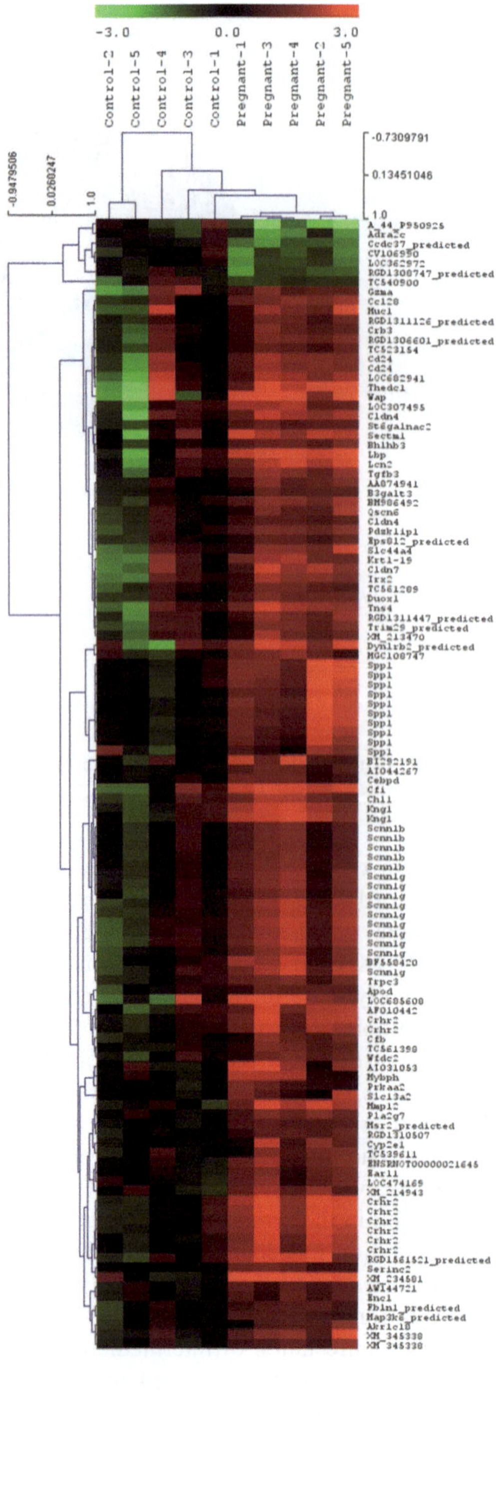

Fig. 3.30 Heat map showing the up- (*red*) and downregulated genes (*green*) of post pregnancy rat mammary glands using a $p<0.01$ and FC of 2.0

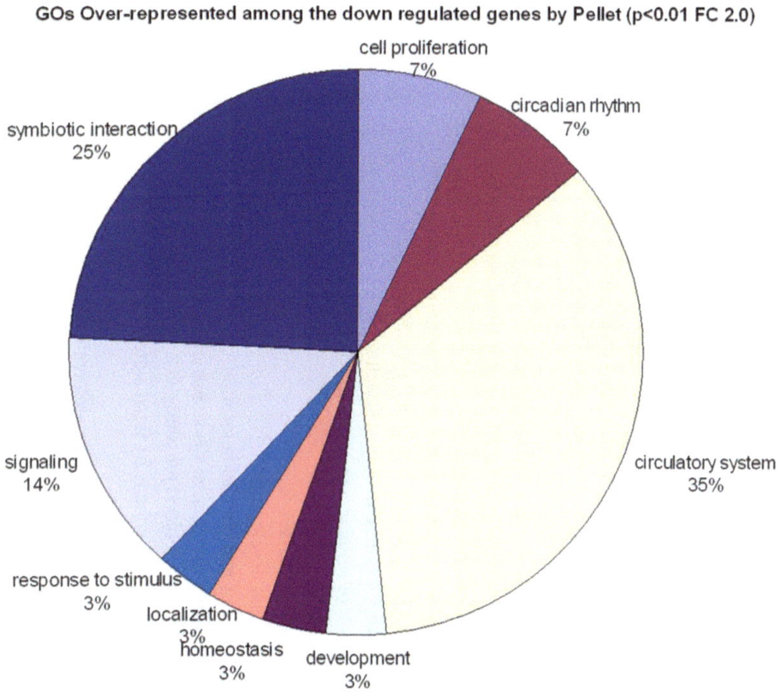

Fig. 3.31 Gene Ontology of the overrepresented genes downregulated in the mammary gland of pellet treated rats using a $p<0.01$ and FC of 2.0

indicate that irx1 and Irx2 are dispensable, whereas irx3 is necessary for intermediate tubule formation in *Xenopus* [182]. Irx1 and Irx2 serve an evolutionary conserved role in the regulation of alpha-cell-specific gene expression regulating pancreatic endocrine development and function [183]. In the stage during which ES cells differentiate into neural stem cells, modulation of nearly 1,000 genes was observed. Most of transcription factors (Otx2, Ebf-3, Ptx3, Sox4, 13, 18, engrailed, Irx2, Pax8, and Lim3), signaling molecules (Wnt, TGF, and Shh family members), and ECM/adhesion molecules (collagens, MAPs, and NCAM) were upregulated. However, some genes which may play important roles in maintaining the pluripotency of ES cells (Kruppel-like factor 2, 4, 5, 9, myeloblast oncogene like2, ZFP 57, and Esg-1) were downregulated [184]. *Therefore it is possible to speculate that Irx2 is involved in the pattern of mammary gland differentiation and that is elicited by the three prevention modalities* (Figs. 3.21 and 3.22).

Claudin 4 (*Cldn4*) is upregulated in the rat mammary gland by the three prevention modalities tested. This gene encodes an integral membrane protein, which belongs to the claudin family [185]. The protein is a component of tight junction strands and may play a role in internal organ development and function during pre- and postnatal life. Expression of adhesion molecules (AM) in the adherens, tight and gap junction pathways in embryonic stem cells subpopulations

Table 3.23 Biological processes overrepresented among the genes downregulated by pellet ($p<0.01$ and FC 2.0)

GOBPID	*P*-value	Odds ratio	Exp count	Count	Size	Term
GO:0003013	0	18.424	0	4	246	Circulatory system process
GO:0003044	0.001	58.89	0	2	33	Regulation of systemic arterial blood pressure mediated by a chemical signal
GO:0042752	0.001	52.137	0	2	37	Regulation of circadian rhythm
GO:0045777	0.001	48.005	0	2	40	Positive regulation of blood pressure
GO:0001907	0.001	Inf	0	1	1	Killing by symbiont of host cells
GO:0001986	0.001	Inf	0	1	1	Negative regulation of the force of heart contraction involved in baroreceptor response to increased systemic arterial blood pressure
GO:0002158	0.001	Inf	0	1	1	Osteoclast proliferation
GO:0019836	0.001	Inf	0	1	1	Hemolysis by symbiont of host erythrocytes
GO:0031547	0.001	Inf	0	1	1	Brain-derived neurotrophic factor receptor signaling pathway
GO:0044179	0.001	Inf	0	1	1	Hemolysis in other organism
GO:0051801	0.001	Inf	0	1	1	Cytolysis in other organism involved in symbiotic interaction
GO:0052025	0.001	Inf	0	1	1	Modification by symbiont of host cell membrane
GO:0052111	0.001	Inf	0	1	1	Modification by symbiont of host structure
GO:0052188	0.001	Inf	0	1	1	Modification of cellular component in other organism involved in symbiotic interaction
GO:0003014	0.002	37.962	0	2	50	Renal system process
GO:0046548	0.003	832.545	0	1	2	Retinal rod cell development
GO:0051659	0.003	832.545	0	1	2	Maintenance of mitochondrion location
GO:0001994	0.004	416.227	0	1	3	Norepinephrine-epinephrine vasoconstriction involved in regulation of systemic arterial blood pressure
GO:0002017	0.004	416.227	0	1	3	Regulation of blood volume by renal aldosterone
GO:0070541	0.004	416.227	0	1	3	Response to platinum ion
GO:0071883	0.004	416.227	0	1	3	Activation of MAPK activity by adrenergic receptor signaling pathway
GO:0035625	0.005	277.455	0	1	4	Epidermal growth factor-activated receptor transactivation by G-protein coupled receptor signaling pathway
GO:0001978	0.007	208.068	0	1	5	Regulation of systemic arterial blood pressure by carotid sinus baroreceptor feedback

GO:0046010	0.007	208.068	0	1	5	Positive regulation of circadian sleep/wake cycle, non-REM sleep
GO:0065008	0.008	5.07	2	6	1,515	Regulation of biological quality
GO:0050880	0.008	17.759	0	2	104	Regulation of blood vessel size
GO:0051818	0.008	166.436	0	1	6	Disruption of cells of other organism involved in symbiotic interaction
GO:0071875	0.008	152.517	0	1	7	Adrenergic receptor signaling pathway
GO:0033688	0.009	138.682	0	1	7	Regulation of osteoblast proliferation

Table 3.24 Biological processes overrepresented among the genes upregulated by pellet ($p<0.01$ and FC 2.0)

GOBPID	*P*-value	Odds ratio	Exp count	Count	Size	Term
GO:0061179	0	456.4	0	2	3	Negative regulation of insulin secretion involved in cellular response to glucose stimulus
GO:0006950	0	3.749	7	18	1,540	Response to stress
GO:0009725	0	4.466	3	11	683	Response to hormone stimulus
GO:0043949	0	91.24	0	2	7	Regulation of cAMP-mediated signaling
GO:0032967	0.001	50.667	0	2	11	Positive regulation of collagen biosynthetic process
GO:0035313	0.001	50.667	0	2	11	Wound healing, spreading of epidermal cells
GO:0045730	0.002	41.445	0	2	13	Respiratory burst
GO:0019725	0.002	4.027	2	8	512	Cellular homeostasis
GO:0043627	0.002	6.127	1	5	202	Response to estrogen stimulus
GO:0009967	0.002	4.387	2	7	405	Positive regulation of signal transduction
GO:0010712	0.002	32.554	0	2	16	Regulation of collagen metabolic process
GO:0048518	0.002	2.621	9	18	2,049	Positive regulation of biological process
GO:0007565	0.002	7.903	1	4	124	Female pregnancy
GO:0007568	0.002	5.956	1	5	213	Aging
GO:0042060	0.003	5.912	1	5	209	Wound healing
GO:0044253	0.003	30.38	0	2	17	Positive regulation of multicellular organismal metabolic process
GO:0002237	0.003	5.524	1	5	223	Response to molecule of bacterial origin
GO:0001818	0.003	10.895	0	3	67	Negative regulation of cytokine production
GO:0006921	0.004	22.773	0	2	22	Cellular component disassembly involved in apoptosis
GO:0007155	0.005	3.813	2	7	462	Cell adhesion
GO:0002232	0.005	Inf	0	1	1	Leukocyte chemotaxis involved in inflammatory response
GO:0007499	0.005	Inf	0	1	1	Ectoderm and mesoderm interaction
GO:0014064	0.005	Inf	0	1	1	Positive regulation of serotonin secretion
GO:0032078	0.005	Inf	0	1	1	Negative regulation of endodeoxyribonuclease activity
GO:0032600	0.005	Inf	0	1	1	Chemokine receptor transport out of membrane raft
GO:0032913	0.005	Inf	0	1	1	Negative regulation of transforming growth factor beta3 production
GO:0034107	0.005	Inf	0	1	1	Negative regulation of erythrocyte clearance

GO:0034119	0.005	Inf	0	1	1	Negative regulation of erythrocyte aggregation
GO:0035482	0.005	Inf	0	1	1	Gastric motility
GO:0042103	0.005	Inf	0	1	1	Positive regulation of T-cell homeostatic proliferation
GO:0046014	0.005	Inf	0	1	1	Negative regulation of T-cell homeostatic proliferation
GO:0048685	0.005	Inf	0	1	1	Negative regulation of collateral sprouting of intact axon in response to injury
GO:0060265	0.005	Inf	0	1	1	Positive regulation of respiratory burst involved in inflammatory response
GO:0060529	0.005	Inf	0	1	1	Squamous basal epithelial stem cell differentiation involved in prostate gland acinus development
GO:2000293	0.005	Inf	0	1	1	Negative regulation of defecation
GO:0010876	0.005	6.522	1	4	149	Lipid localization
GO:0070482	0.006	4.78	1	5	256	Response to oxygen levels
GO:0032844	0.006	6.015	1	4	161	Regulation of homeostatic process
GO:0032755	0.008	16.856	0	2	29	Positive regulation of interleukin-6 production
GO:0034103	0.008	16.856	0	2	29	Regulation of tissue remodeling
GO:0090278	0.008	16.856	0	2	29	Negative regulation of peptide hormone secretion
GO:0022411	0.008	7.903	0	3	91	Cellular component disassembly
GO:0007623	0.008	7.813	0	3	92	Circadian rhythm
GO:0006954	0.009	4.351	1	5	280	Inflammatory response
GO:0045087	0.009	5.417	1	4	178	Innate immune response
GO:0006956	0.009	15.69	0	2	31	Complement activation
GO:0002842	0.009	222.634	0	1	2	Positive regulation of T-cell-mediated immune response to tumor cell
GO:0006922	0.009	222.634	0	1	2	Cleavage of lamin
GO:0010260	0.009	222.634	0	1	2	Organ senescence
GO:0015891	0.009	222.634	0	1	2	Siderophore transport
GO:0015920	0.009	222.634	0	1	2	Lipopolysaccharide transport
GO:0032074	0.009	222.634	0	1	2	Negative regulation of nuclease activity

(continued)

Table 3.24 (continued)

GOBPID	*P*-value	Odds ratio	Exp count	Count	Size	Term
GO:0032594	0.009	222.634	0	1	2	Protein transport within lipid bilayer
GO:0033037	0.009	222.634	0	1	2	Polysaccharide localization
GO:0033212	0.009	222.634	0	1	2	Iron assimilation
GO:0042335	0.009	222.634	0	1	2	Cuticle development
GO:0043932	0.009	222.634	0	1	2	Ossification involved in bone remodeling
GO:0045617	0.009	222.634	0	1	2	Negative regulation of keratinocyte differentiation
GO:0060197	0.009	222.634	0	1	2	Cloacal septation
GO:0070318	0.009	222.634	0	1	2	Positive regulation of G0 to G1 transition
GO:0070483	0.009	222.634	0	1	2	Detection of hypoxia
GO:0071280	0.009	222.634	0	1	2	Cellular response to copper ion
GO:0090281	0.009	222.634	0	1	2	Negative regulation of calcium ion import
GO:2000252	0.009	222.634	0	1	2	Negative regulation of feeding behavior
GO:0031103	0.009	15.165	0	2	32	Axon regeneration
GO:0031346	0.009	7.474	0	3	96	Positive regulation of cell projection organization
GO:0050778	0.01	5.204	1	4	185	Positive regulation of immune response
GO:0071326	0.01	14.674	0	2	33	Cellular response to monosaccharide stimulus
GO:0071333	0.01	14.674	0	2	33	Cellular response to glucose stimulus

Table 3.25 Biological processes and downregulated genes in hCG group ($p<0.01$ and fold change 2)

Symbol	Name
Adhesion (GO:0035759)	
Ccl21	Chemokine (C-C motif) ligand 21
Apoptosis (GO:0043067, GO:0016265, GO:0042981, GO:0060548, GO:0046671)	
Plcg2	Phospholipase C, gamma 2
Cxcr4	Chemokine (C-X-C motif) receptor 4
Cflar	CASP8 and FADD-like apoptosis regulator
Stk17b	Serine/threonine kinase 17b
Cd40	CD40 molecule, TNF receptor superfamily member 5
Bcl2	B-cell CLL/lymphoma 2
Prkcb	Protein kinase C, beta
Cd38	CD38 molecule
Ubd	Ubiquitin D
Ccl21	Chemokine (C-C motif) ligand 21
Clcf1	Cardiotrophin-like cytokine factor 1
Cidec	Cell death-inducing DFFA-like effector c
Ghrl	Ghrelin/obestatin prepropeptide
Birc3	Baculoviral IAP repeat-containing 3
Unc13d	Unc-13 homolog D (*C. elegans*)
Cell activation (GO:0001775, GO:0050867)	
Unc13d	Unc-13 homolog D (*C. elegans*)
Prkcb	Protein kinase C, beta
Ubd	Ubiquitin D
Plcg2	Phospholipase C, gamma 2
Ccl21	Chemokine (C-C motif) ligand 21
Rhoh	Ras homolog gene family, member H
Satb1	SATB homeobox 1
Tnfrsf14	Tumor necrosis factor receptor superfamily, member 14 (herpesvirus entry mediator)
Cxcr4	Chemokine (C-X-C motif) receptor 4
Coro1a	Coronin, actin-binding protein 1A
Cd40	CD40 molecule, TNF receptor superfamily member 5
Bcl2	B-cell CLL/lymphoma 2
Cd38	CD38 molecule
Zap70	Zeta-chain (TCR) associated protein kinase
Clcf1	Cardiotrophin-like cytokine factor 1
Cell communication (GO:0010646)	
Cflar	CASP8 and FADD-like apoptosis regulator
Cd40	CD40 molecule, TNF receptor superfamily member 5
Prkcb	Protein kinase C, beta
Cd38	CD38 molecule
Hcls1	Hematopoietic cell-specific Lyn substrate 1
Ubd	Ubiquitin D
Ccl21	Chemokine (C-C motif) ligand 21
Zap70	Zeta-chain (TCR) associated protein kinase
Rhoh	Ras homolog gene family, member H
Clcf1	Cardiotrophin-like cytokine factor 1

(continued)

Table 3.25 (continued)

Symbol	Name
Ghrl	Ghrelin/obestatin prepropeptide
Kcnn4	Potassium intermediate/small conductance calcium-activated channel, subfamily N, member 4
Cell cycle (GO:0035417)	
Ubd	Ubiquitin D
Cell motility (GO:0010764, GO:2000508, GO:2000529, GO:0040012)	
Arhgap4	Rho GTPase-activating protein 4
Ccl21	Chemokine (C-C motif) ligand 21
Coro1a	Coronin, actin-binding protein 1A
Bcl2	B-cell CLL/lymphoma 2
Ghrl	Ghrelin/obestatin prepropeptide
Cxcr4	Chemokine (C-X-C motif) receptor 4
Cell proliferation (GO:0032946, GO:0032943, GO:0008284)	
Coro1a	Coronin, actin-binding protein 1A
Cd40	CD40 molecule, TNF receptor superfamily member 5
Bcl2	B-cell CLL/lymphoma 2
Cd38	CD38 molecule
Zap70	Zeta-chain (TCR) associated protein kinase
Clcf1	Cardiotrophin-like cytokine factor 1
Satb1	SATB homeobox 1
Tnfrsf14	Tumor necrosis factor receptor superfamily, member 14 (herpesvirus entry mediator)
Cxcr4	Chemokine (C-X-C motif) receptor 4
Hcls1	Hematopoietic cell-specific Lyn substrate 1
Rac2	Ras-related C3 botulinum toxin substrate 2 (rho family, small GTP-binding protein Rac2)
Cellular component organization (GO:0030838, GO:0051126, GO:0008154)	
Coro1a	Coronin, actin-binding protein 1A
Ccl21	Chemokine (C-C motif) ligand 21
Ghrl	Ghrelin/obestatin prepropeptide
Cellular metabolic process (GO:0051174, GO:0060255, GO:0043420, GO:0045937)	
Bcl2	B-cell CLL/lymphoma 2
Cd6	Cd6 molecule
Hcls1	Hematopoietic cell-specific Lyn substrate 1
Ccl21	Chemokine (C-C motif) ligand 21
Rhoh	Ras homolog gene family, member H
Clcf1	Cardiotrophin-like cytokine factor 1
Tnfrsf14	Tumor necrosis factor receptor superfamily, member 14 (herpesvirus entry mediator)
Il22ra2	Interleukin 22 receptor, alpha 2
Ghrl	Ghrelin/obestatin prepropeptide
Cd40	CD40 molecule, TNF receptor superfamily member 5
A2m	Alpha-2-macroglobulin
Prkcb	Protein kinase C, beta
Camk4	Calcium/calmodulin-dependent protein kinase IV
Cd38	CD38 molecule

(continued)

Table 3.25 (continued)

Symbol	Name
Skap1	Src kinase-associated phosphoprotein 1
Plcg2	Phospholipase C, gamma 2
Ell3	Elongation factor RNA polymerase II-like 3
Gria3	Glutamate receptor, ionotrophic, AMPA 3
Tasp1	Taspase, threonine aspartase 1
Satb1	SATB homeobox 1
Rhebl1	Ras homolog enriched in brain like 1
Serpinb6b	Serine (or cysteine) peptidase inhibitor, clade B, member 6b
Kynu	Kynureninase (L-kynurenine hydrolase)
Cellular process (GO:0048522)	
Cflar	CASP8 and FADD-like apoptosis regulator
Stk17b	Serine/threonine kinase 17b
Unc13d	Unc-13 homolog D (*C. elegans*)
Prkcb	Protein kinase C, beta
Camk4	Calcium/calmodulin-dependent protein kinase IV
Cd6	Cd6 molecule
Skap1	Src kinase-associated phosphoprotein 1
Ubd	Ubiquitin D
Hap1	Huntingtin-associated protein 1
Ell3	Elongation factor RNA polymerase II-like 3
Ccl21	Chemokine (C-C motif) ligand 21
Tasp1	Taspase, threonine aspartase 1
Tnfrsf14	Tumor necrosis factor receptor superfamily, member 14 (herpesvirus entry mediator)
Cidec	Cell death-inducing DFFA-like effector c
Ghrl	Ghrelin/obestatin prepropeptide
Cxcr4	Chemokine (C-X-C motif) receptor 4
Kcnn4	Potassium intermediate/small conductance calcium-activated channel, subfamily N, member 4
Circadian rhythm (GO:0042322)	
Ghrl	Ghrelin/obestatin prepropeptide
Development (GO:0030097, GO:0045687, GO:0021747)	
Coro1a	Coronin, actin-binding protein 1A
Bcl2	B-cell CLL/lymphoma 2
Hcls1	Hematopoietic cell-specific Lyn substrate 1
Ubd	Ubiquitin D
Plcg2	Phospholipase C, gamma 2
Zap70	Zeta-chain (TCR) associated protein kinase
Rhoh	Ras homolog gene family, member H
Satb1	SATB homeobox 1
Clcf1	Cardiotrophin-like cytokine factor 1
Cxcr4	Chemokine (C-X-C motif) receptor 4
Homeostasis (GO:0006874, GO:0007204, GO:0055082, GO:0050801, GO:0072507, GO:0055065, GO:0030003, GO:0048873, GO:0030322, GO:0032848, GO:0060249, GO:0048871)	
Bcl2	B-cell CLL/lymphoma 2

(continued)

Table 3.25 (continued)

Symbol	Name
Prkcb	Protein kinase C, beta
Cd38	CD38 molecule
Plcg2	Phospholipase C, gamma 2
Ccl21	Chemokine (C-C motif) ligand 21
Ghrl	Ghrelin/obestatin prepropeptide
Cxcr4	Chemokine (C-X-C motif) receptor 4
Kcnn4	Potassium intermediate/small conductance calcium-activated channel, subfamily N, member 4
Scd	Stearoyl-CoA desaturase (delta-9-desaturase)
Coro1a	Coronin, actin-binding protein 1A
Rac2	Ras-related C3 botulinum toxin substrate 2 (rho family, small GTP-binding protein Rac2)
Immune response (GO:0006955, GO:0002429, GO:0002684, GO:0002764, GO:0002253, GO:0050670, GO:0070663, GO:0030890, GO:0002694, GO:0002520, GO:0050852, GO:0046649, GO:0051251, GO:0050853, GO:0042098, GO:0002312, GO:0050864, GO:0046632, GO:0002366, GO:0043368, GO:0045830, GO:0030098, GO:0030183, GO:0051607, GO:0046640, GO:0002316, GO:0002432, GO:0043375, GO:0002204, GO:0002697, GO:0043029, GO:0048002, GO:0002381)	
Kynu	Kynureninase (L-kynurenine hydrolase)
Cd40	CD40 molecule, TNF receptor superfamily member 5
Unc13d	Unc-13 homolog D (*C. elegans*)
A2m	Alpha-2-macroglobulin
Bcl2	B-cell CLL/lymphoma 2
RT1-EC2	RT1 class Ib, locus EC2
Prkcb	Protein kinase C, beta
Cd38	CD38 molecule
Skap1	Src kinase-associated phosphoprotein 1
Ubd	Ubiquitin D
Plcg2	Phospholipase C, gamma 2
RT1-Db1	RT1 class II, locus Db1
Ccl21	Chemokine (C-C motif) ligand 21
Zap70	Zeta-chain (TCR) associated protein kinase
Clcf1	Cardiotrophin-like cytokine factor 1
Gpsm3	G-protein signaling modulator 3 (AGS3-like, *C. elegans*)
Prg2	Proteoglycan 2, bone marrow
Kcnn4	Potassium intermediate/small conductance calcium-activated channel, subfamily N, member 4
Coro1a	Coronin, actin-binding protein 1A
Tnfrsf14	Tumor necrosis factor receptor superfamily, member 14 (herpesvirus entry mediator)
Hcls1	Hematopoietic cell-specific Lyn substrate 1
Rhoh	Ras homolog gene family, member H
Satb1	SATB homeobox 1
Cxcr4	Chemokine (C-X-C motif) receptor 4
Localization (GO:0032879)	
Coro1a	Coronin, actin-binding protein 1A

(continued)

Table 3.25 (continued)

Symbol	Name
Cd40	CD40 molecule, TNF receptor superfamily member 5
Unc13d	Unc-13 homolog D (*C. elegans*)
Bcl2	B-cell CLL/lymphoma 2
Arhgap4	Rho GTPase-activating protein 4
Prkcb	Protein kinase C, beta
Cd38	CD38 molecule
Plcg2	Phospholipase C, gamma 2
Ccl21	Chemokine (C-C motif) ligand 21
Ghrl	Ghrelin/obestatin prepropeptide
Cxcr4	Chemokine (C-X-C motif) receptor 4
Kcnn4	Potassium intermediate/small conductance calcium-activated channel, subfamily N, member 4
Protein modification process (GO:0018212, GO:0007260, GO:0006464, GO:0050730, GO:0042325, GO:0001934, GO:0042516, GO:0035408)	
Hcls1	Hematopoietic cell-specific Lyn substrate 1
Zap70	Zeta-chain (TCR) associated protein kinase
Clcf1	Cardiotrophin-like cytokine factor 1
Tnfrsf14	Tumor necrosis factor receptor superfamily, member 14 (herpesvirus entry mediator)
Il22ra2	Interleukin 22 receptor, alpha 2
Stk17b	Serine/threonine kinase 17b
B3galt4	UDP-Gal:betaGlcNAc beta 1,3-galactosyltransferase, polypeptide 4
Bcl2	B-cell CLL/lymphoma 2
Prkcb	Protein kinase C, beta
Camk4	Calcium/calmodulin-dependent protein kinase IV
Cd6	Cd6 molecule
Ubd	Ubiquitin D
Ccl21	Chemokine (C-C motif) ligand 21
Usp18	Ubiquitin-specific peptidase 18
Satb1	SATB homeobox 1
Ghrl	Ghrelin/obestatin prepropeptide
Birc3	Baculoviral IAP repeat-containing 3
Rhoh	Ras homolog gene family, member H
Regulation of DNA recombination (GO:0000018)	
Cd40	CD40 molecule, TNF receptor superfamily member 5
Clcf1	Cardiotrophin-like cytokine factor 1
Response to stimulus (GO:0048584, GO:0009605, GO:0010037)	
A2m	Alpha-2-macroglobulin
Bcl2	B-cell CLL/lymphoma 2
Cd38	CD38 molecule
Skap1	Src kinase-associated phosphoprotein 1
Plcg2	Phospholipase C, gamma 2
Ghrl	Ghrelin/obestatin prepropeptide
Kynu	Kynureninase (L-kynurenine hydrolase)
Coro1a	Coronin, actin-binding protein 1A

(continued)

Table 3.25 (continued)

Symbol	Name
Cd40	CD40 molecule, TNF receptor superfamily member 5
Prkcb	Protein kinase C, beta
Ccl21	Chemokine (C-C motif) ligand 21
Satb1	SATB homeobox 1
Rac2	Ras-related C3 botulinum toxin substrate 2 (rho family, small GTP-binding protein Rac2)
Cxcr4	Chemokine (C-X-C motif) receptor 4
Signaling (GO:0035556, GO:0043123, GO:0009967, GO:0023051, GO:0046425, GO:0035023, GO:0032321, GO:0010627)	
Cflar	CASP8 and FADD-like apoptosis regulator
Stk17b	Serine/threonine kinase 17b
Cd40	CD40 molecule, TNF receptor superfamily member 5
Arhgap4	Rho GTPase-activating protein 4
Prkcb	Protein kinase C, beta
Hcls1	Hematopoietic cell-specific Lyn substrate 1
Ubd	Ubiquitin D
Plcg2	Phospholipase C, gamma 2
Ccl21	Chemokine (C-C motif) ligand 21
Zap70	Zeta-chain (TCR) associated protein kinase
Rhoh	Ras homolog gene family, member H
Rhebl1	Ras homolog enriched in brain like 1
Clcf1	Cardiotrophin-like cytokine factor 1
Rac2	Ras-related C3 botulinum toxin substrate 2 (rho family, small GTP-binding protein Rac2)
Il22ra2	Interleukin 22 receptor, alpha 2
Rab19	RAB19, member RAS oncogene family
Ghrl	Ghrelin/obestatin prepropeptide
Kcnn4	Potassium intermediate/small conductance calcium-activated channel, subfamily N, member 4
Cd38	CD38 molecule
Arhgap15	Rho GTPase-activating protein 15
Gria3	Glutamate receptor, ionotrophic, AMPA 3
Transport (GO:0006816, GO:0072511)	
Coro1a	Coronin, actin-binding protein 1A
Bcl2	B-cell CLL/lymphoma 2
Prkcb	Protein kinase C, beta
Plcg2	Phospholipase C, gamma 2
Ccl21	Chemokine (C-C motif) ligand 21
Cxcr4	Chemokine (C-X-C motif) receptor 4
Kcnn4	Potassium intermediate/small conductance calcium-activated channel, subfamily N, member 4

Table 3.26 Biological processes and upregulated genes in hCG group ($p<0.01$ and fold change 2)

Symbol	Name
Cell communication (GO:0007499)	
Tp63	Tumor protein p63
Cell motility (GO:0016477, GO:0006928, GO:0040011)	
Mmp12	Matrix metallopeptidase 12
Gja1	Gap junction protein, alpha 1
Scnn1b	Sodium channel, nonvoltage-gated 1, beta
Scnn1g	Sodium channel, nonvoltage-gated 1, gamma
Igfbp5	Insulin-like growth factor binding protein 5
Lbp	Lipopolysaccharide-binding protein
Pla2g7	Phospholipase A2, group VII (platelet-activating factor acetylhydrolase, plasma)
Bambi	BMP and activin membrane-bound inhibitor, homolog (*Xenopus laevis*)
Cell proliferation (GO:0008283, GO:0050678)	
Serpinb5	Serpin peptidase inhibitor, clade B (ovalbumin), member 5
Mmp12	Matrix metallopeptidase 12
Epcam	Epithelial cell adhesion molecule
Cebpb	CCAAT/enhancer-binding protein (C/EBP), beta
Gja1	Gap junction protein, alpha 1
Hspa1a	Heat shock 70 kDa protein 1A
Tp63	Tumor protein p63
Kng1	Kininogen 1
Igfbp5	Insulin-like growth factor binding protein 5
Tgfb3	Transforming growth factor, beta3
Bambi	BMP and activin membrane-bound inhibitor, homolog (*Xenopus laevis*)
Cellular metabolic process (GO:0019546, GO:0052548, GO:0010466)	
Padi3	Peptidyl arginine deiminase, type III
Serpinb5	Serpin peptidase inhibitor, clade B (ovalbumin), member 5
Hspa1a	Heat shock 70 kDa protein 1A
Kng1	Kininogen 1
Foxq1	Forkhead box Q1
Wap	Whey acidic protein
Cellular process (GO:0048518)	
Mmp12	Matrix metallopeptidase 12
Lcn2	Lipocalin 2
Epcam	Epithelial cell adhesion molecule
C4bpa	Complement component 4 binding protein, alpha
Cebpb	CCAAT/enhancer-binding protein (C/EBP), beta
Gja1	Gap junction protein, alpha 1
Hspa1a	Heat shock 70 kDa protein 1A
Tp63	Tumor protein p63
Kng1	Kininogen 1
Igfbp5	Insulin-like growth factor binding protein 5

(continued)

Table 3.26 (continued)

Symbol	Name
Spp1	Secreted phosphoprotein 1
Tgfb3	Transforming growth factor, beta3
Lbp	Lipopolysaccharide-binding protein
Mapk13	Mitogen-activated protein kinase 13
Pla2g7	Phospholipase A2, group VII (platelet-activating factor acetylhydrolase, plasma)
Cd14	CD14 molecule
Crhr2	Corticotropin releasing hormone receptor 2
Foxq1	Forkhead box Q1
Cfi	Complement factor I
Bambi	BMP and activin membrane-bound inhibitor, homolog (*Xenopus laevis*)
Circulatory system (GO:0008015)	
Gja1	Gap junction protein, alpha 1
Hspa1a	Heat shock 70 kDa protein 1A
Kng1	Kininogen 1
Kng1l1	Kininogen 1-like 1
Crhr2	Corticotropin releasing hormone receptor 2
Development (GO:0031069, GO:0009888, GO:0030855, GO:0048627, GO:0048685, GO:0060529, GO:0048732, GO:0060512)	
Tp63	Tumor protein p63
Igfbp5	Insulin-like growth factor binding protein 5
Foxq1	Forkhead box Q1
Serpinb5	Serpin peptidase inhibitor, clade B (ovalbumin), member 5
Cebpb	CCAAT/enhancer-binding protein (C/EBP), beta
Gja1	Gap junction protein, alpha 1
Apod	Apolipoprotein D
Spp1	Secreted phosphoprotein 1
Tgfb3	Transforming growth factor, beta3
Crhr2	Corticotropin releasing hormone receptor 2
Bambi	BMP and activin membrane-bound inhibitor, homolog (*Xenopus laevis*)
Sdc1	Syndecan 1
Epithelial to mesenchymal transition (GO:0010718)	
Tgfb3	Transforming growth factor, beta3
Bambi	BMP and activin membrane-bound inhibitor, homolog (*Xenopus laevis*)
Growth (GO:0048630, GO:0040007)	
Igfbp5	Insulin-like growth factor binding protein 5
Crhr2	Corticotropin releasing hormone receptor 2
Gja1	Gap junction protein, alpha 1
Hspa1a	Heat shock 70 kDa protein 1A
Apod	Apolipoprotein D
Spp1	Secreted phosphoprotein 1
Tgfb3	Transforming growth factor, beta3

(continued)

Table 3.26 (continued)

Symbol	Name
Lbp	Lipopolysaccharide-binding protein
Immune response (GO:0032755, GO:0001817, GO:0045087, GO:0006954, GO:0006958, GO:0032760, GO:0002232, GO:0060265, GO:0002252, GO:0050776)	
Lbp	Lipopolysaccharide-binding protein
Mapk13	Mitogen-activated protein kinase 13
Crhr2	Corticotropin releasing hormone receptor 2
Cebpb	CCAAT/enhancer-binding protein (C/EBP), beta
Tgfb3	Transforming growth factor, beta3
Cd14	CD14 molecule
Lcn2	Lipocalin 2
C4bpa	Complement component 4 binding protein, alpha
Cfi	Complement factor I
Kng1	Kininogen 1
Sdc1	Syndecan 1
Spp1	Secreted phosphoprotein 1
Kng1l1	Kininogen 1-like 1
Hspa1a	Heat shock 70 kDa protein 1A
Localization (GO:0051674, GO:0032879)	
Mmp12	Matrix metallopeptidase 12
Gja1	Gap junction protein, alpha 1
Scnn1b	Sodium channel, nonvoltage-gated 1, beta
Scnn1g	Sodium channel, nonvoltage-gated 1, gamma
Igfbp5	Insulin-like growth factor binding protein 5
Lbp	Lipopolysaccharide-binding protein
Pla2g7	Phospholipase A2, group VII (platelet-activating factor acetylhydrolase, plasma)
Bambi	BMP and activin membrane-bound inhibitor, homolog (*Xenopus laevis*)
Kcnk2	Potassium channel, subfamily K, member 2
Tgfb3	Transforming growth factor, beta3
Cd14	CD14 molecule
Crhr2	Corticotropin releasing hormone receptor 2
Molting cycle (GO:0022404, GO:0042633)	
Tp63	Tumor protein p63
Igfbp5	Insulin-like growth factor binding protein 5
Foxq1	Forkhead box Q1
Response to stimulus (GO:0071223, GO:0071222, GO:0071216, GO:0050909)	
Lbp	Lipopolysaccharide-binding protein
Cd14	CD14 molecule
Lcn2	Lipocalin 2
Scnn1b	Sodium channel, nonvoltage-gated 1, beta
Scnn1g	Sodium channel, nonvoltage-gated 1, gamma
Response to stress (GO:0006950, GO:0033554)	
Mmp12	Matrix metallopeptidase 12
C4bpa	Complement component 4 binding protein, alpha
Gja1	Gap junction protein, alpha 1

(continued)

Table 3.26 (continued)

Symbol	Name
Scnn1b	Sodium channel, nonvoltage-gated 1, beta
Scnn1g	Sodium channel, nonvoltage-gated 1, gamma
Kng1	Kininogen 1
Sdc1	Syndecan 1
Tgfb3	Transforming growth factor, beta3
Kng1l1	Kininogen 1-like 1
Penk	Proenkephalin
Lbp	Lipopolysaccharide-binding protein
Mapk13	Mitogen-activated protein kinase 13
Cd14	CD14 molecule
Cfi	Complement factor I
Lcn2	Lipocalin 2
Hspa1a	Heat shock 70 kDa protein 1A
Tp63	Tumor protein p63
Apod	Apolipoprotein D
Spp1	Secreted phosphoprotein 1
Duox1	Dual oxidase 1
Ndrg1	N-myc downstream regulated 1
Crhr2	Corticotropin releasing hormone receptor 2
Secretion (GO:0014064)	
Crhr2	Corticotropin releasing hormone receptor 2
Signaling (GO:0030512, GO:0009967)	
Tgfb3	Transforming growth factor, beta3
Bambi	BMP and activin membrane-bound inhibitor, homolog (*Xenopus laevis*)
Gja1	Gap junction protein, alpha 1
Tp63	Tumor protein p63
Kng1	Kininogen 1
Igfbp5	Insulin-like growth factor binding protein 5
Lbp	Lipopolysaccharide-binding protein
Crhr2	Corticotropin releasing hormone receptor 2
Transport (GO:0010232, GO:0035482, GO:2000293, GO:0030001)	
Gja1	Gap junction protein, alpha 1
Crhr2	Corticotropin releasing hormone receptor 2
Lcn2	Lipocalin 2
Kcnk2	Potassium channel, subfamily K, member 2
Scnn1b	Sodium channel, nonvoltage-gated 1, beta
Scnn1g	Sodium channel, nonvoltage-gated 1, gamma
Slc39a8	Solute carrier family 39 (zinc transporter), member 8
Wound healing (GO:0042060, GO:0035313)	
Mmp12	Matrix metallopeptidase 12
Gja1	Gap junction protein, alpha 1
Scnn1b	Sodium channel, nonvoltage-gated 1, beta
Scnn1g	Sodium channel, nonvoltage-gated 1, gamma
Kng1	Kininogen 1
Sdc1	Syndecan 1
Apod	Apolipoprotein D
Tgfb3	Transforming growth factor, beta3

Table 3.27 Biological processes and downregulated genes in pregnancy group ($p<0.01$ and fold change 2)

Symbol	Name
Lipid processes (GO:0019433, GO:0044269, GO:0046461, GO:0046503, GO:0019432, GO:0046460, GO:0046504)	
Pnpla3	Patatin-like phospholipase domain containing 3
Signaling (GO:0071883, GO:0035625, GO:0032148, GO:2000273, GO:0045742, GO:0007176, GO:0061098)	
Adra2c	Adrenergic, alpha-2C-, receptor

identified E-cadherin (E-cad), Claudin-4 (Cldn4), Connexin-43 (Cx43), Zona Occludens-1 (ZO-1), and Zona Occludens-2 (ZO-2) transcript which were differentially expressed during early stages of hematopoietic/endothelial commitment. Stable embryonal stem cell (ESC) lines were generated with reduced expression of E-cad, Cldn4, Cx43, ZO-1, and ZO-2 using shRNA technology. Functional and phenotypic consequences of modulating AM expression were assessed using hematopoietic colony forming assays, endothelial sprouting assays, and surface protein expression. A decrease in E-cad, Cldn4, Cx43, and ZO-1 expression was associated with less commitment to the hematopoietic lineage and increased endothelial differentiation as evidenced by functional and phenotypic analysis. A reduction in ZO-2 expression did not influence endothelial differentiation, but decreased hematopoietic commitment twofold. These data indicate that a subset of AM influence ESC decisions to commit to endothelial and hematopoietic lineages. Furthermore, differentially expressed AM provide novel markers to delineate early stages of ESC commitment to hematopoietic/endothelial lineages [186]. Increased membranous expression of claudin-4 in gastric carcinoma is associated with better patient prognosis, whereas cytoplasmic claudin-4 expression did not show a significant association with prognosis. Consistent with the correlation of increased membranous claudin-4 with favorable clinicopathological factors, claudin-4 overexpression inhibited the migration and invasion of gastric cancer cells; in contrast, it did not affect cell growth. Claudin-4 expression also increased the barrier function of TJs [187]. Claudin-4 upregulation was strongly correlated with DNA hypomethylation in both gastric tissues and gastric cancer cells. Moreover, Cldn4 expression was repressed in normal gastric tissues in association with bivalent histone modifications, and loss of repressive histone methylations and gain of active histone modifications were associated with Cldn4 overexpression in gastric cancer cells. Interestingly, Cdnl4 repression could be markedly derepressed by combined treatments that simultaneously target both histone modifications and DNA demethylation in Cldn4-hypermethylated cells, whereas concomitant changes in histone methylations and acetylations are required for Cldn4 induction in Cldn4-repressed cells with low DNA methylation [188]. Low expression of Cldn4 was significantly associated with shorter survival in patients with pancreatic ductal adenocarcinoma (hazard ratio; 1.362, 95% confidence interval; 1.011–1.873, $p=0.0419$). Patients with high Cldn4 expression survived longer for a median of

Table 3.28 Biological processes and upregulated genes in pregnancy group ($p<0.01$ and fold change 2)

Symbol	Name
Apoptosis (GO:0006921, GO:0006922)	
Cd24	CD24 molecule
Gzma	Granzyme A
Cellular component organization (GO:0031346)	
Lcn2	Lipocalin 2
Cd24	CD24 molecule
Tgfb3	Transforming growth factor, beta3
Cellular metabolic process (GO:0006709, GO:0032078, GO:0032074)	
Akr1c18	Aldo-keto reductase family 1, member C18
Gzma	Granzyme A
Cellular process (GO:0051704)	
Lcn2	Lipocalin 2
Akr1c18	Aldo-keto reductase family 1, member C18
Cd24	CD24 molecule
Tgfb3	Transforming growth factor, beta3
Cfb	Complement factor B
Lbp	Lipopolysaccharide-binding protein
Cldn4	Claudin 4
Circulatory system (GO:0034107, GO:0034119)	
Cd24	CD24 molecule
Development (GO:0031103, GO:0048685, GO:0034103, GO:0042335, GO:0043932)	
Apod	Apolipoprotein D
Spp1	Secreted phosphoprotein 1
Chl1	Cell adhesion molecule with homology to L1CAM
Cd24	CD24 molecule
Duox1	Dual oxidase 1
Tgfb3	Transforming growth factor, beta3
Homeostasis (GO:0033212)	
Lcn2	Lipocalin 2
Immune response (GO:0002682, GO:0001818, GO:0002232, GO:0032913, GO:0042103, GO:0046014, GO:0060265, GO:0032755, GO:0006954, GO:0045087, GO:0002690, GO:0006956, GO:0050778, GO:0002842)	
Kng1	Kininogen 1
Cd24	CD24 molecule
Tgfb3	Transforming growth factor, beta3
Cfb	Complement factor B
Lbp	Lipopolysaccharide-binding protein
Pla2g7	Phospholipase A2, group VII (platelet-activating factor acetylhydrolase, plasma)
Cfi	Complement factor I
Crhr2	Corticotropin releasing hormone receptor 2
Spp1	Secreted phosphoprotein 1
Kng1l1	Kininogen 1-like 1
Lcn2	Lipocalin 2

(continued)

Table 3.28 (continued)

Symbol	Name
Localization (GO:0033037)	
Lbp	Lipopolysaccharide-binding protein
Respiratory burst (GO:0045730)	
Cd24	CD24 molecule
Lbp	Lipopolysaccharide-binding protein
Response to oxygen levels (GO:0070483)	
Tgfb3	Transforming growth factor, beta3
Response to stimulus (GO:0010033, GO:0070887, GO:0050909, GO:0050795, GO:0048545, GO:2000252, GO:0032103)	
Lcn2	Lipocalin 2
Cyp2e1	Cytochrome P450, family 2, subfamily e, polypeptide 1
Cd24	CD24 molecule
Spp1	Secreted phosphoprotein 1
Tgfb3	Transforming growth factor, beta3
Duox1	Dual oxidase 1
Cfb	Complement factor B
Lbp	Lipopolysaccharide-binding protein
Adfp	Adipose differentiation-related protein
Cldn4	Claudin 4
Krt19	Keratin 19
Crhr2	Corticotropin releasing hormone receptor 2
Prkaa2	Protein kinase, AMP-activated, alpha 2 catalytic subunit
Pla2g7	Phospholipase A2, group VII (platelet-activating factor acetylhydrolase, plasma)
Scnn1b	Sodium channel, nonvoltage-gated 1, beta
Scnn1g	Sodium channel, nonvoltage-gated 1, gamma
Response to stress (GO:0006950)	
Mmp12	Matrix metallopeptidase 12
Lcn2	Lipocalin 2
Scnn1b	Sodium channel, nonvoltage-gated 1, beta
Scnn1g	Sodium channel, nonvoltage-gated 1, gamma
Kng1	Kininogen 1
Cd24	CD24 molecule
Apod	Apolipoprotein D
Spp1	Secreted phosphoprotein 1
Tgfb3	Transforming growth factor, beta3
Duox1	Dual oxidase 1
Kng1l1	Kininogen 1-like 1
Cfb	Complement factor B
Lbp	Lipopolysaccharide-binding protein
Crhr2	Corticotropin releasing hormone receptor 2
Prkaa2	Protein kinase, AMP-activated, alpha 2 catalytic subunit
Cfi	Complement factor I
Chl1	Cell adhesion molecule with homology to L1CAM

(continued)

Table 3.28 (continued)

Symbol	Name
Secretion (GO:0014064)	
Crhr2	Corticotropin releasing hormone receptor 2
Transport (GO:0032600, GO:0035482, GO:2000293, GO:0015891, GO:0015920, GO:0032594, GO:0090281)	
Cd24	CD24 molecule
Crhr2	Corticotropin releasing hormone receptor 2
Lcn2	Lipocalin 2
Lbp	Lipopolysaccharide-binding protein
Wound healing (GO:0035313, GO:0042060)	
Mmp12	Matrix metallopeptidase 12
Scnn1b	Sodium channel, nonvoltage-gated 1, beta
Scnn1g	Sodium channel, nonvoltage-gated 1, gamma
Kng1	Kininogen 1
Apod	Apolipoprotein D
Tgfb3	Transforming growth factor, beta3

Table 3.29 Biological processes and downregulated genes in pellet group ($p<0.01$ and fold change 2)

Symbol	Name
Cell proliferation (GO:0002158, GO:0033688)	
Npr3	Natriuretic peptide receptor C/guanylate cyclase C (atrionatriuretic peptide receptor C)
Circadian rhythm (GO:0042752, GO:0046010)	
Alb	Albumin
Arntl	Aryl hydrocarbon receptor nuclear translocator-like
Circulatory system (GO:0003013, GO:0003044, GO:0045777, GO:0001907, GO:0001986, GO:0003014, GO:0001994, GO:0002017, GO:0001978, GO:0050880)	
Alb	Albumin
Hsd11b2	Hydroxysteroid 11-beta dehydrogenase 2
Npr3	Natriuretic peptide receptor C/guanylate cyclase C (atrionatriuretic peptide receptor C)
Adra1d	Adrenergic, alpha-1D-, receptor
Development (GO:0046548)	
Ntrk2	Neurotrophic tyrosine kinase, receptor, type 2
Homeostasis (GO:0065008)	
Alb	Albumin
Ntrk2	Neurotrophic tyrosine kinase, receptor, type 2
Hsd11b2	Hydroxysteroid 11-beta dehydrogenase 2
Npr3	Natriuretic peptide receptor C/guanylate cyclase C (atrionatriuretic peptide receptor C)
Gpr120	G-protein coupled receptor 120
Adra1d	Adrenergic, alpha-1D-, receptor

(continued)

Table 3.29 (continued)

Symbol	Name
Localization (GO:0051659)	
Alb	Albumin
Response to stimulus (GO:0070541)	
Alb	Albumin
Signaling (GO:0031547, GO:0071883, GO:0035625, GO:0071875)	
Ntrk2	Neurotrophic tyrosine kinase, receptor, type 2
Adra2c	Adrenergic, alpha-2C-, receptor
Adra1d	Adrenergic, alpha-1D-, receptor
Symbiotic interaction (GO:0019836, GO:0044179, GO:0051801, GO:0052025, GO:0052111, GO:0052188, GO:0051818)	
Alb	Albumin

Table 3.30 Biological processes and upregulated genes in pellet group ($p<0.01$ and fold change 2)

Symbol	Name
Adhesion (GO:0007155)	
Kng1	Kininogen 1
Cd24	CD24 molecule
Mfge8	Milk fat globule-EGF factor 8 protein
Spp1	Secreted phosphoprotein 1
Msln	Mesothelin
Ctgf	Connective tissue growth factor
Cldn7	Claudin 7
Aging (GO:0007568, GO:0010260)	
Aldoc	Aldolase C, fructose-bisphosphate
Tp63	Tumor protein p63
Apod	Apolipoprotein D
Aqp2	Aquaporin 2 (collecting duct)
Tgfb3	Transforming growth factor, beta3
Ctgf	Connective tissue growth factor
Apoptosis (GO:0006921, GO:0006922)	
Cd24	CD24 molecule
Gzma	Granzyme A
Cell communication (GO:0007499)	
Tp63	Tumor protein p63
Cell cycle (GO:0070318)	
Ctgf	Connective tissue growth factor
Cellular component organization c (GO:0022411, GO:0031346)	
Cd24	CD24 molecule
Aqp2	Aquaporin 2 (collecting duct)
Gzma	Granzyme A
Lcn2	Lipocalin 2
Tgfb3	Transforming growth factor, beta3

(continued)

Table 3.30 (continued)

Symbol	Name
Cellular metabolic process (GO:0044253, GO:0032078, GO:0032074)	
Tgfb3	Transforming growth factor, beta3
Ctgf	Connective tissue growth factor
Gzma	Granzyme A
Circadian rhythm c(GO:0007623)	
LOC259246	Alpha-2u globulin PGCL1
Cldn4	Claudin 4
Per2	Period homolog 2 (*Drosophila*)
Circulatory system c(GO:0034107, GO:0034119)	
Cd24	CD24 molecule
Collagen process (GO:0032967, GO:0010712)	
Tgfb3	Transforming growth factor, beta3
Ctgf	Connective tissue growth factor
Development (GO:0048685, GO:0060529, GO:0034103, GO:0042335, GO:0043932, GO:0045617, GO:0060197, GO:0031103)	
Spp1	Secreted phosphoprotein 1
Tp63	Tumor protein p63
Cd24	CD24 molecule
Duox1	Dual oxidase 1
Tgfb3	Transforming growth factor, beta3
Apod	Apolipoprotein D
Homeostasis (GO:0019725, GO:0032844, GO:0033212)	
Ccl28	Chemokine (C-C motif) ligand 28
Lcn2	Lipocalin 2
Kng1	Kininogen 1
Cd24	CD24 molecule
Aqp2	Aquaporin 2 (collecting duct)
LOC259246	Alpha-2u globulin PGCL1
Crhr2	Corticotropin releasing hormone receptor 2
Qsox1	Quiescin Q6 sulfhydryl oxidase 1
Spp1	Secreted phosphoprotein 1
Immune response (GO:0002237, GO:0001818, GO:0002232, GO:0032913, GO:0042103, GO:0046014, GO:0060265, GO:0032755, GO:0006954, GO:0045087, GO:0006956, GO:0002842, GO:0050778)	
Lcn2	Lipocalin 2
Cd24	CD24 molecule
Aqp2	Aquaporin 2 (collecting duct)
Cfb	Complement factor B
Lbp	Lipopolysaccharide-binding protein
Tgfb3	Transforming growth factor, beta3
Crhr2	Corticotropin releasing hormone receptor 2
Kng1	Kininogen 1
Spp1	Secreted phosphoprotein 1
Kng1l1	Kininogen 1-like 1
Cfi	Complement factor I

(continued)

Table 3.30 (continued)

Symbol	Name
Lipid processes (GO:0010876)	
LOC259246	Alpha-2u globulin PGCL1
Lbp	Lipopolysaccharide-binding protein
Crabp2	Cellular retinoic acid-binding protein 2
Adfp	Adipose differentiation-related protein
Localization (GO:0033037)	
Lbp	Lipopolysaccharide-binding protein
Pregnancy (GO:0007565)	
Aqp2	Aquaporin 2 (collecting duct)
Tgfb3	Transforming growth factor, beta3
Cldn4	Claudin 4
Abcg2	ATP-binding cassette, subfamily G (WHITE), member 2
Regulation of biological process (GO:0048518)	
Mmp12	Matrix metallopeptidase 12
Lcn2	Lipocalin 2
Rasd2	RASD family, member 2
Dbp	D site of albumin promoter (albumin D-box) binding protein
Tp63	Tumor protein p63
Kng1	Kininogen 1
Cd24	CD24 molecule
Mfge8	Milk fat globule-EGF factor 8 protein
Spp1	Secreted phosphoprotein 1
Aqp2	Aquaporin 2 (collecting duct)
Tgfb3	Transforming growth factor, beta3
LOC259246	Alpha-2u globulin PGCL1
Gzma	Granzyme A
Cfb	Complement factor B
Lbp	Lipopolysaccharide-binding protein
Ctgf	Connective tissue growth factor
Crhr2	Corticotropin releasing hormone receptor 2
Cfi	Complement factor I
Respiratory burst (GO:0045730)	
Cd24	CD24 molecule
Lbp li	Popolysaccharide-binding protein
Response to oxygen levels (GO:0070482, GO:0070483)	
Aldoc	Aldolase C, fructose-bisphosphate
Scnn1g	Sodium channel, nonvoltage-gated 1, gamma
Cd24	CD24 molecule
Tgfb3	Transforming growth factor, beta3
Ctgf	Connective tissue growth factor
Response to stimulus (GO:0009725, GO:0043627, GO:0071280, GO:2000252, GO:0071326, GO:0071333)	
Cd24	CD24 molecule
Mfge8	Milk fat globule-EGF factor 8 protein
Spp1	Secreted phosphoprotein 1

(continued)

Table 3.30 (continued)

Symbol	Name
Aqp2	Aquaporin 2 (collecting duct)
Tgfb3	Transforming growth factor, beta3
LOC259246	Alpha-2u globulin PGCL1
Cldn4	Claudin 4
Abcg2	ATP-binding cassette, subfamily G (WHITE), member 2
Krt19	Keratin 19
Ctgf	Connective tissue growth factor
Crhr2	Corticotropin releasing hormone receptor 2
Response to stress (GO:0006950)	
Mmp12	Matrix metallopeptidase 12
Lcn2	Lipocalin 2
Aldoc	Aldolase C, fructose-bisphosphate
Tp63	Tumor protein p63
Scnn1g	Sodium channel, nonvoltage-gated 1, gamma
Kng1	Kininogen 1
Cd24	CD24 molecule
Apod	Apolipoprotein D
Spp1	Secreted phosphoprotein 1
Aqp2	Aquaporin 2 (collecting duct)
Tgfb3	Transforming growth factor, beta3
Duox1	Dual oxidase 1
Kng1l1	Kininogen 1-like 1
Cfb	Complement factor B
Lbp	Lipopolysaccharide-binding protein
Ctgf	Connective tissue growth factor
Crhr2	Corticotropin releasing hormone receptor 2
Cfi	Complement factor I
Secretion (GO:0061179, GO:0014064, GO:0090278)	
LOC259246	Alpha-2u globulin PGCL1
Crhr2	Corticotropin releasing hormone receptor 2
Signaling (GO:0043949, GO:0009967)	
Rasd2	RASD family, member 2
Crhr2	Corticotropin releasing hormone receptor 2
Tp63	Tumor protein p63
Kng1	Kininogen 1
Cd24	CD24 molecule
LOC259246	Alpha-2u globulin PGCL1
Lbp	Lipopolysaccharide-binding protein
Transport (GO:0032600, GO:0035482, GO:2000293, GO:0015891, GO:0015920, GO:0032594, GO:0090281)	
Cd24	CD24 molecule
Crhr2	Corticotropin releasing hormone receptor 2
Lcn2	Lipocalin 2
Lbp	Lipopolysaccharide-binding protein

(continued)

Table 3.30 (continued)

Symbol	Name
Wound healing (GO:0035313, GO:0042060)	
Mmp12	Matrix metallopeptidase 12
Scnn1g	Sodium channel, nonvoltage-gated 1, gamma
Kng1	Kininogen 1
Apod	Apolipoprotein D
Tgfb3	Transforming growth factor, beta3

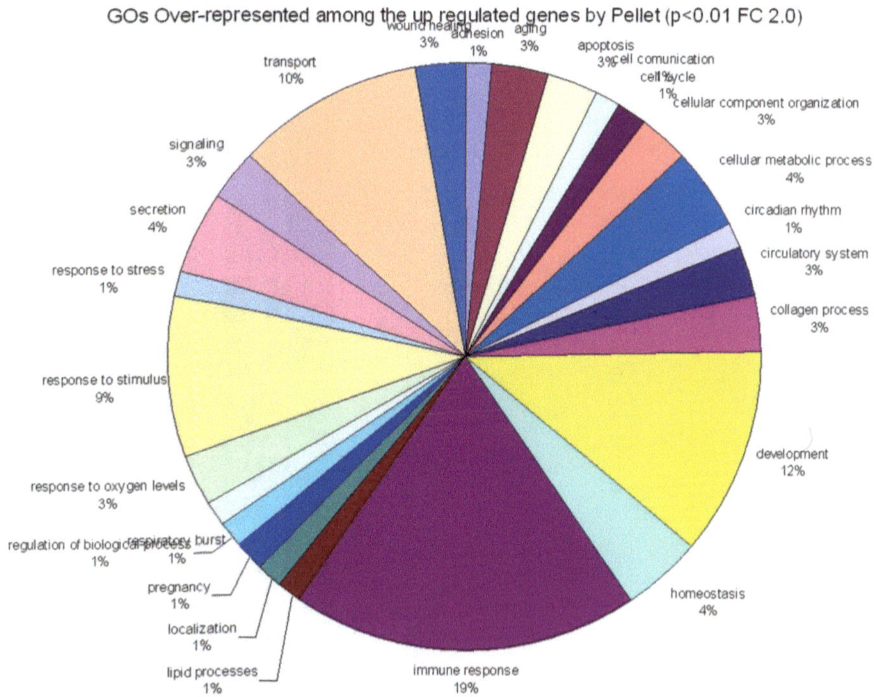

Fig. 3.32 Gene Ontology of the overrepresented genes upregulated in the mammary gland of pellet treated rats using a $p < 0.01$ and FC of 2.0

63.0 months, compared with 14.7 months in patients with low Cldn4 expression ($p = 0.0067$). In immunohistochemical analysis, the level of Cldn4 mRNA expression was significantly correlated with the expression of Cldn4 protein ($p = 0.0168$) [189]. Claudins (Clds) are crucial constituents of tight-junction strands in epithelial cells and have a central role in barrier functions. Cld4 is unexpectedly expressed in normal thymic lymphocytes independently of tight junctions [190]. Differentiation of epithelial cells and morphogenesis of epithelial tubes or layers are closely linked with the establishment and remodeling of the apical junctional complex, which includes adherens junctions and tight junctions. The transcription factor grainyhead-like

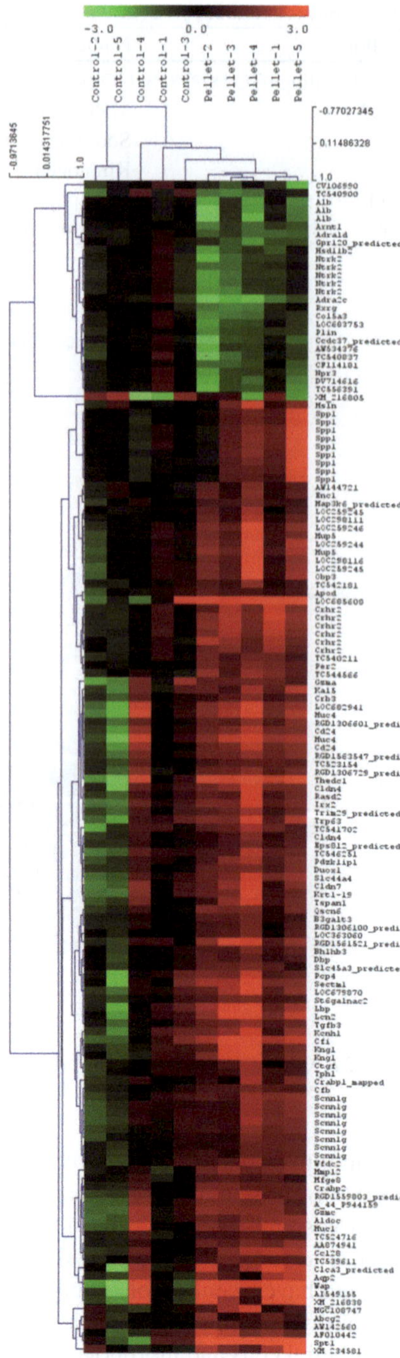

Fig. 3.33 Heat map showing the up- (*red*) and downregulated genes (*green*) of pellet-treated rat mammary glands using a $p < 0.01$ and FC of 2.0

2 (Grhl2), an epithelium-specific mammalian homolog of *Drosophila* Grainyhead, is essential for adequate expression of the adherens junction gene E-cadherin and the tight junction gene claudin 4 in several types of epithelia, including gut endoderm, surface ectoderm, and otic epithelium. Grhl2 mutant mice specifically associate with *cis*-regulatory elements localized at the Cldn4 core promoter and within intron 2 of the E-cadherin gene. Cldn4 promoter activity in epithelial cells is crucially dependent on the availability of Grhl2 and on the integrity of the Grhl2-associated *cis*-regulatory element. At the E-cadherin locus, the intronic Grhl2-associated *cis*-regulatory region contacts the promoter via chromatin looping, while loss of Grhl2 leads to a specific decrease of activating histone marks at the E-cadherin promoter. Grhl2 acts as a target gene-associated transcriptional activator of apical junctional complex components and, thereby, crucially participates in epithelial differentiation [191]. *Altogether these data indicate that overexpression of Cldn4 in the mammary gland is associated with the differentiation pathway elicited by the preventive agents and together with Tgfb3, ApoD, Encl and Wap are markers of cell differentiation* (Fig. 3.22). Supporting evidence of this statement is the fact that breast cancer progression is associated with aberrant DNA methylation and expression of genes that control the epithelial-mesenchymal transition (EMT), a critical step in malignant conversion. Cells that underwent EMT exhibited loss of expression of the CDH1, CGN, CLDN4, and KLK10 genes as a result of hypermethylation of their corresponding promoter regions. Activated TGFbeta-Smad signaling provides an "epigenetic memory" to maintain silencing of critical genes. In support of this hypothesis, disrupting Smad signaling in mesenchymal breast cancer cells resulted in DNA demethylation and reexpression of the genes identified. This epigenetic reversal was accompanied by an acquisition of epithelial morphology and a suppression of invasive properties. Notably, disrupting TGFbeta signaling decreased the DNA binding activity of DNA methyltransferase DNMT1, suggesting that failure to maintain methylation of newly synthesized DNA was the likely cause of DNA demethylation. Hyperactive TGFbeta-TGFbetaR-Smad2 signaling axis needed to maintain epigenetic silencing of critical EMT genes and breast cancer progression [192]. Expression of claudin-3 and claudin-4 is repressed in ovarian epithelial cells in association with promoter "bivalent" histone modifications, containing both the activating trimethylated histone H3 lysine 4 (H3K4me3) mark and the repressive mark of trimethylated histone H3 lysine 27 (H3K27me3). During ovarian tumorigenesis, derepression of CLDN3 and CLDN4 expression correlates with loss of H3K27me3 in addition to trimethylated histone H4 lysine 20 (H4K20me3), another repressive histone modification. Although CLDN4 repression was accompanied by both DNA hypermethylation and repressive histone modifications, DNA methylation was not required for CLDN3 repression in immortalized ovarian epithelial cells. Moreover, activation of both CLDN3 and CLDN4 in ovarian cancer cells was associated with simultaneous changes in multiple histone modifications, whereas H3K27me3 loss alone was insufficient for their derepression. CLDN4 repression was robustly reversed by combined treatment targeting both DNA demethylation and histone acetylation [193, 194].

There is a group of genes that are upregulated in the three preventive modalities tested that are related to the inflammatory response (Table 3.17 and Fig. 3.22).

As depicted in Fig. 3.22 the preventive signature of the mammary gland is related to the upregulation of genes controlling cell differentiation, innate immune defense, inhibition of cell proliferation, angiogenesis, and inflammation, all of them leading to increase in apoptosis. This indicates that the epithelial cells are interacting very actively with the stroma by halting many stressors like inflammation and angiogenesis.

3.6 Concluding Remarks

The transcriptomic profile of the rat mammary gland displays a set of common genes that can explain the protective effect of hCG, pregnancy, and hormones associated with pregnancy like the combined use of estrogen and progesterone. These preventive strategies occurring during a narrow window in the development of the breast would succeed in permanently inducing the molecular changes that will make the mammary gland resistant to develop cancer. Of relevance is that hCG induces specific set of genes and wider transcriptomic changes that could be extremely important to control the progression of the differentiation pathway, and that these changes are permanently imprinted in the genome, regulating the long-lasting refractoriness of the mammary gland to develop cancer.

Acknowledgments This work was supported by a grant from the Komen Foundation for the Cure KG101080 entitled Chromatin Remodeling as a Preventive Strategy in Breast Cancer Prevention granted to JR and IHR. The authors acknowledge the contributions of the many members of the Breast Cancer Research Laboratory, among them Julia Pereira, PhD; Ricardo Lopez de Cicco, PhD; Johana E. Vanegas, MD; and Fathima Sheriff, MD who have worked with us to generate the data incorporated into this chapter and allow us to elaborate it into a unified concept.

References

1. Welsch CW (1985) Host factors affecting the growth of carcinogen-induced rat mammary carcinomas: a review and tribute to Charles Brenton Huggins. Cancer Res 45:3415–3443
2. Russo IH, Russo J (1996) Mammary gland neoplasia in long-term rodent studies. Environ Health Perspect 104:938–967
3. Huggins C, Briziarelli G, Sutton H (1959) Rapid induction of mammary carcinoma in the rat and the influence of hormones on the tumors. J Exp Med 709:25–42
4. Huggins C, Grand L, Fukunishi R (1964) Aromatic influences in the yields of mammary cancers following administration of 7,12-dimethylbenzanthracene. Proc Natl Acad Sci USA 57:737–742
5. Gullino PM, Pettigrew HM, Grantham FH (1975) N-nitrosomethylurea as mammary gland carcinogen in rats. J Natl Cancer Inst 54:401–414
6. Thordarson G, Lee AV, McCarty M, Van Horn K, Chu O, Chou YC et al (2001) Growth and characterization of N-methyl-N-nitrosourea-induced mammary tumors in intact and ovariectomized rats. Carcinogenesis 22:2039–2047

7. Russo IH, Russo J (2011) Pregnancy-Induced changes in breast cancer risk. A review. J Mammary Gland Biol Neoplasia 16:221–233
8. Russo IH, Russo J (2007) Primary prevention of breast cancer by hormone-induced differentiation. Recent Results Cancer Res 174:111–130
9. Russo J, Tait L, Russo IH (1983) Susceptibility of the mammary gland to carcinogenesis: III the cell of origin of rat mammary carcinoma. Am J Pathol 113:50–66
10. Russo J, Russo IH (eds) (2004) Molecular basis of breast cancer: prevention and treatment. Springer, Berlin
11. Blakely CM, Stoddard AJ, Belka GK, Dugan KD, Notarfrancesco KL, Moody SE et al (2006) Hormone-induced protection against mammary tumorigenesis is conserved in multiple rat strains and identifies a core gene expression signature induced by pregnancy. Cancer Res 66:6421–6431
12. Russo IH, Koszalka M, Gimotty PA, Russo J (1990) Protective effect of chorionic gonadotropin on DMBA-induced mammary carcinogenesis. Br J Cancer 62:243–247
13. Russo IH, Koszalka M, Russo J (1991) Comparative study of the influence of pregnancy and hormonal treatment on mammary carcinogenesis. Br J Cancer 64:481–484
14. Russo J, Russo IH (1980) Susceptibility of the mammary gland to carcinogenesis. II. Pregnancy interruption as a risk factor in tumor incidence. Am J Pathol 100:497–512
15. Russo J, Tay LK, Ciocca D, Russo IH (1983) Molecular and cellular basis of the mammary gland susceptibility to carcinogenesis. Environ Health Perspect 49:185–199
16. Vanegas JE, Kocdor M, Pereira JS, Kocdor H, Russo J, Snider K et al (2009) Preventive effect of hCG on rat mammary carcinogenesis. Proc Am Assoc Cancer Res 50:2059a
17. Huang D, Sherman BT, Lempicki RA (2009) Systematic and integrative analysis of large gene lists using DAVID bioinformatics resources. Nat Protoc 4:44–57
18. García-Calero E, Puelles L (2009) Enc1 expression in the chick telencephalon at intermediate and late stages of development. J Comp Neurol 517:564–580
19. Kim SG, Jang SJ, Soh J, Lee K, Park JK, Chang WK et al (2009) Expression of ectodermal neural cortex 1 and its association with actin during the ovulatory process in the rat. Endocrinology 15:3800–3806
20. White EA, Sowa ME, Tan MJ, Jeudy S, Hayes SD, Santha S (2012) Systematic identification of interactions between host cell proteins and E7 oncoproteins from diverse human papillomaviruses. Proc Natl Acad Sci USA 109:E260–E267
21. Wang XJ, Zhang DD (2009) Ectodermal-neural cortex 1 down-regulates Nrf2 at the translational level. PLoS One 4(5):e5492
22. Bonazzi VF, Irwin D, Hayward NK (2009) Identification of candidate tumor suppressor genes inactivated by promoter methylation in melanoma. Genes Chromosomes Cancer 48:10–21
23. Leng X, Wu Y, Arlinghaus RB (2011) Relationships of lipocalin 2 with breast tumorigenesis and metastasis. J Cell Physiol 226:309–314
24. Berger T, Cheung CC, Elia AJ, Mak TW (2010) Disruption of the Lcn2 gene in mice suppresses primary mammary tumor formation but does not decrease lung metastasis. Proc Natl Acad Sci USA 107:2995–3000
25. Mahadevan NR, Rodvold J, Almanza G, Pérez AF, Wheeler MC, Zanetti M (2011) ER stress drives Lipocalin 2 upregulation in prostate cancer cells in an NF-κB-dependent manner. BMC Cancer 11:229
26. Fougère M, Gaudineau B, Barbier J, Guaddachi F, Feugeas JP, Auboeuf D, Jauliac S (2010) NFAT3 transcription factor inhibits breast cancer cell motility by targeting the lipocalin 2 gene. Oncogene 29:2292–2301
27. Leng X, Ding T, Lin H, Wang Y, Hu L, Hu J, Feig B, Zhang W, Pusztai L, Symmans WF, Wu Y, Arlinghaus RB (2009) Inhibition of lipocalin 2 impairs breast tumorigenesis and metastasis. Cancer Res 69:8579–8584
28. Yang J, Moses MA (2009) Lipocalin 2: a multifaceted modulator of human cancer. Cell Cycle 8:2347–2352

29. Shi H, Gu Y, Yang J, Xu L, Mi W, Yu W (2008) Lipocalin 2 promotes lung metastasis of murine breast cancer cells. J Exp Clin Cancer Res 27:83
30. Nilsen-Hamilton M, Liu Q, Ryon J, Bendickson L, Lepont P, Chang Q (2003) Tissue involution and the acute phase response. Ann N Y Acad Sci 995:94–108
31. Devireddy LR, Teodoro JG, Richard FA, Green MR (2001) Induction of apoptosis by a secreted lipocalin that is transcriptionally regulated by IL-3 deprivation. Science 293:829–834
32. Savill JS, Wyllie AH, Henson JE, Walport MJ, Henson PM, Haslett C (1989) Macrophage phagocytosis of aging neutrophils in inflammation. Programmed cell death in the neutrophil leads to its recognition by macrophages. J Clin Invest 83:865–875
33. DiGiovanni J, Juchau MR (1980) Biotransformation and bioactivation of 7, 12-dimethylbenz[a] anthracene (7, 12-DMBA). Drug Metab Rev 11:61–101
34. Josephy PD, Coomber BL (1998) The 1996 Veylien Henderson Award of the Society of Toxicology of Canada. Current concepts: neutrophils and the activation of carcinogens in the breast and other organs. Can J Physiol Pharmacol 76:693–700
35. Anderson RF, Patel KB, Reghebi K, Hill SA (1989) Conversion of xanthine dehydrogenase to xanthine oxidase as a possible marker for hypoxia in tumours and normal tissues. Br J Cancer 60:193–197
36. Chen Y, Sheng H, Xu Y, Zhang Y, Ni X (2012) Activation of CRHR2 exerts an inhibitory effect on the expression of collapsin response mediator protein 3 in hippocampal neurons. Neuropeptides 6:93–98
37. Zohar I, Weinstock M (2011) Differential effect of prenatal stress on the expression of corticotrophin-releasing hormone and its receptors in the hypothalamus and amygdala in male and female rats. J Neuroendocrinol 23:320–328
38. Harris RB (2010) Leptin responsiveness of mice deficient in corticotrophin-releasing hormone receptor type 2. Neuroendocrinology 92:198–206
39. Im E, Rhee SH, Park YS, Fiocchi C, Taché Y, Pothoulakis C (2010) Corticotropin-releasing hormone family of peptides regulates intestinal angiogenesis. Gastroenterology 138:2457–2467, 2467.e1–5
40. Xiao Q, Pepe AE, Wang G, Luo Z, Zhang L, Zeng L, Zhang Z, Hu Y, Ye S, Xu Q (2012) Nrf3-Pla2g7 interaction plays an essential role in smooth muscle cell differentiation from stem cells. Arterioscler Thromb Vasc Biol 32:730–734
41. Vainio P, Lehtinen L, Mirtti T, Hilvo M, Seppänen-Laakso T, Virtanen J, Sankila A, Nordling S, Lundin J, Rannikko A, Orešič M, Kallioniemi O, Iljin K (2011) Phospholipase PLA2G7, associated with aggressive prostate cancer, promotes prostate cancer cell migration and invasion and is inhibited by statins. Oncotarget 2:1176–1190
42. Li L, Qi L, Lv N, Gao Q, Cheng Y, Wei Y, Ye J, Yan X, Dang A (2011) Association between lipoprotein-associated phospholipase A2 gene polymorphism and coronary artery disease in the Chinese Han population. Ann Hum Genet 75:605–611
43. Serão NV, Delfino KR, Southey BR, Beever JE, Rodriguez-Zas SL (2011) Cell cycle and aging, morphogenesis, and response to stimuli genes are individualized biomarkers of glioblastoma progression and survival. BMC Med Genomics 4:49
44. Vainio P, Gupta S, Ketola K, Mirtti T, Mpindi JP, Kohonen P, Fey V, Perälä M, Smit F, Verhaegh G, Schalken J, Alanen KA, Kallioniemi O, Iljin K (2011) Arachidonic acid pathway members PLA2G7, HPGD, EPHX2, and CYP4F8 identified as putative novel therapeutic targets in prostate cancer. Am J Pathol 178:525–536
45. Wu Y, Li Y, Lange EM, Croteau-Chonka DC, Kuzawa CW, McDade TW, Qin L, Curocichin G, Borja JB, Lange LA, Adair LS, Mohlke KL (2010) Genome-wide association study for adiponectin levels in Filipino women identifies CDH13 and a novel uncommon haplotype at KNG1-ADIPOQ. Hum Mol Genet 19:4955–4964
46. Vionnet N, Tregouët D, Kazeem G, Gut I, Groop PH, Tarnow L, Parving HH, Hadjadj S, Forsblom C, Farrall M, Gauguier D, Cox R, Matsuda F, Heath S, Thévard A, Rousseau R, Cambien F, Marre M, Lathrop M (2006) Analysis of 14 candidate genes for diabetic

nephropathy on chromosome 3q in European populations: strongest evidence for association with a variant in the promoter region of the adiponectin gene. Diabetes 55:3166–3174
47. Gautier T, Lagrost L (2011) Plasma PLTP (phospholipid-transfer protein): an emerging role in 'reverse lipopolysaccharide transport' and innate immunity. Biochem Soc Trans 39:984–988
48. Meheus LA, Fransen LM, Raymackers JG, Blockx HA, Van Beeumen JJ, Van Bun SM, Van de Voorde A (1993) Identification by microsequencing of lipopolysaccharide-induced proteins secreted by mouse macrophages. J Immunol 151:1535–1547
49. Balbin M, Fueyo A, Knauper V, Pendás AM, López JM, Jiménez MG, Murphy G, López-Otín C (1998) Collagenase 2 (MMP-8) expression in murine tissue-remodeling processes: analysis of its potential role in postpartum involution of the uterus. J Biol Chem 273:23959–23968
50. Imler JL, Hoffmann JA (2000) Toll and toll-like proteins: an ancient family of receptors signaling infection. Rev Immunogenet 2:294–304
51. O'Neill LA (2002) Wanted: a molecular basis for specificity in toll-like receptor signal transduction. Mol Cell 10:969–971
52. Avirutnan P, Hauhart RE, Somnuke P, Blom AM, Diamond MS, Atkinson JP (2011) Binding of flavivirus nonstructural protein NS1 to C4b binding protein modulates complement activation. J Immunol 187:424–433
53. Grosskinsky S, Schott M, Brenner C, Cutler SJ, Simon MM, Wallich R (2010) Human complement regulators C4b-binding protein and C1 esterase inhibitor interact with a novel outer surface protein of Borrelia recurrentis. PLoS Negl Trop Dis 4:e698
54. Mitterhuemer S, Petzl W, Krebs S, Mehne D, Klanner A, Wolf E, Zerbe H, Blum H (2010) Escherichia coli infection induces distinct local and systemic transcriptome responses in the mammary gland. BMC Genomics 11:138
55. Zadura AF, Theander E, Blom AM, Trouw LA (2009) Complement inhibitor C4b-binding protein in primary Sjögren's syndrome and its association with other disease markers. Scand J Immunol 69:374–380
56. Scieglinska D, Piglowski W, Chekan M, Mazurek A, Krawczyk Z (2011) Differential expression of HSPA1 and HSPA2 proteins in human tissues; tissue microarray-based immunohistochemical study. Histochem Cell Biol 135:337–350
57. Hageman J, van Waarde MA, Zylicz A, Walerych D, Kampinga HH (2011) The diverse members of the mammalian HSP70 machine show distinct chaperone-like activities. Biochem J 435:127–142
58. Pan ZQ, Fang ZQ, Lu WL, Liang C, Wu ZH, Liu XM, Hou L, Zhang H, Zhuo SY, Liao MJ, Gao BF (2008) Differentially expressed genes in adrenal gland of H22 liver cancer mice with different syndromes and in different stages. Zhong Xi Yi Jie He Xue Bao 6:843–851
59. Zhang SX, Garcia-Gras E, Wycuff DR, Marriot SJ, Kadeer N, Yu W, Olson EN, Garry DJ, Parmacek MS, Schwartz RJ (2005) Identification of direct serum-response factor gene targets during Me2SO-induced P19 cardiac cell differentiation. J Biol Chem 280: 19115–19126
60. Natoli M, Leoni BD, D'Agnano I, D'Onofrio M, Brandi R, Arisi I, Zucco F, Felsani A (2011) Cell growing density affects the structural and functional properties of Caco-2 differentiated monolayer. J Cell Physiol 226:1531–1543
61. Dehne T, Schenk R, Perka C, Morawietz L, Pruss A, Sittinger M, Kaps C, Ringe J (2010) Gene expression profiling of primary human articular chondrocytes in high-density micromasses reveals patterns of recovery, maintenance, re- and dedifferentiation. Gene 462:8–17
62. Myers SM, Mulligan LM (2004) The RET receptor is linked to stress response pathways. Cancer Res 64:4453–4463
63. Chen W, Chan AS, Dawson AJ, Liang X, Blazar BR, Miller JS (2005) FLT3 ligand administration after hematopoietic cell transplantation increases circulating dendritic cell precursors that can be activated by CpG oligodeoxynucleotides to enhance T-cell and natural killer cell function. Biol Blood Marrow Transplant 11:23–34

64. Melichar B, Tousková M, Dvorák J, Jandík P, Kopecký O (2001) The peripheral blood leukocyte phenotype in patients with breast cancer: effect of doxorubicin/paclitaxel combination chemotherapy. Immunopharmacol Immunotoxicol 23:163–173
65. Menéndez P, Prósper F, Bueno C, Arbona C, San Miguel JF, García-Conde J, Solá C, Hornedo J, Cortés-Funes H, Orfao A (2001) Sequential analysis of CD34+ and CD34- cell subsets in peripheral blood and leukapheresis products from breast cancer patients mobilized with SCF plus G-CSF and cyclophosphamide. Leukemia 15:430–439
66. Minasian LM, Yao TJ, Steffens TA, Scheinberg DA, Williams L, Riedel E (1995) A phase I study of anti-GD3 ganglioside monoclonal antibody R24 and recombinant human macrophage-colony stimulating factor in patients with metastatic melanoma. Cancer 75:2251–2257
67. Larson JH, Kumar CG, Everts RE, Green CA, Everts-van der Wind A, Band MR, Lewin HA (2006) Discovery of eight novel divergent homologs expressed in cattle placenta. Physiol Genomics 25:405–413
68. Bellomo EA, Meur G, Rutter GA (2011) Glucose regulates free cytosolic Zn^{2+} concentration, Slc39 (ZiP), and metallothionein gene expression in primary pancreatic islet β-cells. J Biol Chem 286:25778–25789
69. Thévenod F (2010) Catch me if you can! Novel aspects of cadmium transport in mammalian cells. Biometals 23:857–875
70. Himeno S, Yanagiya T, Fujishiro H (2009) The role of zinc transporters in cadmium and manganese transport in mammalian cells. Biochimie 91:1218–1222
71. Fujishiro H, Okugaki S, Yasumitsu S, Enomoto S, Himeno S (2009) Involvement of DNA hypermethylation in down-regulation of the zinc transporter ZIP8 in cadmium-resistant metallothionein-null cells. Toxicol Appl Pharmacol 241:195–201
72. Aydemir TB, Liuzzi JP, McClellan S, Cousins RJ (2009) Zinc transporter ZIP8 (SLC39A8) and zinc influence IFN-gamma expression in activated human T cells. J Leukoc Biol 86:337–348
73. Ryu MS, Lichten LA, Liuzzi JP, Cousins RJ (2008) Zinc transporters ZnT1 (Slc30a1), Zip8 (Slc39a8), and Zip10 (Slc39a10) in mouse red blood cells are differentially regulated during erythroid development and by dietary zinc deficiency. J Nutr 138:2076–2083
74. Moore-Scott BA, Opoka R, Lin SC, Kordich JJ, Wells JM (2007) Identification of molecular markers that are expressed in discrete anterior-posterior domains of the endoderm from the gastrula stage to mid-gestation. Dev Dyn 236:1997–2003
75. Liu L, Zacchia M, Tian X, Wan L, Sakamoto A, Yanagisawa M, Alpern RJ, Preisig PA (2010) Acid regulation of NaDC-1 requires a functional endothelin B receptor. Kidney Int 78:895–904
76. Love M, Sandberg JL, Ziarek JJ, Gerarden KP, Rode RR, Jensen DR, McCaslin DR, Peterson FC, Veldkamp CT (2012) Solution structure of CCL21 and identification of a putative CCR7 binding site. Biochemistry 51:733–735
77. Tal O, Lim HY, Gurevich I, Milo I, Shipony Z, Ng LG, Angeli V, Shakhar G (2011) DC mobilization from the skin requires docking to immobilized CCL21 on lymphatic endothelium and intralymphatic crawling. J Exp Med 208:2141–2153
78. Liu J, Zhang L, Wang C (2012) CCL21 modulates the migration of NSCL cancer by changing the concentration of intracellular Ca2+. Oncol Rep 27:481–486
79. Nguyen-Hoai T, Baldenhofer G, Sayed Ahmed MS, Pham-Duc M, Vu MD, Lipp M, Dörken B, Pezzutto A, Westermann J (2012) CCL21 (SLC) improves tumor protection by a DNA vaccine in a Her2/neu mouse tumor model. Cancer Gene Ther 19:69–76
80. Jackaman C, Lansley S, Allan JE, Robinson BW, Nelson DJ (2012) IL-2/CD40-driven NK cells install and maintain potency in the anti-mesothelioma effector/memory phase. Int Immunol 24(6):357–368
81. Li R, Pang XQ, Chen WC, Li L, Tian WY, Zhang XG (2012) Gastric cancer cell lines AGS before and after CD40 signal activating. Mol Biol Rep 39:6615–6623

82. Feldman R, Zagoory-Sharon O, Weisman O, Schneiderman I, Gordon I, Maoz R, Shalev I, Ebstein RP (2012) Sensitive parenting is associated with plasma oxytocin and polymorphisms in the OXTR and CD38 genes. Biol Psychiatry 72(3):175–181
83. Camacho Villa AY, Reyes Maldonado E, Montiel Cervantes LA, Vela Ojeda J (2012) CD133+CD34+ and CD133+CD38+ blood progenitor cells as predictors of platelet engraftment in patients undergoing autologous peripheral blood stem cell transplantation. Transfus Apher Sci 46:239–244
84. Zucchetto A, Vaisitti T, Benedetti D, Tissino E, Bertagnolo V, Rossi D et al (2012) The CD49d/CD29 complex is physically and functionally associated with CD38 in B-cell chronic lymphocytic leukemia cells. Leukemia 26(6):1301–1312
85. Fan J, Cai H, Li Q, Du Z, Tan W (2012) The effects of ROS-mediating oxygen tension on human CD34(+)CD38(−) cells induced into mature dendritic cells. J Biotechnol 158:104–111
86. Ma Y, Jiang J, Wang L, Nie H, Xia W, Liu J, Ying W (2012) CD38 is a key enzyme for the survival of mouse microglial BV2 cells. Biochem Biophys Res Commun 418:714–719
87. Srivastava P, Russo J, Russo IH (1997) Chorionic gonadotropin inhibits mammary carcinogenesis through activation of programmed cell death. Carcinogenesis 18:1799–1808
88. Srivastava P, Russo J, Russo IH (1999) Inhibition of rat mammary tumorigenesis by human chorionic gonadotropin is associated with increased expression of inhibin. Mol Carcinog 26:10–19
89. Tang X, Xing Z, Tang H, Liang L, Zhao M (2011) Human cell-death-inducing DFF45-like effector C induces apoptosis via caspase-8. Acta Biochim Biophys Sin (Shanghai) 43:779–786
90. Ito M, Nagasawa M, Omae N, Ide T, Akasaka Y, Murakami K (2011) Differential regulation of CIDEA and CIDEC expression by insulin via Akt1/2- and JNK2-dependent pathways in human adipocytes. J Lipid Res 52:1450–1460
91. Yonezawa T, Kurata R, Kimura M, Inoko H (2011) Which CIDE are you on? Apoptosis and energy metabolism. Mol Biosyst 7:91–100
92. Li F, Gu Y, Dong W, Li H, Zhang L, Li N, Zhang L, Song Y, Jiang L, Ye J, Li Q (2010) Cell death-inducing DFF45-like effector, a lipid droplet-associated protein, might be involved in the differentiation of human adipocytes. FEBS J 277:4173–4183
93. Wang ZQ, Yu Y, Zhang XH, Floyd EZ, Cefalu WT (2010) Human adenovirus 36 decreases fatty acid oxidation and increases de novo lipogenesis in primary cultured human skeletal muscle cells by promoting Cidec/FSP27 expression. Int J Obes (Lond) 34:1355–1364
94. Lin WH, Wu CH, Chen YC, Chow WY (2006) Embryonic expression of zebrafish AMPA receptor genes: zygotic gria2alpha expression initiates at the midblastula transition. Brain Res 1110:46–54
95. Ripka S, Riedel J, Neesse A, Griesmann H, Buchholz M, Ellenrieder V, Moeller F, Barth P, Gress TM, Michl P (2010) Glutamate receptor GRIA3—target of CUX1 and mediator of tumor progression in pancreatic cancer. Neoplasia 12:659–667
96. Bonneau A, Parmar N (2012) Effects of RhebL1 silencing on the mTOR pathway. Mol Biol Rep 39:2129–2137
97. Yuan J, Shan Y, Chen X, Tang W, Luo K, Ni J, Wan B, Yu L (2005) Identification and characterization of RHEBL1, a novel member of Ras family, which activates transcriptional activities of NF-kappa B. Mol Biol Rep 32:205–214
98. Tee AR, Blenis J, Proud CG (2005) Analysis of mTOR signaling by the small G-proteins, Rheb and RhebL1. FEBS Lett 579:4763–4768
99. Dunlop EA, Dodd KM, Seymour LA, Tee AR (2009) Mammalian target of rapamycin complex 1-mediated phosphorylation of eukaryotic initiation factor 4E-binding protein 1 requires multiple protein-protein interactions for substrate recognition. Cell Signal 21:1073–1084
100. Maeurer C, Holland S, Pierre S, Potstada W, Scholich K (2009) Sphingosine-1-phosphate induced mTOR-activation is mediated by the E3-ubiquitin ligase PAM. Cell Signal 21:293–300

101. Robb VA, Karbowniczek M, Klein-Szanto AJ, Henske EP (2007) Activation of the mTOR signaling pathway in renal clear cell carcinoma. J Urol 177:346–352
102. Robb VA, Astrinidis A, Henske EP (2006) Frequent [corrected] hyperphosphorylation of ribosomal protein S6 [corrected] in lymphangioleiomyomatosis-associated angiomyolipomas. Mod Pathol 19:839–846
103. Lütcke A, Olkkonen VM, Dupree P, Lütcke H, Simons K, Zerial M (1995) Isolation of a murine cDNA clone encoding Rab19, a novel tissue-specific small GTPase. Gene 155:257–260
104. Guo JH, Chen L, Chen S, Liu X, Saiyin H, Deng Q, Zhuang Y, Wan B, Yu L, Zhao SY (2003) Isolation, expression pattern of a novel human RAB gene RAB41 and characterization of its intronless homolog RAB41P. DNA Seq 14:431–435
105. Sinka R, Gillingham AK, Kondylis V, Munro S (2008) Golgi coiled-coil proteins contain multiple binding sites for Rab family G proteins. J Cell Biol 183:607–615
106. Sasaki Y, Negishi H, Koyama R, Anbo N, Ohori K, Idogawa M, Mita H, Toyota M, Imai K, Shinomura Y, Tokino T (2009) p53 family members regulate the expression of the apolipoprotein D gene. J Biol Chem 284:872–883
107. Molnár A, Gyurján I, Korpos E, Borsy A, Stéger V, Buzás Z, Kiss I, Zomborszky Z, Papp P, Deák F, Orosz L (2007) Identification of differentially expressed genes in the developing antler of red deer Cervus elaphus. Mol Genet Genomics 277:237–248
108. Bujalska IJ, Quinkler M, Tomlinson JW, Montague CT, Smith DM, Stewart PM (2006) Expression profiling of 11beta-hydroxysteroid dehydrogenase type-1 and glucocorticoid-target genes in subcutaneous and omental human preadipocytes. J Mol Endocrinol 37:327–340
109. Hummasti S, Laffitte BA, Watson MA, Galardi C, Chao LC, Ramamurthy L, Moore JT, Tontonoz P (2004) Liver X receptors are regulators of adipocyte gene expression but not differentiation: identification of apoD as a direct target. J Lipid Res 45:616–625
110. Alvarez ML, Barbón JJ, González LO, Abelairas J, Boto A, Vizoso FJ (2003) Apolipoprotein D expression in retinoblastoma. Ophthalmic Res 35:111–116
111. Tsui KH, Chang YL, Feng TH, Chang PL, Juang HH (2012) Glycoprotein transmembrane nmb: an androgen-downregulated gene attenuates cell invasion and tumorigenesis in prostate carcinoma cells. Prostate 72:1431–1442
112. Fotovati A, Abu-Ali S, Sugita Y, Nakamura Y (2011) Expression of N-myc downstream regulated gene 1 (NDRG1) in central neurocytoma. J Clin Neurosci 18:1383–1385
113. Lai LC, Su YY, Chen KC, Tsai MH, Sher YP, Lu TP, Lee CY, Chuang EY (2011) Down-regulation of NDRG1 promotes migration of cancer cells during reoxygenation. PLoS One 6(8):e24375
114. McCaig C, Potter L, Abramczyk O, Murray JT (2011) Phosphorylation of NDRG1 is temporally and spatially controlled during the cell cycle. Biochem Biophys Res Commun 411:227–234
115. Liu W, Xing F, Iiizumi-Gairani M, Okuda H, Watabe M, Pai SK, Pandey PR, Hirota S, Kobayashi A, Mo YY, Fukuda K, Li Y, Watabe K (2012) N-myc downstream regulated gene 1 modulates Wnt-β-catenin signalling and pleiotropically suppresses metastasis. EMBO Mol Med 4:93–108
116. Lerner A, Grafi-Cohen M, Napso T, Azzam N, Fares F (2012) The indolic diet-derivative, 3,3′-diindolylmethane, induced apoptosis in human colon cancer cells through upregulation of NDRG1. J Biomed Biotechnol 2:256178
117. Kobayashi A, Okuda H, Xing F, Pandey PR, Watabe M, Hirota S, Pai SK, Liu W, Fukuda K, Chambers C, Wilber A, Watabe K (2011) Bone morphogenetic protein 7 in dormancy and metastasis of prostate cancer stem-like cells in bone. J Exp Med 208:2641–2655
118. Hickok JR, Sahni S, Mikhed Y, Bonini MG, Thomas DD (2011) Nitric oxide suppresses tumor cell migration through N-Myc downstream-regulated gene-1 (NDRG1) expression: role of chelatable iron. J Biol Chem 286:41413–41424
119. Meitzler JL, Brandman R, Ortiz de Montellano PR (2010) Perturbed heme binding is responsible for the blistering phenotype associated with mutations in the Caenorhabditis elegans dual oxidase 1 (DUOX1) peroxidase domain. J Biol Chem 285:40991–41000

120. Senou M, Khalifa C, Thimmesch M, Jouret F, Devuyst O, Col V, Audinot JN, Lipnik P, Moreno JC, Van Sande J, Dumont JE, Many MC, Colin IM, Gérard AC (2010) A coherent organization of differentiation proteins is required to maintain an appropriate thyroid function in the Pendred thyroid. J Clin Endocrinol Metab 95:4021–4030
121. Rigutto S, Hoste C, Grasberger H, Milenkovic M, Communi D, Dumont JE, Corvilain B, Miot F, De Deken X (2009) Activation of dual oxidases Duox1 and Duox2: differential regulation mediated by camp-dependent protein kinase and protein kinase C-dependent phosphorylation. J Biol Chem 284:6725–6734
122. van der Hoeven R, McCallum KC, Cruz MR, Garsin DA (2011) Ce-Duox1/BLI-3 generated reactive oxygen species trigger protective SKN-1 activity via p38 MAPK signaling during Infection in C. elegans. PLoS Pathog 7(12):e1002453
123. Lu CL, Qiu JL, Huang PZ, Zou RH, Hong J, Li BK, Chen GH, Yuan YF (2011) NADPH oxidase DUOX1 and DUOX2 but not NOX4 are independent predictors in hepatocellular carcinoma after hepatectomy. Tumour Biol 32:1173–1182
124. Hirakawa S, Saito R, Ohara H, Okuyama R, Aiba S (2011) Dual oxidase 1 induced by Th2 cytokines promotes STAT6 phosphorylation via oxidative inactivation of protein tyrosine phosphatase 1B in human epidermal keratinocytes. J Immunol 186:4762–4770
125. Donkó A, Ruisanchez E, Orient A, Enyedi B, Kapui R, Péterfi Z, de Deken X, Benyó Z, Geiszt M (2010) Urothelial cells produce hydrogen peroxide through the activation of Duox1. Free Radic Biol Med 49:2040–2048
126. Kennedy KA, Ostrakhovitch EA, Sandiford SD, Dayarathna T, Xie X, Waese EY, Chang WY, Feng Q, Skerjanc IS, Stanford WL, Li SS (2010) Mammalian numb-interacting protein 1/dual oxidase maturation factor 1 directs neuronal fate in stem cells. J Biol Chem 285:17974–17985
127. Ostrakhovitch EA, Li SS (2010) NIP1/DUOXA1 expression in epithelial breast cancer cells: regulation of cell adhesion and actin dynamics. Breast Cancer Res Treat 119:773–786
128. Gattas MV, Forteza R, Fragoso MA, Fregien N, Salas P, Salathe M, Conner GE (2009) Oxidative epithelial host defense is regulated by infectious and inflammatory stimuli. Free Radic Biol Med 47:1450–1458
129. Boots AW, Hristova M, Kasahara DI, Haenen GR, Bast A, van der Vliet A (2009) ATP-mediated activation of the NADPH oxidase DUOX1 mediates airway epithelial responses to bacterial stimuli. J Biol Chem 284:17858–17867
130. Perttilä J, Huaman-Samanez C, Caron S, Tanhuanpää K, Staels B, Yki-Järvinen H, Olkkonen VM (2012) PNPLA3 is regulated by glucose in human hepatocytes and its i148M mutant slows down triglyceride hydrolysis. Am J Physiol Endocrinol Metab 302:E1063–E1069
131. Fuchs C, Claudel T, Kumari P, Haemmerle G, Pollheimer M, Stojakovic T, Scharnagl H, Halilbasic E, Gumhold J, Silbert D, Koefeler H, Trauner M (2012) Absence of adipose triglyceride lipase protects from hepatic ER stress. Hepatology 56(1):270–280. doi:10.1002/hep.25601
132. Hernandez L, Magalhaes MA, Coniglio SJ, Condeelis JS, Segall JE (2011) Opposing roles of CXCR4 and CXCR7 in breast cancer metastasis. Breast Cancer Res 13:R128
133. Chu JH, Lazarus R, Carey VJ, Raby BA (2011) Quantifying differential gene connectivity between disease states for objective identification of disease-relevant genes. BMC Syst Biol 5:89
134. Delassus GS, Cho H, Eliceiri GL (2011) New signaling pathways from cancer progression modulators to mRNA expression of matrix metalloproteinases in breast cancer cells. J Cell Physiol 226:3378–3384
135. Shishido-Hara Y, Kurata A, Fujiwara M, Itoh H, Imoto S, Kamma H (2010) Two cases of breast carcinoma with osteoclastic giant cells: are the osteoclastic giant cells pro-tumoural differentiation of macrophages? Diagn Pathol 5:55
136. Margheri F, Serratì S, Lapucci A, Anastasia C, Giusti B, Pucci M, Torre E, Bianchini F, Calorini L, Albini A, Ventura A, Fibbi G, Del Rosso M (2009) Systemic sclerosis-endothelial

cell antiangiogenic pentraxin 3 and matrix metalloprotease 12 control human breast cancer tumor vascularization and development in mice. Neoplasia 11:1106–1115
137. Aharinejad S, Paulus P, Sioud M, Hofmann M, Zins K, Schäfer R, Stanley ER, Abraham D (2004) Colony-stimulating factor-1 blockade by antisense oligonucleotides and small interfering RNAs suppresses growth of human mammary tumor xenografts in mice. Cancer Res 64:5378–5384
138. Giambernardi TA, Grant GM, Taylor GP, Hay RJ, Maher VM, McCormick JJ, Klebe RJ (1998) Overview of matrix metalloproteinase expression in cultured human cells. Matrix Biol 16:483–496
139. Kretschmer C, Sterner-Kock A, Siedentopf F, Schoenegg W, Schlag PM, Kemmner W (2011) Identification of early molecular markers for breast cancer. Mol Cancer 10:15
140. Chakraborty G, Jain S, Patil TV, Kundu GC (2008) Down-regulation of osteopontin attenuates breast tumour progression in vivo. J Cell Mol Med 12:2305–2318
141. Mi Z, Oliver T, Guo H, Gao C, Kuo PC (2007) Thrombin-cleaved COOH(−) terminal osteopontin peptide binds with cyclophilin C to CD147 in murine breast cancer cells. Cancer Res 67:4088–4097
142. Allan AL, George R, Vantyghem SA, Lee MW, Hodgson NC, Engel CJ, Holliday RL, Girvan DP, Scott LA, Postenka CO, Al-Katib W, Stitt LW, Uede T, Chambers AF, Tuck AB (2006) Role of the integrin-binding protein osteopontin in lymphatic metastasis of breast cancer. Am J Pathol 169:233–246
143. Cook AC, Chambers AF, Turley EA, Tuck AB (2006) Osteopontin induction of hyaluronan synthase 2 expression promotes breast cancer malignancy. J Biol Chem 281:24381–24389
144. Khan SA, Cook AC, Kappil M, Günthert U, Chambers AF, Tuck AB, Denhardt DT (2005) Enhanced cell surface CD44 variant (v6, v9) expression by osteopontin in breast cancer epithelial cells facilitates tumor cell migration: novel post-transcriptional, post-translational regulation. Clin Exp Metastasis 22:663–673
145. Briese J, Schulte HM, Bamberger CM, Löning T, Bamberger AM (2006) Expression pattern of osteopontin in endometrial carcinoma: correlation with expression of the adhesion molecule CEACAM1. Int J Gynecol Pathol 25:161–169
146. Uehara N, Unami A, Kiyozuka Y, Shikata N, Oishi Y, Tsubura A (2006) Parous mammary glands exhibit distinct alterations in gene expression and proliferation responsiveness to carcinogenic stimuli in Lewis rats. Oncol Rep 15:903–911
147. Parsley S, Gazi L, Bobirnac I, Loetscher E, Schoeffter P (1999) Functional alpha2C-adrenoceptors in human neuroblastoma SH-SY5Y cells. Eur J Pharmacol 372:109–115
148. Cayla C, Schaak S, Roquelaine C, Gales C, Quinchon F, Paris H (1999) Homologous regulation of the alpha2C-adrenoceptor subtype in human hepatocarcinoma, HepG2. Br J Pharmacol 126:69–78
149. Pihlavisto M, Sjöholm B, Scheinin M, Wurster S (1998) Modulation of agonist binding to recombinant human alpha2-adrenoceptors by sodium ions. Biochim Biophys Acta 1448:135–146
150. Powe DG, Voss MJ, Habashy HO, Zänker KS, Green AR, Ellis IO, Entschladen F (2011) Alpha- and beta-adrenergic receptor (AR) protein expression is associated with poor clinical outcome in breast cancer: an immunohistochemical study. Breast Cancer Res Treat 130:457–463
151. Vázquez SM, Mladovan AG, Pérez C, Bruzzone A, Baldi A, Lüthy IA (2006) Human breast cell lines exhibit functional alpha2-adrenoceptors. Cancer Chemother Pharmacol 58:50–61
152. Devedjian JC, Schaak S, Gamet L, Denis-Pouxviel C, Paris H (1996) Regulation of alpha 2A-adrenergic receptor expression in the human colon carcinoma cell line HT29: SCFA-induced enterocytic differentiation results in an inhibition of alpha 2C10 gene transcription. Proc Assoc Am Physicians 108:334–344
153. Northcott PA, Korshunov A, Witt H, Hielscher T, Eberhart CG, Mack S, Bouffet E, Clifford SC, Hawkins CE, French P, Rutka JT, Pfister S, Taylor MD (2011) Medulloblastoma comprises four distinct molecular variants. J Clin Oncol 29:1408–1414

154. Heesch S, Schlee C, Neumann M, Stroux A, Kühnl A, Schwartz S, Haferlach T, Goekbuget N, Hoelzer D, Thiel E, Hofmann WK, Baldus CD (2010) BAALC-associated gene expression profiles define IGFBP7 as a novel molecular marker in acute leukemia. Leukemia 24:1429–1436
155. Filipski E, Li XM, Lévi F (2006) Disruption of circadian coordination and malignant growth. Cancer Causes Control 17:509–514
156. Hua H, Wang Y, Wan C, Liu Y, Zhu B, Wang X, Wang Z, Ding JM (2007) Inhibition of tumorigenesis by intratumoral delivery of the circadian gene mPer2 in C57BL/6 mice. Cancer Gene Ther 14:815–818
157. Hrushesky WJ, Grutsch J, Wood P, Yang X, Oh EY, Ansell C, Kidder S, Ferrans C, Quiton DF, Reynolds J, Du-Quiton J, Levin R, Lis C, Braun D (2009) Circadian clock manipulation for cancer prevention and control and the relief of cancer symptoms. Integr Cancer Ther 8:387–397
158. Wood PA, Yang X, Hrushesky WJ (2009) Clock genes and cancer. Integr Cancer Ther 8:303–308
159. Zhang X, Zarbl H (2008) Chemopreventive doses of methylselenocysteine alter circadian rhythm in rat mammary tissue. Cancer Prev Res 1:119–127
160. Boots AW, Hristova M, Kasahara DI, Haenen GR, Bast A, van der Vliet A (2009) ATP-mediated activation of the NADPH oxidase DUOX1 mediates airway epithelial responses to bacterial stimuli. Biol Chem 284:17858–17867
161. Umekita Y, Souda M, Hatanaka K, Hamada T, Yoshioka T, Kawaguchi H, Tanimoto A (2011) Gene expression profile of terminal end buds in rat mammary glands exposed to diethylstilbestrol in neonatal period. Toxicol Lett 205:15–25
162. Wellberg E, Metz RP, Parker C, Porter WW (2010) The bHLH/PAS transcription factor single-minded 2s promotes mammary gland lactogenic differentiation. Development 137:945–952
163. Tiffen PG, Omidvar N, Marquez-Almuina N, Croston D, Watson CJ, Clarkson RW (2008) A dual role for oncostatin M signaling in the differentiation and death of mammary epithelial cells in vivo. Mol Endocrinol 22:2677–2688
164. Wei YY, Chen YJ, Hsiao YC, Huang YC, Lai TH, Tang CH (2008) Osteoblasts-derived TGF-beta1 enhance motility and integrin upregulation through Akt, ERK, and NF-kappaB-dependent pathway in human breast cancer cells. Mol Carcinog 47:526–537
165. Blakely CM, Stoddard AJ, Belka GK, Dugan KD, Notarfrancesco KL, Moody SE, D'Cruz CM, Chodosh L (2006) Hormone-induced protection against mammary tumorigenesis is conserved in multiple rat strains and identifies a core gene expression signature induced by pregnancy. Cancer Res 66:6421–6431
166. Thordarson G, Slusher N, Leong H, Ochoa D, Rajkumar L, Guzman R, Nandi S, Talamantes F (2004) Insulin-like growth factor (IGF)-I obliterates the pregnancy-associated protection against mammary carcinogenesis in rats: evidence that IGF-I enhances cancer progression through estrogen receptor-alpha activation via the mitogen-activated protein kinase pathway. Breast Cancer Res 6:R423–R436
167. Ghellal A, Li C, Hayes M, Byrne G, Bundred N, Kumar S (2000) Prognostic significance of TGF beta 1 and TGF beta 3 in human breast carcinoma. Anticancer Res 20:4413–4418
168. Chakravarthy D, Green AR, Green VL, Kerin MJ, Speirs V (1999) Expression and secretion of TGF-beta isoforms and expression of TGF-beta-receptors I, II and III in normal and neoplastic human breast. Int J Oncol 15:187–194
169. Archey WB, Sweet MP, Alig GC, Arrick BA (1999) Methylation of CpGs as a determinant of transcriptional activation at alternative promoters for transforming growth factor-beta3. Cancer Res 59:2292–2296
170. Scollen S, Luccarini C, Baynes C, Driver K, Humphreys MK, Garcia-Closas M, Figueroa J, Lissowska J, Pharoah PD, Easton DF, Hesketh R, Metcalfe JC, Dunning AM (2011) TGF-β signaling pathway and breast cancer susceptibility. Cancer Epidemiol Biomarkers Prev 20:1112–1119
171. Gauger KJ, Chenausky KL, Murray ME, Schneider SS (2011) SFRP1 reduction results in an increased sensitivity to TGF-β signaling. BMC Cancer 11:59

172. Figueroa JD, Flanders KC, Garcia-Closas M, Anderson WF, Yang XR, Matsuno RK, Duggan MA, Pfeiffer RM, Ooshima A, Cornelison R, Gierach GL, Brinton LA, Lissowska J, Peplonska B, Wakefield LM, Sherman ME (2010) Expression of TGF-beta signaling factors in invasive breast cancers: relationships with age at diagnosis and tumor characteristics. Breast Cancer Res Treat 121:727–735
173. Laverty HG, Wakefield LM, Occleston NL, O'Kane S, Ferguson MW (2009) TGF-beta3 and cancer: a review. Cytokine Growth Factor Rev 20:305–317
174. Flanders KC, Wakefield LM (2009) Transforming growth factor-(beta)s and mammary gland involution; functional roles and implications for cancer progression. J Mammary Gland Biol Neoplasia 14:131–144
175. McDonald LA, Gerrelli D, Fok Y, Hurst LD, Tickle C (2010) Comparison of Iroquois gene expression in limbs/fins of vertebrate embryos. J Anat 216:683–691
176. Rodríguez-Seguel E, Alarcón P, Gómez-Skarmeta JL (2009) The Xenopus Irx genes are essential for neural patterning and define the border between prethalamus and thalamus through mutual antagonism with the anterior repressors Fezf and Arx. Dev Biol 329:258–268
177. Matsumoto K, Nishihara S, Kamimura M, Shiraishi T, Otoguro T, Uehara M, Maeda Y, Ogura K, Lumsden A, Ogura T (2004) The prepattern transcription factor Irx2, a target of the FGF8/MAP kinase cascade, is involved in cerebellum formation. Nat Neurosci 7:605–612
178. Ahn JI, Lee KH, Shin DM, Shim JW, Lee JS, Chang SY, Lee YS, Brownstein MJ, Zülch A, Becker MB, Gruss P (2001) Expression pattern of Irx1 and Irx2 during mouse digit development. Mech Dev 106:159–162
179. Chambers KF, Pearson JF, Pellacani D, Aziz N, Gužvić M, Klein CA, Lang SH (2011) Stromal upregulation of lateral epithelial adhesions: gene expression analysis of signalling pathways in prostate epithelium. J Biomed Sci 22:18–45
180. Kamalakaran S, Varadan V, Giercksky Russnes HE, Levy D, Kendall J, Janevski A, Riggs M, Banerjee N, Synnestvedt M, Schlichting E, Kåresen R, Shama Prasada K, Rotti H, Rao R, Rao L, Eric Tang MH, Satyamoorthy K, Lucito R, Wigler M, Dimitrova N, Naume B, Borresen-Dale AL, Hicks JB (2011) DNA methylation patterns in luminal breast cancers differ from non-luminal subtypes and can identify relapse risk independent of other clinical variables. Mol Oncol 5:77–92
181. Choy SW, Cheng CW, Lee ST, Li VW, Hui MN, Hui CC, Liu D, Cheng SH (2010) A cascade of irx1a and irx2a controls shh expression during retinogenesis. Dev Dyn 239:3204–3214
182. Reggiani L, Raciti D, Airik R, Kispert A, Brändli AW (2007) The prepattern transcription factor Irx3 directs nephron segment identity. Genes Dev 21:2358–2370
183. Petri A, Ahnfelt-Rønne J, Frederiksen KS, Edwards DG, Madsen D, Serup P, Fleckner J, Heller RS (2006) The effect of neurogenin3 deficiency on pancreatic gene expression in embryonic mice. J Mol Endocrinol 37:301–316
184. Rauch TA, Wang Z, Wu X, Kernstine KH, Riggs AD, Pfeifer GP (2012) DNA methylation biomarkers for lung cancer. Tumour Biol 33:287–296
185. Vreeburg RA, van Wezel EE, Ocaña-Calahorro F, Mes JJ (2012) Apple extract induces increased epithelial resistance and claudin 4 expression in Caco-2 cells. J Sci Food Agric 92:439–444
186. Stankovich BL, Aguayo E, Barragan F, Sharma A, Pallavicini MG (2011) Differential adhesion molecule expression during murine embryonic stem cell commitment to the hematopoietic and endothelial lineages. PLoS One 6(9):e23810
187. Gao Z, Xu X, McClane B, Zeng Q, Litkouhi B, Welch WR, Berkowitz RS, Mok SC, Garner EI (2011) C terminus of Clostridium perfringens enterotoxin downregulates CLDN4 and sensitizes ovarian cancer cells to Taxol and Carboplatin. Clin Cancer Res 17:1065–1074
188. Kwon MJ, Kim SH, Jeong HM, Jung HS, Kim SS, Lee JE, Gye MC, Erkin OC, Koh SS, Choi YL, Park CK, Shin YK (2011) Claudin-4 overexpression is associated with epigenetic derepression in gastric carcinoma. Lab Invest 91:1652–1667
189. Tsutsumi K, Sato N, Tanabe R, Mizumoto K, Morimatsu K, Kayashima T, Fujita H, Ohuchida K, Ohtsuka T, Takahata S, Nakamura M, Tanaka M (2011) Claudin-4 expression predicts survival in pancreatic ductal adenocarcinoma. Ann Surg Oncol 2011 Aug 12 [Epub ahead of print]

190. Kawai Y, Hamazaki Y, Fujita H, Fujita A, Sato T, Furuse M, Fujimoto T, Jetten AM, Agata Y, Minato N (2011) Claudin-4 induction by E-protein activity in later stages of CD4/8 double-positive thymocytes to increase positive selection efficiency. Proc Natl Acad Sci USA 108:4075–4080
191. Werth M, Walentin K, Aue A, Schönheit J, Wuebken A, Pode-Shakked N, Vilianovitch L, Erdmann B, Dekel B, Bader M, Barasch J, Rosenbauer F, Luft FC, Schmidt-Ott KM (2010) The transcription factor grainyhead-like 2 regulates the molecular composition of the epithelial apical junctional complex. Development 137:3835–3845
192. Papageorgis P, Lambert AW, Ozturk S, Gao F, Pan H, Manne U, Alekseyev YO, Thiagalingam A, Abdolmaleky HM, Lenburg M, Thiagalingam S (2010) Smad signaling is required to maintain epigenetic silencing during breast cancer progression. Cancer Res 70:968–978
193. Kwon MJ, Kim SS, Choi YL, Jung HS, Balch C, Kim SH, Song YS, Marquez VE, Nephew KP, Shin YK (2010) Derepression of CLDN3 and CLDN4 during ovarian tumorigenesis is associated with loss of repressive histone modifications. Carcinogenesis 31:974–983
194. Yuan X, Lin X, Manorek G, Kanatani I, Cheung LH, Rosenblum MG, Howell SB (2009) Recombinant CPE fused to tumor necrosis factor targets human ovarian cancer cells expressing the claudin-3 and claudin-4 receptors. Mol Cancer Ther 8:1906–1915

Chapter 4
The Use of In Vitro Three-Dimensional System for Studying Breast Cancer and Preventing Agents

4.1 Introduction

Historically, the challenge of recreating tissue architecture in three-dimensions has been the task of those tissue engineers interested in growing implants for the purpose of grafting this tissue into human patients. Part of the challenge has been finding alternatives to tissues derived from animals or humans which may vary from batch to batch. Since 1975, our laboratory has used the very simple concept that the three-dimensional (3D) model must reproduce the morphological appearance of the tissue of origin. Originally, we used collagen-coated cellulose sponges, which provide an excellent technique for the study of 3D expression of tumor morphology and for investigating MCF-7s cellular interrelations [1–5]. The morphologic pattern exhibited by the metastatic human breast cancer cell line MCF-7 grown in the collagen-coated cellulose sponge was similar to the histological pattern found in both the precursor primary tumor and the pleural metastasis from which this cell line was derived [6]. From this seminal work, we have identified that the use of type I collagen matrix is a reproducible extracellular matrix for creating a 3D structure of the tumor tissue and most importantly the normal ductal structures. Primary mammary epithelial cells grown in collagen matrix are able to form tree-like structures resembling in vivo ductulogenesis [7]. The human breast epithelial cells MCF-10F formed tubules when grown in type I collagen. The advantage of an in vitro model of 3D growth is that it allows for modeling of the epithelial architecture of the breast [5, 8–10]. Normal epithelial cells form ducts-like structures, having apical–basal polarity and well-organized tubular structures with stable adherent junctions and cell-basement communications. The malignant transformation is associated with the loss of apical–basal polarity and monolayer morphology and significant deviations from normal epithelial behavior in 3D cultures [10, 11] (see Sect. 4.5). In several studies, basement membrane (BM) like Matrigel has been used to study the growth and differentiation of the breast epithelia. Matrigel is a complex mixture of extracellular matrix proteins and growth factors extracted from a murine tumor (Engelbreth-Holm-Swarm); its components are laminin, type IV collagen, epidermal

J. Russo and I.H. Russo, *Role of the Transcriptome in Breast Cancer Prevention*,
DOI 10.1007/978-1-4614-4884-6_4,

growth factor (EGF), transforming growth factor beta (TGF-β), and insulin like growth factor (IGF) [12, 13]. The advantage of the type I collagen is that it provides the structural support which allows for the expression of the breast epithelial cells intrinsic properties, while the use of BM is best used to study the role of different factors and extracellular matrix components that affect the branching [12]. For example, some cells such as MDCK kidney cells formed tubular structures in type I collagen in the presence of hepatocyte growth factor (HGF), but not in Matrigel. The MDCK cells form multicellular cysts when they are grown suspended in Matrigel, whereas they form branching cords in type I collagen. However, when cultured in a mixture of collagen and Matrigel, these cells give rise to elongated, branched tubules with visible lumen. Studies of the matrix components demonstrated that collagen IV and vitronectin inhibit the branching and tubule formation, whereas collagen I, laminin, and fibronectin promote the process. Furthermore, EGF promotes proliferation and spheroid formation and low TGF concentrations induce tubule formation [10]. Due to the different response of the epithelium to the composition of the extracellular matrix, we have selected to use type I collagen gel matrix which is more appropriate for our study to observe the effect of the carcinogenic or environmental compounds on the breast epithelial cells MCF-10F in the absence of the morphogenetic factors present in the matrigel.

4.2 The Three-dimensional Growth of Human Breast Epithelial Cells

Our observations that ductal carcinomas originate in lobules type 1 (Lob 1) of the immature breast [14] (Fig. 4.1), which are the structures with the highest proliferative activity, provide a mechanistic explanation for the higher susceptibility of these structures to undergo neoplastic transformation when exposed to chemical carcinogens, as demonstrated in in vitro experiments [3]. The cells obtained from the normal lobular structures type 1 proliferate in culture and are ERα negative suggesting that the stem cells that originate from normal ductal structures are the ERα negative proliferating cells. This is supported by our observations that MCF-10F, a spontaneously immortalized ERα negative human breast epithelial cell line derived from breast tissues containing Lob 1 and Lob 2 [1, 2], is able to form normal ductal structures in a 3D collagen matrix system. The ductal structures are lined by a monolayer of well polarized epithelial cells that become malignant after exposure to the chemical carcinogens benz(a)pyrene [3] or 17β-estradiol (E_2) [4, 15]. In this model [4, 5], the immortal MCF-10F cells that are E_2-transformed (trMCF cells) progressively express phenotypes of in vitro cell transformation, including loss of the ductulogenic capacity (Fig. 4.2). Loss of the ductulogenic capacity is the earliest phenotype observed accompanied by increasing cell proliferation and the activation of genes related to DNA cell replication, inhibition of apoptosis, and the expression of genes related to cell polarity, cell positioning, and cellular architecture (Table 4.1). Further selection of these trMCF cells for invasiveness in a Matrigel invasion system identified cells (bcMCF) that

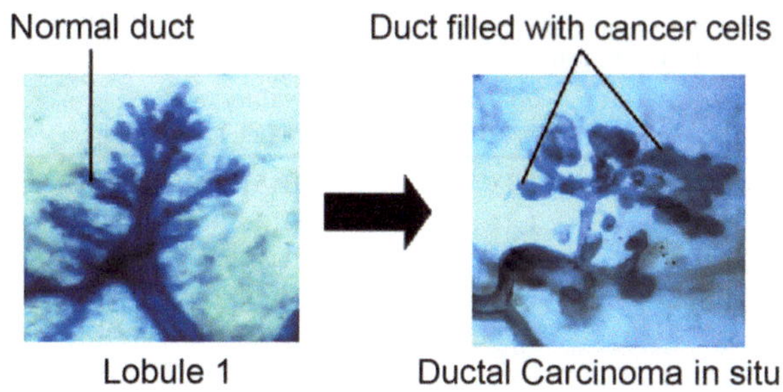

Fig. 4.1 Lobule type 1 or the terminal ductal lobular unit is the site of origin of ductal carcinoma in situ (DCIS) (adapted from Russo et al (2000) J Natl Cancer Inst Monogr 27:17–38)

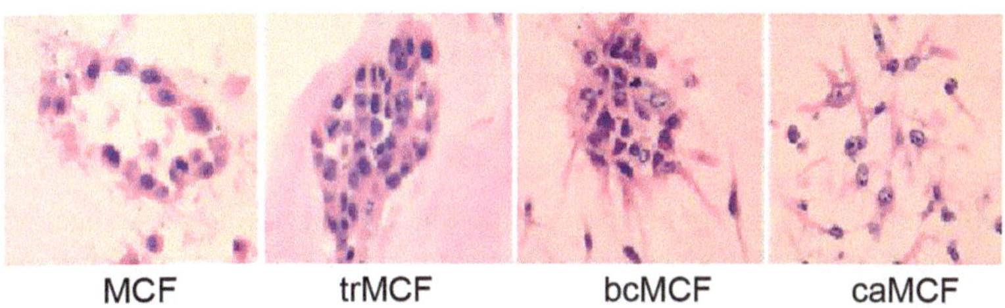

Fig. 4.2 In vitro–in vivo model of cell transformation. MCF-10F, a human breast epithelial cell line spontaneously immortalized and estrogen receptor alpha (ERα)-negative, became transformed after 17b-estradiol treatment. losing their ductulogenic capacity forming the trMCF cells that evolve to bcMCF and caMCF cells. All the cells were cultured in Dulbecco's modified Eagle medium (DMEM/F-12, Gibco®; Formula 90-5212 EF) with 5% horse serum, 2.43 g/L sodium bicarbonate, 20 μg/L epidermal growth factor (EGF), 100 μg/L *Vibrio cholera* toxin, 10 mg/L insulin, 0.5 mg/L hydrocortisone, 1.05 mM calcium, antibiotics, and antimicotic (Gibco, Cat # 15240-062). The cells were resuspended at a final concentration of 7.5×10^3 cells/mL in collagen matrix consisting of 2.68 mg/mL (89.3%) type I collagen (PureCol, Inamed Biomaterials CO., Fremont, CA), 8% 12.5× DMEM-F12 with antibiotics, 0.1 mg/mL insulin, 14 mM $NaHCO_3$, and 0.01 N NaOH. A volume of 400 μL of this mixture was plated into 24-well chambers pre-coated 400 μL collagen base at the same concentration. Eight wells were used and 3,000 cells were plated per well. After the solidification of the collagen, the cells were fed with standard medium which was replaced daily. The cells in collagen matrix were examined under an inverted microscope (Nikon Eclipse, TS100, Japan), and after 8 days, the ductulogenesis process was evaluated. Twenty ducts from each were chosen at random and the length and diameter of the main tubule was measured using an ocular scale; also the number of primary, secondary, and tertiary branching arising from the main duct were counted. Analysis of variance (ANOVA) followed by Tukey's test was be used for comparing architectural parameters (adapted from [4] and Tiezzi et al (2007) Int J Oncol 31:823–827)

formed tumors in severe combined immunodeficient (SCID) mice. The cell lines derived from those tumors (caMCF) were poorly differentiated ERα, PR, and ERBB2 negative adenocarcinomas [4, 5]. These characteristics are similar to the human basal cell-like carcinomas previously described [16]. To better understand the molecular events associated with the progressive phenotypic changes that were observed during estrogen-mediated malignant cell transformation, we analyzed chromosomal copy number (CN), loss of heterozygosity (LOH), and gene expression changes that

Table 4.1 List of genes dysregulated during the neoplastic transformation of human breast epithelial cells and in primary breast cancer

Gene	Fold change (trMCF)	*q*-value (trMCF)	Gene	Fold change (trMCF)	*q*-value (trMCF)
MKI67	1.78	0.0451	POLE2	2.68	0.0123
AURKB	1.84	0.013	RFC3	2.14	0.0473
BIRC5	1.71	0.0475	ARHGDIA	3.41	0.0294
CENPA	1.91	0.0438	TGFB2	−3.64	0.0163
CST6	−4.29	0.0104	TGFBR2	−2.21	0.0112
DUSP1	2.97	0.0641	TRIM22	−40.82	0.00844
E2F2	1.95	0.0395	TP53I3	−4.11	0.00718
KIF2C	2.03	0.0419	USP1	1.81	0.0534
LOX	2.93	0.0507	UBE2S	1.77	0.0413
PLK1	1.7	0.0561	MYBL2	1.95	0.0129

occurred at different stages of cell transformation. By integrating these data, we were able to identify associations between CN changes, LOH, transcript expression, and phenotypes of invasion and tumorigenicity, including a strong gene signature of epithelial to mesenchymal transition (EMT) that was confirmed by immunohistochemistry [5]. The bcMCF (invasive) and caMCF (tumor-derived) cells showed dramatic changes in morphology, losing epithelial characteristics of polarity and acquiring mesenchymal characteristics of a fibroblast-like spindle shape and increased migratory behavior and invasiveness. Changes in gene and protein expression were characteristic of EMT, namely loss of intercellular adhesion (E-cadherin and occludins), downregulation of epithelial makers (cytokeratins), and upregulation of mesenchymal markers (vimentin and smooth muscle actin) [4, 5].

4.3 Importance of an In Vitro Model

Among all the human diseases, breast cancer offers unique challenges due to its preponderance among the cause-related death in women, the heterogeneity in clinical course, and our lack of understanding of a specific etiologic agents of the disease. Environmental factors derived from both lifestyle practices and industrial toxins remain an area of intense public and scientific concerns, even though few factors beyond ionizing radiation are of proven of setiologic significance. Therefore, it is rational and imperative to develop experimental models that mimic the human disease and that allow us to identify not only a more precise relation between causative agents and disease, but also that the disease thus produced has the same phenotype and genomic profile of primary breast cancer. The development of animal models for testing carcinogenicity as well as therapeutic and preventive agents is quite extended; however, these models, although crucial, are not economically practical in order to test carcinogenic substances for having a potential role as causative agents of breast cancer. In addition. extrapolation to humans needs to be done with caution due to the significant difference in response that exists between animals species and human. Therefore, it is in this context that the challenge to develop 3D or virtual models to reduce use of animals in research needs to be considered. Breast cancer incidence rates in the United States have increased at a rate of 1% per year since 1940. Despite considerable advances in early detection and in therapeutic modalities, the mortality caused by this disease has remained almost unchanged for the past five decades. This already dismal picture is worsened by the gradual increase in breast cancer incidence in most Western countries and in societies that have recently become westernized or are in the process of westernization. Furthermore, daughters of women who migrate from low-incidence to high-incidence countries acquire the breast cancer risk prevailing in the new country [4], suggesting that aspects of lifestyle or the environment are the major determinants of breast cancer. Many environmental chemicals are weakly estrogenic and are therefore hypothesized to increase breast cancer risk by mimicking 17β-estradiol. Furthermore, they are excreted in breast milk, suggesting that ductal and other cells in the breast are exposed directly. Thus, many of these compounds bioaccumulate in the food chain and persist in the body and in the environment. The concentrations of these chemicals can be measured in breast milk, adipose tissue, and blood. Most of the epidemiologic literature on organochlorines focuses on DDT, DDE (1,1-dichloro-2,2,-bis (*p*-dichlorophenyl) ethylene, the main metabolite of DDT), and PCBs because they are among the most persistent in humans. In addition to the compounds described above, there are environmental pollutants that can mimic estrogens in vitro and in vivo and are called xenoestrogens. Xenoestrogens are part of a larger group of synthetic and naturally occurring agents termed endocrine disruptors because of their capacity to perturb normal hormonal actions. It has been suggested that some endocrine disruptors may contribute to the development of hormone-dependent cancers, such as breast and endometrial cancers. The widely used industrial monomer bisphenol A (BPA) is a xenoestrogen that has been used since the 1950s as a monomer that is polymerized to manufacture polycarbonate plastic and epoxy resins. BPA derivatives are widely used as industrial materials and found as environmental contaminants. Human exposure occurs by the leaching of BPA from plastic-lined food and beverage cans and from some dental sealants. BPA also is used as an additive in many other products, with global capacity at >6 billion lb/year. Polycarbonate is less durable than commonly believed because the ester bond linking polymerized BPA molecules can be hydrolyzed, and hydrolysis increases dramatically at high or low pH and as temperature increases. BPA thus leaches into food and beverages with use of tin cans and polycarbonate plastic containers under normal conditions and the rate of leaching greatly increases when polycarbonate is scratched and discolored. Evidence for estrogenic effects of BPA has been reported in several studies showing that it activates estrogen receptors alpha (ERα) and beta (ERβ) and stimulates MCF-7 breast cancer cell growth. Although BPA mimics E_2 by competitively binding and activating endogenous ERs, its affinity is at least 10,000-fold less than that of E_2 for both ERα and ERβ. There is significant exposure of women of reproductive age and pregnant women to BPA, as indicated by its presence in serum and follicular fluid, and of biologically active (unconjugated) BPA in human fetuses, whose mean blood levels at parturition are in the range of 2–3 ng/mL (approximately 10 nM) and in amniotic fluid during fetal reproductive tract differentiation levels are even higher, at 8 ng/mL. There is some uncertainly as to the level and risk of exposure to BPA, but evidence suggests that BPA can disrupt normal reproductive tract development in male and female rodents. BPA exposure during perinatal periods has been shown to inhibit testosterone synthesis in adult rats and promote feminization of *Xenopus laevis* tadpoles. Urinary levels of BPA and its conjugates have been found in 88–92% of males in Japan and 53–100% of females in Japan and Korea [17]. BPA was found in 95% of urinary samples tested in a larger study in United States. Butyl benzyl phthalate (BBP) is another endocrine disruptor that has been reported to be an estrogenic compound. It is used as a plasticizer and is widely used in food wraps and cosmetic formulations. The International Program of Chemical Safety (IPCS) concluded that BBP exposure among the general population is based almost entirely on food intake, because the concentrations of BBP in air, drinking water, and soil are very low and intakes from these routes are essentially negligible. Adult intake has been estimated at 2 μg/kg body weight/day and exposure to infants and children could be up to threefold higher. Studies in rats have described that prenatal exposure to 500, or 1,000 mg/kg of BBP, or 250 or 375 mg/kg of its major metabolite, monobenzyl phthalate, induced significant alterations in the reproductive system of male offspring, including undescended testes and decrease in the ano-genital distance. When administered during sexual differentiation, BBP also causes male reproductive tract malformation of the external genitalia, sex accessory glands, epididymides, and testes. Several in vitro tests, such as MCF-7 cell proliferation, ER binding in the rat uterus, and yeasts transfected with human ER gene, have demonstrated the estrogenic activity of BBP. However, there is poor evidence on the mechanism mediating its effect on cell proliferation. It is likely that the estrogenic response is not only elicited via the ER, but also through the activation of other still unknown pathways. The role of BPA and BBP as estrogenic substances is of relevance to breast cancer because this estrogen-dependent malignancy is steadily increasing in incidence in most western societies and in countries that are becoming industrialized.

4.3.1 Developing a Carcinogenicity Index for Testing the Carcinogenicity of Environmental Agents

Based on previous data, we have *developed a carcinogenicity index* using four different approaches: (a) Ductulogenesis assay in a 3D matrix; (b) Confirmation of the 3D structures by histological and immunocytochemical studies; (c) the invasion index in a matrigel membrane; and (d) expression analysis using RT-PCR of the genes listed in Table 4.1. These genes are representative of the transformation event in MCF-10F by 17β-estradiol, but are also related to the behavior and progression of primary breast cancer. To evaluate the carcinogen effect in the ductulogenesis, we measure the following parameters: (1) Presence or absence of ducts; (2) Presence or absence of solid masses (i.e., the maximal expression of carcinogenicity); (3) If ducts are found then we determine: (a) number of branches; (b) length of the ducts; and (c) thickness. (4) If solid masses are formed, we determine their distribution in size. All these parameters are measured using an automatic imaging system consisting of an IX81 motorized inverted microscope (Olympus, Inc.) equipped with a cooled CCD camera, an incubator, and a motorized stage in the *XYZ* dimensions control by Metamorph Software (Molecular Devices). A ×2 objective is used to tabulate the type and number of structures for the image analysis using Metamorph. The final values of a carcinogenicity index are compared to our standard which is the MCF-10F transformed with 17β-estradiol. We evaluate the structures on collagen at day eighth because the tubules show a complete lumen formation and branching at this time. It has been reported that the lumen formation is completed between days 6 and 8 [8]. In our work, we showed that MCF-10F cells produce tubules with secondary branches that can be quantitated and measured. For example, when we use 17β-estradiol, there is a significant increase in width with an incomplete lumen formation and this effect was associated with increased cellular proliferation (Ki67 positive cells). It has been suggested that the filling of the lumen would be the result of a decrease in central apoptosis, enhanced cellular proliferation, or a combination of both. Luminal filling is the earliest morphologic alteration and is commonly reported in neoplastic processes. Luminal filling is commonly seen in atypical ductal hyperplasia and ductal carcinoma in situ (DCIS).

4.3.2 Construction of an Index of Carcinogenesis

We apply image analysis to cells in a matrix culture. Such cells may form clumps or masses which are counted and measured. Short of that, they may exhibit ducts whose thicknesses and lengths are measured as well as their numbers of branches. These variables are used to construct the required index. First, each variable is tested singly for association with the rank order of the tested carcinogens. Variables that are significantly associated with carcinogenesis are entered into a multivariable regression in an attempt to improve the association. We also cast these variables into multidimensional space to visualize their joint effect in discriminating the several compounds. Simple linear discriminant analyses are applied with the compounds grouped into a smaller number of similar carcinogenic levels. In collaboration with Drs. E. Ross and S. Litwin from FCCC, Philadelphia, and Dr. P. Gutierrez Diez from the Univ. Valladolid, Spain, we attempted to improve the results of linear discriminant analysis by using special surfaces that follow classes of similar carcinogenicity more closely than hyperplanes are able to do. For further refinement of the index, we consider two possible functional forms for the index. We focus our attention on functions that will most likely be useful in this role. Namely: Let C be the carcinogenicity index. Let x denote the total number of solid masses; let y_i be the size of i-solid mass, $i = 1,2,\ldots,x$; let z be the total number of ducts; let w_j denote the thickness of the j-duct, $j=1,2,\ldots,z$; let u_j be the number of branches of the j-duct, $j=1,2,\ldots,z$; and let v_j denote the length of j-duct, $j=1,2,\ldots,z$. The carcinogenicity index must be defined as a real valued function $C(x,y_1,y_2,\ldots,y_x,z,w_1,w_2,\ldots,w_z,u_1,u_2,\ldots,u_z,v_1,v_2,\ldots,v_z)$ satisfying: p1. $\partial C/\partial x>0$ and $\partial C/\partial y_i>0$ (number and size of solid masses are signs of cancer strength and increase the carcinogenicity index). p2. $\partial C/\partial z>0$ and $\partial C/\partial w_j>0$ (number and thickness of thick ducts are signs of precancerous state severity and increase the carcinogenicity index). p3. $\partial C/\partial u_j<0$ and $\partial C/\partial v_j<0$ (number of branches of the ducts and length of the ducts are signs of normal ductulogenesis and decrease the carcinogenicity index). Among the possible carcinogenicity indexes verifying p1–p3, we select that with the best behavior from the mathematical and biological points of view, finding the appropriate constant values involved in the carcinogenicity index through the experimentation results with cultured cells. This selection starts from the simplest indexes, such as those linear or log-linear in the variables and of logistic type. Denoting by y, w, u, and v to the average values for y_i, w_j, u_j, and v_j, respectively, good and simple initial proposals satisfying p1–p3 are the following:

$$C(x,y_1,\ldots,y_x,z,w_1,\ldots,w_z,u_1,\ldots,u_z,v_1,\ldots,v_z)=A+Bx+Cy+Dz+Ew+Fu+Gv,$$

$$C(x,y_1,\ldots,y_x,z,w_1,\ldots,w_z,u_1,\ldots,u_z,v_1,\ldots v_z)=Ax^By^Cz^Dw^Eu^Fv^G,$$

$$C(x,y_1,\ldots,y_x,z,w_1,\ldots,w_z,u_1,\ldots,u_z,v_1,\ldots,v_z)=A+\frac{Bx}{x+b}+\frac{Cy}{y+c}+\frac{Dz}{z+d}+\frac{Ew}{w+e}+\frac{Fu}{u-f}+\frac{Gv}{v-g},$$

$$C(x,y_1,\ldots,y_x,z,w_1,\ldots,w_z,u_1,\ldots,u_z,v_1,\ldots,v_z)=A\left(\frac{Bx}{x+b}\right)\left(\frac{Cy}{y+c}\right)\left(\frac{Dz}{z+d}\right)\left(\frac{Ew}{w+e}\right)\left(\frac{Fu}{u-f}\right)\left(\frac{Gv}{v-g}\right),$$

where A, B, b, C, c, D, d, E, e, F, f, G, and g are the constants to be determined. Other statistics of the data such as variances and outliers may also be incorporated as variables if found to be significant.

4.3.3 Design

In collaboration with Dr. E. Ross at the FCCC in Philadelphia we applied the *Play the winner* methods to determine the most carcinogenic level for each compound. To this end, we test at least five levels of each agent and select the one that is maximally carcinogenic. Five replicate plates are used to estimate the carcinogenic potential of each compound at its selected dose level. We estimate the carcinogenic index of each compound using a test index function obtained as above. We then submit the carcinogenic indices of the tested compounds along with their surrogate estimates of carcinogenic potential to Pearson's to test for correlation. With ten agents, for example, this test is able to distinguish a correlation coefficient of 0.66 from 1 of 0 with 80% power and 5% type I error. Using variables that are singly significant, we determine index parameters, as in Sect. 4.3.2 above, and that maximize the correlation of the index with the surrogate endpoint rank order. We apply the above methods to each of our surrogate endpoints, namely: invasiveness, gene expression, and histology. Each endpoint is fitted with its own special function. Thus, there are 23 special functions, 20 of which are for gene expression. The set of 22 functions are subjected to principal component analysis for final index construction, although some of the individual functions may themselves be appropriate indices. We consider various composites of the 22 functions as they occur to improve the performance of our index.

4.4 An In Vitro In Vivo Model for Studying the Basal Breast Cancer

Invasive breast cancer that leads to metastasis is a heterogeneous disease that encompasses a variety of pathological features that are associated with specific clinical behavior. The discovery that the morphological heterogeneity of breast cancer is reflected at the transcriptome level has allowed for the classification of breast cancer into five main groups: luminal A, luminal B, normal breast-like, ERBB2 (HER2), and basal-like breast carcinomas [18]. The luminal-like subtypes display moderate to high expression of ERα and luminal cytokeratins. The basal-like carcinomas, which have been reported to have a more aggressive clinical behavior, are composed of cells that consistently express genes usually found in normal basal/myoepithelial cells of the breast, including basal cytokeratins (5/6, 14 and 17), p-cadherin, and caveolin 1 and p53. Molecular analyses of basal-like carcinomas have confirmed the frequent lack of expression of estrogen (ER) and progesterone (PR) receptors and HER2, high levels of expression of proliferation-related genes, and frequent mutation of the TP53 gene. Morphologically, basal-like breast carcinomas present with high histological grade, high mitotic indices, central necrotic zones, pushing borders, and a conspicuous lymphocytic infiltrate. In addition, metaplastic elements and medullary/atypical medullary features have been reported. Similarities have been found between basal-like tumors and breast carcinomas occurring in *BRCA1* mutation carriers in a premenopausal population of African American (AA) women and in the younger breast cancer patient population in general. Since basal-like breast cancer confers a poor prognosis [5], a great percentage of these tumors could be prevented by interventions that eliminate the causative agents if they are properly identified. Therefore, the 3D model of the human breast has allowed us to test the carcinogenic potential of environmental agents that can be applied directly to this type of breast cancer.

Ductulognesis of MCF-10F cells grown in collagen matrix (3D-cultures) and after the cells are treated with E_2, the ductulogenesis is quantitatively evaluated by estimating

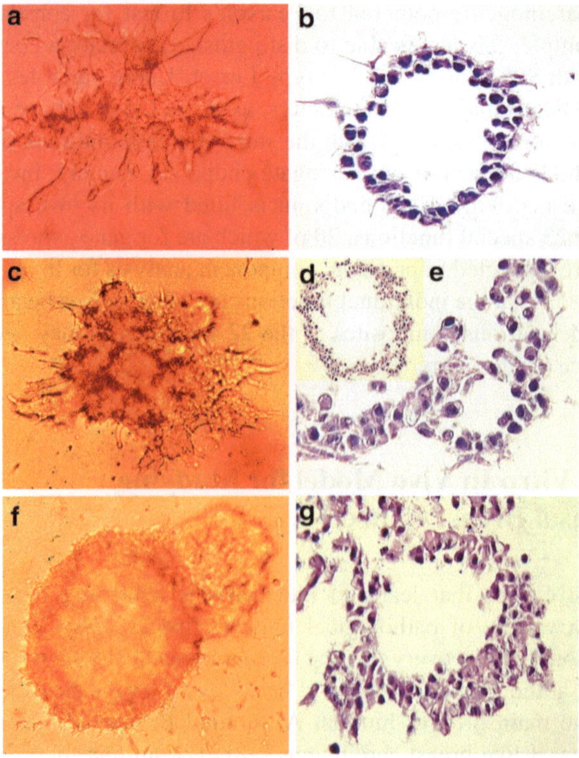

Fig. 4.3 Loss of branching by treatment of MCF-10F cells with 17β-estradiol (E_2). (**a**, **c**, **f**) Cells in collagen matrix. Phase contrast (×10); (**b**, **d**, **e**, **g**) cross section of the corresponding structures shown in the *left side panel*. (**a**, **b**) MCF-10F cells treated with DMSO (control) forming ductules lined by a double layer of low cuboidal epithelial cells; (**c**, **d**, **e**) MCF-10F cells treated with 0.007 nM estradiol tend to form spheres lined by a multilayerd epithelium with secondary lumina; (**f**, **g**) MCF-10F cells treated with 70 nM estradiol form large sherical masses lined by a hyperplastic epithelium (reprinted from Russo J, Russo IH (2004) Biological and molecular basis of breast cancer. Springer, Heidelberg, Chapter 4, p 104, Figure 4.13a–g)

the ability of the cell to form tubules. When MCF-10F cells grow in regular media or in media with DMSO and plated in collagen, the cells formed tubules (Fig. 4.3a). When the cells are treated with E_2 alone and plated in collagen, cells form semi solid masses of 178 ± 33.16 μm in diameter (Fig. 4.3f). The treatment with E_2 increased cell proliferation evaluated using an antibody against Ki67 antigen. The Ki67 antigen is a cell cycle-related nuclear protein, expressed by proliferating cells in all phases of the active cell cycle (G_1, S, G_2, and M phases) and it is absent in resting (G_0) cells. The cross sections of the tubular structures showed a monolayer of epithelial cells around the lumen (Fig. 4.3b), whereas in the E_2 treated cells, the cross section of the tubules showed an increase of both number of epithelial layers (Fig. 4.3d, e, g) and

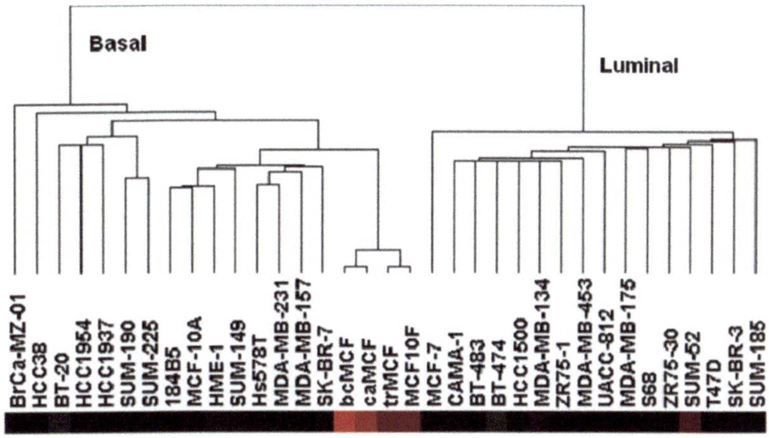

Fig. 4.4 MCF-10F and derived cell lines (trMCF, bcMCF, and caMCF) classify as basal cell lines. The expression data for these cell lines was combined with the published expression values of a 364 gene set and used to classify the breast cell lines by hierarchical clustering. The MCF-10F and derived cell lines occupy a distinct branch of the basal subtype (*left branch*) because the expression values were calculated independently from different batches of normalized genechips (reprinted from Russo J, Russo IH (2011) The role of the basal stem cell of the human breast in normal development and cancer. Adv Exp Med Biol 720:121–134)

Ki67 positive cells (Proliferative index=91.16). The epithelial cells layering the ducts showed to be estrogen receptor alpha (ERα) negative and they have a significantly low expression of cadherins, laminin, and fibronectin. The filling of the lumen is the result of a decrease in central apoptosis, enhanced cellular proliferation, or a combination of the two. Luminal filling is the earliest morphologic alteration and is commonly reported in neoplastic processes. Luminal filling is seen in atypical ductal hyperplasia and DCIS. These phenotypical changes occur in the MCF-10F which is representative of the basal cell type breast tumors. This type of tumor is characterized by exhibiting EMT that is predominately regulated by the TGF-β and Wnt signaling pathways. The Immortal MCF-10F cells are non-transformed, non-tumorigenic, and ER negative. Because malignant cell transformation of these cells produced poorly differentiated tumors characteristic of basal-like carcinomas, we chose to classify these cells relative to the breast cell lines described by Charafe-Jauffret et al. [19]. As shown in Fig. 4.4, these MCF-10F and derived cell lines clustered in the branch containing the basal breast cell lines. In our molecular characterization of malignant cell transformation [6], we identified the "intermediate filament" component enriched in Gene Ontology (GO) analysis, separating the non-tumorigenic MCF-10F and trMCF cells from the tumorigenic bcMCF and caMCF cells. Numerous cytokeratins were suppressed or absent, whereas vimentin was strongly induced in bcMCF (7.0-fold) and caMCF (8.1-fold).

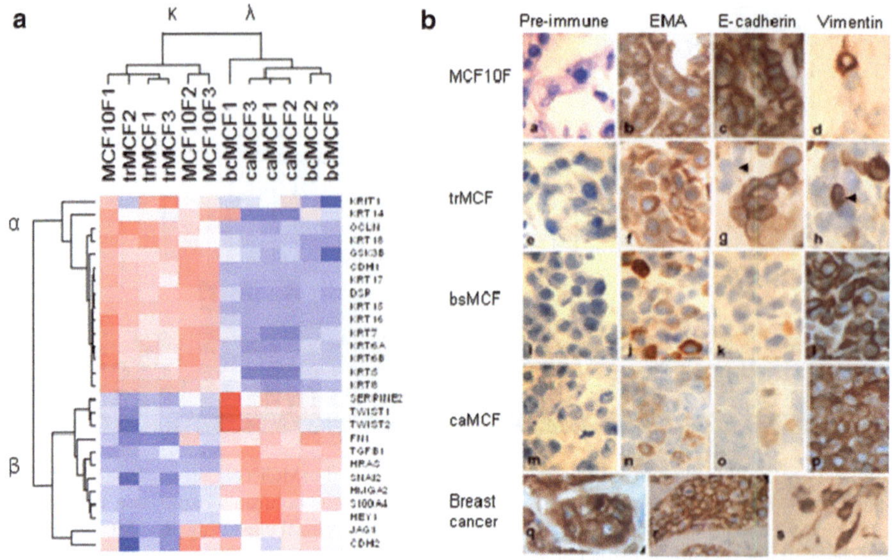

Fig. 4.5 Expression profile of epithelial to mesenchymal transition (EMT) markers and their regulators during malignant cell transformation. (**a**) A list of EMT markers and promoting genes was generated a priory by literature search [4]. Hierarchical clustering of cell lines and genes was performed using dChip software. Two sample clusters (κ and λ) and two gene clusters (α and β) were identified. The *red*, *white*, and *blue* colors represent level above, at, and below mean expression, respectively. (**b**) Detection of epithelial and mesenchymal markers by immunocytochemistry (×100). *a:* Histological sections of MCF-10F cells, reacted with pre-immune mouse serum, were used as the negative control; *b*, *c*, *d*: MCF-10F reacted for EMA, E-cadherin, vimentin, respectively; *e*: trMCF cells reacted with pre-immune mouse serum used as negative control; *f*, *g*, *h*: trMCF cells reacted for EMA, E-cadherin, and vimentin, respectively; *i*: bsMCF cells reacted with pre-immune mouse serum as a negative control; *j*, *k*, *l*: bsMCF cells reacted for EMA, E-cadherin, and vimentin, respectively; *m*: caMCF tumor cell line cells reacted with pre-immune mouse serum used as negative control; *n*, *o*, *p*: caMCF tumor cell lines reacted for EMA, E-cadherin, and vimentin, respectively; *q*, *r*: invasive ductal carcinoma of the breast as positive control and immunoreacted for EMA and E-cadherin, respectively; *s*: histological section of an invasive adenocarcinoma immunoreacted for vimentin (reprinted from [5])

Because of these findings, we generated a gene list from published literature for EMT markers and their regulators [5]. The 52 genes in this list were filtered by low stringency criteria of combined coefficient of variation >0.3 and "Present calls" in more than 30% of the samples. The 27 genes passing these criteria were used for sample and gene clustering (Fig. 4.5a). Two sample groups and two gene groups were identified. The nontumorigenic MCF-10F and trMCF cells were grouped into sample cluster κ, while the tumorigenic bcMCF and caMCF cells were grouped into cluster λ. On the other side, the genes were grouped into cluster α and β based on their expression pattern. The epithelial markers *E-cadherin, occludin, desmoplakin,* and *cytokeratins* were decreased, while the mesenchymal markers *fibronectin, vimentin,* and *N-cadherin* were increased in bcMCF and caMCF cells (Fig. 4.5a). It was confirmed by real time RT-PCR that the expression of FN1, S100A4, SNAI2, HRAS, and TGF-β1 was increased, while CDH1 (E-cadherin) was decreased in bcMCF and caMCF cells [5]. Immunocytochemical analysis using antibodies against epithelial membrane antigen EMA (also called MUC1) and E-cadherin displayed significant loss of these epithelial markers and increased expression of the mesenchymal marker vimentin in tumorigenic cells (Fig. 4.5b). These findings confirmed the EMT phenotype revealed by gene expression profile in Fig. 4.5a.

In order to determine whether there is a relationship between our EMT gene signature (Fig. 4.5a) and the classification of the Basal A and Basal B breast cell lines reported by Neve et al., we identified nine genes present in both our EMT gene signature and Neve et al. 396 gene classifier set [20]. By Prediction Analysis of Microarray (PAM), we show that the parent MCF-10F cells and trMCF cells can be classified as Basal A, whereas the bcMCF (invasive) and caMCF (tumor-derived) cells classified as Basal B (Table 4.2). Based on these data, we hypothesize that both Basal subtypes A and B can arise from the same cell of origin and may reflect differing degrees of EMT and invasive potential. To explore this hypothesis further, we extracted our EMT gene signature from the GeneChip expression files of the 30 cell lines that were characterized for invasiveness in a modified Boyden chamber assay [20]. As shown in Fig. 4.6, this EMT gene signature classified, with complete concordance to [20], the cell lines into luminal, Basal A, and Basal B subtypes. The Basal B cell lines that scored as invasive grouped to the far left (Fig. 4.6). This result along with the recent report showing that EMT occurs more frequently in basal-like tumors indicates the relevance of these breast cell lines for molecular analysis of the networks regulating EMT and that the Basal A that originates B is the stem cell involved in the early stage of cell transformation or trMCF.

CD44^{+}*/CD24*$^{-/low}$ is the cell surface marker of tumorigenic breast cancer cells in which the tumorigenic capacity is further increased by additional expression of *ESA* [21]. These cells are characterized by a 186-gene "invasiveness" gene signature that is associated with risk of death and metastasis in breast cancer [21]. *CD24* encodes a small, heavily glycosylated cell-surface adhesion protein. *CD44* undergoes extensive alternative splicing within its central region spanning exon 6a to 14, also termed as variable exon v1 to v10. The two variants expressed in our model are mRNA precursor variant 3 with exon 6a to 11 spliced out and variant 4 with exon 6a to 14 spliced out, corresponding to *CD44E* and *CD44H*, respectively. The *CD44H* is mainly expressed on cells of lymphohematopoietic origin; it plays an important role in cell adhesion and its expression promotes tumor cell migration. *CD44E* is preferentially expressed on epithelial cells and it is involved in the recognition of a common determinant in *CD44H* and *CD44E* promoting homotypic cellular aggregation. Microarray and RT-PCR analysis of *CD44* and *CD24* revealed an expression pattern of *CD44H*^{high}*/CD44E*$^{-}$*/*

Table 4.2 EMT-genes discriminate Basal A and Basal B cell lines

Upregulated EMT gene				Downregulated EMT gene			
Gene symbol	Basal A score	Basal B score	Luminal score	Gene symbol	Basal A score	Basal B score	Luminal score
TWIST1	0	0.0353	0	KRT6B	0.0377	0	0
SNAI2	0	0.3775	0	KRT5	0.1797	0	0
FGFB1	0	0.1225	0	KRT16	0.5258	0	0
JAG1	0.0458	0	0	KRT17	0.0722	0	0
				KRT8	0	−0.5887	0.0332

In order to link our EMT genes with the genes classified as Luminal, Basal A, or Basal B, we used the PAM method for the 396 gene set of classifiers identified by Neve et al. [20]. Note that a positive or negative score indicates a significant association with cell subtype. We found 4 of our 11 downregulated EMT genes are among 396 genes list, and 3 out of 4 (75%) show Basal B subtype (upregulated); while 5 of our 15 upregulated EMT genes are among 396 genes list, and 4 of 5 (80%) show Basal A subtype (downregulated). Thus, our previously identified EMT gene signature [5] can clearly discriminate the Basal A and Basal B subtypes of breast cell lines

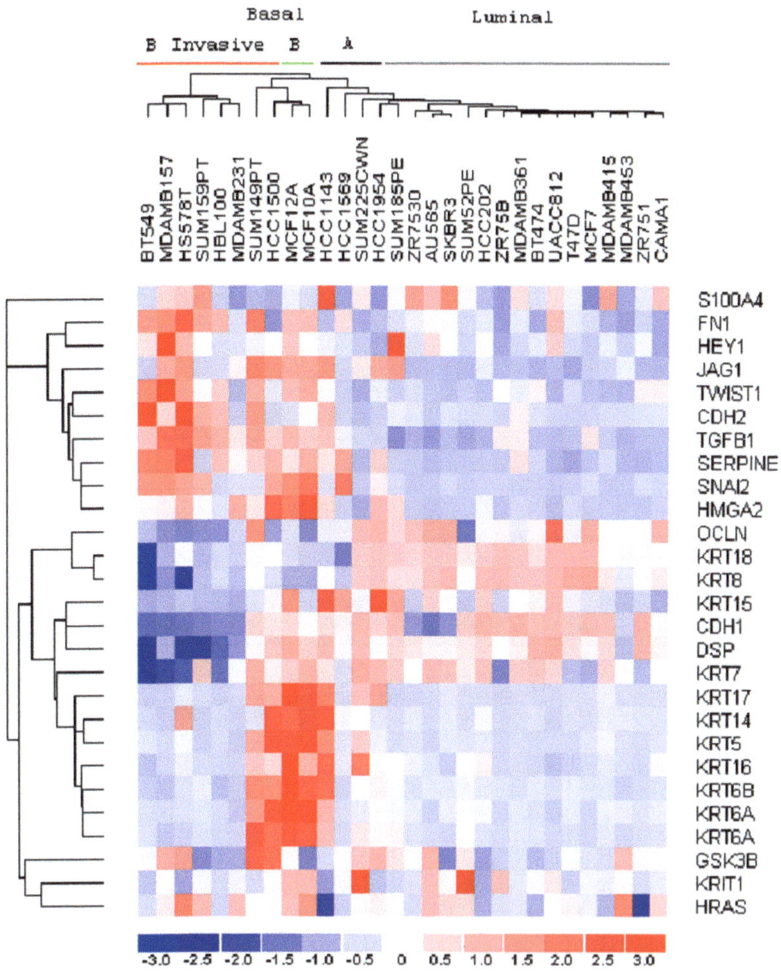

Fig. 4.6 Classification of breast cell lines using an EMT gene signature identifies subtype and invasiveness. Gene expression values were extracted from the CEL files of the 30 cell line subset of breast cancer cell lines that were previously characterized for invasive potential. The invasive Basal B cell lines are indicated by the *red bar*; noninvasive by a *green bar* (reprinted from Russo J, Russo IH (2011) The role of the basal stem cell of the human breast in normal development and cancer. Adv Exp Med Biol 720:121–134)

CD24⁻ in bcMCF and caMCF. The increased ratio of CD44H/CD44E in trMCF cells might represent an early marker for E_2-transformed HBECs (Fig. 4.7a–d). The significant increase of CD44H and complete loss of CD44E might be a novel phenotype associated with the tumorigenic capacity. In addition, the loss of *ESA* in bcMCF and caMCF indicated that *ESA* expression is not required for the tumorigenic capacity in our model.

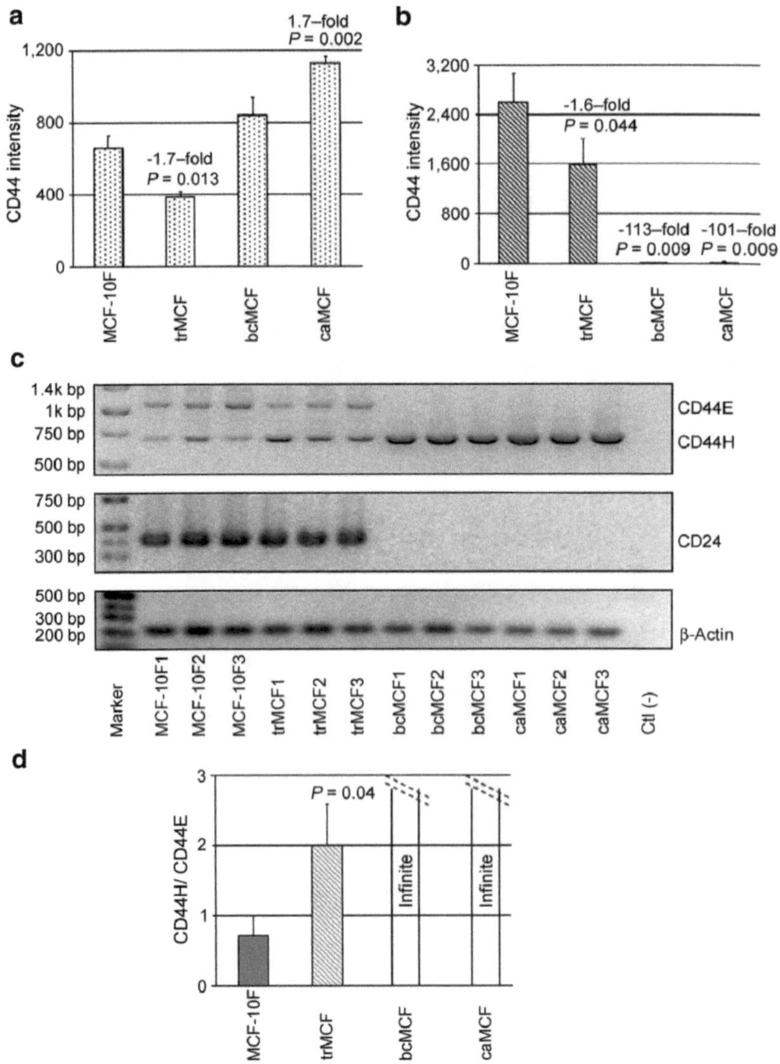

Fig. 4.7 Characterization of the expression of CD44 and CD24. (**a**, **b**) Microarray expression values of CD44 and CD24, respectively. Significance: $p<0.05$ in unpaired t test compared with MCF-10F. (**c**) RT-PCR validation for CD44 (*top*) and CD24 (*middle*) expression levels. (**d**) Densitometry ratio of CD44H to CD44E detected in RT-PCR (reprinted from [5])

4.5 Stem Cell and the Asymmetric Cell Division

One unresolved challenging question in breast cancer is whether the cancer stem cell originates from normal stem/progenitor cells or from mature cells that acquired the stem cell phenotype because of a transformation event or subsequent mutations. There is evidence that in the human breast there is a stem cell population that can give rise to many different cell types and are important for breast development, pregnancy-induced differentiation, lactation, and involution [22]. Stem cells have the unique potential to divide asymmetrically to generate daughters of distinct fates, one of which remains a stem cell and the other turns into a cell committed to differentiation. By dividing asymmetrically, stem cells maintain the stem cell pool and simultaneously generate committed cells that reconstitute the organ, for example, to prepare the breast for a new pregnancy after the involution from a previous pregnancy and lactation process [23, 24]. However, in this cumulative knowledge we still do not know if the cancer stem cell originates from normal stem/progenitor cells or from mature cells that acquired the stem cell phenotype because of a transformation event or subsequent mutations. Our starting hypothesis is that the normal stem cell divides asymmetrically and that the carcinogenic event disrupts this process leading to a neoplastic breast cancer stem cell. Furthermore, the main challenge has been to demonstrate that the asymmetric cell division takes place as part of the normal process of ductulogenesis and that the carcinogenic agent (17β-estradiol) modifies this process [4, 5, 25].

Our model offers a stem cell with the characteristic of the basal cell type that differentiates normally in a tridimensional in vitro system forming ductular structures mimicking the lobules type 1 of the human breast [4, 5, 25]. This in turn offers a structural model to understand how the normal cellular architecture is modified during the asymmetric cell division as the main driver of this normal morphogenetic process. In addition, the basal stem cell when challenged by a carcinogenic agent loses the ability to form ductal structures and becomes neoplastic mimicking the histological appearance of the early neoplastic process like carcinoma in situ and forming an epithelial multilayer with loss of polarity and increased cell proliferation [4, 5]. Therefore, in this unique system we have been able to demonstrate that the normal stem cell is the one that under a carcinogenic insult switch the process of asymmetric cell division. Altogether, this model is offering a way to understand the mechanism of asymmetric cell division that is still elusive in the breast cells and to demonstrate how the disruption of this phenomenon by estrogen can trigger the initial step of cell transformation. The supporting evidence for this hypothesis is in the *genomic alterations in the transformed cells (trMCF), which indicate that the asymmetric cell division is the target mechanism of neoplastic transformation.*

4.5.1 Genomic Alterations in the trMCF Cells Indicate That the Asymmetric Cell Division Is the Target Mechanism of Neoplastic Transformation

Loss of the ductulogenic capacity is the earliest phenotype observed during the neoplastic transformation of MCF-10F cells by 17β-estradiol. Asymmetric cell division takes place in the normal process of ductulogenesis and this process is modified by the carcinogenic agent. Specifically we have demonstrated that

17β-estradiol acting on the basal cell type induces architectural changes in the stemness, the cell polarity, the partitioning of the cell component and the mitotic apparatus, and the interaction with the niche or extracellular matrix.

4.5.2 Cell Partitioning in Asymmetric Cell Division

In Table 4.3 and Figs. 4.8 and 4.9 are listed some of the genes that may contribute in altering the cell partitioning during the asymmetric cell division. Among them is *NOTCH3*, which is significantly downregulated in the estrogen-transformed cells that have lost the ability to form ductal components in the collagen matrix. As it is depicted in Fig. 4.10, NOTCH3 is polarized in its localization in MCF-10F cells; when the cell divides, one of the daughter cells carries the expression of NOTCH3 and the other one does not. Instead, in the E_2-treated cells or trMCF, most of the cells have very low or not expression of NOTCH3. Therefore, we conclude that NOTCH3 could be asymmetrically partitioned in the breast epithelial cells and that daughter cells that are transformed by estradiol will have a loss of the expression of this gene. There is supporting evidence in the literature indicating that Notch-1 and Notch-3 have been shown to affect stem cell fates, suggesting that Notch function in specifying cell fate might also be evolutionarily conserved [26–29]. Interestingly, the Notch pathway plays multiple roles in hematopoiesis, including differentiation, proliferation, and survival, and may be critical for human stem cell (HSC) activity [30, 31]. Notch-1 was found in the $CD34^{+}CD38^{-}Lin^{-}$ subpopulation of human bone marrow cells (SAGE) and in two enriched stem cell populations derived from the fetal liver ($Sca\text{-}1^{+}AA4.1^{+}Lin^{lo/-}cKit^{+}$ cells) (SCDb) [32, 33]. In the *Drosophila,* it is suggested that asymmetrical localization/segregation of Numb in neural precursors enables sibling cells to respond differently to extrinsic Notch signaling and, thus, to adopt distinct fates (A or B). During the asymmetric precursor division, Numb segregates exclusively into one daughter cell, the future B cell. The Notch ligand Delta signals both progenies to adopt the A-cell fate. In the A cell, Delta activation of Notch induces the cleavage of the Notch receptor and the subsequent translocation of the Notch intracellular domain to the nucleus, where it regulates transcription of specific target genes and allows the cell to adopt the A fate. In the B cell, Numb blocks reception and/or transduction of the Notch signal, possibly through its endocytosis. The absence of active Notch signaling in these cells is deterministic for B-cell fate [34]. The silencing of NOTCH3 in the trMCF or the daughter cell generated in the transformation of MCF could be due to degradation. Protein ubiquitination and deubiquitination are dynamic processes implicated in the regulation of numerous cellular pathways. Table 4.3 lists genes that are modified during the transformation induced by 17β-estradiol. Among them are TRIM22 and TRIM5 [35–40], SLPI [41–43], USP1 [44], UBE2Q2 [45, 46], and UBE2S, all components of the ubiquitin pathway leading to proteosome degradation that is significantly dysregulated in the trMCF cells. This supports the interpretation that the localization of this complex could be asymmetrically located in the trMCF cells under the treatment with estradiol disrupting the asymmetrical process.

Table 4.3 Dysregulated genes in the trMCF cells

Symbol	Fold change	q-value	Symbol	Fold change	q-value	Symbol	Fold change	q-value
Downregulated genes								
BMP1	2.14	0.042	FXYD3	2.25	0.025	NTN4	2.59	0.009
BMPR2	2.01	0.019	GSN	3.77	0.014	PACS1	2.00	0.010
CDC42	1.74	0.047	ITGAV	1.81	0.034	SEC14L2	3.37	0.005
COL17A1	3.69	0.009	ITGB4	1.93	0.010	SLITRK6	6.14	0.016
COL1A1	6.12	0.030	ITGB6	2.64	0.010	SLPI	1.82	0.048
COL4A5	1.81	0.015	KIF13B	2.24	0.038	TNC	4.87	0.010
DSC2	1.85	0.014	LAMA3	3.48	0.021	TRIM22	40.82	0.008
EPLIN	1.71	0.029	LAMB3	2.70	0.048	TRIM5	2.74	0.019
EPS8L2	2.04	0.006	LAMC2	3.61	0.013	TRIOBP	1.88	0.009
EVA1	1.79	0.041	NEBL	2.25	0.032	TSPAN1	3.24	0.005
FLNB	2.12	0.036	NOTCH3	3.81	0.012	UBE2Q2	1.75	0.056
FN1	18.88	0.011	NRP2	2.40	0.034	YPEL5	2.18	0.011
Upregulated genes								
AURKB	1.84	0.013	MKI67	1.78	0.045	RFC3	2.14	0.047
BIRC5	1.71	0.048	MLF1	3.16	0.009	TOP2A	1.76	0.019
CENPA	1.91	0.044	PLK1	1.70	0.056	UBE2S	1.77	0.041
COL12A1	1.99	0.073	POLE2	2.68	0.012	USP1	1.81	0.053
KIF2C	2.03	0.042	PSIP1	1.82	0.030			

List of genes showed to be dysregulated in the trMCF cells in the microarrays. Fold change is related to the MCF-10F cells

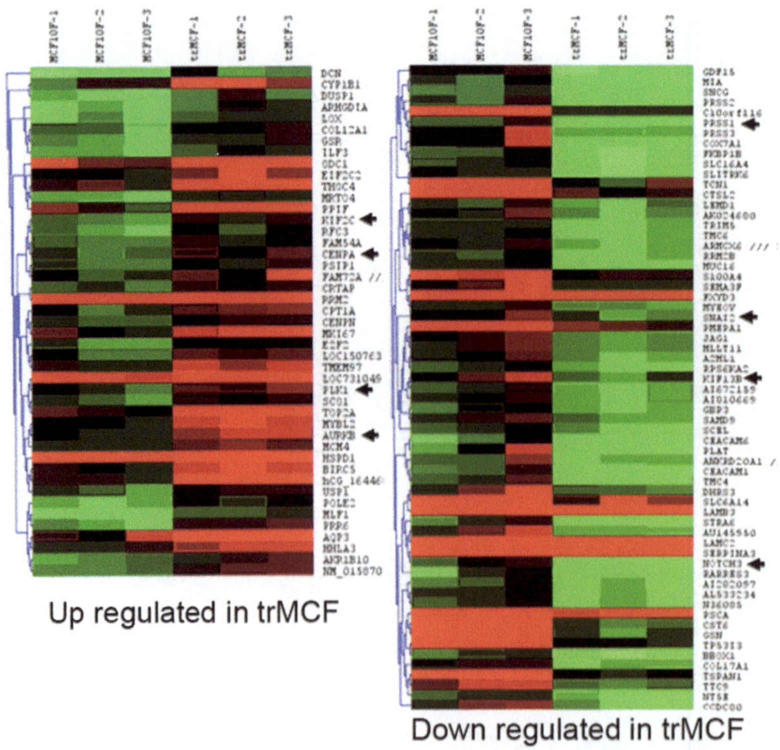

Fig. 4.8 Heat maps showing clusters of genes upregulated (on the *left*) or downregulated (on the *right*) in the trMCF cells. *Arrows* indicate some of the genes that were validated through real time RT-PCR, *red* represents higher values of expression and *green* lower expression

Of great interest is TRIM22, a functional E3 ubiquitin ligase, which is also ubiquitinated itself and is downregulated in the trMCF cells indicating a possible role in the partitioned position in the stem cells MCF (Table 4.3). There is 41-fold downregulation of TRIM22 in trMCF when compared to the stem cell MCF. Its potential role in the cell asymmetry is suggested to us by the work of Herr et al. [36], which shows that human and rhesus TRIM22 localize to different sub cellular compartments and that this difference can be assigned to the positively selected B30.2 domain. It is possible that TRIM22 is asymmetrically located in the MCF cells and that during transformation the daughter cells trMCF lose or alternatively silence the expression of this gene. Further support is the fact that TRIM22 underwent self-ubiquitylation in vitro in combination with the E_2 enzyme UbcH5B and the ubiquitylation was dependent on its RING finger domain. Further evidences showed that TRIM22 could also be self-ubiquitylated in vivo. Importantly, TRIM22 was conjugated with poly-ubiquitin chains and stabilized by the proteasome inhibitor in 293T cells, suggesting that TRIM22 targeted itself for proteasomal degradation through

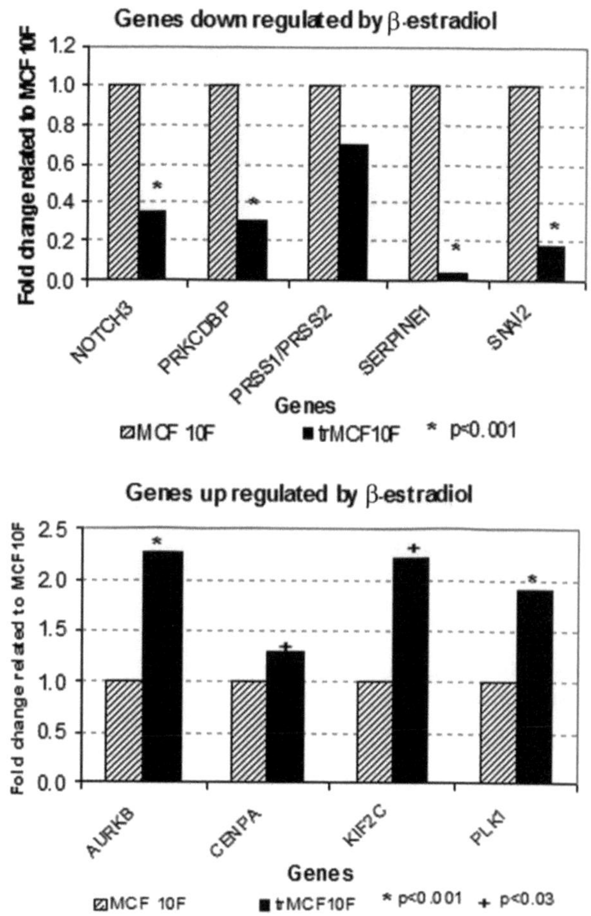

Fig. 4.9 Graphs showing the results from the real time RT-PCR of some of the genes listed in Table 4.3. Gene expressions are relative to the MCF-10F cells. Graph on the *top* shows the downregulated genes and the graph *below* shows the upregulated genes; *Asterisks* represent the genes that had $p < 0.001$ compared to control and *plus symbol* $p < 0.03$

the poly-ubiquitylation [37]. Another piece of evidence showing that it could be involved in the asymmetry of cell division is the finding that interferon induces TRIM22 as a p53 target gene, with possible involvement in proliferation and differentiation of leukemia cells in which expression of TRIM22 correlates inversely to differentiation, as TRIM22 is highly expressed in $CD34^+$ human bone marrow progenitor cells, but declines in mature populations. The erythroid lineage appears as a special case, as TRIM22 expression shows an extreme decrease during late erythroid maturation and is completely undetectable in nucleated erythroid populations in contrast to other lineages [38, 39]. A similar phenomenon has been reported in T cells [40].

Besides NOTCH3, there are other candidate proteins coded by the genes MLF1 [47–50], NEBL [51–54], PACS1 [55–57], SEC14L2 [58], TRIOBP [59–61],

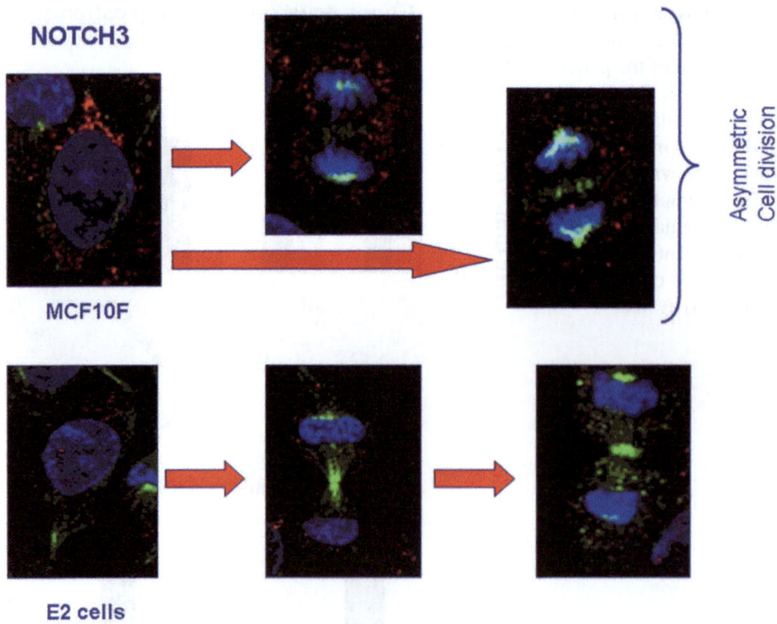

Fig. 4.10 Immunofluorescence studies of NOTCH3. MCF-10F and E_2 cells were plated onto round cover slips and grown overnight at 37 °C. Cells were fixed using 4% Formaldehyde and incubated with the primary antibody (anti-NOTCH3, Abcam 2 μg/mL) for 50 min at room temperature. Slides were viewed and images recorded using the Nikon Eclipse 2000-U C1 LSCM and a ×40-NA 1.3 oil objective lens. Nikon EZ-C1 software was used to view images (reprinted from Russo J, Pereira J, Snider K, Russo IH (2010) Estrogen-induced breast cancer is the result in the disruption of the asymmetric cell division of the stem cell. Horm Mol Biol Clin Investig 1(2):53–65)

TSPAN1, and PSIP1 (Table 4.3) which may have a regulatory effect on the partition distribution of proteins and organelles affecting the asymmetric cell division. For example, the Myeloid leukemia factor 1 (MLF1) expresses normally in a variety of tissues including hematopoietic stem cells and also in the MCF cells, but it is unregulated several folds in the trMCF cells (Table 4.3). MFL1 is a negative regulator of cell cycle progression functioning upstream of the tumor suppressor p53 [47, 49, 50], stabilizing the activity of the tumor suppressor p53 by suppressing E3 ubiquitin ligase and the shuttling of MFL1 is critical for the regulation of cell proliferation and a disturbance in the shuttling balance increases the cell's susceptibility to oncogenic transformation [48]. Therefore, this gene product is a target for evaluation in the loss of asymmetric division induced by E_2 in the MCF cells. There are also three genes, PACS1 [55–57], SEC14L2 [58], and TRIOBP [59–61], that play a role in cell sorting and interaction with actin filaments, and are significantly downregulated in trMCF cells, suggesting that they may play an unsuspected role in asymmetric cell division.

4.5.3 Mitotic Apparatus

A significant amplification in the expression of Aurora Kinase B (AURKB), polo-like kinase 1 (PLK1), centromere protein A (CENPA), and kinesin family member C(KIF2C) are observed in the E_2 cells with respect to the MCF-10 cells (Table 4.2; Fig. 4.9). This could indicate that the dysregulation of theses genes by the carcinogenic agent 17β-estradiol contribute to the alteration of the asymmetric pattern of cell division of the stem cell MCF. Supporting evidence for this is the knowledge that the binding of kinetochores to spindle microtubules during mitosis regulates the trafficking of macropinosomes to the cytoskeleton during antigen presentation. The CENPA is a histone H3-like protein that is thought to be involved in the nucleosomal packaging of centromeric DNA. It is a marker of embryonic stem cells [62, 63] and highly expressed in breast cancer cells. CENPA interacts with poly(ADP-ribose) polymerase 2 (PARP-2) in a cell cycle-dependent manner, accumulating at centromeres during prometaphase and metaphase, disassociating during anaphase, and disappearing from the centromeres by telophase [64, 65]. The KIF2C/mitotic centromere-associated kinesin (MCAK) is associated to the growth of breast cancer cells. It is expressed at undetectable levels in normal human tissues and upregulated in the trMCF cells as well as in breast cancer tissue. Treatment of breast cancer cells with small interfering RNA (siRNA) against KIF2C/MCAK effectively suppressed KIF2C/MCAK expression and inhibited the growth of the breast cancer cell lines T47D and HBC5 [66]. The importance of these kinetochore-related proteins is that few-fold reductions in kinetochore-microtubule turnover, particularly in early mitosis, induce severe chromosome segregation defects. Enough stimulation of microtubule dynamics at kinetochores restores stability to chromosomally unstable tumor cell lines, establishing a causal relationship between deregulation of kinetochore-microtubule dynamics and chromosomal instability. Thus, temporal control of microtubule attachment to chromosomes during mitosis is central to genome stability in human cells [67]. In the *Drosophila* sensory organ precursor cells, Aurora A regulates the asymmetrical localization of Numb [68]. Mammalian Auroras (member of the serine/threonine kinase family) regulate centrosome separation, chromosome segregation, and cytokinesis. Auroras are overexpressed in many cancers and high protein levels correlated with chromosomal instability [69–71]. A key regulator in the process of cell division is the PLK1. It controls cytokinesis, the final stage of cell division, and is a novel player in maintaining genomic stability during DNA replication and is an important modulator of the DNA damage checkpoint. Importantly, it has been shown to be a link between developmental processes and the cell cycle machinery during asymmetric cell division in flies and worms [72, 73].

Two genes YPEL5 and EPLIN identified by our group may have an unsuspected role in the control of asymmetric cell division in the human breast epithelial cells. YPEL5 gene is downregulated in the 17β-estradiol transformed cells and the coded protein is localized to the centrosome and nucleus during interphase and at the mitotic spindle during mitosis. This sub cellular localization in association with centrosome or mitotic spindle suggests a novel function involved in the cell division [74].

The second gene EPLIN (epithelial protein lost in neoplasm; also known as Lima-1) (Table 4.3) [75] is also significantly downregulated in the trMCF cells and plays an important role in the first phase of the cytokinesis that is the membrane ingression. The ingression phase generates a cleavage furrow and this requires co-operative function of the actin-myosin II contractile ring and septin filaments [76]. Therefore, it is possible that EPLIN plays an important role in the asymmetric cell division of the stem cell MCF and is silenced in the trMCF cells. This concept is supported by data showing low level of EPLIN in tumor tissues [77]. Of interest is that EPLIN couples with alpha-catenin and, in turn, links the cadherin-catenin complex to F-actin [78]. EPLIN is a substrate for ERK. ERK phosphorylates Ser360, Ser602, and Ser692 on EPLIN in vitro and in intact cells. Phosphorylation of the C-terminal region of EPLIN reduces its affinity for actin filaments [79]. EPLIN increases the number and size of actin stress fibers and inhibits membrane ruffling induced by Rac and the reduced expression may contribute to the motility of invasive tumor cells [80, 81]. All of these data point toward a need for detailed analysis of the architectural localization of these gene products in the MCF cells during the normal process of ductulogenesis and during the loss of the asymmetric properties of these cells induced by 17β-estradiol.

4.5.4 Cell Polarity and Asymmetric Cell Division

As is depicted in Table 4.3, there are several genes that are significantly deregulated in the trMCF such as CDC42, EPSL8L2, FLNB, FXYD3, and NRP2. Whereas the role of EPSL8L2, FLNB, FXYD3, and NRP2 is less clear, the CDC42 is known to regulate the generation of cell polarity from yeast to man and in a wide range of biological contexts and the downstream target Par6 [82, 83]. Epithelial morphogenesis involves the establishment of an apical surface in an individual cell and the formation of cadherin-based adherents junctions and claudin-based tight junctions between adjacent cells. Accompanying reorganization of the actin and microtubule cytoskeletons and polarized vesicle trafficking reinforces these interactions, leading to a stable tissue of polarized cells. Expression of dominant-negative or constitutively active versions of Cdc42 in the dog kidney epithelial cell line MDCK grown on a two-dimensional (2D) surface leads to defective tight junction formation (typically a delay) as well as mislocalized delivery of basolateral proteins [83–86]. Similar experiments performed with MDCK grown in three dimensions to provide a more physiological growth context have concluded that Cdc42 is required to form an apical surface through regulated trafficking of a vacuolar apical compartment [87, 88]. In Caco-2, a human intestinal epithelial cell line, which, when grown in a 3D matrix, generates polarized cysts with a single central lumen. CDC42 is not required for the formation of an apical surface, but instead is required to position the apical surface with respect to the growing 3D structure. CDC42 regulates apical surface positioning by controlling spindle orientation during cell division.

4.5.5 Cell Positioning and Asymmetric Cell Division

The interrelation between extrinsic determinants (niche), stem cells, and the regulation of cell fate is better characterized in germline cells of lower organisms [89, 90]. In mammalian cells such as the breast epithelia, this interrelation could be determined by the extracellular matrix. Among the proteins that are involved in the breast epithelial cells are the E-cadherin and the bone morphogenetic protein. Both of them are expressed in the normal cells and lost in the trMCF cells. In the *Drosophila* germinal stem cell of the female gonads, DE-cadherin-mediated cell adhesion was shown to be essential for anchoring ovarian gonadal stem cells to their niches and stimulating their proliferation [91]. Decapentaplegic (Dpp) (the *Drosophila* homolog of human bone morphogenetic protein 2/4) is expressed in anterior somatic cells of the gonad and is essential for PGC proliferation. PGC mutants for *thick veins*, an essential Dpp receptor, are impaired in their ability to clonally populate a niche, further suggesting that Dpp is one of the extrinsic mitotic signals that promote the clonal expansion of gonadal stem cells in the niche [92]. Recent studies identify the osteoblasts and the BMP signaling pathway as potential in vivo regulators of the HSC niches [93, 94]. In mice BMP signaling promotes the generation of astrocytes and mature, myelinating oligodendrocytes in vivo, but does not affect oligodendrocyte precursor development, thus suggesting tight regulation of BMP signaling to ensure proper gliogenesis [95].

The concept of asymmetric cell division also needs to be studied in the context of the activation of cell proliferation, apoptosis, and cell junction gene products that are significantly modified during the transformation of MCF cells. Some of these genes are listed in Table 4.3 and among them are TOP2A [96, 97], MK62, RFC3 [98, 99], BIRC5, and GSN. Of interest is the upregulation of BIRC5 or Survivin (Table 4.3; Fig. 4.11), a member of inhibitor of apoptosis family protein. A vector-based siRNAs silenced Survivin expression in prostate cancer cells, resulting in significantly reduced cell proliferation and enhanced apoptosis, and increased the sensitivity of prostate cancer cells to the apoptosis-inducing agent, platinol [98]. Signal transducer and activator of transcription 3 (Stat3) and survivin have been shown to exert oncogenic effects in various human neoplasms [99]. Global gene expression analysis shows that BIRC5 or Survivin, an anti-apoptotic oncofetal gene, is highly expressed in human embryonic stem (hES) cells and teratomas but not in embryoid bodies. Genetic and pharmacological ablation of Survivin induces apoptosis in hES cells and in teratomas both in vitro and in vivo [7]. Treatment with Ochratoxin A (OTA), a potent renal carcinogen, resulted in overexpression of key regulators of mitosis, including the mitotic protein kinases PLK1, Aurora B and cyclin-dependent-kinase 1 (Cdk1(Cdc2)), several cyclins and cyclin-dependent-kinase inhibitors, topoisomerase II, and survivin. Immunohistochemical analysis confirmed upregulation of Cdk1, p21(WAF1/CIP1), topoisomerase II, and survivin in S3 proximal tubule cells, from which OTA-induced tumors in rats arise, and demonstrated increased phosphorylation of histone H3, a target of Aurora B. Importantly, many of the genes found to be deregulated in response to OTA have been linked to

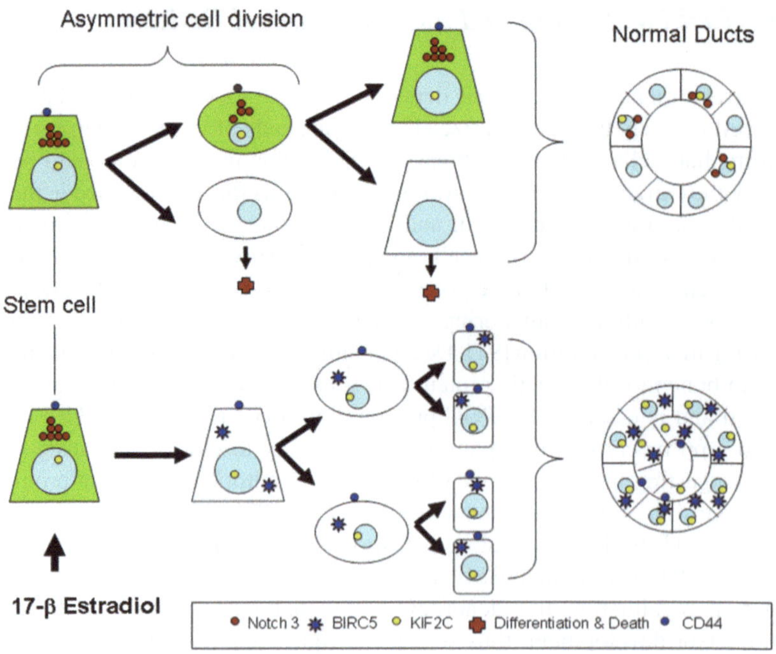

Fig. 4.11 Schematic representation showing the role of asymmetric cell division in ductulogenesis and the effect of estradiol in the loss of this property (reprinted from Russo J, Pereira J, Snider K, Russo IH (2010) Estrogen-induced breast cancer is the result in the disruption of the asymmetric cell division of the stem cell. Horm Mol Biol Clin Investig 1(2):53–65)

chromosomal instability and malignant transformation, supporting the hypothesis that aberrant mitosis, resulting in blocked or asymmetric cell division, accompanied by an increased risk of aneuploidy acquisition, may play a critical role in OTA carcinogenicity [8]. There is a similarity in the behavior of this carcinogen with 17β-estradiol.

4.6 The Molecular Pathway of Epithelial Mesenchymal Transition

While the regulation of epithelial mesenchymal transition (EMT) is not fully understood, a network of several signaling pathways affecting the expression and/or function of a complex hierarchical network of transcription factors (TFs) has been partially elaborated [100, 101]. Known signaling pathways include multiple tyrosine kinase receptors leading to Ras-mediated activation of MAPK and PI3K pathways, TGF-β, Notch, and Wnt. From our studies, we have evidence that enhanced TGF-β and Wnt signaling pathways are found in the EMT expressing bcMCF and caMCF cells [5]. TGF-β acting through Smad transcriptional complexes can repress expression of the Id TFs (Id1, Id2, Id3) and activate HMGA2, a DNA binding protein important for chromatin architecture [99]. Expression of HMGA2 is known to regulate several EMT controlling TFs including TWIST1, SNAI1, and SNAI2 (Slug) [5, 100, 101] (Figs. 4.5 and 4.6). TGF-β and Wnt signaling also affect the expression of several additional EMT-regulating TFs including ZEB1 (TCF8), TCF3 (E2A encoding E12 and E47), and LEF1 [101].

Analysis of the EMT expressing bcMCF cell line revealed the absence of expression of the secreted frizzled-related protein 1 (SFRP1), a repressor of Wnt signaling [5]. One allele of SFRP1 was deleted in these cells, with the remaining apparently silenced by methylation, accounting for the 28-fold reduction of this transcript. Loss and epigenetic inactivation of SFRP1 occurs often in invasive breast cancer and is associated with poor prognosis [102]. Inspection of the SFRP1 expression levels in Basal B cell lines [5] showed absent calls for four of the eight invasive cell lines and eightfold decreases in another three invasive cell lines relative to the non-invasive MCF-10A cells. Inspection of the expression files for bcMCF cells and the eight invasive Basal B cell lines [5] revealed that LEF1 was always absent, while TCF3 and TCF8 were expressed.

4.7 The Metastatic Phenotype

As indicated above, the bsMCF cells induced tumors in SCID mice that were poorly differentiated adenocarcinomas that were ESRα, progesterone receptor (PR) and ERBB2 negatives. When bsMCF or caMCF (T4 or T5) cells are inoculated in the tail of SCID mice, they induced metastatic foci in the lung (Figs. 4.12 and 4.13). This unique model allows us: (a) to study the genomic and epigenomic changes present in the cell with metastatic capabilities, (b) to use metastatic and nonmetastatic cells from the same genetic background, and (c) to elucidate the functional role of each of the genes thus identified. We have found that more than 74 genes are either down- or upregulated in the invasive and metastatic phenotype of the bsMCF (Fig. 4.14; Tables 4.4 and 4.5). Several genes controlling invasion and metastasis are significantly downregulated in bsMCF (C5) cells (Fig. 4.14; Table 4.5). Many of these genes are silenced by methylation in specific GpC islands and their role in the process of invasion and metastasis has been already determined or suspected. For example, AZGP1 is known to be downregulated in malignant prostate epithelium [103, 104], but its precise role in metastasis is not clear. CLDN7 or Claudin 7 is significantly downregulated in bsMCF cells as well as in breast [105, 106] and other types of cancer [107]. Hypermethylation at the CLDN7 promoter was detected in 20% of colon cancer cells with low CLDN7 expression. EPB41L5 erythrocyte membrane protein band 4.1 like 5 is involved in cell polarity and in maintaining by separation of the apical and basolateral domains through specialized cell–cell junctions [108, 109] and could be an early marker of metastasis. GPR56 or G protein-coupled receptor 56 is downregulated in bsMCF cells and is markedly downregulated in the

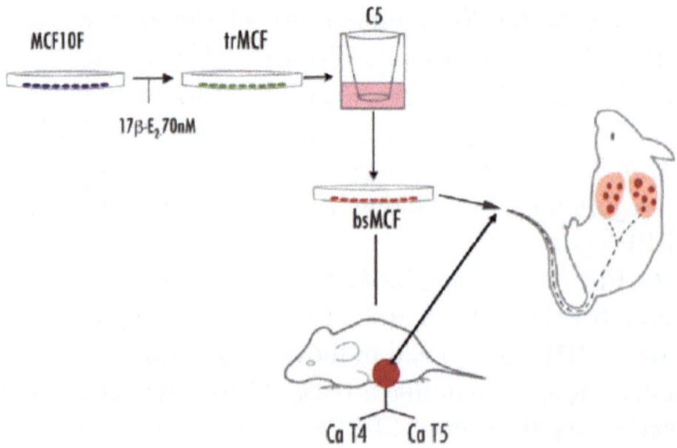

Fig. 4.12 Transformation of MCF-10F cells by 17β-estradiol treatment. Experimental protocol: MCF-10F cells treated with 70 nM 17β-estradiol (E_2) that expressed high colony efficiency (CE) and loss of ductulogenic capacity in collagen-matrix were classified as transformed (trMCF). Transformed cells that were invasive in a Matrigel Boyden type invasion chambers were selected (bsMCF) and plated at low density for cloning (bcMCF). MCF-10F, trMCF, bsMCF, and bcMCF were tested for carcinogenicity by injecting them into the mammary fat pad of 45-day-old female SCID mice. MCF-10F and trMCF cells did not induce tumors; bsMCF formed solid tumors from which four cell lines, identified as caMCF, were derived and cells proven to be tumorigenic in SCID mice. bsMCF or caMCF when injected in the tail of SCID mice develop metastatic foci in the lung (reprinted from Russo J, Russo IH (2011) The role of the basal stem cell of the human breast in normal development and cancer. Adv Exp Med Biol 720:121–134)

metastatic variants of melanoma. Functional studies have shown that overexpression of GPR56 suppresses tumor growth and metastasis, whereas reduced expression of GPR56 enhances tumor progression [110, 111]. KLF5 Kruppel-like factor 5 is downregulated also in bsMCF cells and reduced in expression in many types of human tumor [112].

FRMD3 is a member of the protein 4.1 superfamily and is a putative tumor suppressor [113] significantly downregulated in bsMCF cells. Grbl4, a growth factor receptor-bound protein 14 member of the Grb7 family of adapters, is an inhibitor of FGFR signaling. Grbl4 induces an arrest of the signaling transduction cascades in the MDA-MB-231cells by blocking PLCy, ERK2, JNK1, and AKT [114, 115]. Another role of GRB14 is as a binding partner of tankyrase 2. Tankyrase is an ankyrin repeat-containing poly [ADP-ribose] polymerase originally isolated as a binding partner for the telomeric protein TRF1. MEST or mesoderm-specific transcript homolog is a hypermethylated gene that is highly enriched for targets of the PRC2 (Polycomb repressive complex 2) in embryonic stem cells. MTUS1 or microtubule associated tumor suppressor 1 is downregulated in bsMCF cells and is significantly downregulated in colon cancer and in a breast cancer [116–118] and in the triple negative (ER− PR− HER2−) breast carcinomas, a subgroup of highly proliferative tumors with poor outcome and no available targeted therapy. Functional studies indicate that silencing MTUS1 expression by siRNA increases cellular

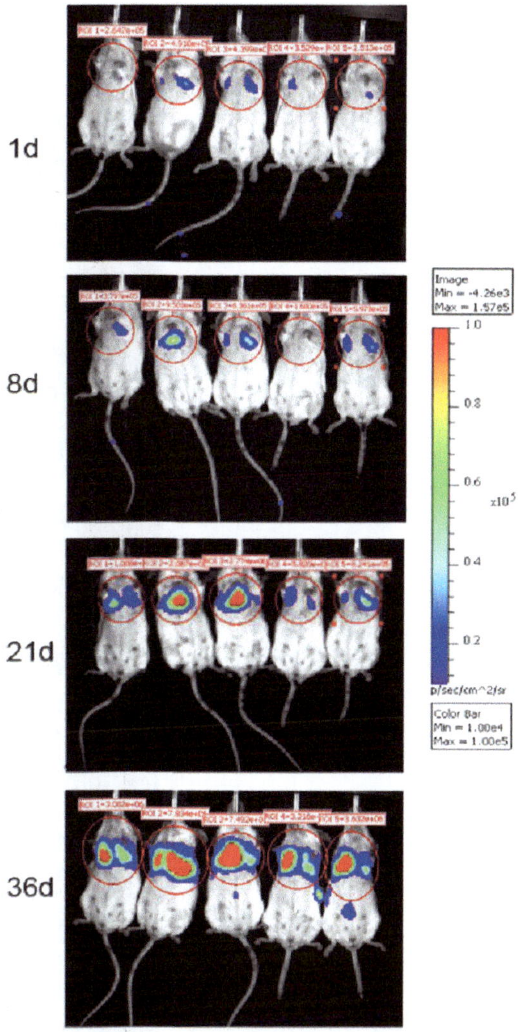

Fig. 4.13 bcMCF cells were transfected by Lipofectamine/Plus Reagent from Life Technologies. The plasmids that were used for the cotransfection were pGL3 control red (SV40-luc) from Promega/C. Contag, Stanford University, and pSV40/Zeo from Invitrogen. After the cells were transfected, selection occurred over a period of 10–12 days using 1 μg/mL of Zeocin (Invitrogen). After selection, the cells were allowed a period of time to recover after which they were expanded. To ensure the presence of luciferase in the cells, a Luciferase Assay (Promega) was performed using the EnVision Workstation plate reader. Mice were placed in a plastic restraining device equipped with a hole from which we could access the tail. The tails of the mice were placed in warm water in order to dilate the lateral tail veins and to allow easy visualization. Two million (2×10^6) cells suspended in PBS were injected into the lateral tail vein using a 26 gauge needle. The animals were followed over a period of 5 weeks by Bioluminescence Imaging using the Caliper LS/Xenogen IVIS Spectrum System to determine the location of the bcMCF cells (reprinted from Russo J, Russo IH (2011) The role of the basal stem cell of the human breast in normal development and cancer. Adv Exp Med Biol 720:121–134)

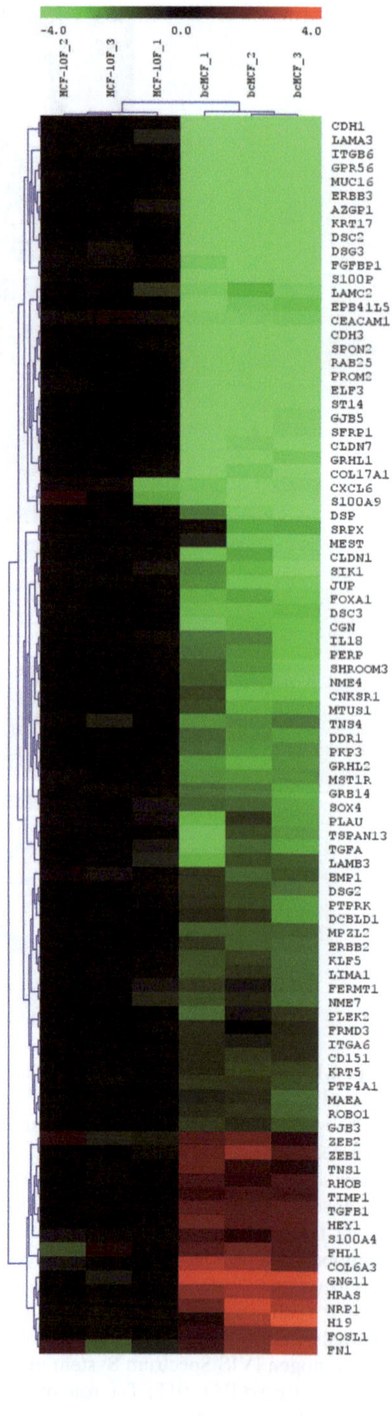

Fig. 4.14 Heat map of the bcMCF cells compared with the MCF-10F cells (reprinted from Russo J, Russo IH (2011) The role of the basal stem cell of the human breast in normal development and cancer. Adv Exp Med Biol 720:121–134)

Table 4.4 Genes differentially expressed genes in bcMCF compared to MCF-10F

Symbol	Gene name	Fold change
AZGP1	Alpha-2-glycoprotein 1, zinc-binding	–31.8
CDH1	Cadherin 1, type 1, E-cadherin (epithelial)	–497.8
EPB41L5	Erythrocyte membrane protein band 4.1 like 5	–17.7
FRMD3	FERM domain containing 3	–3.3
GRB14	Growth factor receptor-bound protein 14	–4.1
GPR56	G protein-coupled receptor 56	–27.8
KLF5	Kruppel-like factor 5 (intestinal)	–2.9
MEST	Mesoderm-specific transcript homolog (mouse)	–4.3
MTUS1	Mitochondrial tumor suppressor 1	–2.4
RAB25	RAB25, member RAS oncogene family	–46.2
SFRP1	Secreted frizzled-related protein 1	–5.8
SFRP1	Secreted frizzled-related protein 1	–5.5
SFRP1	Secreted frizzled-related protein 1	–4.8
SRPX	Sushi-repeat-containing protein, X-linked	–6.4
ST14	Suppression of tumorigenicity 14 (colon carcinoma)	–5.8
ST14	Suppression of tumorigenicity 14 (colon carcinoma)	–4.2
S100A9	S100 calcium binding protein A9	–18.2
SIK1	Salt-inducible kinase 1	–6.9

Table 4.5 Upregulated genes differentially expressed genes in bcMCF compared to MCF-10F

Symbol	Gene name	Fold change
FHL1	Four and a half domains 1	6.5
HEY1	Hairy/enhancer-of-split related with YRPW motif 1	5.4
ZEB1	Zinc finger E-box binding homeobox 1	12.0
ZEB2	Zinc finger E-box binding homeobox 2	11.5
COL6A3	Collagen, type VI, alpha 3	77.1
FN1	Fibronectin 1	4.9
FOSL1	FOS-like antigen 1	3.8
GNG11	Guanine nucleotide binding protein (G protein), gamma 11	10.5
HRAS	V-Ha-ras Harvey rat sarcoma viral oncogene homolog	6.0
NRP1	Neuropilin 1	6.9
RHOB	Ras homolog gene family, member B	5.7
S100A4	S100 calcium binding protein A4	18.8
TGFB1	Transforming growth factor, beta 1	3.1
TIMP1	TIMP metallopeptidase inhibitor 1	2.9
TNS1	Tensin 1	14.9

proliferation. Conversely, restoring endogenous levels of MTUS1 expression leads to reduced cancer cell proliferation, clonogenicity, and anchorage-independent growth and reduces the incidence and size of xenografts grown in vivo [119]. Loss of SFRP1, secreted frizzled-related protein 1, expression is observed in breast, along with several other cancers [120–124], and is associated with poor patient prognosis. SFRP1 is significantly downregulated in bsMCF cells and it has been shown to be methylated in many pre and neoplastic breast cancer cell lines. SFRP1 antagonizes the Wnt/β-catenin signaling pathway by competing with the Frizzled receptor for Wnt ligands, resulting in an attenuation of the signal transduction cascade leading to the development of several human cancers, including breast cancer. SRPX sushi-repeat-containing protein, X-linked is downregulated in bsMCF cells and is also markedly reduced in carcinomas of colon, bladder, and ovary and closely linked to the progression of T-cell leukemia/lymphoma. The SRPX gene was originally isolated as a novel suppressor gene of v-src transformation and was shown to induce apoptosis in human cancer cells. It has been observed by us and others that TWIST, which is an important transcription factor during embryonic development and has recently been found to promote the EMT phenomenon seen during the initial steps of tumor metastasis, is upregulated in bsMCF cells, whereas SRPX is downregulated. The siRNA-mediated depletion of TWIST results in upregulation of SRPX, indicating an important role of the SRPX gene in invasion and metastasis. Another gene downregulated in bsMCF cells is SNF1LK or the serine-threonine kinase SIK1 (salt-inducible kinase 1) as a regulator of p53-dependent anoikis. Inactivation of SIK1 compromised p53 function in anoikis and allowed cells to grow in an anchorage-independent manner. In vivo, SIK1 loss facilitated metastatic spread and survival of disseminated cells as micrometastases in lungs. The presence of functional SIK1 was required for the activity of the kinase LKB1 in promoting p53-dependent anoikis and suppressing anchorage-independent growth, matrigel invasion, and metastatic potential. Decreased expression of the gene encoding SIK1 closely correlated with development of distal metastases in breast cancers from three independent cohorts. Together, these findings indicate that SIK1 links LKB1 to p53-dependent anoikis and suppresses metastasis [125, 126]. SIK is an inducible gene target of TGF-β/Smad signaling. Loss of endogenous SIK results in enhanced gene responses of the fibrotic and cytostatic programs of TGF-β [127].

Among the upregulated genes in the bsMCF cells are the one listed in Table 4.5, FHL1, HEY1, ZEB1, ZEB2, FOSL1, and S100A4. FHL1 (four and a half LIM domains 1) may play an important role in ER signaling as well as breast cancer cell growth regulation [128, 129]. HEY1 hairy/enhancer-of-split related with YRPW motif 1 and NOTCH3 are upregulated also in bsMCF cells and may be involved in the EMT process [129–131]. TGF-β is upregulated in bsMCF cells and is involved in the EMT through activation of Smad and non-Smad signaling pathways. EMT is the differentiation switch by which polarized epithelial cells differentiate into contractile and motile mesenchymal cells. Cell motility and invasive capacity are activated upon EMT. Multiple transcription factors, including deltaEF1/ZEB1, SIP1/ZEB2, and Snail/SNAI1, are induced by TGF-β-Smad signaling and play critical roles in TGF-β-induced EMT. In addition, both non-Smad signaling activated by TGF-β and cross-talk with other signaling pathways play important roles in induction of EMT. Of these, Ras signaling synergizes with TGF-β-Smad signaling and plays an important role in the induction of EMT. FOSL1 is upregulated in bsMCF cells and has been shown to be overexpressed in MCF-7 cells after development of antiestrogen resistance. Fos is a component of the dimeric transcription factor activator protein-1 (Ap-1), which is composed mainly of Fos (c-Fos, FosB, Fra-1, and Fra-2) and Jun proteins (c-Jun, JunB, and JunD). Unlike Fra-1 (encoded by FOSL1), c-Fos contains transactivation domains required for oncogenesis and cellular transformation [132]. The Fos-related antigen-1 (Fra-1) is activated in multiple cancers and gene ablation can suppress the invasive phenotypes of many tumor cell lines [132–134]. S100A4 calcium binding protein A4 is upregulated in bsMCF cells and many other cancers [135, 136]. This protein promotes metastasis in several experimental animal models, and S100A4 protein expression is associated with patient outcome in a number of tumor types and possesses a wide range of biological functions, such as regulation of angiogenesis, cell survival, motility, and invasion [137, 138]. *From these data, we concluded that the EMT occurring in the breast basal cells depends predominately on TGF-β and Wnt signaling pathways, which increase the expression and function of transcription and chromatin organization factors that repress the epithelial and enhance the mesenchymal phenotype, thus favoring increased invasion and metastatic activity.*

4.8 Human Chorionic Gonadotropin Prevents the Transformed Phenotypes Induced by 17β-Estradiol in Human Breast Epithelial Cells

Clinical and epidemiological studies have shown that prolonged or cumulative estrogenic exposure such as early menarche or late menopause are associated with increased breast cancer incidence [139–141]. Moreover, these effects continue even after menopause due to local tissue estrogen production [142]. We have demonstrated that estrogen-induced neoplastic transformation in vitro is characterized by the loss of the ductulogenic pattern in collagen matrix with disruption of the normal breast epithelial architecture [4, 143]. At early stages in the transformation process, estrogen produces a downregulation in the expression of genes related to cell adhesion such as *ITGB6* (integrin β6), *LAMA3* (laminin α3), *LAMC2* (laminin γ2), and *FN1* (fibronectin 1) and downregulation of other genes by epigenetic modifications [5, 144]. Unlike estrogen, parity at early age, especially before age 24, decreases the incidence of breast cancer [12, 145] compared to nulliparous women. Women with at least one full-term pregnancy have 25% reduction in breast cancer risk and increasing number of pregnancies confers further protection [146, 147]. This can be explained by comparing the morphology of the breast of nulliparous and parous women. The breast of a normally cycling woman contains three types of lobules described as type 1 (Lob 1), type 2 (Lob 2), and type 3 (Lob 3) by the degree of their increasing complexity, defined as the number of alveoli per lobule [148–150]. The breast attains its maximum development during pregnancy when there is a progression of Lob 2 to Lob 3; this growth phase is followed by the secretory phase in fully differentiated lobules type 4 (Lob 4). With the progressive maturation of Lob 1 to Lob 2, Lob 3, and Lob 4, there is a progressive decrease in the percentage of proliferating cells and a reduction in the susceptibility of the cells to be transformed by carcinogens [150]. After post-lactational involution, Lob 4 regress to Lob 3, which remains present as the predominant structures in the breast until a woman reaches the fourth decade of life, at which point the structures decrease due to their involution to Lob 2 and Lob 1. As opposed to the breasts of parous women, the nulliparous breast contains a great number of Lob 1, whose percentage remains almost constant throughout their lifespan; in nulliparous women, Lob 2 are present in moderate numbers and Lob 3 are almost totally absent. After menopause, the breast regresses in both nulliparous and parous women and this is manifested as an increase in the number of Lob 1, and a concomitant decline in the number of Lob 2 and Lob 3. At the end of the fifth decade of life, the breast of both nulliparous and parous postmenopausal women contains predominantly Lob 1, although the Lob 1 in parous women are refractory to carcinogenesis and they have a "genomic signature" or gene expression profile that is different from the Lob 1 of nulliparous women [150, 151]. We further demonstrated in a model of mammary carcinogenesis in rats that a full-term pregnancy results in substantial protection against DMBA-induced malignant transformation [152]. Moreover, short-term treatment of virgin rats with hCG induces the same differentiation than pregnancy, as described in Chap. 3. Thus, the mammary epithelium is able to gain resistance to carcinogenesis by hCG pretreatment [153]. In an experiment in which virgin rats were treated with human chorionic gonadotropin (hCG) for 21 days (the length of a pregnancy), followed by a 21-day rest period and then administration of DMBA, a dramatic dose-dependent decline incidence was observed [148, 152, 154]. Based on these observations, it was proposed that in the breast, pregnancy or hCG is able to shift the stem cells 1 that are susceptible to transformation by a carcinogen to stem cells 2 that are refractory [150, 155]. Stem cells 2 are progenitor cells originated after post-lactation involution of the breast and they can proliferate and differentiate under the stimulus of a new pregnancy [150, 155]. This concept, known as *terminal differentiation hypothesis of breast cancer prevention*, predicts that the loss of stem cells 1 through differentiation to stem cells 2 and the general increase in the mammary gland differentiation following pregnancy or hCG treatment results in protection from tumorigenesis [155, 156] (Fig. 4.15). Furthermore, previous studies from our laboratory have shown that full-term pregnancy induces a permanent genomic signature in the breast epithelial cells associated with lower cell proliferation and

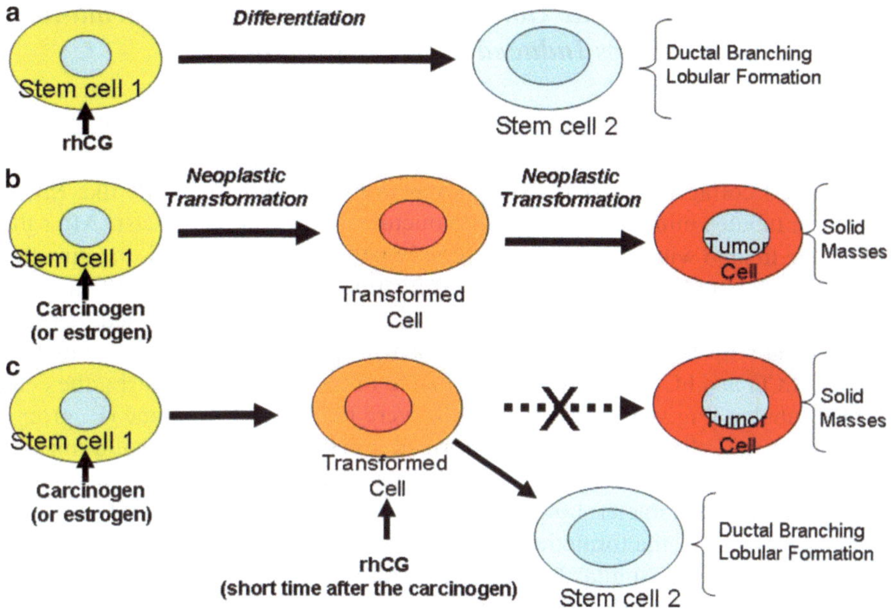

Fig. 4.15 The terminal differentiation hypothesis of breast cancer prevention. Stem cells 1 are susceptible to be transformed by carcinogens (or E_2), although stem cells 2 are refractory. This hypothesis predicts that: (**a**) the loss of a population of susceptible stem cells 1 through differentiation to stem cells 2 and a general increase in the differentiation of the cells in the mammary gland following recombinant human chorionic gonadotropin (rhCG) treatment results in protection from tumorigenic changes. (**b**) Stem cells 1 exposed to carcinogens (or E_2) give origin to early transformed cells that progress to tumor cells. (**c**) In the case of carcinogen (or E_2) administration followed by rhCG treatment, transformed cells are inhibited from progressing to the tumorigenic stages (reprinted from Kocdor H, Kocdor MA, Russo J, Snider KE, Vanegas JE, Russo IH, Fernandez SV (2009) Human chorionic gonadotropin (hCG) prevents the transformed phenotypes induced by 17 β-estradiol in human breast epithelial cells. Cell Biol Int 33:1135–1143)

efficient DNA repair capacity, creating a differentiated breast epithelium that is more resistant to carcinogenesis [155, 157]. The disruption of the tubular structures of the breast epithelial cells, including loss of apico-basal polarity and filling of the luminal space, are considered a hallmark in epithelial cancers [8]. The architectural features and branching morphogenesis during neoplastic transformation have critical importance for better understanding the mechanisms behind mammary epithelial carcinogenesis and its prevention. Presumably, early parity and/or hCG play critical roles in preventing the neoplastic process in the breast epithelium by preserving the normal 3D epithelial architecture. We further demonstrated in vitro that rhCG was able to prevent the transformation phenotypes induced by E_2 and stimulated the ductulogenesis by increasing the length of the ducts and producing tertiary branching of the breast epithelial cells.

4.8.1 Human Chorionic Gonadotropin Prevented the Formation of Solid Masses Induced by 17β-Estradiol (E_2)

The effect of the rhCG on the transformation induced by E_2 was studied using MCF-10F cells grown in collagen matrix (3D-cultures). One of the advantages of using type I collagen matrix is that the human breast epithelial cells like MCF-10F form tubules mimicking the normal ductules of the human breast. After the cells were treated with E_2 or rhCG or a combination of E_2 and rhCG, the ductulogenesis was quantitatively evaluated by estimating the ability of the cells to form tubules. When MCF-10F cells were grown in regular media (regular media group) or in media with DMSO (DMSO group) or with rhCG alone or in combination with E_2 (hCG and hCG + E_2 groups) and plated in type I collagen matrix, the cells formed tubules (Fig. 4.16). When the cells were treated with E_2 alone (E_2 group) and plated in collagen, some cells formed tubules and others solid masses (Figs. 4.16, 4.17 and 4.18). E_2 induced the formation of solid masses of 178 ± 33.16 μm in diameter; however, when the cells were treated with E_2 in combination with rhCG, the formation of solid masses was prevented (Fig. 4.18). The number of ducts was similar between the groups except between the control in regular media and hCG + E_2 group in which the difference was significant ($p = 0.01$ Tukey's test) (Fig. 4.18).

4.8.2 Human Chorionic Gonadotropin Induced Longer Tubules with Tertiary Branching

The tubules formed in collagen showed different morphology between the groups; the length and diameter of the main duct and the number of primary, secondary, and tertiary branching arising from the main tubule were different according to the treatments (Fig. 4.16). The ducts were significantly longer and had more branches when the cells were treated with rhCG (hCG alone or in combination with E_2) (Fig. 4.19). In Fig. 4.16, the length, width, and branching of the tubules from each group are represented. The tubules formed by the cells treated with rhCG (hCG group) were significantly longer compared to the other groups ($p < 0.001$, Tukey's test) (Fig. 4.19a). In addition, the tubules formed by the cells treated with rhCG in combination with E_2 (hCG + E_2 group) were longer compared to other groups ($p < 0.001$; Tukey's test) (Fig. 4.19a). The diameter of the main tubules was also measured; the tubules showed a significant increase in width when the cells were treated with E_2 alone (E_2 group) ($p < 0.001$; ANOVA) and no significant differences were found among the other groups (Fig. 4.19a). Also, the primary, secondary, and tertiary branching was evaluated (Fig. 4.19b). All the tubules showed primary and secondary branches and the differences were not significant between the treatments; only when the cells were treated with rhCG (alone or in combination with E_2), the ducts

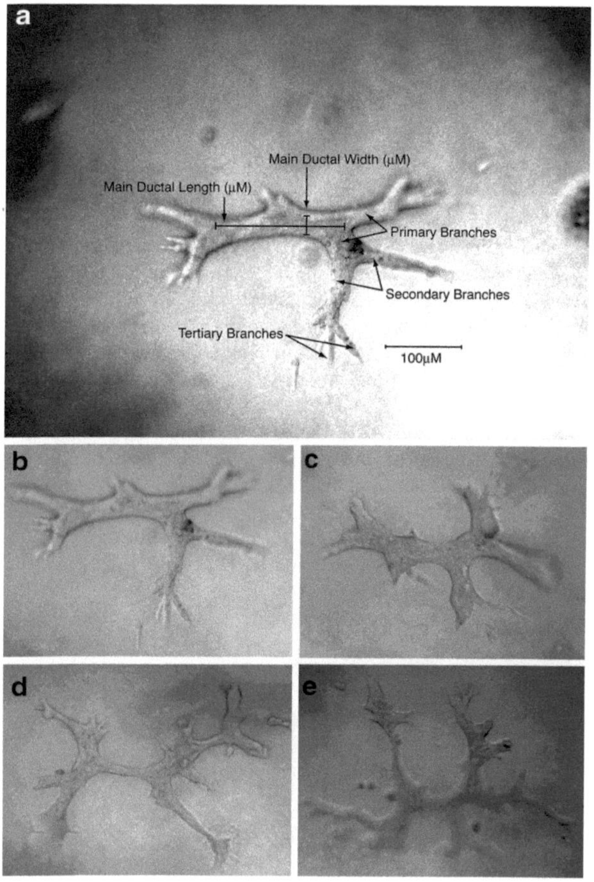

Fig. 4.16 Tubules on collagen matrix. (**a**) Parameters for the evaluation of 3D growth of human breast epithelial cells MCF-10F in collagen. The main ductal length, main ductal width and primary, secondary, and tertiary branches are indicated; (**b**) tubule formed by MCF-10F cells growing in collagen after treatment with DMSO; (**c**) tubule formed by MCF-10F cells after treatment with 70 nM 17β-estradiol (E_2): the tubules are shorter and increased in width; (**d**) tubule formed by MCF-10F after treatment with rhCG: the ducts are longer, thinner and present a significant higher number of secondary and tertiary branches; (**e**) tubule formed by MCF-10F cells after treatment with rhCG in combination with 17β-estradiol (hCG+E_2 group): the presence of hCG prevents the alterations induced by E_2 (reprinted from Kocdor H, Kocdor MA, Russo J, Snider KE, Vanegas JE, Russo IH, Fernandez SV (2009) Human chorionic gonadotropin (hCG) prevents the transformed phenotypes induced by 17 β-estradiol in human breast epithelial cells. Cell Biol Int 33:1135–1143)

showed tertiary branching (Fig. 4.19b). All the ducts from the hCG group and 60% of the hCG+E_2 group showed tertiary branching. The number of tertiary branches per duct was higher when the cells were treated with rhCG alone (hCG group) than when they were treated with rhCG in combination with E_2 (hCG+E_2 group) (Student's *t* test, $p<0.001$).

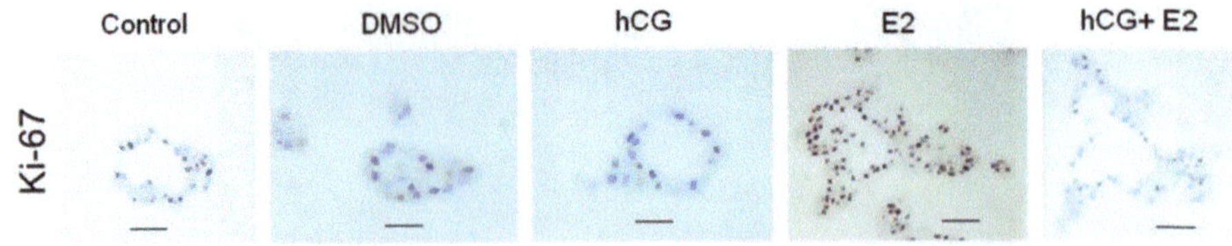

Fig. 4.17 Cell proliferation study by immunohistochemistry. The cross sections of the tubules grown in collagen matrix after the different treatments are presented. Only some cells were positive for Ki67 antigen in the control in regular media (Control), DMSO, hCG, E2 and hCG+E_2. In a cross section, the MCF-10F breast epithelial cells were arranged forming a monolayer around the lumen of the duct except in the cells treated with estradiol (E_2). E_2 impairs not only ductal morphology and lumen formation, but also causes loss of epithelial characteristics and proliferation as consequences of neoplastic transformation. An increased number of cells showed to be positive for Ki67 antigen in the tubules formed by the cells treated with E_2 (bar = 50 μm) (reprinted from Kocdor H, Kocdor MA, Russo J, Snider KE, Vanegas JE, Russo IH, Fernandez SV (2009) Human chorionic gonadotropin (hCG) prevents the transformed phenotypes induced by 17 β-estradiol in human breast epithelial cells. Cell Biol Int 33:1135–1143)

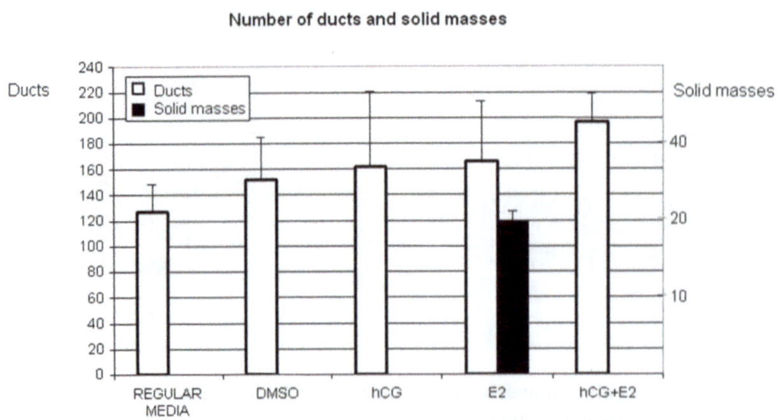

Fig. 4.18 Number of tubules and solid masses on type I collagen matrix. MCF-10F cells were treated during 2 weeks with 70 nM (E_2 group); 50 IU/mL rhCG (hCG group) or 50 IU/mL rhCG in combination with 70 nM E_2 (hCG+E_2 group); as controls cells were treated with DMSO (DMSO group) or maintained in the regular media (regular media group). After the treatments, the ductulogenesis assay was performed and the number of ducts and solid masses were counted. Solid masses with a mean diameter of 178 μm appeared after treatment with E_2, although when E_2 was used in combination with rhCG, solid masses did not appear on the collagen. The mean and the standard deviation (SD) are indicated (reprinted from Kocdor H, Kocdor MA, Russo J, Snider KE, Vanegas JE, Russo IH, Fernandez SV (2009) Human chorionic gonadotropin (hCG) prevents the transformed phenotypes induced by 17 β-estradiol in human breast epithelial cells. Cell Biol Int 33:1135–1143)

4.8.3 The 17β-Estradiol (E_2) Treatment Increased Cell Proliferation

The cell proliferation was evaluated using an antibody against Ki67 antigen. The Ki67 antigen is a cell cycle-related nuclear protein, expressed by proliferating cells in all phases of the active cell cycle (G_1, S, G_2 and M phase) and it is absent in resting

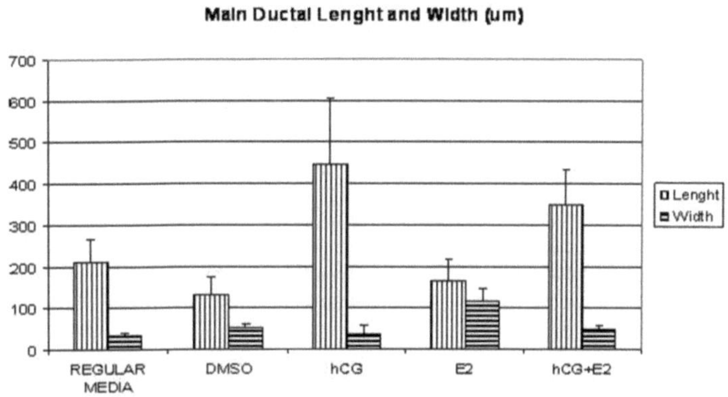

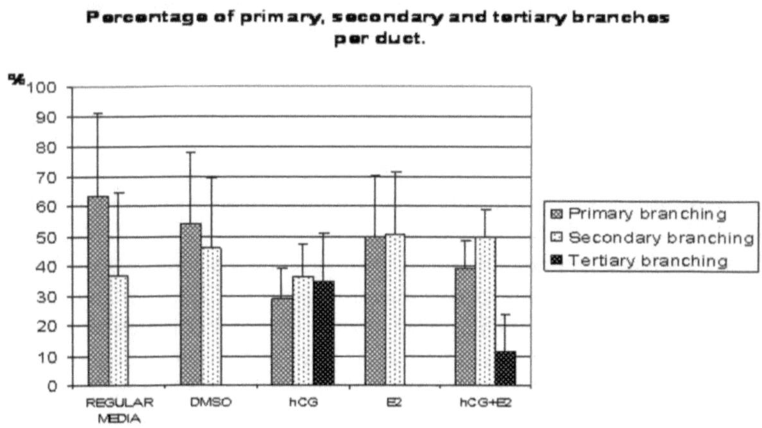

Fig. 4.19 *Upper histogram:* Ductal length and width. The ducts were longer in the hCG groups (hCG and hCG+E_2 groups). The tubules showed increased width in the E_2 group. The ducts in hCG group are significantly longer than in DMSO, E_2, control in regular media and hCG+E_2 group ($p<0.001$; $p<0.001$; $p<0.001$ and $p=0.008$ respectively, Tukey's test); furthermore, the tubules are longer in the hCG+E_2 group than in the DMSO ($p<0.001$ Tukey's test), E_2 ($p<0.001$ Tukey's test), and control in regular media ($p<0.001$ Tukey's test) groups. The differences in the length of the tubules were no significant between control in regular media vs. DMSO, control in regular media vs. E_2, and E_2 vs. DMSO ($p=0.064$, $p=0.052$, and $p=0.79$, respectively; Tukey's test). The treatment with E_2 (E_2 group) increased the width of the ducts when compared to other groups ($p<0.001$ ANOVA followed by Tukey's test). *Lower histogram:* Percentage of primary, secondary, and tertiary branching per duct. Tertiary branching was only observed in the rhCG groups (hCG alone or hCG+E_2) (reprinted from Kocdor H, Kocdor MA, Russo J, Snider KE, Vanegas JE, Russo IH, Fernandez SV (2009) Human chorionic gonadotropin (hCG) prevents the transformed phenotypes induced by 17 β-estradiol in human breast epithelial cells. Cell Biol Int 33:1135–1143)

(G_0) cells. The cross sections of the tubular structures showed a monolayer of epithelial cells around the lumen in all the groups except in the E_2 group (Fig. 4.17). In the E_2 treated group, the cross section of the tubules showed an increase of both number of epithelial layers and Ki67 positive cells (Proliferative index = 54.9),

Table 4.6 Proliferative index

Group		Percentage of positive Ki67cells on ductal structures (Average ± SD)
1	Control in regular media	36.8 ± 6.7
2	DMSO	32 ± 3.45
3	hCG	31.63 ± 11.6
4	hCG + E_2	29.34 ± 7.35
5	E_2	54.9 ± 8.1

In the ducts, the number of cells Ki67 positive was counted from approximately 100 cells that formed the ducts. The proliferative index with the standard deviation is indicated in each case

indicating an increase in the cell proliferation rate; no difference in the proliferation rate was observed in the other groups (Table 4.6). Interestingly, there was no increase in the cell proliferation rate when the cells were treated with E_2 in combination with rhCG (hCG + E_2 group) (PI = 29.34) compared to the control in regular media (PI = 36.8) or DMSO (PI = 32) (Table 4.1). The epithelial cells layering the ducts showed to be estrogen receptor alpha (ERα) negative and positive for E-cadherin, laminin, vimentin, and keratin shown, but no differences were found between the groups.

Primary mammary epithelial cells grown in collagen matrix are able to form tree-like structures resembling in vivo ductulogenesis [7]. The human breast epithelial cells MCF-10F formed tubules when grown in type I collagen and we demonstrated that treatment of these cells with E_2 induces phenotypical changes indicative of neoplastic transformation [4, 143]. We have demonstrated that the transformation of MCF-10F by E_2, which is associated with impaired ductal morphogenesis, can be abrogated by the hCG; the treatment of the human breast epithelial cells MCF-10F with E_2 induced formation of solid masses of 178 μm in diameter, although treatment with E_2 in combination with hCG prevented their formation. Treatment with E_2 in combination with rhCG produced the differentiation of the cells and branching formation in collagen; the rhCG prevents the action of E_2 acting as antagonist. Also, we demonstrated that rhCG has a direct effect on the branching of breast epithelium; significant ductal elongation was observed in hCG-treated groups and tertiary branches only appear in the presence of hCG (alone or in combination with E_2). Furthermore, the increase in the width of the tubules produced by E_2 was prevented by the rhCG. In conclusion, the loss of differentiation and disorganized growth of transformed MCF-10F cells caused by estrogen was abrogated by hCG. Altogether our data clearly showed that estrogen-induced neoplastic transformation associated with altered ductal morphology and solid masses formation and hCG was able to abrogate them. These results further support the *terminal differentiation hypothesis of breast cancer protection*. MCF-10F cells which are ERα negative and $CD44^+$ form ductules in collagen and can be transformed by carcinogens [4, 5, 150] and it was proposed that these cells exhibit characteristics of stem cells 1 [150].

The ducts formed a significant increase in width with an incomplete lumen formation when the cells were treated with E_2 (E_2 group) and this effect was associated with increased cellular proliferation (Ki67 positive cells). It has been suggested that the filling of the lumen would be the result of a decrease in central apoptosis, enhanced cellular proliferation, or a combination of the two [158]. Luminal filling is the earliest morphologic alteration and is commonly reported in neoplastic processes [158]. Luminal filling is commonly seen in atypical ductal hyperplasia and DCIS.

4.9 Concluding and Summary Remarks

The advantage of an in vitro model of 3D growth (3D-cultures) is that it allows modeling of the epithelial architecture of the breast [8, 10, 159]. Normal epithelial cells form duct-like structures with apical–basal polarity and well-organized tubular structures with stable adherens junctions and cell-basement communications. Malignant transformation is associated with the loss of apical–basal polarity and monolayer morphology and significant deviations from normal epithelial behavior in 3D-cultures [10, 11]. In several studies, basement membrane (BM) like Matrigel was used to study the growth and differentiation of the breast epithelia instead of type I collagen matrix. Matrigel is a complex mixture of extracellular matrix proteins and growth factors [12, 13]. At difference of type I collagen that provide the structural support allowing the expression of the intrinsic properties of the breast epithelial cells, the use of BM has allowed to study the role of different factors and extracellular matrix components that affect the branching [12, 13, 160–163]. Therefore, the usage of type I collagen gel matrix was more appropriate for our study which involved observing the paracrine effect of the hCG on the breast epithelial cells MCF-10F in the absence of these morphogenetic factors.

Although the cellular and molecular mechanisms of tubulogenesis are still incompletely understood, a number of polypeptide growth factors have been shown to stimulate the formation and branching of epithelial tubes [164]. In the present work, we showed that rhCG produced longer tubules with tertiary branches even in the presence of estradiol. It has been reported that hCG treatment resulted in branching and lobulo-alveolar development of the human breast epithelia, although these effects were not observed in ovariectomized animals [165]. Other factors shown to affect the branching morphogenesis are the hepatocyte growth factor/scatter factor (HGF/SF) [12, 166, 167] and several members of the fibroblast growth factor family [168]. Also, it was shown that heregulin and retinoids stimulated the branching [169].

Both LH (luteinizing hormone) and hCG bind to the LH/hCG receptor and they stimulate adenylate cyclase on the internal membrane converting adenosine triphosphate (ATP) into cyclic adenosine monophosphate (cAMP); cAMP stimulates the activation of a protein kinase, which among other actions stimulates steroidogenesis in the mitochondria of the target cell by transforming cholesterol into pregnenolone. Other actions include the induction of proteolytic enzymes, prostaglandine synthesis, inhibin production, induction of 17β-hydroxysteroid dehydrogenase, and changes in gene metabolism [170]. It was shown that LH/hCG receptors are present in human breast tissue, rat breast tissue, and different cell lines [171–174]. Gene expression profile studies of rats have shown that the genomic signature induced by rhCG treatment was similar to the one induced by pregnancy and these data indicated that hCG like pregnancy induce genomic changes that control a specific differentiation pathway that it is capable of changing stem cells 1 to stem cells 2, although other compounds that induce branching were not able to induce that specific signature [151, 155].

A population-based case-control study of breast cancer among women 40 years of age or younger showed that women who received hCG, as a part of a weight loss program popular during the 1960s and 1970s or as a component of infertility treatment, were at lower risk to developing breast cancer [175]. Another population-based cohort study of serum collected from first-trimester pregnant women showed that women with high levels of hCG had lower risk of breast cancer than women with low hCG levels [176]. The fact that parous women at early ages also develop breast cancer at early ages could be explained if the hCG did not reach sufficient levels to be able to change the stem cell 1 population to stem cell 2; it was proposed by Russo and Russo [155] that Lob 1 found in the breast of nulliparous women and parous women with breast cancer never went through the process of differentiation, retaining stem cells 1 that are targets for carcinogens and therefore susceptible to undergo neoplastic transformation. Mutagenic insults or protective factors specifically operating before or during puberty are likely to have profound consequences for breast cancer later in life [177–181]. Different studies have suggested that at puberty during the mammary gland development associated with stem cell 1 expansion, the gland is more sensitive to cancer causing agents. As stem cells 1 are targets of tumorigenesis, reducing this population through a direct effect of hCG treatment would be beneficial.

In conclusion, the rhCG was able to abrogate the transforming abilities of E_2 and it was shown to have a differentiating property on the human breast epithelial cells MCF-10F by increasing the branching, a phenotype indicative of cell differentiation. Our results suggested that rhCG has significant potential as chemopreventive agent, protecting the normal cells from becoming malignant.

References

1. Soule HD, Maloney TM, Wolman SR, Peterson WD Jr, Brenz R, McGrath CM, Russo J, Pauley RJ, Jones RF, Brooks SC (1990) Isolation and characterization of a spontaneously immortalized human breast epithelial cell line, MCF-10. Cancer Res 50:6075–6086
2. Tait L, Soule HD, Russo J (1990) Ultrastructural and immunocytochemical characterization of an immortalized human breast epithelial cell line, MCF-10. Cancer Res 50:6087–6094
3. Calaf G, Russo J (1993) Transformation of human breast epithelial cells by chemical carcinogens. Carcinogenesis 14:483–492
4. Russo J, Fernandez SV, Russo PA, Fernbaugh R, Sheriff FS, Lareef HM, Garber J, Russo IH (2006) 17-Beta-estradiol induces transformation and tumorigenesis in human breast epithelial cells. FASEB J 20:1622–1634

5. Huang Y, Fernandez SV, Goodwin S, Russo PA, Russo IH, Sutter TR, Russo J (2007) Epithelial to mesenchymal transition in human breast epithelial cells transformed by 17beta-estradiol. Cancer Res 67:11147–11157
6. Russo J, Bradley RH, McGrath C, Russo IH (1977) Scanning and transmission electron microscopy study of a human breast carcinoma cell line (MCF-7) cultured in collagen-coated cellulose sponge. Cancer Res 37:2004–2014
7. Yang J, Guzman R, Richards J, Jentoft V, DeVault MR, Wellings SR, Nandi S (1980) Primary culture of human mammary epithelial cells embedded in collagen gels. J Natl Cancer Inst 65:337–343
8. Debnath J, Muthuswamy SK, Brugge JS (2003) Morphogenesis and oncogenesis of MCF-10A mammary epithelial acini grown in three-dimensional basement membrane cultures. Methods 30:256–268
9. O'Brien LE, Zegers MM, Mostov KE (2002) Opinion: building epithelial architecture: insights from three-dimensional culture models. Nat Rev Mol Cell Biol 3:531–537
10. Shaw KR, Wrobel CN, Brugge JS (2004) Use of three-dimensional basement membrane cultures to model oncogene-induced changes in mammary epithelial morphogenesis. J Mammary Gland Biol Neoplasia 9:297–310
11. Bissell MJ, Radisky D (2001) Putting tumours in context. Nat Rev Cancer 1:46–54
12. Fata JE, Werb Z, Bissell MJ (2004) Regulation of mammary gland branching morphogenesis by the extracellular matrix and its remodeling enzymes. Breast Cancer Res 6:1–11
13. Kleinman HK, Martin GR (2005) Matrigel: basement membrane matrix with biological activity. Semin Cancer Biol 15:378–386
14. Russo J, Gusterson BA, Rogers AE, Russo IH, Wellings SR, van Zwieten MJ (1990) Comparative study of human and rat mammary tumorigenesis. Lab Invest 62:244–278
15. Fernandez SV, Russo IH, Russo J (2006) Estradiol and its metabolites 4-hydroxyestradiol and 2-hydroxyestradiol induce mutations in human breast epithelial cells. Int J Cancer 118:1862–1868
16. Sorlie T, Tibshirani R, Parker J, Hastie T, Marron JS, Nobel A, Deng S, Johnsen H, Pesich R, Geisler S, Demeter J, Perou CM, Lonning PE, Brown PO, Borresen-Dale AL, Botstein D (2003) Repeated observation of breast tumor subtypes in independent gene expression data sets. Proc Natl Acad Sci U S A 100:8418–8423
17. Yang M, Kim SY, Lee SM, Chang SS, Kawamoto T, Jang JY, Ahn YO (2003) Biological monitoring of bisphenol A in a Korean population. Arch Environ Contam Toxicol 44:546–551
18. Perou CM, Sorlie T, Eisen MB, van de Rijn M, Jeffrey SS, Rees CA, Pollack JR, Ross DT, Johnsen H, Akslen LA, Fluge O, Pergamenschikov A, Williams C, Zhu SX, Lonning PE, Borresen-Dale AL, Brown PO, Botstein D (2000) Molecular portraits of human breast tumours. Nature 406:747–752
19. Charafe-Jauffret E, Ginestier C, Monville F, Finetti P, Adelaide J, Cervera N, Fekairi S, Xerri L, Jacquemier J, Birnbaum D, Bertucci F (2006) Gene expression profiling of breast cell lines identifies potential new basal markers. Oncogene 25:2273–2284
20. Neve RM, Chin K, Fridlyand J, Yeh J, Baehner FL, Fevr T, Clark L, Bayani N, Coppe JP, Tong F, Speed T, Spellman PT, DeVries S, Lapuk A, Wang NJ, Kuo WL, Stilwell JL, Pinkel D, Albertson DG, Waldman FM, McCormick F, Dickson RB, Johnson MD, Lippman M, Ethier S, Gazdar A, Gray JW (2006) A collection of breast cancer cell lines for the study of functionally distinct cancer subtypes. Cancer Cell 10:515–527
21. Al-Hajj M, Wicha MS, Benito-Hernandez A, Morrison SJ, Clarke MF (2003) Prospective identification of tumorigenic breast cancer cells. Proc Natl Acad Sci U S A 100:3983–3988
22. Russo J, Russo IH (1987) Development of human mammary gland. In: Neville MC, Daniel CW (eds) The mammary gland development, regulation, and function. Plenum, New York, pp 67–93
23. Russo J, Rivera R, Russo IH (1992) Influence of age and parity on the development of the human breast. Breast Cancer Res Treat 23:211–218

24. Russo J, Romero AL, Russo IH (1994) Architectural pattern of the normal and cancerous breast under the influence of parity. Cancer Epidemiol Biomarkers Prev 3:219–224
25. Russo J, Lareef MH, Tahin Q, Hu YF, Slater C, Ao X, Russo IH (2002) 17-Beta-estradiol is carcinogenic in human breast epithelial cells. J Steroid Biochem Mol Biol 80:149–16226
26. Baker NE (2000) Notch signaling in the nervous system. Pieces still missing from the puzzle. Bioessays 22:264–273
27. Beatus P, Lundkvist J, Oberg C, Lendahl U (1999) The notch 3 intracellular domain represses notch 1-mediated activation through Hairy/Enhancer of split (HES) promoters. Development 126:3925–3935
28. Furukawa T, Mukherjee S, Bao ZZ, Morrow EM, Cepko C (2000) rax, Hes1, and notch1 promote the formation of Muller glia by postnatal retinal progenitor cells. Neuron 26:383–394
29. Morrison SJ, Perez SE, Qiao Z, Verdi JM, Hicks C, Weinmaster G, Anderson DJ (2000) Transient Notch activation initiates an irreversible switch from neurogenesis to gliogenesis by neural crest stem cells. Cell 101:499–510
30. Allman D, Aster JC, Pear WS (2002) Notch signaling in hematopoiesis and early lymphocyte development. Immunol Rev 187:75–86
31. Radtke F, Wilson A, Ernst B, MacDonald HR (2002) The role of Notch signaling during hematopoietic lineage commitment. Immunol Rev 187:65–74
32. Cayouette M, Raff M (2002) Asymmetric segregation of Numb: a mechanism for neural specification from Drosophila to mammals. Nat Neurosci 5:1265–1269
33. Shen Q, Temple S (2002) Creating asymmetric cell divisions by skewing endocytosis. Sci STKE 2002:pe52
34. O'Connor-Giles KM, Skeath JB (2003) Numb inhibits membrane localization of Sanpodo, a four-pass transmembrane protein, to promote asymmetric divisions in Drosophila. Dev Cell 5:231–243
35. Eldin P, Papon L, Oteiza A, Brocchi E, Lawson TG, Mechti N (2009) TRIM22 E3 ubiquitin ligase activity is required to mediate antiviral activity against encephalomyocarditis virus. J Gen Virol 90:536–545
36. Herr AM, Dressel R, Walter L (2009) Different subcellular localisations of TRIM22 suggest species-specific function. Immunogenetics 61:271–280
37. Duan Z, Gao B, Xu W, Xiong S (2008) Identification of TRIM22 as a RING finger E3 ubiquitin ligase. Biochem Biophys Res Commun 374:502–506
38. Obad S, Olofsson T, Mechti N, Gullberg U, Drott K (2007) Expression of the IFN-inducible p53-target gene TRIM22 is downregulated during erythroid differentiation of human bone marrow. Leuk Res 31:995–1001
39. Obad S, Brunnstrom H, Vallon-Christersson J, Borg A, Drott K, Gullberg U (2004) Staf50 is a novel p53 target gene conferring reduced clonogenic growth of leukemic U-937 cells. Oncogene 23:4050–4059
40. Gongora C, Tissot C, Cerdan C, Mechti N (2000) The interferon-inducible Staf50 gene is downregulated during T cell costimulation by CD2 and CD28. J Interferon Cytokine Res 20:955–961
41. Taggart CC, Greene CM, McElvaney NG, O'Neill S (2002) Secretory leucoprotease inhibitor prevents lipopolysaccharide-induced IkappaBalpha degradation without affecting phosphorylation or ubiquitination. J Biol Chem 277:33648–33653
42. Viatour P, Dejardin E, Warnier M, Lair F, Claudio E, Bureau F, Marine JC, Merville MP, Maurer U, Green D, Piette J, Siebenlist U, Bours V, Chariot A (2004) GSK3-mediated BCL-3 phosphorylation modulates its degradation and its oncogenicity. Mol Cell 16:35–45
43. Urso ML, Chen YW, Scrimgeour AG, Lee PC, Lee KF, Clarkson PM (2007) Alterations in mRNA expression and protein products following spinal cord injury in humans. J Physiol 579(pt 3):877–892
44. Nijman SM, Huang TT, Dirac AM, Brummelkamp TR, Kerkhoven RM, D'Andrea AD, Bernards R (2005) The deubiquitinating enzyme USP1 regulates the Fanconi anemia pathway. Mol Cell 17:331–339

45. Banerjee S, Brooks WS, Crawford DF (2007) Inactivation of the ubiquitin conjugating enzyme UBE2Q2 causes a prophase arrest and enhanced apoptosis in response to microtubule inhibiting agents. Oncogene 26:6509–6517
46. Melner MH, Haas AL, Klein JM, Brash AR, Boeglin WE, Nagdas SK, Winfrey VP, Olson GE (2006) Demonstration of ubiquitin thiolester formation of UBE2Q2 (UBCi), a novel ubiquitin-conjugating enzyme with implantation site-specific expression. Biol Reprod 75:395–406
47. Winteringham LN, Endersby R, Kobelke S, McCulloch RK, Williams JH, Stillitano J, Cornwall SM, Ingley E, Klinken SP (2006) Myeloid leukemia factor 1 associates with a novel heterogeneous nuclear ribonucleoprotein U-like molecule. J Biol Chem 281:38791–38800
48. Yoneda-Kato N, Kato JY (2008) Shuttling imbalance of MLF1 results in p53 instability and increases susceptibility to oncogenic transformation. Mol Cell Biol 28:422–434
49. Yoneda-Kato N, Tomoda K, Umehara M, Arata Y, Kato JY (2005) Myeloid leukemia factor 1 regulates p53 by suppressing COP1 via COP9 signalosome subunit 3. EMBO J 24:1739–1749
50. Suzuki H, Arakawa Y, Ito M, Saito S, Takeda N, Yamada H, Horiguchi-Yamada J (2007) MLF1-interacting protein is mainly localized in nucleolus through N-terminal bipartite nuclear localization signal. Anticancer Res 27:1423–1430
51. Bonzo JR, Norris AA, Esham M, Moncman CL (2008) The nebulette repeat domain is necessary for proper maintenance of tropomyosin with the cardiac sarcomere. Exp Cell Res 314:3519–3530
52. Deng XA, Norris A, Panaviene Z, Moncman CL (2008) Ectopic expression of LIM-nebulette (LASP2) reveals roles in cell migration and spreading. Cell Motil Cytoskeleton 65:827–840
53. Holmes WB, Moncman CL (2008) Nebulette interacts with filamin C. Cell Motil Cytoskeleton 65:130–142
54. Panaviene Z, Moncman CL (2007) Linker region of nebulin family members plays an important role in targeting these molecules to cellular structures. Cell Tissue Res 327:353–369
55. Scott GK, Gu F, Crump CM, Thomas L, Wan L, Xiang Y, Thomas G (2003) The phosphorylation state of an autoregulatory domain controls PACS-1-directed protein traffic. EMBO J 22:6234–6244
56. Crump CM, Hung CH, Thomas L, Wan L, Thomas G (2003) Role of PACS-1 in trafficking of human cytomegalovirus glycoprotein B and virus production. J Virol 77:11105–11113
57. Wan L, Molloy SS, Thomas L, Liu G, Xiang Y, Rybak SL, Thomas G (1998) PACS-1 defines a novel gene family of cytosolic sorting proteins required for trans-Golgi network localization. Cell 94:205–216
58. Zingg JM, Kempna P, Paris M, Reiter E, Villacorta L, Cipollone R, Munteanu A, De Pascale C, Menini S, Cueff A, Arock M, Azzi A, Ricciarelli R (2008) Characterization of three human sec14p-like proteins: alpha-tocopherol transport activity and expression pattern in tissues. Biochimie 90:1703–1715
59. Seipel K, O'Brien SP, Iannotti E, Medley QG, Streuli M (2001) Tara, a novel F-actin binding protein, associates with the Trio guanine nucleotide exchange factor and regulates actin cytoskeletal organization. J Cell Sci 114(pt 2):389–399
60. Yu J, Lan J, Zhu Y, Li X, Lai X, Xue Y, Jin C, Huang H (2008) The E3 ubiquitin ligase HECTD3 regulates ubiquitination and degradation of Tara. Biochem Biophys Res Commun 367:805–812
61. Hamada T, Murasawa S, Yokoyama A, Hayashi S, Kobayashi Y, Asahara T (2009) Changing modified regions in the genome in hematopoietic stem cell differentiation. Biochem Biophys Res Commun 381:135–138
62. Biermann K, Heukamp LC, Nettersheim D, Steger K, Zhou H, Franke FE, Guetgemann I, Sonnack V, Brehm R, Berg J, Bastian PJ, Muller SC, Wang-Eckert L, Schorle H, Buttner R (2007) Embryonal germ cells and germ cell tumors. Verh Dtsch Ges Pathol 91:39–48
63. Biermann K, Heukamp LC, Steger K, Zhou H, Franke FE, Guetgemann I, Sonnack V, Brehm R, Berg J, Bastian PJ, Muller SC, Wang-Eckert L, Schorle H, Buttner R (2007) Gene expression profiling identifies new biological markers of neoplastic germ cells. Anticancer Res 27:3091–3100

64. Wang IC, Chen YJ, Hughes D, Petrovic V, Major ML, Park HJ, Tan Y, Ackerson T, Costa RH (2005) Forkhead box M1 regulates the transcriptional network of genes essential for mitotic progression and genes encoding the SCF (Skp2-Cks1) ubiquitin ligase. Mol Cell Biol 25:10875–10894
65. Saxena A, Wong LH, Kalitsis P, Earle E, Shaffer LG, Choo KH (2002) Poly(ADP-ribose) polymerase 2 localizes to mammalian active centromeres and interacts with PARP-1, Cenpa, Cenpb and Bub3, but not Cenpc. Hum Mol Genet 11:2319–2329
66. Ueki T, Nishidate T, Park JH, Lin ML, Shimo A, Hirata K, Nakamura Y, Katagiri T (2008) Involvement of elevated expression of multiple cell-cycle regulator, DTL/RAMP (denticleless/RA-regulated nuclear matrix associated protein), in the growth of breast cancer cells. Oncogene 27:5672–5683
67. Bakhoum SF, Thompson SL, Manning AL, Compton DA (2009) Genome stability is ensured by temporal control of kinetochore-microtubule dynamics. Nat Cell Biol 11:27–35
68. Macarulla T, Ramos FJ, Tabernero J (2008) Aurora kinase family: a new target for anticancer drug. Recent Pat Anticancer Drug Discov 3:114–122
69. Takaki T, Trenz K, Costanzo V, Petronczki M (2008) Polo-like kinase 1 reaches beyond mitosis—cytokinesis, DNA damage response, and development. Curr Opin Cell Biol 20:650–660
70. Wianny F, Tavares A, Evans MJ, Glover DM, Zernicka-Goetz M (1998) Mouse polo-like kinase 1 associates with the acentriolar spindle poles, meiotic chromosomes and spindle midzone during oocyte maturation. Chromosoma 107:430–439
71. Hosono K, Sasaki T, Minoshima S, Shimizu N (2004) Identification and characterization of a novel gene family YPEL in a wide spectrum of eukaryotic species. Gene 340:31–43
72. Meng X, Wilkins JA (2005) Compositional characterization of the cytoskeleton of NK-like cells. J Proteome Res 4:2081–2087
73. Chircop M, Oakes V, Graham ME, Ma MP, Smith CM, Robinson PJ, Khanna KK (2009) The actin-binding and bundling protein, EPLIN, is required for cytokinesis. Cell Cycle 8:757–764
74. Jiang WG, Martin TA, Lewis-Russell JM, Douglas-Jones A, Ye L, Mansel RE (2008) Eplin-alpha expression in human breast cancer, the impact on cellular migration and clinical outcome. Mol Cancer 7:71
75. Abe K, Takeichi M (2008) EPLIN mediates linkage of the cadherin catenin complex to F-actin and stabilizes the circumferential actin belt. Proc Natl Acad Sci U S A 105:13–19
76. Han MY, Kosako H, Watanabe T, Hattori S (2007) Extracellular signal-regulated kinase/mitogen-activated protein kinase regulates actin organization and cell motility by phosphorylating the actin cross-linking protein EPLIN. Mol Cell Biol 27:8190–8204
77. Maul RS, Song Y, Amann KJ, Gerbin SC, Pollard TD, Chang DD (2003) EPLIN regulates actin dynamics by cross-linking and stabilizing filaments. J Cell Biol 160:399–407
78. Song Y, Maul RS, Gerbin CS, Chang DD (2002) Inhibition of anchorage-independent growth of transformed NIH3T3 cells by epithelial protein lost in neoplasm (EPLIN) requires localization of EPLIN to actin cytoskeleton. Mol Biol Cell 13:1408–1416
79. Etienne-Manneville S (2004) Cdc42—the centre of polarity. J Cell Sci 117:1291–1300
80. Welchman DP, Mathies LD, Ahringer J (2007) Similar requirements for CDC-42 and the PAR-3/PAR-6/PKC-3 complex in diverse cell types. Dev Biol 305:347–357
81. Kroschewski R, Hall A, Mellman I (1999) Cdc42 controls secretory and endocytic transport to the basolateral plasma membrane of MDCK cells. Nat Cell Biol 1:8–13
82. Rojas R, Ruiz WG, Leung SM, Jou TS, Apodaca G (2001) Cdc42-dependent modulation of tight junctions and membrane protein traffic in polarized Madin-Darby canine kidney cells. Mol Biol Cell 12:2257–2274
83. Wells CD, Fawcett JP, Traweger A, Yamanaka Y, Goudreault M, Elder K, Kulkarni S, Gish G, Virag C, Lim C, Colwill K, Starostine A, Metalnikov P, Pawson T (2006) A Rich1/Amot complex regulates the Cdc42 GTPase and apical-polarity proteins in epithelial cells. Cell 125:535–548
84. Vega-Salas DE, Salas PJ, Rodriguez-Boulan E (1987) Modulation of the expression of an apical plasma membrane protein of Madin-Darby canine kidney epithelial cells: cell-cell

interactions control the appearance of a novel intracellular storage compartment. J Cell Biol 104:1249–1259
85. Martin-Belmonte F, Gassama A, Datta A, Yu W, Rescher U, Gerke V, Mostov K (2007) PTEN-mediated apical segregation of phosphoinositides controls epithelial morphogenesis through Cdc42. Cell 128:383–397
86. Lin H (2002) The stem-cell niche theory: lessons from flies. Nat Rev Genet 3:931–940
87. Fuchs E, Tumbar T, Guasch G (2004) Socializing with the neighbors: stem cells and their niche. Cell 116:769–778
88. Song X, Xie T (2002) DE-cadherin-mediated cell adhesion is essential for maintaining somatic stem cells in the Drosophila ovary. Proc Natl Acad Sci U S A 99:14813–14818
89. Zhu CH, Xie T (2003) Clonal expansion of ovarian germline stem cells during niche formation in Drosophila. Development 130:2579–2588
90. Calvi LM, Adams GB, Weibrecht KW, Weber JM, Olson DP, Knight MC, Martin RP, Schipani E, Divieti P, Bringhurst FR, Milner LA, Kronenberg HM, Scadden DT (2003) Osteoblastic cells regulate the haematopoietic stem cell niche. Nature 425:841–846
91. Zhang J, Niu C, Ye L, Huang H, He X, Tong WG, Ross J, Haug J, Johnson T, Feng JQ, Harris S, Wiedemann LM, Mishina Y, Li L (2003) Identification of the haematopoietic stem cell niche and control of the niche size. Nature 425:836–841
92. See J, Mamontov P, Ahn K, Wine-Lee L, Crenshaw EB III, Grinspan JB (2007) BMP signaling mutant mice exhibit glial cell maturation defects. Mol Cell Neurosci 35:171–182
93. Liang Z, Zeng X, Gao J, Wu S, Wang P, Shi X, Zhang J, Liu T (2008) Analysis of EGFR, HER2, and TOP2A gene status and chromosomal polysomy in gastric adenocarcinoma from Chinese patients. BMC Cancer 8:363
94. Pode-Shakked N, Metsuyanim S, Rom-Gross E, Mor Y, Fridman E, Goldstein I, Amariglio N, Rechavi G, Keshet G, Dekel B (2009) Developmental tumorigenesis: NCAM as a putative marker for the malignant renal stem/progenitor cell population. J Cell Mol Med 13:1792–1808
95. Shen J, Liu J, Long Y, Miao Y, Su M, Zhang Q, Han H, Hao X (2009) Knockdown of survivin expression by siRNAs enhances chemosensitivity of prostate cancer cells and attenuates its tumorigenicity. Acta Biochim Biophys Sin 41:223–230
96. Nikitakis NG, Scheper MA, Papanikolaou VS, Sklavounou A, Sauk JJ (2009) Immunohistochemical expression of the oncogenic molecules active Stat3 and survivin in benign and malignant salivary gland tumors. Oral Surg Oral Med Oral Pathol Oral Radiol Endod 107:837–843
97. Blum B, Bar-Nur O, Golan-Lev T, Benvenisty N (2009) The anti-apoptotic gene survivin contributes to teratoma formation by human embryonic stem cells. Nat Biotechnol 27:281–287
98. Adler M, Muller K, Rached E, Dekant W, Mally A (2009) Modulation of key regulators of mitosis linked to chromosomal instability is an early event in ochratoxin A carcinogenicity. Carcinogenesis 30:711–719
99. Han HJ, Russo J, Kohwi Y, Kohwi-Shigematsu T (2008) SATB1 reprogrammes gene expression to promote breast tumour growth and metastasis. Nature 452:187–193
100. Moustakas A, Heldin C-H (2007) Signaling networks guiding epithelial-mesenchymal transitions during embryogenesis and cancer progression. Cancer Sci 98:1512–1520
101. Peinado H, Olmeda D, Cano A (2007) Snail, ZEB and bHLH factors in tumor progression: an alliance against the epithelial phenotype? Nat Rev 7:415–428
102. Klopocki E, Kristiansen G, Wild PJ, Klaman I, Castanos-Velez E, Singer G, Stohr R, Sauter G, Leibiger H, Essers L, Weber B, Hermann K, Rosenthal A, Hartmann A, Dahl E (2004) Loss of SFRP1 is associated with breast cancer progression and poor prognosis in early stage tumors. Int J Oncol 25:641–649
103. Henshall SM, Horvath LG, Quinn DI, Eggleton SA, Grygiel JJ, Stricker PD, Biankin AV, Kench JG, Sutherland RL (2006) Zinc-alpha2-glycoprotein expression as a predictor of metastatic prostate cancer following radical prostatectomy. J Natl Cancer Inst 98:1420–1424

104. Lapointe J, Li C, Higgins JP, van de Rijn M, Bair E, Montgomery K, Ferrari M, Egevad L, Rayford W, Bergerheim U, Ekman P, DeMarzo AM, Tibshirani R, Botstein D, Brown PO, Brooks JD, Pollack JR (2004) Gene expression profiling identifies clinically relevant subtypes of prostate cancer. Proc Natl Acad Sci U S A 101:811–816
105. Park D, Kåresen R, Axcrona U, Noren T, Sauer T (2007) Expression pattern of adhesion molecules (E-cadherin, alpha-, beta-, gamma-catenin and claudin-7), their influence on survival in primary breast carcinoma, and their corresponding axillary lymph node metastasis. APMIS 115:52–65
106. Sauer T, Pedersen MK, Ebeltoft K, Naess O (2005) Reduced expression of Claudin-7 in fine needle aspirates from breast carcinomas correlate with grading and metastatic disease. Cytopathology 16:193–198
107. Usami Y, Chiba H, Nakayama F, Ueda J, Matsuda Y, Sawada N, Komori T, Ito A, Yokozaki H (2006) Reduced expression of claudin-7 correlates with invasion and metastasis in squamous cell carcinoma of the esophagus. Hum Pathol 37:569–577
108. Usami Y, Satake S, Nakayama F, Matsumoto M, Ohnuma K, Komori T, Semba S, Ito A, Yokozaki H (2008) Snail-associated epithelial-mesenchymal transition promotes oesophageal squamous cell carcinoma motility and progression. J Pathol 215:330–339
109. Gosens I, Sessa A, den Hollander AI, Letteboer SJ, Belloni V, Arends ML, Le Bivic A, Cremers FP, Broccoli V, Roepman R (2007) FERM protein EPB4iL5 is a novel member of the mammalian CRB-MPP5 polarity complex. Exp Cell Res 313:3959–3970
110. Xu L, Begum S, Hearn JD, Hynes RO (2006) GPR56, an atypical G protein-coupled receptor, binds tissue transglutaminase, TG2, and inhibits melanoma tumor growth and metastasis. Proc Natl Acad Sci U S A 103:9023–9028
111. Xu L, Hynes RO (2007) GRP56 and TG2: possible roles in suppression of tumor growth by the microenvironment. Cell Cycle 6:160–165
112. Kwak MK, Lee HJ, Hur K, Park do J, Lee HS, Kim WH, Lee KU, Choe KJ, Guilford P, Yang HK (2008) Expression of Krüppel-like factor 5 in human gastric carcinomas. J Cancer Res Clin Oncol 134:163–167
113. Haase D, Meister M, Muley T, Hess J, Teurich S, Schnabel P, Hartenstein B, Angel P (2007) FMRD3, a novel putative tumour suppressor in NSCLC. Oncogene 26:4464–4468
114. Kairouz R, Parmar J, Lyons RJ, Swarbrick A, Musgrove EA, Daly RJ (2005) Hormonal regulation of the Grb14 signal modulator and its role in cell cycle progression of MCF-7 human breast cancer cells. J Cell Physiol 203:85–93
115. Lyons RJ, Deane R, Lynch DK, Ye ZS, Sanderson GM, Eyre HJ, Sutherland GR, Daly RJ (2001) Identification of a novel human tankyrase through its interaction with the adaptor protein Grb14. J Biol Chem 276:17172–171780
116. Rodrigues-Ferreira S, Di Tommaso A, Dimitrov A, Cazaubon S, Gruel N, Colasson H, Nicolas A, Chaverot N, Molinié V, Reyal F, Sigal-Zafrani B, Terris B, Delattre O, Radvanyi F, Perez F, Vincent-Salomon A, Nahmias C (2009) 8p22 MTUS1 gene product ATIP3 is a novel anti-mitotic protein underexpressed in invasive breast carcinoma of poor prognosis. PLoS One 4:e7239
117. Frank B, Bermejo JL, Hemminki K, Sutter C, Wappenschmidt B, Meindl A, Kiechle-Bahat M, Bugert P, Schmutzler RK, Bartram CR, Burwinkel B (2007) Copy number variant in the candidate tumor suppressor gene MTUS1 and familial breast cancer risk. Carcinogenesis 28:1442–1445
118. Di Benedetto M, Bièche I, Deshayes F, Vacher S, Nouet S, Collura V, Seitz I, Louis S, Pineau P, Amsellem-Ouazana D, Couraud PO, Strosberg AD, Stoppa-Lyonnet D, Lidereau R, Nahmias C (2006) Structural organization and expression of human MTUS1, a candidate 8p22 tumor suppressor gene encoding a family of angiotensin II AT2 receptor-interacting proteins, ATIP. Gene 380:127–136
119. Zuern C, Heimrich J, Kaufmann R, Richter KK, Settmacher U, Wanner C, Galle J, Seibold S (2010) Down-regulation of MTUS1 in human colon tumors. Oncol Rep 23:183–189
120. Huang D, Yu B, Deng Y, Sheng W, Peng Z, Qin W, Du X (2010) SFRP4 was overexpressed in colorectal carcinoma. J Cancer Res Clin Oncol 136:395–401

121. Saini S, Liu J, Yamamura S, Majid S, Kawakami K, Hirata H, Dahiya R (2009) Functional significance of secreted Frizzled-related protein 1 in metastatic renal cell carcinomas. Cancer Res 69:6815–6822
122. Hu J, Dong A, Fernandez-Ruiz V, Shan J, Kawa M, Martínez-Ansó E, Prieto J, Qian C (2009) Blockade of Wnt signaling inhibits angiogenesis and tumor growth in hepatocellular carcinoma. Cancer Res 69:6951–6959
123. Lin YW, Chung MT, Lai HC, De Yan M, Shih YL, Chang CC, Yu MH (2009) Methylation analysis of SFRP genes family in cervical adenocarcinoma. J Cancer Res Clin Oncol 135:1665–1674
124. Gauger KJ, Hugh JM, Troester MA, Schneider SS (2009) Down-regulation of sfrp1 in a mammary epithelial cell line promotes the development of a cd44high/cd24low population which is invasive and resistant to anoikis. Cancer Cell Int 9:11
125. Cheng H, Liu P, Wang ZC, Zou L, Santiago S, Garbitt V, Gjoerup OV, Iglehart JD, Miron A, Richardson AL, Hahn WC, Zhao JJ (2009) SIK1 couples LKB1 to p53-dependent anoikis and suppresses metastasis. Sci Signal 2:ra35
126. Takemori H, Katoh Hashimoto Y, Nakae J, Olson EN, Okamoto M (2009) Inactivation of HDAC5 by SIK1 in AICAR-treated C2C12 myoblasts. Endocr J 56:121–130
127. Kowanetz M, Lönn P, Vanlandewijck M, Kowanetz K, Heldin CH, Moustakas A (2008) TGFbeta induces SIK to negatively regulate type I receptor kinase signaling. J Cell Biol 182:655–662
128. Ding L, Niu C, Zheng Y, Xiong Z, Liu Y, Lin J, Sun H, Huang K, Yang W, Li X, Ye Q (2009) FHL1 interacts with estrogen receptors and regulates breast cancer cell growth. J Cell Mol Med 15:72–85
129. Lin J, Ding L, Jin R, Zhang H, Cheng L, Qin X, Chai J, Ye Q (2009) Four and a half LIM domains 1 and receptor interacting protein of 140kDa (RIP140) interact and cooperate in estrogen signaling. Int J Biochem Cell Biol 41:1613–1618
130. Engin F, Bertin T, Ma O, Jiang MM, Wang L, Sutton RE, Donehower LA, Lee B (2009) Notch signaling contributes to the pathogenesis of human osteosarcomas. Hum Mol Genet 18:1464–1470
131. Miyazono K (2009) Transforming growth factor-beta signaling in epithelial-mesenchymal transition and progression of cancer. Proc Jpn Acad Ser B Phys Biol Sci 85:314–323
132. Pennanen PT, Sarvilinna NS, Ylikomi TJ (2009) Gene expression changes during the development of estrogen-independent and antiestrogen-resistant growth in breast cancer cell culture models. Anticancer Drugs 20:51–58
133. Matsuo K, Owens JM, Tonko M, Elliott C, Chambers TJ, Wagner EF (2000) Fosl1 is a transcriptional target of c-Fos during osteoclast differentiation. Nat Genet 24:184–187
134. Young MR, Colburn NH (2006) Fra-1 a target for cancer prevention or intervention. Gene 379:1–11
135. Wang HY, Zhang JY, Cui JT, Tan XH, Li WM, Gu J, Lu YY (2010) Expression status of S100A14 and S100A4 correlates with metastatic potential and clinical outcome in colorectal cancer after surgery. Oncol Rep 23:45–52
136. Hua J, Chen D, Fu H, Zhang R, Shen W, Liu S, Sun K, Sun X (2010) Short hairpin RNA-mediated inhibition of S100A4 promotes apoptosis and suppresses proliferation of BGC823 gastric cancer cells in vitro and in vivo. Cancer Lett 292:41–47
137. Boye K, Maelandsmo GM (2010) S100A4 and metastasis: a small actor playing many roles. Am J Pathol 176:528–535
138. Ismail TM, Zhang S, Fernig DG, Gross S, Martin-Fernandez ML, See V, Tozawa K, Tynan CJ, Wang G, Wilkinson MC, Rudland PS, Barraclough R (2010) Self-association of calcium-binding protein S100A4 and metastasis. J Biol Chem 285:914–922
139. Dorgan JF, Longcope C, Stephenson HE Jr, Falk RT, Miller R, Franz C, Kahle L, Campbell WS, Tangrea JA, Schatzkin A (1996) Relation of prediagnostic serum estrogen and androgen levels to breast cancer risk. Cancer Epidemiol Biomarkers Prev 5:533–539
140. Toniolo PG, Levitz M, Zeleniuch-Jacquotte A, Banerjee S, Koenig KL, Shore RE, Strax P, Pasternack BS (1995) A prospective study of endogenous estrogens and breast cancer in postmenopausal women. J Natl Cancer Inst 87:190–197

141. Greenlee RT, Murray T, Bolden S, Wingo PA (2000) Cancer statistics. CA Cancer J Clin 50:7–33
142. Geisler J (2003) Breast cancer tissue estrogens and their manipulation with aromatase inhibitors and inactivators. J Steroid Biochem Mol Biol 86:245–253
143. Russo J, Lareef MH, Balogh GA, Guo S, Russo IH (2002) 17 Beta-estradiol is carcinogenic in human breast epithelial cells. J Steroid Biochem Mol Biol 80:149–162
144. Fernandez SV, Wu Y-Z, Russo IH, Plass C, Russo J (2006) The role of DNA methylation in estrogen-induced transformation of human breast epithelial cells. Proc Am Assoc Cancer Res 47:375
145. Lambe M, Hsieh CC, Chan HW, Ekbom A, Trichopoulos D, Adami HO (1996) Parity, age at first and last birth, and risk of breast cancer: a population-based study in Sweden. Breast Cancer Res Treat 38:305–311
146. Hinkula M, Pukkala E, Kyyronen P, Kauppila A (2001) Grand multiparity and the risk of breast cancer: population-based study in Finland. Cancer Causes Control 12:491–500
147. Key TJ, Verkasalo PK, Banks E (2001) Epidemiology of breast cancer. Lancet Oncol 2:133–140
148. Russo J, Russo IH (1994) Toward a physiological approach to breast cancer prevention. Cancer Epidemiol Biomarkers Prev 3:353–364
149. Balogh GA, Heulings R, Mailo DA, Russo PA, Sheriff F, Russo IH, Moral R, Russo J (2006) Genomic signature induced by pregnancy in the human breast. Int J Oncol 28:399–410
150. Russo J, Balogh GA, Chen J, Fernandez SV, Fernbaugh R, Heulings R, Mailo DA, Moral R, Russo PA, Sheriff F, Vanegas JE, Wang R, Russo IH (2006) The concept of stem cell in the mammary gland and its implication in morphogenesis, cancer and prevention. Front Biosci 11:151–172
151. Russo J, Balogh GA, Russo IH (2008) Full-term pregnancy induces a specific genomic signature in the human breast. Cancer Epidemiol Biomarkers Prev 17:51–66
152. Russo IH, Koszalka M, Russo J (1991) Comparative study of the influence of pregnancy and hormonal treatment on mammary carcinogenesis. Br J Cancer 64:481–484
153. Russo J, Moral R, Balogh GA, Mailo D, Russo IH (2005) The protective role of pregnancy in breast cancer. Breast Cancer Res 7:1–12
154. Russo IH, Koszalka M, Russo J (1990) Human chorionic gonadotropin and rat mammary cancer prevention. J Natl Cancer Inst 82:1286–1289
155. Russo J, Russo IH (1997) Role of differentiation in the pathogenesis and prevention of breast cancer. Endocr Relat Cancer 4:7–12
156. Russo J, Russo IH (1987) Biological and molecular bases of mammary carcinogenesis. Lab Invest 57:112–137
157. Russo IH, Russo J (2007) Primary prevention of breast cancer by hormone-induced differentiation. Recent Results Cancer Res 174:111–130
158. Hebner C, Weaver VM, Debnath J (2008) Modeling morphogenesis and oncogenesis in three-dimensional breast epithelial cultures. Annu Rev Pathol 3:313–339
159. O'Brien LE, Zegers MM, Moskow KE (2002) Opinion: building epithelial architecture: insights from three-dimensional culture models. Nat Rev Mol Cell Biol 3:531–537
160. Lu P, Sternlicht MD, Werb Z (2006) Comparative mechanisms of branching morphogenesis in diverse systems. J Mammary Gland Biol Neoplasia 11:213–228
161. Santos OFP, Nigan SK (1993) HGF-induced tubulogenesis and branching of epithelial cells is modulated by extracellular matrix and TGF-beta. Dev Biol 160:293–302
162. Karihaloo A, Nickel C, Cantley LG (2005) Signals which build a tubule. Nephron Exp Nephrol 100:e40–e45
163. Montesano R, Matsumoto K, Nakamura T, Orci L (1991) Identification of a fibroblast-derived epithelial morphogen as hepatocyte growth factor. Cell 67:901–908
164. Hogan BL, Kolodziej PA (2002) Organogenesis: molecular mechanisms of tubulogenesis. Nat Rev Genet 3:513–523
165. Popnikolov N, Yang J, Liu A, Guzman R, Nandi S (2001) Reconstituted normal human breast in nude mice: effect of host pregnancy environment and human chorionic gonadotropin on proliferation. J Endocrinol 168:487–496

166. Berdichevsky F, Alford D, D'Souza B, Taylor-Papadimitriou J (1994) Branching morphogenesis of human epithelial cells in collagen gels. J Cell Sci 107:3557–3568
167. Trusolino L, Comoglio PM (2002) Scatter-factor and semaphoring receptors. Nat Rev Cancer 2:289–300
168. Bellusci S, Grindley J, Emoto H, Itoh N, Hogan B (1997) Fibroblast growth factor 10 (FGF10) and branching morphogenesis in the embryonic mouse lung. Development 124:4867–4878
169. Offterdinger M, Schneider SM, Grunt TW (2003) Heregulin and retinoids synergistically induce branching morphogenesis of breast cancer cells cultivated in 3D collagen gels. J Cell Physiol 195:260–275
170. Guo S, Russo IH, Lareef MH, Russo J (2004) Effect of human chorionic gonadotropin in the gene expression profile of MCF-7 cells. Int J Oncol 24:399–407
171. Lojun S, Bao S, Lei ZM, Rao CV (1997) Presence of functional luteinizing hormone/chorionic gonadotropin (hCG) receptors in human breast cell lines: implications supporting the premise that hCG protects women against breast cancer. Biol Reprod 57:1202–1210
172. Meduri G, Charnaux N, Loosfelt H, Jolivet A, Spyratos F, Brailly S, Milgrom E (1997) Luteinizing hormone/human chorionic gonadotropin receptors in breast cancer. Cancer Res 57:857–864
173. Tao YX, Lei ZM, Rao CV (1997) The presence of luteinizing hormone/human chorionic gonadotropin receptors in lactating rat mammary glands. Life Sci 60:1297–1303
174. Gromoll J, Eiholzer U, Nieschlag E, Simoni M (2000) Male hypogonadism caused by homozygous deletion of exon 10 of the luteinizing hormone (LH) receptor: differential action of human chorionic gonadotropin and LH. J Clin Endocrinol Metab 85:2281–2286
175. Bernstein L, Hanisch R, Sullivan-Halley J, Ross RK (1995) Treatment with human chorionic gonadotropin and risk of breast cancer. Cancer Epidemiol Biomarkers Prev 4:437–440
176. Lukanova A, Andersson R, Wulff M, Zeleniuch-Jacquotte A, Grankvist K, Dossus L, Afanasyeva Y, Johansson R, Arslan AA, Lenner P, Wadell G, Hallmans G, Toniolo P, Lundin E (2008) Human chorionic gonadotropin and alpha-fetoprotein concentrations in pregnancy and maternal risk of breast cancer: a nested case-control study. Am J Epidemiol 168:1284–1291
177. Tokunaga M, Land CE, Tokuoka S, Nishimori I, Soda M, Akiba S (1994) Incidence of female breast cancer among atomic bomb survivors, 1950–1985. Radiat Res 138:209–223
178. Aisenberg AC, Finkelstein DM, Doppke KP, Koerner FC, Boivin JF, Willett CG (1997) High risk of breast carcinoma after irradiation of young women with Hodgkin's disease. Cancer 79:1203–1210
179. Wu AH, Wan P, Hankin J, Tseng CC, Yu MC, Pike MC (2002) Adolescent and adult soy intake and risk of breast cancer in Asian-Americans. Carcinogenesis 23:1491–1496
180. Land CE, Tokunaga M, Koyama K, Soda M, Preston DL, Nishimori I, Tokuoka S (2003) Incidence of female breast cancer among atomic bomb survivors, Hiroshima and Nagasaki, 1950–1990. Radiat Res 160:707–717
181. Horwich A, Swerdlow AJ (2004) Second primary breast cancer after Hodgkin's disease. Br J Cancer 90:294–298

Chapter 5
Methodological Approach for Studying the Human Breast

5.1 Introduction

This chapter has been designed in answer to the need of unifying methodological, analytical, and clinical procedures for studying the normal human breast [1–7]. We describe standard operating procedures, guidance on specimen collection and handling, data collection and analysis, and to serve as a unique source of reference for all the researchers using this source. The information contained in this work provides guidelines for the coordination of procedures that include breast core biopsies (CB), sample identification, preservation, and storage, laser capture microdissection (LCM), RNA extraction, and cDNA microarray [8–19].

5.2 Recruitment and Consent Process

The recruitment of women willing to donate normal breast tissue samples requires the full participation of institutions, hospitals, physicians, nurses, and the women donating their tissue [6]. In general the recruitment starts by selecting potentially eligible participants by mail. A letter giving a full description of the study, how it will be performed and what data and material will be collected should be first read and approved by the prospective donor. The study nurse completes an Eligible Participant Study Log containing the name of the potentially eligible participant, date letter sent, telephone contact (yes/no) for verification of participation, date called, willingness to participate (yes/no); if no, reason for decline, age, and parity status (Tables 5.1 and 5.2). For each subject who elects to participate in the study, the nurse fills out a questionnaire collecting information on reproductive, lifestyle, and medical history (including all current medications). The study nurse checks the eligibility criteria and if eligible the participant signs an informed consent [6]. The study nurse registers each participant and assigns a unique ID; she obtains anthropometrical measurements (height, weight, waist, and hip), a mammography exam and

J. Russo and I.H. Russo, *Role of the Transcriptome in Breast Cancer Prevention*, DOI 10.1007/978-1-4614-4884-6_5, © Springer Science+Business Media New York 2013

Table 5.1 Women's Gene Expression Study-eligibility questionnaire

Participant's Name ____

First MI Last

Date __ __ /__ __ /__ __
mon day year

What is your current home address?

____
Street Apt. #

____
City State Zip Code

What is your home telephone number? __ __ __ - __ __ __ - __ __ __ __

Do you mind giving us your work telephone number?

❑ __ __ __ - __ __ __ - __ __ __ __

❑ I do not work outside my home

❑ I prefer not to give you my work number

1. How old are you? _______ years (*If < 50 yrs. Not eligible*)
2. Did a doctor ever tell you that you have cancer?

❑ No

❑ Yes *(Not eligible, except non-melanoma skin cancer)*

❑ Unknown

If yes, what cancer did the doctor say you had?____________________

3. Did you ever have a hysterectomy (uterus or womb removed)?

❑ No

❑ Yes *(If currently < 60 years old not eligible unless blood is provided for FSH)*

❑ Unknown

4. Did you ever have surgery on your ovaries?

❑ No

❑ Yes

❑ Unknown

If yes, was one or both of your ovaries removed?

❑ No

❑ Yes, one ovary removed

❑ Yes, two ovaries removed *(Not eligible)*

If no, could you describe what the surgery was?

____

____

(continued)

Table 5.1 (continued)

5. Did you have a menstrual period during the last year?

   ❑ No
   ❑ Yes (*Not eligible*)

6. Are you currently using or have you in the past month used Tamoxifen or Evista?

   ❑ No
   ❑ Yes (*Not eligible*)

7. Has a doctor ever told you that you have Alzheimer's disease or severe memory loss?

   ❑ No
   ❑ Yes (Not eligible)

Table 5.2 Women's Gene Expression Study questionnaire

A. Instructions
Please clearly print your answers on the lines provided or put an **x** in the box next to the answer that best describes you.

Name ____

i. ***First, Middle, Last***

Today's Date ____________________

Thank you for your willingness to participate in this research study. Please answer the questions that follow to the best of your ability. Medical terms can be confusing, so if you do not understand a question please ask for clarification.

Section A – Personal History

1. When were you born? __________ _____ ____
   Month Day Year
2. Were you born in the United States?
   - ❑ No
   - ❑ Yes

   If no,

   a. Where were you born?

   ____

   b. How old were you when you come to live in the United States?

   ________ years old

3. What is your current marital status?
   - ❑ Never married
   - ❑ Married or living as married
   - ❑ Separated
   - ❑ Divorced
   - ❑ Widowed

4. What is the highest level of education you completed?
   - ❑ Less than 8 years
   - ❑ 8 - 11 years (without graduation)
   - ❑ High school graduate or G.E.D.
   - ❑ Vocational or technical school after high school
   - ❑ Some college or university
   - ❑ Bachelor's degree
   - ❑ Graduate degree

(continued)

Table 5.2 (continued)

5. Are you Hispanic or Latino?
   - ❑ No
   - ❑ Yes, Mexican, Mexican Am., Chicano
   - ❑ Yes, Puerto Rican
   - ❑ Yes, Cuban
   - ❑ Yes, Other Hispanic, Latino, Spanish

   If other, please specify ________________

6. What is your race? *(check one or more)*
   - ❑ White
   - ❑ Black, African American, or Negro
   - ❑ Asian
   - ❑ American Indian or Alaska Native
   - ❑ Native Hawaiian or Pacific Islander
   - ❑ Other______________________________ *(specify)*

7. What is your ancestry or ethnic origin?

____

For example: Italian, Jamaican, Dominican, Puerto Rican, Irish, French, Mexican, Korean, Thai, Chinese etc.

8. What is your religion?
   - ❑ Christian
   - ❑ Muslim
   - ❑ Jewish
   - ❑ None
   - ❑ Other ______________________________ *(specify)*

Section B - Medical and Reproductive History

9. What is your height?______________
10. What is your weight?_____________
11. Have you ever had a breast biopsy before now?
    - ❑ No
    - ❑ Yes, surgical biopsy
    - ❑ Yes, needle biopsy

If yes, what was the result?

____

(continued)

Table 5.2 (continued)

12. Were you ever treated by radiation that included the chest area (do not include diagnostic chest xrays)?
    - ❑ No
    - ❑ Yes
    - ❑ Unknown

If yes:

a. Why were you treated by radiation to the chest area?

____

b. How old were you when you were first treated by radiation to the chest area?

_______ **years old**

13. Have you ever been treated by radiation that included your lower abdomen or pelvis
    - ❑ No
    - ❑ Yes
    - ❑ Unknown

If yes:

a. Why were you treated by radiation to the lower abdomen or pelvis?

____

____

b. How old were you when you were first treated by radiation to the abdomen or pelvis?

_______ years old

14. How old were you when you had your first menstrual period?

_______ years old

15. During your twenties and thirties, were your periods regular? That is, when you were not pregnant or breastfeeding was the number of days between your periods usually about the same each month?
    - ❑ No
    - ❑ Yes

16. During your twenties and thirties, how many days were there usually between your periods, that is from the start of one period to the start of the next?

_________ days

(continued)

Table 5.2 (continued)

17. How many times have you been pregnant? *(Please include all pregnancies regardless of whether they ended by miscarriage, induced abortion, live birth, or stillbirth)*
_______ times

If 1 or more pregnancies, please provide information about each of your pregnancies

a. Pregnancy Number	How old were you?	How did this pregnancy end?	***If live birth,*** did you breastfeed?
1		❑ Live birth ❑ Stillbirth ❑ Miscarriage ❑ Induced abortion	❑ No ❑ Yes ________ (How long?)
2		❑ Live birth ❑ Stillbirth ❑ Miscarriage ❑ Induced abortion	❑ No ❑ Yes ________ (How long?)
3		❑ Live birth ❑ Stillbirth ❑ Miscarriage ❑ Induced abortion	❑ No ❑ Yes ________ (How long?)
4		❑ Live birth ❑ Stillbirth ❑ Miscarriage ❑ Induced abortion	❑ No ❑ Yes ________ (How long?)
5		❑ Live birth ❑ Stillbirth ❑ Miscarriage ❑ Induced abortion	❑ No ❑ Yes ________ (How long?)
6		❑ Live birth ❑ Stillbirth ❑ Miscarriage ❑ Induced abortion	❑ No ❑ Yes ________ (How long?)
7		❑ Live birth ❑ Stillbirth ❑ Miscarriage ❑ Induced abortion	❑ No ❑ Yes ________ (How long?)

If you need additional space, please use back of page.

(continued)

Table 5.2 (continued)

18. Have you <u>ever</u> used birth control pills or other hormonal contraceptives including implants and injections for birth control or other reasons?
    - ☐ No *(Go to #19)*
    - ☐ Yes

    If yes,

    a. Why did you use hormonal contraceptives?

	No	Yes	Unk
Birth control	☐	☐	☐
Regulate periods	☐	☐	☐
Treat acne	☐	☐	☐
Menopause	☐	☐	☐
Other	☐	☐	☐

If yes *to any of above,* please describe

____

b. How old were you when you first used hormonal contraceptives?
____ years

c. If you used hormonal contraceptives to treat menopausal symptoms, were you still having periods when you first began using hormonal contraceptives for those symptoms?
- ☐ No
- ☐ Yes

d. How long did you use hormonal contraceptives? (Please do not include occasional breaks in use. For example, if you stopped use for three months, don't include those three months.)
____years

e. Are you currently using hormonal contraceptives?
- ☐ No
- ☐ Yes

If yes, What are you taking? ______________________________

If no, When did you last use hormonal contraceptives?

____
- ☐ weeks ago
- ☐ months ago
- ☐ years ago

(continued)

Table 5.2 (continued)

19. Did you have a menstrual period during the past year?
   - ☐ No
   - ☐ Yes

   If no,

   a. When did you have your last period?
   ________ years ago ***or*** _______ years old

   b. Why did your periods stop?
   - ☐ Pregnancy
   - ☐ Natural menopause
   - ☐ Hysterectomy (uterus or womb removed)
   - ☐ Both ovaries removed
   - ☐ Radiation or chemotherapy
   - ☐ Depropovera or other medication
   - ☐ Other _________________ *(specify)*
   - ☐ Don't know

20. Have you <u>ever</u> taken tamoxifen?
   - ☐ No *(Go to #21)*
   - ☐ Yes

   If yes:

   a. How old were you when you first took tamoxifen? ____ years

   b. Were you still having periods when you first took tamoxifen?
   - ☐ No
   - ☐ Yes

   c. How long did you take tamoxifen? (Please do not include occasional breaks in use. For example, if you stopped use for three months, don't include those three months.)
   _____ years

   d. Are you currently using Tamoxifen?
   - ☐ No
   - ☐ Yes

   If no, When did you last use tamoxifen?

   _____ ☐ weeks ago ☐ months ago ☐ years ago

21. Have you <u>ever</u> taken raloxifene or Evista?
   - ☐ No *(Go to #22)*
   - ☐ Yes

   If yes:

   a. How old were you when you first took raloxifene or Evista?
   ______ years

   b. Were you still having periods when you first took raloxifene or Evista?
   - ☐ No
   - ☐ Yes

   c. How long did you take raloxifene or Evista? (Please do not include occasional breaks in use. For example, if you stopped use for three months, don't include those three months.)
   ______ years

(continued)

Table 5.2 (continued)

d. Are you currently using raloxifen or Evista?

- ❑ No
- ❑ Yes

If no, When did you last use raloxifen or Evista?

_____ ❑ weeks ago
❑ months ago
❑ years ago

22. Have you ever used estrogen, progesterone or other female hormones for menopause? *(Please do not include oral contraceptives, Tamoxifen, Evista.)*
    - ❑ No *(go to #23)*
    - ❑ Yes

    If yes,

    a. What have you used?

	No	Yes	Unk
Premarin..	☐	☐	☐
Other pills..	☐	☐	☐
Estrogen skin patch..........................	☐	☐	☐
Hormone Shots or injections............	☐	☐	☐
Hormone implants............................	☐	☐	☐
Vaginal creams or suppositories that contain hormones.....................	☐	☐	☐
Facial creams with estrogen or progesterone..................................	☐	☐	☐
Other..	☐	☐	☐

If yes to any of the above, please specify

____

b. How old were you when you first took female hormones for menopause?

_____ years

c. Were you still having periods when you first took female hormones for menopause?

- ❑ No
- ❑ Yes

d. How long did you take female hormones for menopause? (Please do not include occasional breaks in use. For example, if you stopped use for three months, don't include those three months.)

_____ years

e. Are you currently using any female hormones?

- ❑ No
- ❑ Yes

(continued)

Table 5.2 (continued)

If yes, please specify ______________________________

If no, When did you last use any female hormones?

_________ ❑ weeks ago
❑ months ago
❑ years ago

23. Are you currently taking any steroids, androgens or drugs to make you more muscular, increase your sex drive, make you feel better, or for any other reasons?

❑ No
❑ Yes

If yes, what are you taking?

	No	Yes	Unk
Testosterone	☐	☐	☐
Androstenedione	☐	☐	☐
Dehydroepiandrosterone, DHEA, DHEAS	☐	☐	☐
Pregnenolone	☐	☐	☐
Any other drugs to make you more muscular or increase your sex drive	☐	☐	☐

If yes to any of above, could you tell me the name of the product you are using?

____

24. Are you currently taking any of the following medications:

	No	Yes	Unk
Prednisone or cortisone	☐	☐	☐
Thyroid hormones	☐	☐	☐
Insulin	☐	☐	☐
Asthma drugs (including inhalers)	☐	☐	☐
Pills to lower blood sugar	☐	☐	☐

If yes to any of the above, could you tell me the name of the product you are using?

____

25. Do you currently take any other drugs including both prescription and non-prescription med cations?

❑ No
❑ Yes

If yes,

Could you tell me what you take?	How often do you take it?

(continued)

Table 5.2 (continued)

26. Has a doctor ever told you that you have any of the following conditions?

	No	Yes	Unk
Diabetes	☐	☐	☐
Thyroid problems	☐	☐	☐
Adrenal gland problem, Cushings disease, or Addison's disease	☐	☐	☐
Hypertension or High Blood pressure	☐	☐	☐
Stroke	☐	☐	☐
Liver disease or Hepatitis	☐	☐	☐
Gall bladder disease	☐	☐	☐
Kidney disease	☐	☐	☐
Seizure Disorder or epilepsy	☐	☐	☐
Asthma	☐	☐	☐
Depression	☐	☐	☐
Arthritis	☐	☐	☐
Any Other conditions	☐	☐	☐

If yes to any condition, please describe

____

27. Have you ever been hospitalized for a reason other than pregnancy?

☐ No

☐ Yes

If, yes,

Why were you hospitalized?	When?

(continued)

Table 5.2 (continued)

Section C – Diet and Activity

28. Do you eat soy products?

☐ No
☐ Yes

If yes:

a. How often do you usually eat soy products?

__________ times per ☐ day ☐ week ☐ year

b. Which soy products do you usually eat?

	No	Yes	Unk
Tofu	☐	☐	☐
Soy milk	☐	☐	☐
Soy burgers	☐	☐	☐
Other	☐	☐	☐

If other, please specify

____

c. Why do you eat soy products?

	No	Yes	Unk
Enjoy the taste	☐	☐	☐
Vegetarian diet	☐	☐	☐
Menopausal symptoms	☐	☐	☐
Other reason	☐	☐	☐

If other, please specify

(continued)

Table 5.2 (continued)

29. Not including herbs used in cooking, do you take any herbs like ginko, black cohash (Remifemin), or red clover?

❑ No
❑ Yes

If yes,

What herbs do you take?	How often do you take it?	Why do you take it?

30. Do you drink beer?

❑ No
❑ Yes

If yes, how many 12 ounce cans or bottles of beer do you usually drink?

__________ beers per ❑ day ❑ week ❑ year

31. Do you drink wine or wine coolers?

❑ No
❑ Yes

If yes, how many glasses of wine or wine coolers do you usually drink?

__________ glasses per ❑ day ❑ week ❑ year

32. Do you drink liquor or spirits?

❑ No
❑ Yes

If yes, how many shots of liquor or spirits do you usually drink?

__________ shots per ❑ day ❑ week ❑ year

33. During the past year, on average how often did you participate in vigorous physical activities like jogging, swimming laps, singles tennis, skiing, kick boxing?

❑ Never
❑ Less than once a month
❑ 1 – 3 times a month
❑ 4 times a month or once a week
❑ More than once a week but not daily
❑ Daily

(continued)

Table 5.2 (continued)

34. During the past year, on average how often did you participate in moderate physical activities like aerobics, doubles tennis, social dancing, leisurely bike riding, horseback riding, canoeing?
    - ❑ Never
    - ❑ Less than once a month
    - ❑ 1 – 3 times a month
    - ❑ 4 times a month or once a week
    - ❑ More than once a week but not daily
    - ❑ Daily
35. During the past year, on average how often did you participate in light physical activities like golf, fishing, bowling, sailing, yoga, gardening, walking for exercise?
    - ❑ Never
    - ❑ Less than once a month
    - ❑ 1 – 3 times a month
    - ❑ 4 times a month or once a week
    - ❑ More than once a week but not daily
    - ❑ Daily
36. Have you smoked 100 or more cigarettes during your life?
    - ❑ No *(please go to #37)*
    - ❑ Yes

    If yes,

    a. Do you currently smoke cigarettes?
    - ❑ No
    - ❑ Yes

    If current smoker,

    i. How long have you smoked cigarettes? ____ years

    ii. How much do you usually smoke?

    _______ cigarettes per ❑ day ❑ week ❑ year

    If past smoker,

    i. How long ago did you quit? ____ years

    ii. How long did you smoke cigarettes before quitting? ____ years

    ii. How much did you usually smoke?

    _______ cigarettes per ❑ day ❑ week ❑ year

(continued)

Table 5.2 (continued)

37. What was your total household income last year? Please include from all sources including wages, salary, investments, public assistance, social security, retirement, alimony, child support, and any other sources.
    - ❑ Less than 15,000
    - ❑ 15,000-24,999
    - ❑ 25,000-34,999
    - ❑ 35,000-49,999
    - ❑ 50,000-74,999
    - ❑ 75,000-99,999
    - ❑ 100,000 or more
    - ❑ unknown

D. Section D – Family History Questions in this section refer only to your biologic (blood) relatives. Please do not include step mothers, half-sisters, or adopted daughters,

38. Is your biological mother living?
    - ❑ No
    - ❑ Yes
    - ❑ Unknown

If alive, how old is she? ________ years old

❑ Unknown

If deceased, how old was she when she died? ________ years old

❑ Unknown

39. Did your biologic mother have breast cancer?
    - ❑ No
    - ❑ Yes
    - ❑ Unknown

If yes, how old was she when she was first diagnosed with breast cancer? ________ years old

❑ Unknown

(continued)

Table 5.2 (continued)

40. How many full sisters do you have? ________ full sisters

If 1 or more full sisters, please provide information in the chart on their health status

Sister	Is your sister alive?	***If living,*** how old is she now? ***If deceased,*** how old was she when she died?	Was this sister ever diagnosed with breast cancer?	If she had breast cancer, how old was she at the time of diagnosis?
1	❑ No ❑ Yes ❑ Unknown	______ years	❑ No ❑ Yes ❑ Unknown	______ years
2	❑ No ❑ Yes ❑ Unknown	______ years	❑ No ❑ Yes ❑ Unknown	______ years
3	❑ No ❑ Yes ❑ Unknown	______ years	❑ No ❑ Yes ❑ Unknown	______ years
4	❑ No ❑ Yes ❑ Unknown	______ years	❑ No ❑ Yes ❑ Unknown	______ years
5	❑ No ❑ Yes ❑ Unknown	______ years	❑ No ❑ Yes ❑ Unknown	______ years
6	❑ No ❑ Yes ❑ Unknown	______ years	❑ No ❑ Yes ❑ Unknown	______ years

If you need additional space, please use back of page.

(continued)

Table 5.2 (continued)

41. How many biologic daughters do you have? ______ biologic daughters

If 1 or more, please provide information in the chart on their health status

Daughter	Is your daughter alive?	***If living,*** how old is she now? ***If deceased,*** how old was she when she died?	Was this daughter ever diagnosed with breast cancer?	If she had breast cancer, how old was she at the time of diagnosis?
1	❑ No ❑ Yes ❑ Unknown	______ years	❑ No ❑ Yes ❑ Unknown	______ years
2	❑ No ❑ Yes ❑ Unknown	______ years	❑ No ❑ Yes ❑ Unknown	______ years
3	❑ No ❑ Yes ❑ Unknown	______ years	❑ No ❑ Yes ❑ Unknown	______ years
4	❑ No ❑ Yes ❑ Unknown	______ years	❑ No ❑ Yes ❑ Unknown	______ years
5	❑ No ❑ Yes ❑ Unknown	______ years	❑ No ❑ Yes ❑ Unknown	______ years
6	❑ No ❑ Yes ❑ Unknown	______ years	❑ No ❑ Yes ❑ Unknown	______ years

If you need additional space, please use back of page.

42. Did any of your biologic male relatives ever have breast cancer? *(If you do not have any full brothers or biologic sons, please check the box in the column marked **NA** for not applicable.)*

	No	**Yes**	**Unk**	**NA**
Biologic father....................................	☐	☐	☐	
Full brothers....................................	☐	☐	☐	☐
Biologic sons....................................	☐	☐	☐	☐

43. Please tell us anything else about you that you think we should know but did not ask about specifically.

THE END – Thank you

enrolls new subjects consecutively until the required number of study subjects is filled and collects biological specimens described in Sect. 5.3. When an accrual report shows that the database includes the number assigned for the particular study a training set is created and the same when the adequate number has been recruited, to create the validation set.

5.3 Specimen Collection Procedures

Every sample received in our laboratory is logged in a database and stored in −80°C freezer. Each breast sample consists of four core biopsies. One core is processed for histopathological analysis and the other three for genomic analysis (Fig. 5.1). All breast core biopsies must be obtained by a qualified physician and specimens are obtained after an authorization for use and disclosure of protected health information for research has been approved by the Institutional Review Board (IRB) in compliance with the US HIPAA regulations (Fig. 5.1). All breast core biopsies and corresponding participant's data are de-identified following the safe harbor method recommended by the institution's De-Identification of Protected Health Information policies. In the protocol used in our studies four core biopsies with a 10G biopsy needle were taken from the upper outer quadrant (UOQ) of the right or the left

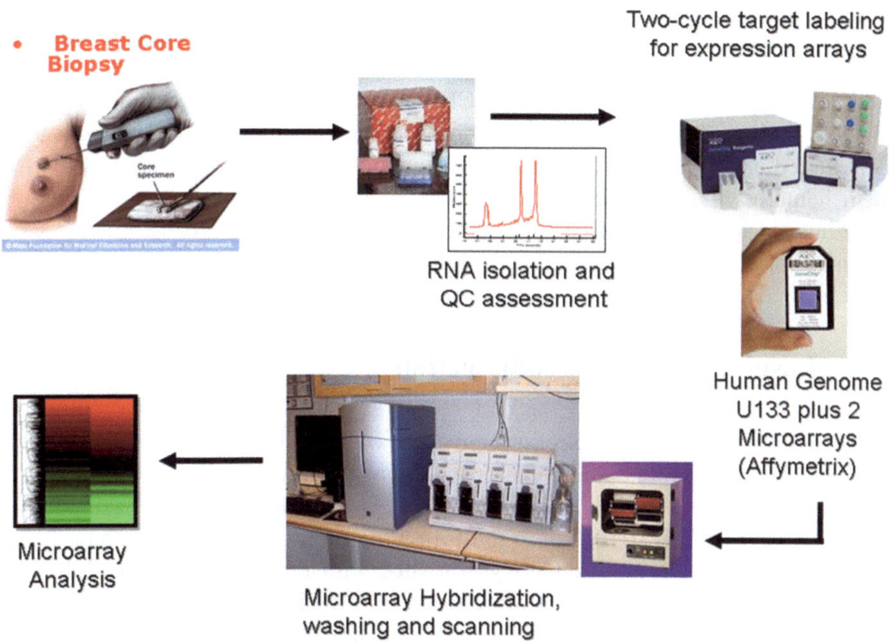

Fig. 5.1 Diagrammatic representation of the steps followed for the isolation of mRNA from the core biopsy sample for performing Affymetrix analysis

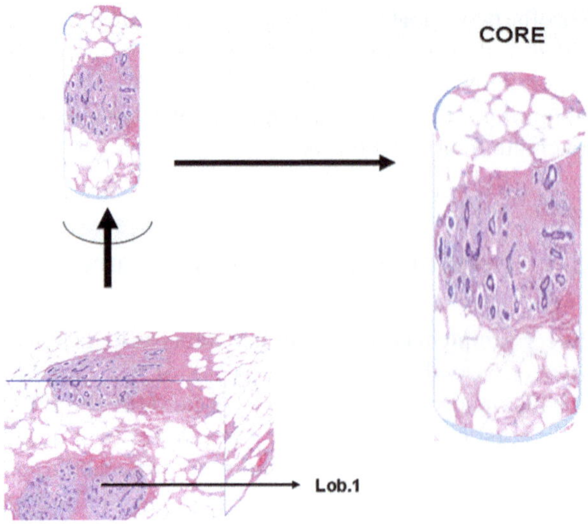

Fig. 5.2 Histological processing of the core biopsy

breast, preferentially sampling dense or gritty areas in the breast tissue which may be appreciated on the mammogram. From the four core biopsies collected, the first one is preserved in 70% ethanol for histopathological evaluation; the second, third, and fourth passes are separately preserved in an RNA-preserving fluid (RNAlater®, Ambion) for genomic analysis.

The first core specimen from each CNB is stored in 70% ethanol at 4°C. Cell clusters or tissue fragments are tightly positioned in a tissue cassette, which is then dehydrated and embedded in paraffin and sectioned at 4 μm thickness and stained with hematoxylin-eosin (H&E), or processed for immunocytochemical studies utilizing an automated cell stainer (Optimax Plus Automatic Consolidated Cell Stainer, Biogenex, San Ramon, CA) following standard procedures (Fig. 5.2).

5.4 Laser Capture Microdissection

LCM is performed on frozen sections cut approximately 1 h prior to staining. Slides are placed on dry ice immediately after sectioning and remained there until staining commenced. Slides are then stained using the Arcturus HistoGene Frozen Section Staining Kit (cat# KIT0401) with the following method: 30″, 70% ethanol; dip in nuclease-free water; 1′, hematoxylin treated with ProtectRNA Rnase Inhibitor (Sigma, cat# R7397); dip in bluing reagent; 30″, eosin treated with ProtectRNA Rnase Inhibitor; 30″, 70% ethanol; 30″, 95% ethanol; 5′, 100% ethanol; 5′, xylene. Slides are allowed to air dry for about 1 min before beginning the LCM. Each

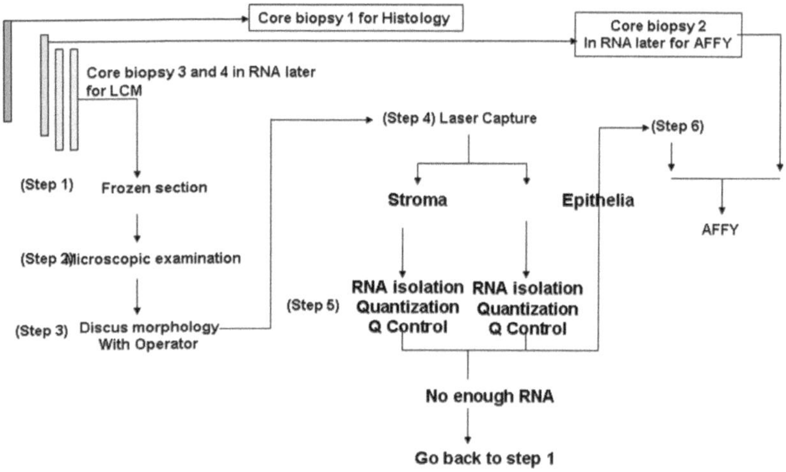

Fig. 5.3 Laser capture microdissection (LCM) processing

Arcturus HistoGene Frozen Section Staining Kit has enough reagents to process 120 slides [6]. LCM is performed using the Arcturus Veritas automated system. Cells are captured onto CapSure® Macro LCM Caps (cat# LCM0211). RNA is isolated from the captured cells with the PicoPure RNA Isolation Kit (Arcturus cat# KIT0202/KIT0204) and DNA extracted with the PicoPure DNA Extraction Kit (Arcturus cat# KIT0103) according to manufacturer's protocols. Each section provided enough cell material for two caps. In average, 40–45 min are required to collect cells on each cap. RNA extraction from Macro LCM caps requires 30 min of incubation time, and the RNA purification process takes 20 min. The success rate in obtaining high-quality RNA as measured by bioanalyzer is 64%. DNA extraction from Macro LCM caps requires 3:30 h of incubation time and final DNA purification. The success rate in obtaining high-quality RNA as measured by bioanalyzer is (4/4) 100% (Figs. 5.3, 5.4 and 5.5).

5.5 RNA Preservation for Affymetrix Studies

For RNA preservation the second and third breast core biopsies are immersed in 500 μL of RNAlater® (Ambion cat# AM7020), in an Eppendorf tube that are identified specifying the name, ID, date, and solution lot number. The subject number is the unique identifier used in our laboratory for specimen archiving, assay tracking, and results reporting. It is linked back to the slide, the date the sample was obtained, the type of sample, the preservatives used, and all information related to

RNA

Sample ID	Epi/Stroma	ng/ul	Total RNA (ng)	260/280	260/230	Laser Pulses	Bioanalyzer	LCM Images
Cap 1 (2/16/10)	E	1.93	21.23	3.49	0.25	2412		
Cap 3 (2/16/10)	E	3.76	41.36	1.44	0.64	2589		
Cap 4 (2/16/10)	S	2.24	24.64	1.8	0.59	1993		
Cap 3 (2.12.10)	E	28.34	311.74	1.39	0.64	596		
Cap 4 (2.12.10)	E	4.36	47.96	1.15	0.41	1362		
Cap5 (2.12.10)	E	5.5	60.5	1.49	0.63	1313		

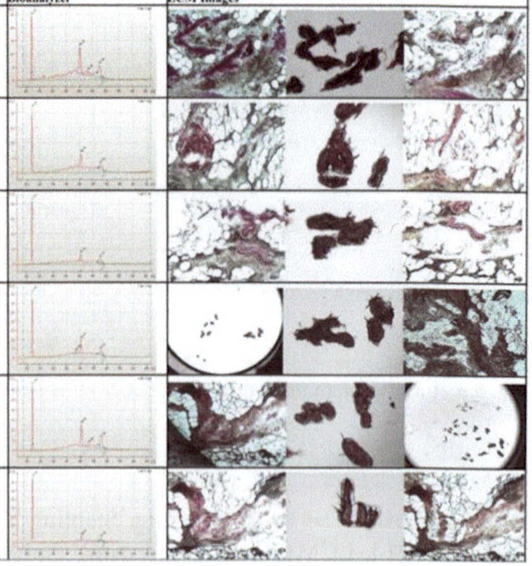

Fig. 5.4 Procurement of mRNA from LCM and kits quality control

DNA

Sample ID		ng/ul	Total DNA	260/280	260/230	Laser Pulses	
cap 1 DNA	E	61.17	3.08μg	1.05	0.14	1458	
cap 2 DNA	E	62.28	3.1μg	1.04	0.14	3045	
cap 3 DNA	E	61.48	3.07μg	1.02	0.14	1462	
cap 4 DNA	S	57.92	2.9μg	1.02	0.13	2918	

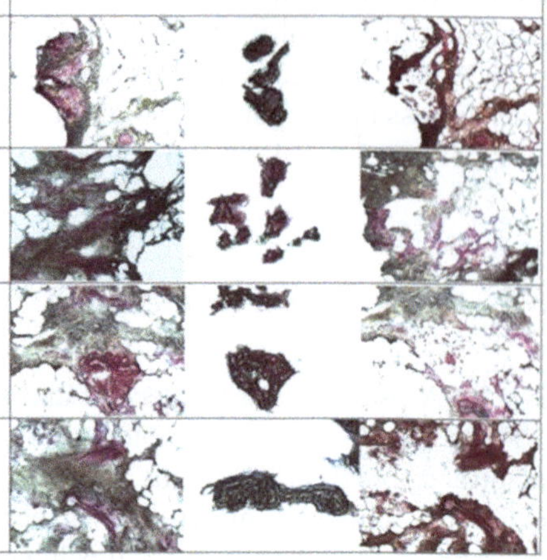

Fig. 5.5 Procurement of DNA from LCM and kits quality control

assay dates, quality control parameters, lot numbers of reagents, and results. All the tubes containing breast core biopsies will be kept at 4°C before shipping. As an additional measure each sample tube should be wrapped with Parafilm to prevent possible leakage during shipment. The samples have to be shipped in a Styrofoam box with frozen ice packs by overnight express mail. The samples need to be packed tightly so they do not move during shipping.

5.6 RNA Extraction for mRNA Sequencing

5.6.1 Total RNA Isolation

The protocol that we use is suitable for 1–10 μg of total RNA because lower amounts may result in inefficient ligation and low yield. The protocol has been optimized using 1 μg of high-quality universal human reference total RNA as input. It is very important to use high-quality RNA as the starting material. Use of degraded RNA can result in low yield, overrepresentation of the 5′ ends of the RNA molecules, or failure of the protocol. Illumina recommends that you check total RNA integrity following isolation using an Agilent Technologies 2100 Bioanalyzer with an RNA Integrity Number (RIN) value greater than 8.

Total RNA is extracted from Macro LCM caps using the PicoPure RNA Isolation Kit. The kit enables the recovery of total cellular RNA from pico-scale samples. The PicoPure RNA Isolation Kit is optimized for use with cells acquired using LCM on CapSure Macro LCM. Total cellular RNA isolated using the PicoPure RNA Isolation Kit produces RNA in a small volume of low ionic strength buffer, ready for use in diverse downstream applications. In summary, total cell extract is loaded onto a preconditioned purification column and the total RNA is captured on the column membrane. The column is washed and the RNA is eluted in low ionic strength buffer.

5.7 PicoPure® DNA Extraction Kit

Extraction Kit provides a fast and easy genomic DNA extraction procedure. No organic extractions or spin columns are needed, enabling very high DNA recovery from samples and single-tube DNA extraction and subsequent amplification. This streamlined method makes the kit ideal for processing small samples, of as few as ten cells, where maximum DNA recovery is critical. The DNA extraction protocol requires a 3 h incubation of the LCM caps in proteinase K. After proteinase K is denatured, sample is spun and DNA is ready for downstream applications.

5.8 RNA Processing and Quality Control for cDNA Microarray Analysis

All specimens that have been collected in RNAlater and kept at room temperature for no more than 30 min and then stored at 4°C are used for total RNA isolation Trizol (Invitrogen, Inc.). The concentration and the quality of each RNA is confirmed through electrophoresis by capillarity using Agilent 2100 Bioanalyzer (Agilent Technologies, Inc., Wilmington, DE, USA) before the RNA is used for amplification and labeling (Fig. 5.1). When this process is concluded, the efficiency of the amplification and incorporation of dye into the RNA is measured and hybridization proceeds only if the values indicated by the manufacturer have been reached. The two-Cycle Eukaryotic Target Labeling Assay will be used. Total RNA (10–100 ng) is first reverse transcribed using a T7-Oligo(dT) Promoter Primer in the first-strand cDNA synthesis reaction. Following RNase H-mediated second-strand cDNA synthesis, the double-stranded cDNA is purified and serves as a template in the subsequent in vitro transcription (IVT) reaction. The IVT reaction is carried out in the presence of T7 RNA Polymerase and a biotinylated nucleotide analog/ribonucleotide mix for complementary RNA (cRNA) amplification and biotin labeling. The biotinylated cRNA targets are then cleaned up, fragmented, and hybridized to GeneChip expression arrays. Because we will start with an initial low amount of total RNA, an additional cycle of cDNA synthesis and IVT amplification is required to obtain sufficient amounts of labeled cRNA target for analysis with arrays. After cDNA synthesis in the first cycle, an unlabeled ribonucleotide mix is used in the first cycle of IVT amplification. The unlabeled cRNA is then reverse transcribed in the first-strand cDNA synthesis step of the second cycle using random primers. Subsequently, the T7-Oligo(dT) Promoter Primer is used in the second-strand cDNA synthesis to generate double-stranded cDNA template containing T7 promoter sequences. The resulting double-stranded cDNA is then amplified and labeled using a biotinylated nucleotide analog/ribonucleotide mix in the second IVT reaction. The labeled cRNA is then cleaned up, fragmented, and hybridized to Affymetrix GeneChip expression arrays (GeneChip® Human Genome U133 Plus 2.0; Part# 900470). The GeneChip® Human Genome U133 Plus 2.0 Array offers a comprehensive analysis of genome-wide expression on a single array. It also provides comprehensive coverage of the transcribed human genome on a single array and analyzes the expression level of over 47,000 transcripts and variants, including 38,500 well-characterized human genes. It comprises more than 54,000 probe sets and 1,300,000 distinct oligonucleotide features.

cDNA Microarray QA/QC: The scanned images of the microarrays are submitted to the software Feature Extraction v9.5.1 (Agilent Technologies, Inc., Wilmington, DE, USA), which measures quality parameters, qualifies each spot based on intensity of signal, background, shape, saturation, and also identifies areas with problems of hybridization or wash. Those slides that don't present a satisfactory quality are excluded from the analysis to assure the most trustful results (Fig. 5.1).

5.9 Blood Collection for Hormone Determination

After proper participant identification and verification of informed consent form signature, whole blood is collected from the median cubital vein for extraction and storage of serum and plasma. Serum obtained from postmenopausal women is utilized for blood level determination of follicle-stimulating hormone (FSH) for confirmation of postmenopausal condition.

5.10 Blood Collection for Genomic Analysis

For whole blood RNA extraction, the PreAnalytiX PAXgene Blood RNA System which stabilizes the gene transcription profile at the point of sample collection and provides highly purified cellular RNA is used. PAXgene Blood RNA Tubes stabilize cellular RNA for up to 3 days at 18–25°C or up to 5 days at 2–8°C or 6 months at −20°C.

Acknowledgements We, the authors, acknowledge the contributions of the many members of the Breast Cancer Research Laboratory at the Fox Chase Cancer Center among them Drs. R. Lopez, F. Sheriff, and Ms P. A. Russo who have contributed to generate the methods incorporated into this chapter and allowed us to elaborate it into a unified concept.

References

1. Balogh GA, Heulings R, Mailo DA, Russo PA, Sheriff F, Russo IH, Moral R, Russo J (2006) Genomic signature induced by pregnancy in the human breast. Int J Oncol 28:399–410
2. Russo J, Balogh GA, Heulings R, Mailo DA, Moral R, Russo PA, Sheriff F, Vanegas J, Russo IH (2006) Molecular basis of pregnancy-induced breast cancer protection. Eur J Cancer Prev 15:306–342
3. Russo J, Tay LK, Russo IH (1982) Differentiation of the mammary gland and susceptibility to carcinogenesis. Breast Cancer Res Treat 2:5–73
4. Balogh GA, Russo J, Mailo DA, Heulings R, Russo PA, Morrison P, Sheriff F, Russo IH (2007) The breast of parous women without cancer has a different genomic profile compared to those with cancer. Int J Oncol 31:1165–1175
5. Russo J, Balogh G, Russo IH (2007) Breast cancer prevention. Climacteric 10(suppl 2):47–53
6. Russo J, Balogh GA, Russo IH (2008) Full-term pregnancy induces a specific genomic signature in the human breast. Cancer Epidemiol Biomarkers Prev 17:51–66
7. Russo J, Russo IH (1995) Hormonally induced differentiation: a novel approach to breast cancer prevention. J Cell Biochem Suppl 22:58–64
8. Anderson K, Hess KR, Kapoor M, Tirrell S, Courtemanche J, Wang B, Wu Y, Gong Y, Hortobagyi GN, Symmans WF, Pusztai L (2006) Reproducibility of gene expression signature-based predictions in replicate experiments. Clin Cancer Res 12:1721–1727
9. Anderson NL, Anderson NG (2002) The human plasma proteome: history, character, and diagnostic prospects. Mol Cell Proteomics 1:845–867
10. Bair E, Tibshirani R (2003) Improved detection of differential gene expression through the singular value decomposition. Technical Report, Department of Statistics, Stanford University, Stanford

11. Brunet JP, Tamayo P, Golub TR, Mesirov JP (2004) Metagenes and molecular pattern discovery using matrix factorization. Proc Natl Acad Sci USA 101:4164–4169
12. Development Core Team, R (2005) A language and environment for statistical computing. R Foundation for Statistical Computing, Vienna, Austria. http://www.R-project.org
13. Gentleman RC, Carey VJ, Bates DM, Bolstad B, Dettling M, Dudoit S, Ellis B, Gautier L, Ge Y, Gentry J, Hornik K, Hothorn T, Huber W, Iacus S, Irizarry R, Leisch F, Li C, Maechler M, Rossini AJ, Sawitzki G, Smith C, Smyth G, Tierney L, Yang JY, Zhang J (2004) Bioconductor: open software development for computational biology and bioinformatics. Genome Biol 5:R80
14. Pascual-Montano A, Carmona-Saez P, Chagoyen M, Tirado F, Carazo JM, Pascual-Marqui RD (2006) bioNMF: a versatile tool for non-negative matrix factorization in biology. BMC Bioinformatics 7:366
15. Roy J (1995) Controlling the false discovery rate: a practical and powerful approach to multiple testing. J R Stat Soc Series B Stat Methodol 57:289–300
16. Simon RM, Dobbin K (2003) Experimental design of DNA microarray experiments. Biotechniques (suppl):16–21
17. Storey JD, Tibshirani R (2003) Statistical significance for genomewide studies. Proc Natl Acad Sci USA 100:9440–9445
18. Tusher VG, Tibshirani R, Chu G (2001) Significance analysis of microarrays applied to the ionizing radiation response. Proc Natl Acad Sci USA 98:5116–5121
19. Devarajan K (2008) Nonnegative matrix factorization: an analytical and interpretive tool in computational biology. PLoS Comput Biol 4:e1000029

Chapter 6
The Transcriptome of Breast Cancer Prevention

6.1 Introduction

More than 300 years have elapsed since a striking excess in breast cancer mortality was reported in nuns, in whom the increased risk was attributed to their childlessness [1] until MacMahon et al. [2] in a landmark case-control study found an almost linear relationship between a woman's risk and the age at which she bore her first child (see Chap. 1). This work, which included areas of high, intermediate and low breast cancer risk in seven parts of the world, confirmed that pregnancy had a protective effect that was evident from the early teen years and persisted until the middle 20s [2]. Other studies have reported that additional pregnancies and breastfeeding confer greater protection to young women, including a statistically significantly reduced risk of breast cancer in women with deleterious *BRCA1* mutations who breast-fed for a cumulative total of more than 1 year [3, 4]. Our studies, designed to unravel what specific changes occurred in the breast during pregnancy that confer a lifetime protection from developing cancer, led us to the discovery that endogenous endocrinological or environmental influences affecting breast development before the first full-term pregnancy (FFTP) were important modulators of the susceptibility of the breast to undergo neoplastic transformation. The fact that exposure of the breast of young nulliparous females to environmental physical agents [5] or chemical toxicants [6, 7] results in a greater rate of cell transformation suggests that the immature breast possesses a greater number of susceptible cells that can become the site of origin of cancer, similarly to what has been reported in experimental animal models [8–11]. In these models, the initiation of cancer is prevented by the differentiation of the mammary gland induced by pregnancy [11, 12]. The molecular changes involved in this phenomenon are just starting to be unraveled [13–18]. The protection conferred by pregnancy is age-specific since a delay in childbearing after age 24 progressively increases the risk of cancer development. Eventually, this risk becomes greater than that of nulliparous women when the FFTP occurs after 35 years of age [2]. The higher breast cancer risk that has been associated with early menarche further emphasizes the importance of the length of the susceptibility

J. Russo and I.H. Russo, *Role of the Transcriptome in Breast Cancer Prevention*,
DOI 10.1007/978-1-4614-4884-6_6, © Springer Science+Business Media New York 2013

"window" that encompasses the period of breast development occurring between menarche and the first pregnancy, when the organ is more susceptible to undergo complete differentiation under physiological hormonal stimuli. Differentiation is a hallmark that protects the breast from developing cancer by lessening the risk of suffering genetic or epigenetic damages. This postulate is supported by our observations that the architectural pattern of lobular development in parous women with cancer differs from that of parous women without cancer; the former being similar to the architectural pattern of lobular development of nulliparous women with or without cancer. Thus, the higher breast cancer risk in parous women might have resulted from either a failure of the breast to fully differentiate under the influence of the hormones of pregnancy and/or proliferation of transformed cells initiated by early damage or genetic predisposition [18].

Numerous studies have been performed to understand how the dramatic modifications that occur during pregnancy in the pattern of lobular development and differentiation, cell proliferation, and steroid hormone receptor content of the breast [18] influence cancer risk. Studies at the molecular level using different platforms for global genome analysis have confirmed the universality of this phenomenon in various strains of rats and mice [13–18]. Studies in experimental animal models have been useful for uncovering the sequential genomic changes occurring in the mammary gland in response to multiple hormonal stimuli of pregnancy that lead to the imprinting of a permanent genomic signature. Work reported herein was designed with the purpose of testing whether a similar phenomenon occurs in the breast of postmenopausal parous women. Our results support our hypothesis that postmenopausal parous women exhibit a genomic "signature" that differs from the expression present in the breast of nulliparous women, who traditionally represent a high breast cancer risk group.

6.2 Methodologic Approach

The study participants consisted of postmenopausal women who were grouped according to their reproductive history into parous (P) and nulliparous (NP). The nulliparous group included both, nulligravida nulliparous (NN) and gravida nulliparous (GN); both NN and GN women were considered within the NP as a single group for most analyses, unless indicated otherwise. Breast core needle biopsies (CNBs) were first analyzed histopathologically in order to determine the adequacy of tissue, presence of ductal and lobular structures, and the characteristics of the stroma. A total of 126 biopsies obtained from 82 P and 44 NP women were eligible for final genomic analysis. In order to gain insight into the functional and molecular events that differ between parous and nulliparous breast samples, we applied data mining methods to identify biological processes, pathways, and gene networks that are statistically significant. The up- and downregulated genes for these analyses were selected as described in Table 6.1. Ingenuity Pathways Analysis (IPA) provides a rich functional annotation of genes and proteins, protein–protein interactions, and the roles of genes in various diseases. The genes differentially

Table 6.1 Probesets differentially expressed in parous vs. nulliparous ($p<0.001$ and log2 fold change of at least 0.3)

Gene symbol	Probe ID	Log ratio	*p* Value	Adj. *p* value	Gene name
ABAT	209460_at	0.31	0.0005	0.02	4-Aminobutyrate aminotransferase
ABAT	209459_s_at	0.34	0.0001	0.01	4-Aminobutyrate aminotransferase
ABHD5	213805_at	–0.32	0.0003	0.01	Abhydrolase domain containing 5
AFG3L1	1552287_s_at	0.35	0.0002	0.01	AFG3 ATPase family gene 3-like 1 (*Saccharomyces cerevisiae*)
AGBL3	232395_x_at	0.48	0.0005	0.02	ATP/GTP binding protein-like 3
AHSA2	230148_at	0.42	0.0006	0.02	AHA1, activator of heat shock 90 kDa protein ATPase homolog 2 (yeast)
AHSA2	226334_s_at	0.44	0.0007	0.02	AHA1, activator of heat shock 90 kDa protein ATPase homolog 2 (yeast)
AHSA2	226665_at	0.65	0.0003	0.01	AHA1, activator of heat shock 90 kDa protein ATPase homolog 2 (yeast)
ANKRD10	223251_s_at	0.32	0.0001	0.01	Ankyrin repeat domain 10
ANXA9	211712_s_at	0.37	0.0003	0.01	Annexin A9
AP1G2	201613_s_at	0.33	0.0001	0.01	Adaptor-related protein complex 1, gamma 2 subunit
ARGLU1	228477_at	0.33	0.0001	0.01	Arginine and glutamate rich 1
ARGLU1	218067_s_at	0.34	0.0002	0.01	Arginine and glutamate rich 1
ARHGAP8	232567_at	0.33	0.0008	0.02	Rho GTPase activating protein 8
ATHL1	219359_at	0.35	0.0006	0.02	ATH1, acid trehalase-like 1 (yeast)
BZRAP1	205839_s_at	0.33	0.0000	0.01	Benzodiazapine receptor (peripheral) associated protein 1
C11orf31	228331_at	0.49	0.0000	0.01	Chromosome 11 open reading frame 31
C1orf168	238625_at	0.80	0.0000	0.01	Chromosome 1 open reading frame 168
C1orf63	209007_s_at	0.51	0.0010	0.02	chromosome 1 open reading frame 63
C1orf63	209006_s_at	0.52	0.0006	0.02	chromosome 1 open reading frame 63
C2orf63	228316_at	0.31	0.0004	0.01	Chromosome 2 open reading frame 63
C3orf15	236222_at	0.30	0.0003	0.01	Chromosome 3 open reading frame 15
C4orf19	235350_at	–0.32	0.0005	0.02	Chromosome 4 open reading frame 19

(continued)

Table 6.1 (continued)

Gene symbol	Probe ID	Log ratio	p Value	Adj. p value	Gene name
C6orf170	232038_at	0.38	0.0001	0.01	Chromosome 6 open reading frame 170
C8orf79	239297_at	0.32	0.0002	0.01	Chromosome 8 open reading frame 79
C8orf84	235209_at	0.40	0.0008	0.02	Chromosome 8 open reading frame 84
CAPN3	210944_s_at	0.40	0.0006	0.02	Calpain 3 (p94)
CAPN8	229030_at	0.55	0.0000	0.01	Calpain 8
CASP4	213596_at	0.37	0.0003	0.01	Caspase 4, apoptosis-related cysteine peptidase
CBX3	1555920_at	0.53	0.0003	0.01	Chromobox homolog 3 (HP1 gamma homolog, *Drosophila*)
CCDC14	225017_at	0.35	0.0002	0.01	Coiled-coil domain containing 14
CCDC45	225705_at	0.32	0.0002	0.01	Coiled-coil domain containing 45
CCNL1	1555411_a_at	0.35	0.0009	0.02	Cyclin L1
CCNL1	220046_s_at	0.40	0.0001	0.01	Cyclin L2
CCNL2	222999_s_at	0.47	0.0002	0.01	Cyclin L2
CD69	209795_at	0.32	0.0006	0.02	CD69 molecule
CDCA7	224428_s_at	0.31	0.0005	0.02	Cell division cycle associated 7
CDK12	213557_at	0.37	0.0001	0.01	Cyclin-dependent kinase 12
CDK5RAP3	218740_s_at	0.31	0.0000	0.00	CDK5 regulatory subunit associated protein 3
CENPK	222848_at	0.34	0.0001	0.01	Centromere protein K
CGN	223233_s_at	0.35	0.0004	0.01	Cingulin
CGN	223232_s_at	0.41	0.0002	0.01	Cingulin
CHD2	228999_at	0.33	0.0001	0.01	Chromodomain helicase DNA binding protein 2
CIRBP	230142_s_at	0.45	0.0000	0.01	Cold inducible RNA binding protein
CIRBP	225191_at	0.55	0.0002	0.01	Cold inducible RNA binding protein
CLGN	205830_at	0.47	0.0003	0.01	Calmegin
CLK4	210346_s_at	0.36	0.0004	0.02	CDC-like kinase 4
CMYA5	233520_s_at	0.46	0.0000	0.01	Cardiomyopathy associated 5
COL16A1	204345_at	0.31	0.0000	0.01	Collagen, type XVI, alpha 1
COL27A1	225293_at	0.44	0.0002	0.01	Collagen, type XXVII, alpha 1
COL27A1	225288_at	0.55	0.0000	0.01	Collagen, type XXVII, alpha 1

COL4A5	213110_s_at	0.38	0.0004	0.01	Collagen, type IV, alpha 5
COL4A6	213992_at	0.36	0.0008	0.02	Collagen, type IV, alpha 6
COL7A1	204136_at	0.33	0.0002	0.01	Collagen, type VII, alpha 1
CREBZF	225595_at	0.45	0.0005	0.02	CREB/ATF bZIP transcription factor
CREBZF	225594_at	0.48	0.0001	0.01	CREB/ATF bZIP transcription factor
CSNK1A1	1556006_s_at	0.46	0.0000	0.01	Casein kinase 1, alpha 1
CXorf50B	242292_at	0.35	0.0001	0.01	Non-protein coding RNA 246B
D4S234E	209570_s_at	0.34	0.0008	0.02	DNA segment on chromosome 4 (unique) 234 expressed sequence
DDX17	213998_s_at	0.49	0.0001	0.01	DEAD (Asp-Glu-Ala-Asp) box polypeptide 17
DDX26B	227485_at	0.36	0.0003	0.01	DEAD/H (Asp-Glu-Ala-Asp/His) box polypeptide 26B
DIDO1	213213_at	0.30	0.0007	0.02	Death inducer-obliterator 1
DKFZp667E0512	236079_at	0.47	0.0003	0.01	Hypothetical protein DKFZp667E0512
DNAH5	232381_s_at	0.36	0.0009	0.02	Dynein, axonemal, heavy chain 5
DNALI1	227081_at	0.37	0.0001	0.01	Dynein, axonemal, light intermediate chain 1
DOCK9	232874_at	–0.38	0.0001	0.01	Dedicator of cytokinesis 9
DOPEY1	213267_at	0.35	0.0009	0.02	Dopey family member 1
DSC3	206032_at	0.51	0.0000	0.01	Desmocollin 3
DSC3	206033_s_at	0.55	0.0000	0.01	Desmocollin 3
DYX1C1	235273_at	0.31	0.0000	0.01	Dyslexia susceptibility 1 candidate 1
EBF1	232204_at	–0.33	0.0005	0.02	Early B-cell factor 1
ECHDC2	235305_s_at	0.33	0.0009	0.02	Enoyl CoA hydratase domain containing 2
EED	210656_at	0.35	0.0007	0.02	Embryonic ectoderm development
EFHC1	219833_s_at	0.31	0.0001	0.01	EF-hand domain (C-terminal) containing 1
ELMO3	219411_at	0.30	0.0003	0.01	Engulfment and cell motility 3
ENOSF1	213645_at	0.47	0.0001	0.01	Enolase superfamily member 1
ENPP5	237054_at	0.37	0.0006	0.02	Ectonucleotide pyrophosphatase/phosphodiesterase 5 (putative function)

(continued)

Table 6.1 (continued)

Gene symbol	Probe ID	Log ratio	*p* Value	Adj. *p* value	Gene name
EPM2AIP1	236314_at	0.48	0.0005	0.02	EPM2A (laforin) interacting protein 1
EZH2	203358_s_at	0.44	0.0000	0.01	Enhancer of zeste homolog 2 (*Drosophila*)
FAM101A	227320_at	0.33	0.0000	0.00	Family with sequence similarity 101, member A
FLJ25006	1553292_s_at	0.35	0.0008	0.02	Uncharacterized serine/threonine-protein kinase SgK494
FLJ40330	1569040_s_at	0.73	0.0002	0.01	Hypothetical LOC645784
FNBP4	212232_at	0.36	0.0003	0.01	Formin binding protein 4
FRMD3	230645_at	−0.32	0.0005	0.02	FERM domain containing 3
FUBP1	214093_s_at	0.47	0.0002	0.01	Far upstream element (FUSE) binding protein 1
GALNT6	219956_at	0.44	0.0007	0.02	UDP-*N*-acetyl-alpha-D-galactosamine:polypeptide-*N*-acetylgalactosaminyltransferase 6 (GalNAc-T6)
GAS5	227517_s_at	0.70	0.0001	0.01	Growth arrest-specific 5 (non-protein coding)
GATA3	209602_s_at	0.35	0.0009	0.02	GATA binding protein 3
GATA3	209603_at	0.38	0.0009	0.02	GATA binding protein 3
GOLGA2B	233198_at	0.32	0.0001	0.01	Golgin A2 family, member B
GOLGA8A	208798_x_at	0.75	0.0002	0.01	Golgin A8 family, member A
GOLGA8B	210425_x_at	0.61	0.0003	0.01	Golgin A8 family, member B
HINT1	1555960_at	0.40	0.0002	0.01	Histidine triad nucleotide binding protein 1
HNRNPA1	221919_at	0.50	0.0003	0.01	Heterogeneous nuclear ribonucleoprotein A1
HNRNPA2B1	225932_s_at	0.32	0.0003	0.01	Heterogeneous nuclear ribonucleoprotein A2/B1
HNRNPA2B1	225107_at	0.56	0.0003	0.01	Heterogeneous nuclear ribonucleoprotein A2/B1
HNRNPD	213359_at	0.59	0.0003	0.01	Heterogeneous nuclear ribonucleoprotein D (AU-rich element RNA binding protein 1, 37 kDa)
HNRPDL	212454_x_at	0.65	0.0001	0.01	Heterogeneous nuclear ribonucleoprotein D-like
HSPB11	214163_at	0.46	0.0002	0.01	Heat shock protein family B (small), member 11
IGF1	209540_at	−0.35	0.0002	0.01	Insulin-like growth factor 1 (somatomedin C)
IL28RA	244261_at	0.34	0.0003	0.01	Interleukin 28 receptor, alpha (interferon, lambda receptor)
IL7R	226218_at	0.53	0.0001	0.01	Interleukin 7 receptor
INTU	228946_at	0.51	0.0001	0.01	Inturned planar cell polarity effector homolog (*Drosophila*)

IPW	221974_at	0.42	0.0001	0.01	Imprinted in Prader–Willi syndrome (non-protein coding)
IQCA1	238584_at	0.50	0.0000	0.01	IQ motif containing with AAA domain 1
KCNE1	236407_at	0.46	0.0008	0.02	Potassium voltage-gated channel, Isk-related family, member 1
KIAA0907	202220_at	0.33	0.0007	0.02	KIAA0907
KLHL29	229310_at	0.31	0.0000	0.01	Kelch-like 29 (*Drosophila*)
KLK7	239381_at	0.44	0.0007	0.02	Kallikrein-related peptidase 7
KRT15	204734_at	0.55	0.0001	0.01	Keratin 15
KRT5	201820_at	0.41	0.0002	0.01	Keratin 5
L3MBTL	210306_at	0.40	0.0001	0.01	l(3)mbt-like (*Drosophila*)
LAMA3	203726_s_at	0.30	0.0008	0.02	Laminin, alpha 3
LAMC2	202267_at	0.34	0.0008	0.02	Laminin, gamma 2
LNPEP	231866_at	−0.30	0.0001	0.01	Leucyl/cystinyl aminopeptidase
LOC100127980	242462_at	0.30	0.0010	0.02	Hypothetical protein LOC100127980
LOC100130360	243179_at	0.31	0.0008	0.02	Hypothetical LOC100130360
LOC100286909	228528_at	0.41	0.0007	0.02	Hypothetical protein LOC100286909
LOC150759	213703_at	0.55	0.0003	0.01	Hypothetical protein LOC150759
LOC153682	232794_at	0.37	0.0001	0.01	Hypothetical protein LOC153682
LOC221442	236832_at	0.40	0.0003	0.01	Adenylate cyclase 10 pseudogene
LOC284513	1556597_a_at	0.38	0.0003	0.01	Hypothetical protein LOC284513
LOC339047	221501_x_at	0.40	0.0001	0.01	Hypothetical protein LOC339047
LOC399491	214035_x_at	0.36	0.0001	0.01	GPS, PLAT, and transmembrane domain-containing protein
LOC642587	226755_at	0.64	0.0000	0.01	NPC-A-5
LUC7L3	220044_x_at	0.32	0.0001	0.01	LUC7-like 3 (*S. cerevisiae*)
LUC7L3	203804_s_at	0.34	0.0002	0.01	LUC7-like 3 (*S. cerevisiae*)
MALAT1	224558_s_at	0.56	0.0000	0.01	Metastasis-associated lung adenocarcinoma transcript 1 (non-protein coding)
MARCH3	213256_at	−0.30	0.0003	0.01	Membrane-associated ring finger (C3HC4) 3
MBD4	214048_at	0.36	0.0003	0.01	Methyl-CpG binding domain protein 4

(continued)

Table 6.1 (continued)

Gene symbol	Probe ID	Log ratio	p Value	Adj. p value	Gene name
MCTS1	230235_at	0.31	0.0004	0.01	Malignant T cell amplified sequence 1
MDM1	213761_at	0.31	0.0001	0.01	Mdm1 nuclear protein homolog (mouse)
METTL3	213653_at	0.69	0.0000	0.01	Methyltransferase like 3
MGP	238481_at	0.53	0.0003	0.01	Matrix Gla protein
MPPED2	205413_at	0.39	0.0000	0.00	Metallophosphoesterase domain containing 2
MREG	232682_at	0.35	0.0005	0.02	Melanoregulin
MREG	219648_at	0.45	0.0001	0.01	Melanoregulin
N4BP2L2	235547_at	0.33	0.0002	0.01	NEDD4 binding protein 2-like 2
NANOS1	228523_at	–0.38	0.0002	0.01	Nanos homolog 1 (*Drosophila*)
NCRNA00173	237591_at	0.39	0.0002	0.01	Non-protein coding RNA 173
NCRNA00201	225786_at	0.47	0.0004	0.01	Non-protein coding RNA 201
NDUFB8	214241_at	0.31	0.0004	0.01	NADH dehydrogenase (ubiquinone) 1 beta subcomplex, 8, 19 kDa
NFKBIZ	223217_s_at	0.42	0.0002	0.01	Nuclear factor of kappa light polypeptide gene enhancer in B-cells inhibitor, zeta
NFKBIZ	223218_s_at	0.48	0.0001	0.01	Nuclear factor of kappa light polypeptide gene enhancer in B-cells inhibitor, zeta
NKTR	202380_s_at	0.34	0.0009	0.02	Natural killer-tumor recognition sequence
NLRC3	236295_s_at	0.32	0.0001	0.01	NLR family, CARD domain containing 3
NPHP3	235432_at	0.34	0.0006	0.02	Nephronophthisis 3 (adolescent)
NPHP3	235410_at	0.38	0.0001	0.01	Nephronophthisis 3 (adolescent)
NPIP	204538_x_at	0.38	0.0001	0.01	Nuclear pore complex interacting protein
NRXN1	228547_at	0.60	0.0001	0.01	Neurexin 1
NSMCE4A	228506_at	0.62	0.0002	0.01	Non-SMC element 4 homolog A (*S. cerevisiae*)
NTF4	231785_at	0.36	0.0001	0.01	Neurotrophin 4
OGT	207564_x_at	0.33	0.0001	0.01	O-linked *N*-acetylglucosamine (GlcNAc) transferase (UDP-*N*-acetylglucosamine:polypeptide-*N*-acetylglucosaminyl transferase)

OGT	212307_s_at	0.35	0.0001	0.01	O-linked *N*-acetylglucosamine (GlcNAc) transferase (UDP-*N*-acetylglucosamine:polypeptide-*N*-acetylglucosaminyl transferase)
OGT	229787_s_at	0.37	0.0001	0.01	O-linked *N*-acetylglucosamine (GlcNAc) transferase (UDP-*N*-acetylglucosamine:polypeptide-*N*-acetylglucosaminyl transferase)
OXTR	206825_at	0.54	0.0006	0.02	Oxytocin receptor
PABPC1L	231838_at	0.37	0.0005	0.02	Poly(A) binding protein, cytoplasmic 1-like
PABPN1	213046_at	0.35	0.0007	0.02	Poly(A) binding protein, nuclear 1
PALM2	1554640_at	−0.32	0.0001	0.01	Paralemmin 2
PDLIM4	211564_s_at	0.35	0.0002	0.01	PDZ and LIM domain 4
PDZD2	233025_at	−0.35	0.0004	0.01	PDZ domain containing 2
PIGL	232262_at	0.38	0.0005	0.02	Phosphatidylinositol glycan anchor biosynthesis, class L
PILRB	220954_s_at	0.51	0.0000	0.01	Paired immunoglobin-like type 2 receptor beta
PILRB	225321_s_at	0.64	0.0001	0.01	Paired immunoglobin-like type 2 receptor beta
PNN	1567214_a_at	0.37	0.0003	0.01	Pinin, desmosome-associated protein
PNN	212036_s_at	0.37	0.0001	0.01	Pinin, desmosome-associated protein
PPM1K	235061_at	0.33	0.0004	0.01	protein phosphatase, Mg2+/Mn2+ dependent, 1K
PRPF39	220553_s_at	0.31	0.0000	0.01	PRP39 pre-mRNA processing factor 39 homolog (*S. cerevisiae*)
PRPF4B	202127_at	0.44	0.0005	0.02	PRP4 pre-mRNA processing factor 4 homolog B (yeast)
PTN	209465_x_at	0.55	0.0005	0.02	Pleiotrophin
PTN	211737_x_at	0.66	0.0002	0.01	Pleiotrophin
PTN	209466_x_at	0.67	0.0002	0.01	Pleiotrophin
RALGAPA2	232500_at	−0.30	0.0002	0.01	Ral GTPase activating protein, alpha subunit 2 (catalytic)
RASD1	223467_at	−0.31	0.0009	0.02	RAS, dexamethasone-induced 1
RBBP8	203344_s_at	0.32	0.0000	0.01	Retinoblastoma binding protein 8
RBM25	1557081_at	0.38	0.0009	0.02	RNA binding motif protein 25

(continued)

Table 6.1 (continued)

Gene symbol	Probe ID	Log ratio	p Value	Adj. p value	Gene name
RBMX	225310_at	0.38	0.0000	0.01	RNA binding motif protein, X-linked
RDH13	1559190_s_at	0.35	0.0001	0.01	Retinol dehydrogenase 13 (all-*trans*/9-*cis*)
RGS1	216834_at	0.45	0.0005	0.02	Regulator of G-protein signaling 1
RNF183	235153_at	0.49	0.0001	0.01	Ring finger protein 183
RPL10	221989_at	0.59	0.0000	0.01	Ribosomal protein L10
RPL37A	213459_at	0.50	0.0004	0.01	Ribosomal protein L37a
RPS24	1555878_at	0.55	0.0004	0.02	Ribosomal protein S24
RUNX3	204198_s_at	0.31	0.0001	0.01	Runt-related transcription factor 3
RUNX3	204197_s_at	0.36	0.0000	0.01	Runt-related transcription factor 3
RYR3	206306_at	0.40	0.0003	0.01	Ryanodine receptor 3
SCARNA15	228930_at	0.33	0.0000	0.01	Small Cajal body-specific RNA 15
SCNN1A	203453_at	0.40	0.0003	0.01	Sodium channel, nonvoltage-gated 1 alpha
SCUBE2	219197_s_at	0.42	0.0009	0.02	Signal peptide, CUB domain, EGF-like 2
SFI1	36545_s_at	0.32	0.0000	0.01	Sfi1 homolog, spindle assembly associated (yeast)
SFPQ	214016_s_at	0.46	0.0002	0.01	Splicing factor proline/glutamine-rich
SFPQ	221768_at	0.47	0.0006	0.02	Splicing factor proline/glutamine-rich
SFRS1	201742_x_at	0.30	0.0001	0.01	Splicing factor, arginine/serine-rich 1
SFRS18	212179_at	0.39	0.0003	0.01	Splicing factor, arginine/serine-rich 18
SFRS18	212176_at	0.39	0.0002	0.01	Splicing factor, arginine/serine-rich 18
SFRS18	212177_at	0.40	0.0002	0.01	Splicing factor, arginine/serine-rich 18
SFRS5	203380_x_at	0.31	0.0001	0.01	Splicing factor, arginine/serine-rich 5
SFRS5	212266_s_at	0.36	0.0000	0.01	Splicing factor, arginine/serine-rich 5
SFRS7	213649_at	0.40	0.0004	0.01	Splicing factor, arginine/serine-rich 7, 35 kDa
SGSM2	217538_at	0.50	0.0001	0.01	Small G-protein signaling modulator 2
SLC16A6	230748_at	0.38	0.0009	0.02	Solute carrier family 16, member 6 (monocarboxylic acid transporter 7)
SLC25A27	1554161_at	0.36	0.0008	0.02	Solute carrier family 25, member 27
SLC25A27	230624_at	0.55	0.0006	0.02	Solute carrier family 25, member 27

SLC27A6	219932_at	0.48	0.0005	0.02	Solute carrier family 27 (fatty acid transporter), member 6
SLC4A7	209884_s_at	0.31	0.0001	0.01	Solute carrier family 4, sodium bicarbonate cotransporter, member 7
SLFN13	1553423_a_at	0.31	0.0002	0.01	Schlafen family member 13
SNHG10	244786_at	0.62	0.0000	0.01	small nucleolar RNA host gene 10 (non-protein coding)
SNHG12	228990_at	0.43	0.0000	0.01	Small nucleolar RNA host gene 12 (non-protein coding)
SNHG12	223773_s_at	0.53	0.0000	0.01	Small nucleolar RNA host gene 12 (non-protein coding)
SNORD104	228879_at	0.43	0.0000	0.01	Small nucleolar RNA, C/D box 104
SOX6	227498_at	−0.33	0.0007	0.02	SRY (sex determining region Y)-box 6
SOX6	228214_at	−0.31	0.0000	0.01	SRY (sex determining region Y)-box 6
STC2	203439_s_at	0.49	0.0008	0.02	Stanniocalcin 2
SYCP2	206546_at	0.45	0.0000	0.01	Synaptonemal complex protein 2
SYTL1	227134_at	0.37	0.0005	0.02	Synaptotagmin-like 1
TCTE3	1557945_at	0.35	0.0004	0.01	t-Complex-associated-testis-expressed 3
TNMD	220065_at	−0.58	0.0009	0.02	Tenomodulin
TRAF3IP3	213888_s_at	0.31	0.0006	0.02	TRAF3 interacting protein 3
TTC14	225180_at	0.37	0.0002	0.01	Tetratricopeptide repeat domain 14
TTC18	229170_s_at	0.41	0.0002	0.01	Tetratricopeptide repeat domain 18
TTC6	1556666_a_at	0.76	0.0001	0.01	Tetratricopeptide repeat domain 6
UQCC	229672_at	0.35	0.0001	0.01	Ubiquinol-cytochrome c reductase complex chaperone
UROD	222074_at	0.33	0.0000	0.01	Uroporphyrinogen decarboxylase
VAMP1	213326_at	0.40	0.0000	0.01	Vesicle-associated membrane protein 1 (synaptobrevin 1)
WDR52	230152_at	0.39	0.0005	0.02	WD repeat domain 52
WDR90	227894_at	0.32	0.0000	0.01	WD repeat domain 90
WSB1	210561_s_at	0.35	0.0003	0.01	WD repeat and SOCS box-containing 1
XIST	224589_at	0.39	0.0000	0.01	X (inactive)-specific transcript (non-protein coding)
XIST	221728_x_at	0.57	0.0000	0.01	X (inactive)-specific transcript (non-protein coding)
XIST	214218_s_at	0.57	0.0000	0.01	X (inactive)-specific transcript (non-protein coding)

(continued)

Table 6.1 (continued)

Gene symbol	Probe ID	Log ratio	*p* Value	Adj. *p* value	Gene name
ZDHHC11	1552283_s_at	0.37	0.0000	0.01	Zinc finger, DHHC-type containing 11
ZDHHC11	221646_s_at	0.42	0.0000	0.01	Zinc finger, DHHC-type containing 11
ZMAT1	226344_at	0.47	0.0005	0.02	Zinc finger, matrin type 1
ZNF107	205739_x_at	0.37	0.0001	0.01	Zinc finger protein 107
ZNF207	1556035_s_at	0.41	0.0007	0.02	Zinc finger protein 207
ZNF207	228157_at	0.59	0.0002	0.01	Zinc finger protein 207
ZNF692	220661_s_at	0.34	0.0000	0.00	Zinc finger protein 692
ZNF711	228988_at	0.41	0.0003	0.01	Zinc finger protein 711
ZNF767	219627_at	0.41	0.0002	0.01	Zinc finger family member 767
ZNF785	1554769_at	0.32	0.0003	0.01	Zinc finger protein 785
ZNF789	235231_at	0.32	0.0005	0.02	Zinc finger protein 789
ZNF814	60794_f_at	0.34	0.0006	0.02	Zinc finger protein 814
ZNF83	221645_s_at	0.42	0.0001	0.01	Zinc finger protein 83
	215768_at	−0.49	0.0003	0.01	
	244876_at	−0.47	0.0000	0.01	
	1556935_at	−0.44	0.0004	0.02	
	233648_at	−0.44	0.0006	0.02	
	242736_at	−0.43	0.0002	0.01	
	1560049_at	−0.43	0.0000	0.01	
	1568920_at	−0.42	0.0001	0.01	
	1570246_at	−0.42	0.0006	0.02	
	239220_at	−0.42	0.0008	0.02	
	232331_at	−0.40	0.0009	0.02	
	242868_at	−0.40	0.0000	0.01	
	240772_at	−0.38	0.0000	0.01	
	232882_at	−0.37	0.0003	0.01	
	231644_at	−0.35	0.0009	0.02	
	228731_at	−0.33	0.0008	0.02	

243819_at	–0.33	0.0008	0.02
234224_at	–0.33	0.0003	0.01
234074_at	–0.33	0.0001	0.01
243039_at	–0.31	0.0001	0.01
232582_at	–0.30	0.0002	0.01
239102_s_at	–0.30	0.0005	0.02
232852_at	–0.30	0.0007	0.02
230664_at	0.31	0.0002	0.01
238466_at	0.32	0.0001	0.01
230314_at	0.32	0.0001	0.01
228539_at	0.32	0.0001	0.01
229654_at	0.32	0.0005	0.02
223528_s_at	0.32	0.0000	0.01
229830_at	0.33	0.0003	0.01
229926_at	0.33	0.0004	0.01
1557383_a_at	0.35	0.0003	0.01
239624_at	0.35	0.0007	0.02
235611_at	0.36	0.0003	0.01
239644_at	0.36	0.0002	0.01
244663_at	0.37	0.0002	0.01
226316_at	0.37	0.0002	0.01
239209_at	0.38	0.0001	0.01
244271_at	0.38	0.0003	0.01
214870_x_at	0.38	0.0001	0.01
228464_at	0.39	0.0002	0.01
230304_at	0.39	0.0001	0.01
229111_at	0.39	0.0003	0.01
235892_at	0.40	0.0001	0.01

(continued)

Table 6.1 (continued)

Gene symbol	Probe ID	Log ratio	*p* Value	Adj. *p* value	Gene name
	213212_x_at	0.41	0.0006	0.02	
	235607_at	0.41	0.0001	0.01	
	222018_at	0.41	0.0008	0.02	
	214291_at	0.42	0.0005	0.02	
	235535_x_at	0.43	0.0008	0.02	
	238501_at	0.44	0.0010	0.02	
	240405_at	0.44	0.0001	0.01	
	240182_at	0.45	0.0000	0.01	
	226444_at	0.45	0.0010	0.02	
	214683_s_at	0.48	0.0004	0.01	
	228465_at	0.51	0.0001	0.01	
	221973_at	0.55	0.0001	0.01	
	241863_x_at	0.55	0.0000	0.01	
	229455_at	0.55	0.0001	0.01	
	235771_at	0.55	0.0001	0.01	
	230333_at	0.59	0.0003	0.01	
	235902_at	0.60	0.0001	0.01	
	1556839_s_at	0.62	0.0000	0.01	
	229795_at	0.64	0.0001	0.01	

Total RNA from the core biopsy samples was isolated using the Qiagen Allprep RNA/DNA Mini Kit according to the manufacturer's instructions (Qiagen, Alameda, CA, USA). Total RNA was eluted in a final volume of 60 mL (H2O) and stored at −80 °C until further processing. RNA quantity and quality was assessed by means of the Agilent 2100 Bioanalyzer (Agilent Technologies, Palo Alto, CA, USA). The amount of total RNA yielded from the core biopsies 2 and 3 ranged from 150 ng to 4 mg depending on the ratio of stroma to epithelial tissue. The GeneChip Expression 3¢-Amplification Two-Cycle cDNA Synthesis Kit was used (Affymetrix, Santa Clara, CA). Double-stranded cDNA was synthesized from 100 ng of total RNA. An in vitro transcription (IVT) reaction was then performed to produce biotin-labeled cRNA from the cDNA. The cRNA was fragmented before hybridization. A hybridization cocktail, which included the fragmented target, was prepared. The hybridization cocktail was then hybridized to Affymetrix HG_U133 Plus 2.0 oligonucleotide arrays containing probes to 54,675 transcripts. A total of 169 chips were run. Nine chips were rejected based on standard Affymetrix quality control measures (average background, scale factors, percent present calls). Twenty-eight chips were removed based on probe-level model (PLM) analysis (i.e., in the normalized unscaled standard error (NUSE) plot, the overall median value was below the first quartile of the chip). Nineteen chips represented technical replicates of other (good quality) chips and were excluded from the parous/nulliparous comparison. This left 113 chips (71 parous, 42 nulliparous) in the differential expression analysis of parous vs. nulliparous. Affymetrix gene chips were processed in unbalanced batches of approximately 8 each, and systematic variations in gene expression intensities related to batch were observed. Due to differences in the batch sizes and proportions of parous samples in each batch, we used a permutation test based on the sum of within-batch Mann–Whitney U statistics. The statistic was computed as follows. For each batch, the number of parous–nulliparous pairs in which the intensity of the parous sample exceeded that of the nulliparous sample was calculated. The sum of these counts (Ci) across all applicable batches for probeset i was used as a statistic for consistency of differential expression. The null distribution of the statistic was calculated by repeating the calculation over a large number of permutations of the parity-status vector, with batch membership maintained. This null distribution was then used to derive the p-value for the observed value of Ci. A standardized version of the statistic obtained by rescaling it to take values between −1 and 1 was used as a metric for ranking probesets for downstream analysis. The genes were selected based on a p-value cut-off of 0.001 for further bioinformatics analyses. The standardized score derived from the within-batch Mann–Whitney U statistics was used as a metric to rank differentially expressed genes. Gene ontology (GO) functional categories enriched in differentially expressed genes were identified using conditional hyper-geometric tests in the GOstats package (R/BioConductor). A p-value cut-off of 0.01 was used in selecting GO terms. Ingenuity Pathways Analysis (IPA version 8.5) (http://www.ingenuity.com/) was used to search for underlying biological pathways and molecular networks. IPA provides a rich functional annotation of genes and proteins, protein–protein interactions, and the roles of genes in various diseases. The genes differentially expressed between parous and nulliparous breast samples were uploaded into IPA along with the ranking metrics. These genes were searched in the IPA's functional annotation database, the IPKB. Depending on the input gene list, Ingenuity software models networks and pathways through a statistical computation using functional relationships such as interaction, activation, and localization, between proteins, genes, complexes, cells, tissues, drugs, and diseases. Given a list of genes and their expression values or fold change metrics, IPA computes a score for network eligible genes that were uploaded. The score is simply the negative exponent of this p-value calculation which calculates the likelihood that the Network Eligible Molecules that are part of a network are found therein by random chance alone. A higher score implies a significant composition of genes in a network. Finally, to identify canonical pathways and associations to other knowledge datasets, Gene Set Enrichment Analysis (GSEA) was performed against the lists of differentially expressed genes between parous and nulliparous samples. For GSEA, we did not apply any fold change filter. Canonical pathways were tested for enrichment and pathways were obtained from MSigDB, which is a database of gene sets provided by GSEA. Default parameters were chosen, except that the maximum intensity of probes was only selected while collapsing probe sets for a single gene. To depict the genes that are enriched by GSEA methods as a heatmap, we used the RMA expression values and performed an average linkage hierarchical clustering on selected genes and all the 113 samples (adapted with permission from [45])

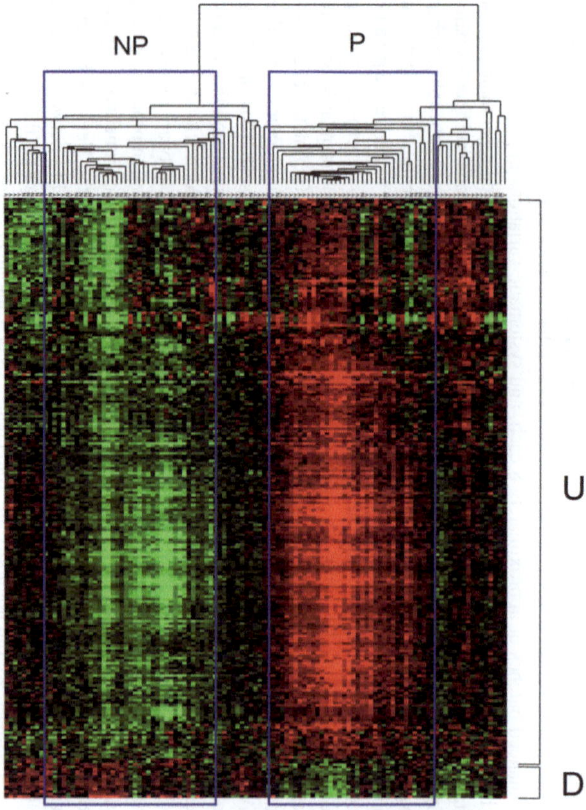

Fig. 6.1 Hierarchical clustering of differentially expressed probesets in parous and nulliparous women. *Red* represents expression values above the median across all samples, and *green* represents values below the median. In the two top-level clusters of samples, the right cluster is composed mainly of parous samples and the left cluster is composed mainly of nulliparous samples. *U* represents the intensity of upregulated probesets among parous samples, whereas *D* represents the intensity of downregulated probesets (reprinted with permission from [45])

expressed between parous and nulliparous breast samples were uploaded into IPA along with the ranking metrics. These genes were searched in the IPA's functional annotation database, the Ingenuity Pathways Knowledge Database (IPKB). Depending on the input gene list, Ingenuity software models networks and pathways through a statistical computation using functional relationships such as interaction, activation, and localization, between proteins, genes, complexes, cells, tissues, drugs, and diseases. Given a list of genes and their expression values or fold change metrics, IPA computes a score for network eligible genes that were uploaded. The score is simply the negative exponent of this *p*-value calculation which calculates the likelihood that the Network Eligible Molecules that are part of a network are found therein by random chance alone. A higher score implies a significant composition of genes in a network. Finally, to identify canonical pathways and associations to other knowledge datasets, Gene Set Enrichment Analysis (GSEA) was performed against the lists of differentially expressed genes between parous and nulliparous samples. For GSEA, we did not apply any fold change filter. Canonical pathways were tested for enrichment and pathways were obtained from MSigDB, which is a database of gene sets provided by GSEA. Default parameters were chosen, except that the maximum intensity of probes was only selected while collapsing probe sets for a single gene. To depict the genes that are enriched by GSEA methods as a heatmap, we used the RMA expression values and performed an average linkage hierarchical clustering on selected genes (Fig. 6.1).

6.3 The Genomic Analysis

From the 126 samples hybridized to Affymetrix HG_U133 Plus 2.0 oligonucleotide arrays, 113 chips (71 P, 42 NP) satisfied quality control thresholds. Using empirical Bayes moderated t-statistics with p-value less than 0.001 and a minimum log2 fold change of 0.3 thresholds as criteria of significance, we identified 305 differentially expressed probesets (corresponding to 208 distinct genes) between P and NP women (Table 6.1). Of these, 267 were upregulated and 38 were downregulated (Fig. 6.1). To understand the biological theme of the observed gene expression differences, we carried out bioinformatics-based analysis of microarray data. Gene ontology (GO) enrichment analysis revealed biological processes that were categorized into groups including RNA metabolic processes, differentiation and development of epidermis and ectoderm, and cell-substrate junction assembly (Table 6.2), findings that are in agreement with existing knowledge that pregnancy hormones promote the differentiation of mammary epithelial cells [4]. Highly represented in the parous breast were biological processes involving both mRNA and RNA metabolic processes and RNA splicing machinery. Important genes that were upregulated within these categories were: RBMX, HNRNPA1, HNRNPA2B1, HNRNPD, LUC7L3, PNN, PRPF39, RBM25, SFPQ, SFRS1, SFRS5, SFRS7, PABPN1, and PRPF4B. Biological processes such as differentiation and development of epithelial and ectodermal cells were represented by the up-regulation of COL7A1, KRT5, KRT15, LAMA3, LAMC2, NTF4, and KLK7. We also found that genes which are pivotal in two biological processes that are critical to the anchoring of epithelial cells to the basement membrane, hemidesmosome, and cell-substrate junction assembly, such as KRT5, LAMA3 and LAMC2, were upregulated in the P group (Table 6.2).

Among the downregulated genes, insulin-like growth factor 1 (IGF1) was enriched in 19 biological processes that comprised cell proliferation, regulation of IGF-like growth factor receptor signaling, somatic stem cell maintenance, muscle cell differentiation and apoptosis, among others. Other downregulated genes were RALGAPA2, SOX6, ABHD5, EBF1, and RASD1 (Table 6.2).

We used GSEA to compare differentially expressed genes from this study to 3,717 curated gene sets of specific pathways, processes, and profiles of previous profiling experiments obtained through MSigDB [19]. Pathways enriched by upregulated genes included breast cancer estrogen signaling, cell communication, and mRNA processing (Table 6.3). The breast cancer estrogen signaling pathway encompassed a set of genes that were dysregulated in estrogen receptor-dependent breast cancers. Among these genes were SCGB2A1, SCGB2A2, GATA3, TP53, TFF1, STC2, SerpinB5, and SerpinA3. Since full-term pregnancy involves the influx of several hormones including estrogen, we postulated that several downstream targets of estrogen would be co-regulated in parous subjects (Table 6.4). Other pathways that were enriched by upregulated genes were cell communication (DSC3 and KRT5) and the mRNA processing reactome (Table 6.3). Of great interest was the significant number of genes related to the mRNA processing reactome that were differentially expressed by parity. This pathway was comprised of those genes involved in key molecular mechanisms that encompass mRNA and pre-mRNA

Table 6.2 Overrepresented GO biological processes for differentially expressed genes*

GO term ID	GO term	Genes upregulated in parous samples
GO:0007044	Cell-substrate junction assembly	KRT5, LAMA3, LAMC2
GO:0007398	Ectoderm development	COL7A1, KRT5, KRT15, LAMA3, LAMC2, NTF4, KLK7
GO:0008544	Epidermis development	COL7A1, KRT5, KRT15, LAMA3, LAMC2, NTF4, KLK7
GO:0010160	Formation of organ boundary	NTF4
GO:0031581	Hemidesmosome assembly	KRT5, LAMA3, LAMC2
GO:0016071	mRNA metabolic process	CIRBP, RBMX, HNRNPA1, HNRNPA2B1, HNRNPD, LUC7L3, PNN, PRPF39, RBM25, SFPQ, SFRS1, SFRS5, SFRS7, PABPN1, PRPF4B
GO:0006397	mRNA processing	RBMX, HNRNPA1, HNRNPA2B1, LUC7L3, PNN, PRPF39, RBM25, SFPQ, SFRS1, SFRS5, SFRS7, PABPN1, PRPF4B
GO:0034059	Response to anoxia	OXTR
GO:0016070	RNA metabolic process	DDX17, CHD2, CBX3, CIRBP, ZNF785, EZH2, L3MBTL, GATA3, RBMX, ZNF789, HNRNPA1, HNRNPA2B1, HNRNPD, LUC7L3, PNN, PRPF39, ZNF83, METTL3, CREBZF, RBM25, RBBP8, RPS24, CENPK, SFPQ, SFRS1, SFRS5, SFRS7, ZNF814, ZNF207, PABPN1, RUNX3, FUBP1, PRPF4B, HNRPDL
GO:0006396	RNA processing	DDX17, RBMX, HNRNPA1, HNRNPA2B1, HNRNPD, LUC7L3, PNN, PRPF39, RBM25, RPS24, SFPQ, SFRS1, SFRS5, SFRS7, PABPN1, PRPF4B, HNRPDL
GO:0008380	RNA splicing	RBMX, HNRNPA1, HNRNPA2B1, HNRNPD, LUC7L3, PNN, PRPF39, RBM25, SFPQ, SFRS1, SFRS5, SFRS7, PABPN1, PRPF4B
GO term ID	**GO term**	**Genes downregulated in parous samples**
GO:0032859	Activation of Ral GTPase activity	RALGAPA2
GO:0021534	Cell proliferation in hindbrain	IGF1
GO:0009441	Glycolate metabolic process	IGF1
GO:0042692	Muscle cell differentiation	IGF1, SOX6
GO:0051450	Myoblast proliferation	IGF1
GO:0006654	Phosphatidic acid biosynthetic process	ABHD5

(continued)

Table 6.2 (continued)

GO term ID	GO term	Genes downregulated in parous samples
GO:0031325	Positive regulation of cellular metabolic process	EBF1, IGF1, ABHD5, SOX6
GO:0045821	Positive regulation of glycolysis	IGF1
GO:0051006	Positive regulation of lipoprotein lipase activity	ABHD5
GO:0042523	Positive regulation of tyrosine phosphorylation of Stat5 protein	IGF1
GO:0031329	Regulation of cellular catabolic process	IGF1, ABHD5
GO:0043567	Regulation of insulin-like growth factor receptor signaling pathway	IGF1
GO:0010660	Regulation of muscle cell apoptosis	IGF1
GO:0032485	Regulation of Ral protein signal transduction	RALGAPA2
GO:0010889	Regulation of sequestering of triglyceride	ABHD5
GO:0033143	Regulation of steroid hormone receptor signaling pathway	IGF1
GO:0090207	Regulation of triglyceride metabolic process	ABHD5
GO:0043403	Skeletal muscle tissue regeneration	IGF1
GO:0007264	Small GTPase mediated signal transduction	IGF1, RASD1, RALGAPA2
GO:0035019	Somatic stem cell maintenance	IGF1

*Adapted with permission from [45].

Table 6.3 Overrepresented GSEA gene sets for differentially expressed genes*

Pathways enriched by upregulated genes	NES	FDR q-value	Genes
Breast cancer estrogen signaling	2.217	0.002	SCGB2A1, TFF1, SCGB2A2, SCGB1D2, STC2, GATA3, SERPINB5, SERPINA3, AZGP1, TP53, CCNA2, CCNE2, EGFR, PTEN, DLC1, FHL5
HSA01430 cell communication	1.711	0.075	KRT15, DSC3, DSG3, KRT5, COL4A6, KRT17, KRT14, LAMC2, LAMA3, LAMB3, THBS3, LAMA5, LAMC1, GJA4, LAMA4, VWF, COL4A1, COL4A2
mRNA processing reactome	1.626	0.093	METTL3, HNRPD, HNRPA2B1, PRPF4B, SFRS7, CLK4, SFRS5, PABPN1, CSTF3, HNRPU, RBM5, SNRP70, SFRS14, SNRPA1, CLK2, NXF1, SFRS8, SFRS2, PTBP2, FUS, SFRS6, SFRS16, SF3B1, HNRPA3, SNRPB, PRPF3, SFRS12, U2AF1, PHF5A, TXNL4A, CUGBP2

Pathways enriched by downregulated genes	NES	FDR q-value	Genes
HSA04910 insulin signaling pathway	−2.242	0.004	CALML3, SHC4, IKBKB, PKM2, PIK3CD, PHKA1, CALM1, CBL, MAPK9, GSK3B, SKIP, MAP2K1, PIK3R3, CRK, IRS2, SORBS1, SOS1, PDE3A, PDE3B, PRKAR2B, MAPK10, PCK1
HSA04080 neuroactive ligand receptor interaction	−2.148	0.007	NPY2R, OXTR, PARD3, GABBR1, LTB4R, NR3C1, EDNRA, EDNRB, EDG1, CALCRL, ADRB2, AGTRL1, ADRA2A, GHR, PTGER3, ADRA1A
HSA04530 tight junction	−2.053	0.012	CGN, INADL, EXOC3, LLGL2, PARD3, PARD6G, TJP1, EPB41L1, ZAK, PPP2R1B, PTEN, GNAI1, RRAS2, CTNNA1, MAGI1, CLDN10
HSA04010 MAPK signaling pathway	−2.018	0.013	NTF5, FGFR3, CACNA1D, RASGRP1, MAP3K14, TP53, CACNA1G, FAS, PDGFA, IKBKB, CACNA2D2, DAXX, GNA12, MAPK9, EGFR, GADD45A, DUSP10, CHP, DUSP3, MAP2K1, CRK, MEF2C, ZAK, EVI1, TGFBR1, SOS1, FGF10, RAPGEF2, RRAS2, RASGRF2, MAPK10, ACVR1C
HSA05210 colorectal cancer	−1.972	0.013	TP53, IGF1R, FZD8, RALGDS, PIK3CD, FZD6, CYCS, MAPK9, EGFR, GSK3B, MAP2K1, PIK3R3, TGFBR1, SOS1, TCF7L2, FZD4, MAPK10, ACVR1C
HSA04510 focal adhesion	−1.913	0.016	PAK7, COL4A6, LAMC2, LAMA3, SHC4, PAK6, ITGA10, LAMB3, ITGA4, PDGFA, IGF1R, THBS3, LAMA5, ZYX, PPP1R12A, ITGA2, PIK3CD, MAPK9, CAV1, EGFR, PARVA, GSK3B, LAMC1, MAP2K1, PIK3R3, CRK, FLT1, FYN, CCND2, PTEN, LAMA4, SOS1, VWF, IGF1, CAV2, TLN2, COL4A1, PDGFC, COL4A2, MAPK10
Integrin mediated cell adhesion KEGG	−1.661	0.062	CAPN3, PAK6, ITGA10, ITGA4, ZYX, ITGA2, CAV1, MAP2K1, CRK, SORBS1, FYN, SOS1, CAV2, TNS1, MAPK10

(continued)

Table 6.3 (continued)

Pathways enriched by downregulated genes	NES	FDR q-value	Genes
HSA04310 Wnt signaling pathway	−1.423	0.161	CSNK1A1, NFATC3, TP53, WNT5A, VANGL2, FZD8, FZD6, MAPK9, GSK3B, CHP, DAAM1, DAAM2, SOX17, PPP2R1B, CCND2, TCF7L2, FZD4, MAPK10
ST integrin signaling pathway	−1.400	0.160	PAK7, PAK6, ITGA10, ITGA4, ZYX, ITGA2, MAPK9, CAV1, CRK, ARHGEF7, FYN, PTEN, SOS1, TLN2, MAPK10
HSA04060 cytokine–cytokine receptor interaction	−1.383	0.152	CXCL6, IL28RA, CCL5, IFNGR2, FAS, IL4R, TNFSF15, PF4V1, TNFRSF14, IL2RB, IFNAR1, EGFR, LIFR, FLT1, BMPR2, TGFBR1, PDGFC, GHR, BMP2

*Adapted with permission from [45]

Table 6.4 Genes differentially expressed by full-term pregnancy (P) when compared to women who did not have a full-term pregnancy (GN) ($p < 0.001$ and log2 fold change of at least 0.3)*

Gene symbol	Gene name	Probe ID	Log ratio	*p* Value	Adj. *p* value
ADCYAP1R1	Adenylate cyclase activating polypeptide 1 (pituitary) receptor type I	226690_at	−0.35	0.0005	0.41
BMPR1B	Bone morphogenetic protein receptor, type IB	229975_at	1.17	0.0001	0.41
C8orf84	Chromosome 8 open reading frame 84	235209_at	0.67	0.0007	0.41
C8orf84	Chromosome 8 open reading frame 84	235210_s_at	0.68	0.0009	0.41
C9orf5	Chromosome 9 open reading frame 5	223007_s_at	−0.31	0.0005	0.41
CDK5RAP3	CDK5 regulatory subunit associated protein 3	218740_s_at	0.34	0.0007	0.41
CLN5	Ceroid-lipofuscinosis, neuronal 5	214252_s_at	0.33	0.0001	0.41
CYTSB	Cytospin B	228900_at	−0.35	0.0009	0.41
FAM101A	Family with sequence similarity 101, member A	227320_at	0.39	0.0007	0.41
MIA	Melanoma inhibitory activity	206560_s_at	0.66	0.0008	0.41
MPPED2	Metallophosphoesterase domain containing 2	205413_at	0.53	0.0001	0.41
SPRY4	Sprouty homolog 4 (*Drosophila*)	221489_s_at	−0.38	0.0005	0.41
XIST	X (inactive)-specific transcript (non-protein coding)	224589_at	0.53	0.0005	0.41
		236373_at	−0.42	0.0001	0.41
		237190_at	−0.32	0.0002	0.41
		232626_at	0.35	0.0010	0.41
		235762_at	0.39	0.0010	0.41
		241600_at	0.40	0.0009	0.41

*Adapted with permission from [45].

Table 6.5 Genes differentially expressed in parous (P) vs. nulligravidas (NG) ($p<0.001$ and log2 fold change of at least 0.3)*

Gene symbol	Gene name	Probe ID	Log ratio	*p* Value	Adj. *p* value
ABAT	4-Aminobutyrate aminotransferase	209459_s_at	0.35	0.0005	0.03
ABHD5	Abhydrolase domain containing 5	213805_at	−0.33	0.0009	0.03
AGBL2	ATP/GTP binding protein-like 2	220390_at	0.32	0.0001	0.02
ANKRD10	Ankyrin repeat domain 10	223251_s_at	0.31	0.0008	0.03
ANXA9	Annexin A9	211712_s_at	0.41	0.0004	0.03
AP1G2	Adaptor-related protein complex 1, gamma 2 subunit	201613_s_at	0.37	0.0002	0.02
ARGLU1	Arginine and glutamate rich 1	228477_at	0.33	0.0005	0.03
BZRAP1	Benzodiazapine receptor (peripheral) associated protein 1	205839_s_at	0.31	0.0004	0.03
C11orf31	Chromosome 11 open reading frame 31	228331_at	0.47	0.0004	0.03
C1orf168	Chromosome 1 open reading frame 168	238625_at	0.82	0.0000	0.02
CAPN8	Calpain 8	229030_at	0.61	0.0001	0.02
CCNL1	Cyclin L1	220046_s_at	0.42	0.0003	0.03
CCNL2	Cyclin L2	222999_s_at	0.47	0.0009	0.03
CDK12	Cyclin-dependent kinase 12	213557_at	0.41	0.0001	0.02
CELF2	CUGBP, Elav-like family member 2	242268_at	−0.36	0.0004	0.03
CGN	Cingulin	223233_s_at	0.41	0.0003	0.03
CGN	Cingulin	223232_s_at	0.46	0.0002	0.02
CHD2	Chromodomain helicase DNA binding protein 2	228999_at	0.31	0.0006	0.03
CIRBP	Cold inducible RNA binding protein	230142_s_at	0.41	0.0003	0.03
CIRBP	Cold inducible RNA binding protein	225191_at	0.57	0.0005	0.03
CMYA5	Cardiomyopathy associated 5	233520_s_at	0.50	0.0000	0.01
COL27A1	Collagen, type XXVII, alpha 1	225288_at	0.55	0.0002	0.02
CREBZF	CREB/ATF bZIP transcription factor	225594_at	0.47	0.0008	0.03
CSNK1A1	Casein kinase 1, alpha 1	1556006_s_at	0.44	0.0003	0.03
CXorf50B	Chromosome X open reading frame 50B	242292_at	0.34	0.0009	0.04
DLC1	Deleted in liver cancer 1	220512_at	−0.35	0.0008	0.03
DNAH5	Dynein, axonemal, heavy chain 5	232381_s_at	0.42	0.0005	0.03
DNALI1	Dynein, axonemal, light intermediate chain 1	227081_at	0.35	0.0006	0.03

DOCK9	Dedicator of cytokinesis 9	232874_at	−0.45	0.0000	0.01
DPP7	Dipeptidyl-peptidase 7	238012_at	0.31	0.0001	0.02
DSC3	Desmocollin 3	206032_at	0.47	0.0007	0.03
DSC3	Desmocollin 3	206033_s_at	0.55	0.0000	0.02
DYX1C1	Dyslexia susceptibility 1 candidate 1	235273_at	0.34	0.0000	0.02
EBF1	Early B-cell factor 1	233261_at	−0.50	0.0007	0.03
ELMO3	Engulfment and cell motility 3	219411_at	0.31	0.0006	0.03
ENOSF1	Enolase superfamily member 1	213645_at	0.50	0.0002	0.02
EPS8L2	EPS8-like 2	218180_s_at	0.32	0.0002	0.02
EZH2	Enhancer of zeste homolog 2 (*Drosophila*)	203358_s_at	0.42	0.0002	0.02
FAM101A	Family with sequence similarity 101, member A	227320_at	0.31	0.0001	0.02
FNBP4	Formin binding protein 4	212232_at	0.37	0.0009	0.03
FYB	FYN binding protein (FYB-120/130)	227266_s_at	0.33	0.0002	0.02
GALNT6	UDP-*N*-acetyl-alpha-D-galactosamine:polypeptide-*N*-acetylgalactosaminyltransferase 6 (GalNAc-T6)	219956_at	0.49	0.0006	0.03
GAS5	Growth arrest-specific 5 (non-protein coding)	227517_s_at	0.70	0.0003	0.03
GATA3	GATA binding protein 3	209602_s_at	0.39	0.0009	0.03
GATA3	GATA binding protein 3	209603_at	0.44	0.0005	0.03
GOLGA2B	Golgin A2 family, member B	233198_at	0.31	0.0006	0.03
GOLGA8A	Golgin A8 family, member A	208798_x_at	0.77	0.0007	0.03
HINT1	Histidine triad nucleotide binding protein 1	1555960_at	0.41	0.0006	0.03
HNRPDL	Heterogeneous nuclear ribonucleoprotein D-like	212454_x_at	0.65	0.0004	0.03
IGF1	Insulin-like growth factor 1 (somatomedin C)	209540_at	−0.37	0.0004	0.03
IL7R	Interleukin 7 receptor	226218_at	0.56	0.0002	0.02
INTU	Inturned planar cell polarity effector homolog (*Drosophila*)	228946_at	0.53	0.0005	0.03
IPW	Imprinted in Prader–Willi syndrome (non-protein coding)	221974_at	0.43	0.0002	0.02
IQCA1	IQ motif containing with AAA domain 1	238584_at	0.46	0.0001	0.02
KRT5	Keratin 5	201820_at	0.41	0.0010	0.04

(continued)

Table 6.5 (continued)

Gene symbol	Gene name	Probe ID	Log ratio	*p* Value	Adj. *p* value
L3MBTL	l(3)mbt-like (*Drosophila*)	210306_at	0.37	0.0010	0.04
LAMC2	Laminin, gamma 2	202267_at	0.38	0.0008	0.03
LNPEP	Leucyl/cystinyl aminopeptidase	231866_at	−0.31	0.0003	0.03
LOC100286909	Hypothetical protein LOC100286909	228528_at	0.45	0.0009	0.03
LOC153682	Hypothetical protein LOC153682	232794_at	0.37	0.0004	0.03
LOC220594	TL132 protein	213510_x_at	0.30	0.0006	0.03
LOC221442	Adenylate cyclase 10 pseudogene	236832_at	0.42	0.0007	0.03
LOC284513	Hypothetical protein LOC284513	1556597_a_at	0.40	0.0009	0.03
LOC339047	Hypothetical protein LOC339047	221501_x_at	0.45	0.0001	0.02
LOC399491	GPS, PLAT, and transmembrane domain-containing protein	214035_x_at	0.39	0.0001	0.02
LOC642587	NPC-A-5	226755_at	0.64	0.0000	0.02
LUC7L3	LUC7-like 3 (*S. cerevisiae*)	220044_x_at	0.32	0.0005	0.03
LUC7L3	LUC7-like 3 (*S. cerevisiae*)	203804_s_at	0.33	0.0010	0.04
MALAT1	Metastasis-associated lung adenocarcinoma transcript 1 (non-protein coding)	224558_s_at	0.57	0.0001	0.02
MARCH3	Membrane-associated ring finger (C3HC4) 3	213256_at	−0.36	0.0001	0.02
MDM1	Mdm1 nuclear protein homolog (mouse)	213761_at	0.31	0.0004	0.03
METTL3	Methyltransferase like 3	213653_at	0.66	0.0001	0.02
MGC24103	Hypothetical MGC24103	232568_at	−0.38	0.0005	0.03
MPPED2	Metallophosphoesterase domain containing 2	205413_at	0.35	0.0001	0.02
MREG	Melanoregulin	219648_at	0.48	0.0001	0.02
MRI1	Methylthioribose-1-phosphate isomerase homolog (*S. cerevisiae*)	228077_at	0.30	0.0009	0.03
NDUFB8	NADH dehydrogenase (ubiquinone) 1 beta subcomplex, 8, 19 kDa	214241_at	0.34	0.0005	0.03
NFKBIZ	Nuclear factor of kappa light polypeptide gene enhancer in B-cells inhibitor, zeta	223217_s_at	0.45	0.0003	0.03
NFKBIZ	Nuclear factor of kappa light polypeptide gene enhancer in B-cells inhibitor, zeta	223218_s_at	0.50	0.0002	0.02
NINL	Ninein-like	207705_s_at	0.30	0.0000	0.02
NLRC3	NLR family, CARD domain containing 3	236295_s_at	0.35	0.0001	0.02
NPHP3	Nephronophthisis 3 (adolescent)	235410_at	0.37	0.0005	0.03
NPIP	Nuclear pore complex interacting protein	204538_x_at	0.42	0.0001	0.02

NRXN1	Neurexin 1	228547_at	0.58	0.0008	0.03
OGT	O-linked *N*-acetylglucosamine (GlcNAc) transferase (UDP-*N*-acetylglucosamine:polypeptide-*N*-acetylglucosaminyl transferase)	207564_x_at	0.33	0.0008	0.03
OGT	O-linked *N*-acetylglucosamine (GlcNAc) transferase (UDP-*N*-acetylglucosamine:polypeptide-*N*-acetylglucosaminyl transferase)	212307_s_at	0.36	0.0005	0.03
OGT	O-linked *N*-acetylglucosamine (GlcNAc) transferase (UDP-*N*-acetylglucosamine:polypeptide-*N*-acetylglucosaminyl transferase)	229787_s_at	0.36	0.0007	0.03
OXTR	Oxytocin receptor	206825_at	0.63	0.0003	0.03
PALM2	Paralemmin 2	1554640_at	−0.37	0.0001	0.02
PAN2	PAN2 poly(A) specific ribonuclease subunit homolog (*S. cerevisiae*)	203117_s_at	0.31	0.0004	0.03
PDZD2	PDZ domain containing 2	233025_at	−0.41	0.0002	0.02
PILRB	Paired immunoglobin-like type 2 receptor beta	220954_s_at	0.51	0.0001	0.02
PILRB	Paired immunoglobin-like type 2 receptor beta	225321_s_at	0.66	0.0004	0.03
PNN	Pinin, desmosome-associated protein	212036_s_at	0.36	0.0008	0.03
PPP1R16B	Protein phosphatase 1, regulatory (inhibitor) subunit 16B	233813_at	−0.33	0.0008	0.03
RALGAPA2	Ral GTPase activating protein, alpha subunit 2 (catalytic)	232500_at	−0.38	0.0000	0.02
RASAL2	RAS protein activator like 2	1557432_at	−0.45	0.0003	0.03
RBBP8	Retinoblastoma binding protein 8	203344_s_at	0.35	0.0000	0.01
RBMX	RNA binding motif protein, X-linked	225310_at	0.38	0.0001	0.02
RDH13	Retinol dehydrogenase 13 (all-*trans*/9-*cis*)	1559190_s_at	0.39	0.0001	0.02
RPL10	Ribosomal protein L10	221989_at	0.59	0.0003	0.03
RUNX3	Runt-related transcription factor 3	204198_s_at	0.32	0.0004	0.03
RUNX3	Runt-related transcription factor 3	204197_s_at	0.36	0.0001	0.02
RYR3	Ryanodine receptor 3	206306_at	0.41	0.0009	0.03
SCARNA15	Small Cajal body-specific RNA 15	228930_at	0.31	0.0004	0.03
SCNN1A	Sodium channel, nonvoltage-gated 1 alpha	203453_at	0.43	0.0005	0.03
SFI1	Sfi1 homolog, spindle assembly associated (yeast)	36545_s_at	0.35	0.0000	0.01

(continued)

Table 6.5 (continued)

Gene symbol	Gene name	Probe ID	Log ratio	p Value	Adj. p value
SFRS18	Splicing factor, arginine/serine-rich 18	212176_at	0.40	0.0007	0.03
SFRS5	Splicing factor, arginine/serine-rich 5	212266_s_at	0.33	0.0006	0.03
SLC16A1	Solute carrier family 16, member 1 (monocarboxylic acid transporter 1)	202234_s_at	–0.31	0.0004	0.03
SLC4A7	Solute carrier family 4, sodium bicarbonate cotransporter, member 7	209884_s_at	0.31	0.0003	0.03
SLFN13	Schlafen family member 13	1553423_a_at	0.32	0.0009	0.04
SNHG10	Small nucleolar RNA host gene 10 (non-protein coding)	244786_at	0.59	0.0005	0.03
SNHG12	Small nucleolar RNA host gene 12 (non-protein coding)	228990_at	0.38	0.0009	0.03
SNHG12	Small nucleolar RNA host gene 12 (non-protein coding)	223773_s_at	0.50	0.0001	0.02
SNORD104	Small nucleolar RNA, C/D box 104	228879_at	0.41	0.0002	0.02
SNRK	SNF related kinase	207474_at	–0.32	0.0006	0.03
SOX6	SRY (sex determining region Y)-box 6	228214_at	–0.31	0.0001	0.02
SYCP2	Synaptonemal complex protein 2	206546_at	0.49	0.0000	0.01
TGFBR1	Transforming growth factor, beta receptor 1	236561_at	–0.31	0.0007	0.03
THSD7A	Thrombospondin, type I, domain containing 7A	213894_at	–0.32	0.0004	0.03
TTC14	Tetratricopeptide repeat domain 14	225180_at	0.37	0.0007	0.03
TTC18	Tetratricopeptide repeat domain 18	229170_s_at	0.42	0.0007	0.03
TTC6	Tetratricopeptide repeat domain 6	1556666_a_at	0.82	0.0002	0.02
UQCC	Ubiquinol-cytochrome c reductase complex chaperone	229672_at	0.35	0.0005	0.03
VAMP1	Vesicle-associated membrane protein 1 (synaptobrevin 1)	213326_at	0.41	0.0002	0.02
WDR90	WD repeat domain 90	227894_at	0.34	0.0001	0.02
XIST	X (inactive)-specific transcript (non-protein coding)	214218_s_at	0.57	0.0003	0.03
XIST	X (inactive)-specific transcript (non-protein coding)	221728_x_at	0.58	0.0001	0.02
ZDHHC11	Zinc finger, DHHC-type containing 11	1552283_s_at	0.38	0.0001	0.02
ZDHHC11	Zinc finger, DHHC-type containing 11	221646_s_at	0.45	0.0001	0.02
ZNF107	Zinc finger protein 107	205739_x_at	0.40	0.0001	0.02
ZNF207	Zinc finger protein 207	228157_at	0.59	0.0007	0.03
ZNF432	Zinc finger protein 432	219848_s_at	0.32	0.0001	0.02
ZNF692	Zinc finger protein 692	220661_s_at	0.34	0.0000	0.01

ZNF767	Zinc finger family member 767	219627_at	0.42	0.0007	0.03
ZNF814	Zinc finger protein 814	60794_f_at	0.37	0.0009	0.03
ZNF83	Zinc finger protein 83	221645_s_at	0.40	0.0009	0.03
		215768_at	−0.64	0.0000	0.01
		233648_at	−0.54	0.0001	0.02
		244876_at	−0.54	0.0000	0.01
		1568920_at	−0.52	0.0000	0.01
		242736_at	−0.51	0.0001	0.02
		240772_at	−0.50	0.0000	0.01
		1560049_at	−0.50	0.0000	0.01
		1556935_at	−0.49	0.0005	0.03
		242868_at	−0.45	0.0000	0.01
		232882_at	−0.45	0.0001	0.02
		234224_at	−0.45	0.0000	0.01
		231644_at	−0.43	0.0002	0.02
		239519_at	−0.43	0.0010	0.04
		1556590_s_at	−0.42	0.0002	0.02
		215791_at	−0.42	0.0004	0.03
		1558410_s_at	−0.41	0.0007	0.03
		234074_at	−0.40	0.0000	0.01
		239102_s_at	−0.40	0.0000	0.02
		241681_at	−0.40	0.0001	0.02
		242457_at	−0.38	0.0005	0.03
		234563_at	−0.38	0.0001	0.02
		1566825_at	−0.38	0.0000	0.01
		1563467_at	−0.38	0.0004	0.03
		232852_at	−0.38	0.0001	0.02
		243819_at	−0.37	0.0006	0.03

(continued)

Table 6.5 (continued)

Gene symbol	Gene name	Probe ID	Log ratio	p Value	Adj. p value
		1556658_a_at	–0.36	0.0007	0.03
		242025_at	–0.36	0.0000	0.02
		233689_at	–0.35	0.0000	0.02
		237778_at	–0.34	0.0002	0.02
		232582_at	–0.34	0.0002	0.02
		242188_at	–0.34	0.0002	0.02
		239809_at	–0.34	0.0004	0.03
		242699_at	–0.34	0.0000	0.01
		243039_at	–0.33	0.0002	0.02
		236355_s_at	–0.33	0.0002	0.02
		233455_at	–0.33	0.0007	0.03
		234118_at	–0.33	0.0000	0.01
		234033_at	–0.33	0.0006	0.03
		236395_at	–0.33	0.0006	0.03
		1556989_at	–0.32	0.0001	0.02
		232776_at	–0.32	0.0006	0.03
		239661_at	–0.32	0.0006	0.03
		1566482_at	–0.31	0.0004	0.03
		241435_at	–0.31	0.0000	0.02
		242664_at	–0.31	0.0005	0.03
		232472_at	–0.30	0.0007	0.03
		244387_at	–0.30	0.0004	0.03
		230314_at	0.31	0.0006	0.03
		228539_at	0.32	0.0008	0.03
		223528_s_at	0.33	0.0001	0.02
		230664_at	0.33	0.0003	0.03
		229654_at	0.35	0.0007	0.03
		238466_at	0.35	0.0000	0.02

239644_at	0.37	0.0007	0.03
226316_at	0.38	0.0007	0.03
230304_at	0.38	0.0005	0.03
239209_at	0.39	0.0003	0.03
244663_at	0.39	0.0004	0.03
235607_at	0.40	0.0005	0.03
240182_at	0.42	0.0005	0.03
214870_x_at	0.42	0.0002	0.02
228465_at	0.50	0.0006	0.03
241863_x_at	0.54	0.0002	0.02
221973_at	0.54	0.0004	0.03
235771_at	0.55	0.0004	0.03
229455_at	0.55	0.0004	0.03
235902_at	0.58	0.0004	0.03
1556839_s_at	0.62	0.0002	0.02

*Adapted with permission from [45]

Table 6.6 Gene validation by real time RT-PCR*

ABI assay	Gene symbol	Gene name	RT-PCR Log ratio	*p*-value	95 % CI
Hs00221881_m1	CREBZF	CREB/ATF bZIP transcription factor	1.59	0.000	[0.705, 2.545]
Hs00300535_s1	XIST	X (inactive)-specific transcript (non-protein coding)	1.19	0.006	[0.375, 1.95]
Hs01085988_m1	CCNL2	Cyclin L2	0.75	0.030	[0.055, 1.42]
Hs00419658_m1	C1orf168	Chromosome 1 open reading frame 168	0.60	0.069	[−0.14, 1.365]
Hs00264525_m1	SOX6	SRY (sex determining region Y)-box 6	−0.59	0.118	[−1.215, 0.13]
Hs00273907_s1	MALAT1	Metastasis-associated lung adenocarcinoma transcript 1 (non-protein coding)	0.54	0.139	[−0.08, 1.265]
Hs00245657_m1	HNRPDL	Heterogeneous nuclear ribonucleoprotein D-like	0.62	0.156	[−0.2, 1.555]
Hs00231122_m1	GATA3	GATA binding protein 3	0.69	0.170	[−0.19, 1.345]
Hs00428757_m1	DDX17	DEAD (Asp-Glu-Ala-Asp) box polypeptide 17	0.45	0.196	[−0.375, 1.08]
Hs01008264_s1	NEAT1	Nuclear paraspeckle assembly transcript 1 (non-protein coding)	0.39	0.236	[−0.2, 1.075]
Hs00414754_m1	SNHG12	Small nucleolar RNA host gene 12 (non-protein coding)	0.50	0.308	[−0.425, 1.435]
Hs01547656_m1	IGF1	Insulin-like growth factor 1 (somatomedin C)	−0.50	0.335	[−1.585, 0.595]
Hs01086912_m1	HNRNPD	Heterogeneous nuclear ribonucleoprotein D (AU-rich element RNA binding protein 1, 37 kDa)	0.19	0.584	[−0.595, 0.96]
Hs00740805_g1	PABPN1	Poly(A) binding protein, nuclear 1	0.17	0.650	[−0.61, 0.89]
Hs00242600_m1	HNRNPA2B1	Heterogeneous nuclear ribonucleoprotein A2/B1	0.17	0.779	[−0.65, 0.805]

*Adapted with permission from [45]

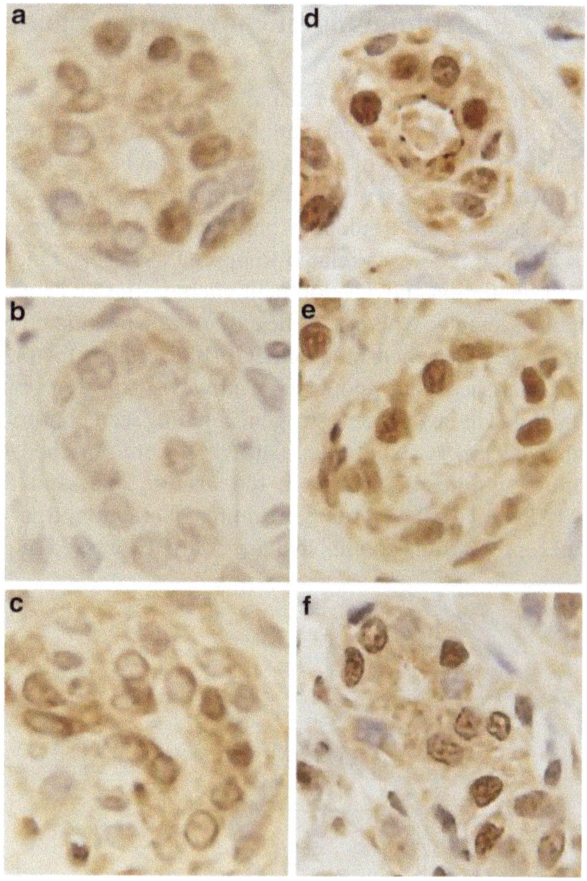

Fig. 6.2 Immunohistochemistry of cyclin–cyclin L2 protein (CCNL2) performed in paraffin embedded tissues of nulliparous and parous samples. CCNL2 protein was overexpressed in the nucleus of epithelial cells of lobules type 1 in parous breast (**d–f**) when compared to nulliparous women (**a–c**) (×40) (reprinted with permission from [45]

processing reactions, as well as splicing of mRNAs, whose representative genes include METTL3, HNRPD, HNRPA2B1, PABPN1, PRPF4B, SRSF7, CLK4, and SFRS5 (Table 6.5). Among the key pathways that were enriched by downregulated genes, the most significant ones were the insulin signaling pathway, MAPK, cytokine–cytokine receptor interaction, and Wnt signaling pathways (Table 6.3). In Table 6.6, we depict the genes that were validated using RT-PCR. The genes XIST, CREBZF, CCNL2, AHSA2, CIRBP, PILRB, OXTR, and TNMD displayed the same expression behavior in both microarray and real time RT-PCR. XIST, CREBZF, and CCNL2 were significantly ($p < 0.05$) upregulated in the parous women. In addition, the level of expression and localization of CCNL2 was verified by immunohistochemistry in nulliparous and parous breasts (Fig. 6.2). CCNL2 protein was significantly overexpressed in the nucleus of epithelial cells of lobules type 1 of the parous breast (Fig. 6.2d–f) when compared with similar structures found in the breast of nulliparous women (Fig. 6.2a–c). These observations confirm the localization of this protein in the splicing factor compartment (nuclear speckles) [20].

6.4 Functional Significance of the Signature of Pregnancy

Differentiation of the breast induced by an early pregnancy imprints a specific genomic signature that can be detected in postmenopausal women (Fig. 6.3; Table 6.7). Using bioinformatics methods, we found transcriptomic differences between the breasts of parous and nulliparous women. These differentially expressed genes were used to identify enriched biological processes and pathways. Enriched biological processes related to upregulated genes included RNA-related processes, differentiation and development of epidermis and ectoderm, and cell-substrate junction assembly; whereas in the case of downregulated genes the biological processes that were enriched included IGF-like growth factor signaling, somatic stem cell maintenance, and apoptosis. Pathways that were enriched by upregulated genes included breast cancer estrogen signaling, cell communication, and mRNA processing machinery. Numerous pathways were enriched by downregulated genes; the most significant ones were the insulin, Wnt and integrins signaling pathways, MAPK, cytokine–cytokine receptor interaction, tight junction, and focal adhesion, all representing proteins that are highly expressed in malignancies.

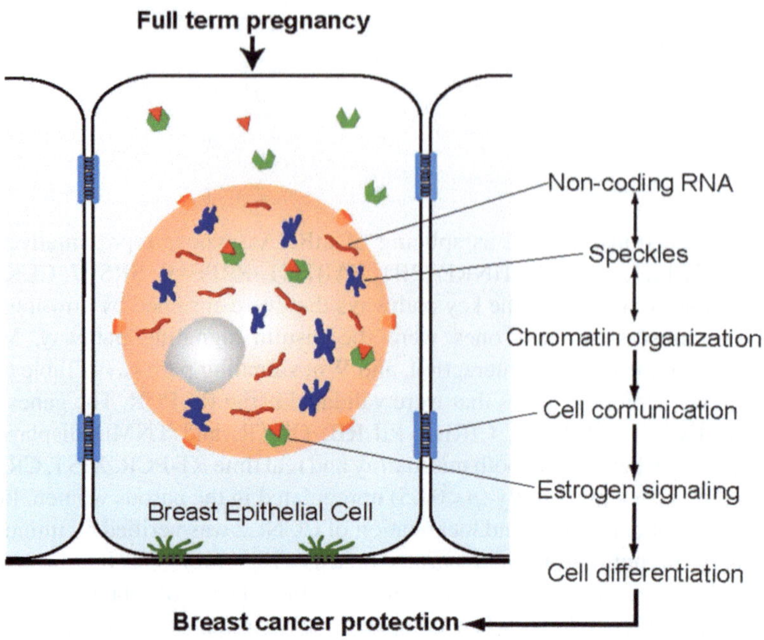

Fig. 6.3 Proposed model of the biological processes involved in differentiation of breast epithelial cells of postmenopausal parous women (reprinted with permission from [45]

6.4.1 The Spliceosome Machinery

The main components of the spliceosome machinery, including RNA and proteins that undergo dynamic changes during the splicing reaction, were upregulated in the parous breast. Among them were the heterogeneous nuclear ribonucleoproteins (HNRPs) that include HNRPA3, HNRPA2B1, HNRPD, and HNRPU [21], which are implicated in the regulation of mRNA stability, as well as other functions, such as mammary gland involution [22], negative regulation of telomere length maintenance [23], and regulation of mRNA trafficking from the nucleus to distal processes in neural cells [24]. Although further studies are needed to define their precise functional role in the postmenopausal breast, we postulate that they may play an important regulatory function as transcriptional regulators. In addition, post-transcriptional methylation of internal adenosine residues in eukaryotic mRNAs by METTL3 (methyltransferase like 3), which is upregulated in the parous breast, could play a role in the efficiency of mRNA splicing, transport, or translation in the differentiated breast epithelium. Other members of the spliceosome complex are the proteins encoded by the genes SF3B1, SFRS2, SFRS7, SFRS8, SFRS14, SFRS16, SNRP70, SNRPB, SNRPA1, PRF3, and PHF5A, all of which are overexpressed in the parous breast. In the case of the small nuclear ribonucleoproteins (snRNPs), there is evidence that they suppress tumor cell growth and may have major implications as cancer therapeutic targets. The pre-mRNA splicing factors are enriched in nuclear domains termed interchromatin granule clusters or nuclear speckles. Among the members of the splicing factor compartment are CCNL1 and CCNL2 that participate in the pre-mRNA splicing process and are located in the nuclear speckles [25, 26]. These two genes are upregulated in the parous breast and the CCNL2 protein is also overexpressed in the nucleus of breast epithelial cells. CCNL1 and CCNL2 are transcriptional regulators [25–28] that modulate the expression of critical factors leading to cell apoptosis, possibly through the Wnt signal transduction pathway [27], a signaling pathway that is enriched by downregulated genes in the parous breast (Table 6.2). In our previously published preclinical and clinical studies [4, 5, 7, 11], we have reported that pregnancy confers protection from breast cancer development by inducing gland differentiation, which imprints a specific and permanent genomic signature in this organ. A similar phenomenon was demonstrated in the involuted breast of postmenopausal parous women [4]. We previously described a case-control study of transcriptomic analysis of normal breast tissues obtained from parous and nulliparous women free of breast pathology and parous and nulliparous women with history of breast cancer that served as controls and cases, respectively [4]. In order to investigate the degree of commonality between the previous case-control and the present study, we applied GO enrichment analysis to the gene lists generated from both studies. We found that processes involved in RNA metabolism and RNA processing were similar in both studies (Table 6.8).

Table 6.7 Important differentially expressed genes in parous vs. nulliparous ($p<0.001$ and log2 fold change of at least 0.3)*

Gene symbol	Log ratio	Gene name
ABHD5	−0.32	Abhydrolase domain containing 5
C1orf168	0.80	Chromosome 1 open reading frame 168
CBX3	0.53	Chromobox homolog 3 (HP1 gamma homolog, *Drosophila*)
CCNL1	0.40	Cyclin L2
CCNL2	0.47	Cyclin L2
CREBZF	0.48	CREB/ATF bZIP transcription factor
DDX17	0.49	DEAD (Asp-Glu-Ala-Asp) box polypeptide 17
DSC3	0.55	Desmocollin 3
EBF1	−0.33	Early B-cell factor 1
EZH2	0.44	Enhancer of zeste homolog 2 (*Drosophila*)
GATA3	0.38	GATA binding protein 3
HNRNPA1	0.50	Heterogeneous nuclear ribonucleoprotein A1
HNRNPA2B1	0.56	Heterogeneous nuclear ribonucleoprotein A2/B1
HNRNPD	0.59	Heterogeneous nuclear ribonucleoprotein D (AU-rich element RNA binding protein 1, 37 kDa)
HNRPDL	0.65	Heterogeneous nuclear ribonucleoprotein D-like
IGF1	−0.35	Insulin-like growth factor 1 (somatomedin C)
KRT15	0.55	Keratin 15
KRT5	0.41	Keratin 5
LAMA3	0.30	Laminin, alpha 3
LAMC2	0.34	Laminin, gamma 2
MALAT1	0.56	Metastasis-associated lung adenocarcinoma transcript 1 (non-protein coding)
METTL3	0.69	Methyltransferase like 3
MGP	0.53	Matrix Gla protein
NCRNA00173	0.39	Non-protein coding RNA 173
NCRNA00201	0.47	Non-protein coding RNA 201
OXTR	0.54	Oxytocin receptor
RALGAPA2	−0.30	Ral GTPase activating protein, alpha subunit 2 (catalytic)
RASD1	−0.31	RAS, dexamethasone-induced 1
RBMX	0.38	RNA binding motif protein, X-linked
SFPQ	0.47	Splicing factor proline/glutamine-rich
SFRS1	0.30	Splicing factor, arginine/serine-rich 1
SFRS18	0.40	Splicing factor, arginine/serine-rich 18
SFRS5	0.36	Splicing factor, arginine/serine-rich 5
SFRS7	0.40	Splicing factor, arginine/serine-rich 7, 35 kDa
SNHG10	0.62	Small nucleolar RNA host gene 10 (non-protein coding)
SNHG12	0.53	Small nucleolar RNA host gene 12 (non-protein coding)
SNORD104	0.43	Small nucleolar RNA, C/D box 104
SOX6	−0.33	SRY (sex determining region Y)-box 6
XIST	0.57	X (inactive)-specific transcript (non-protein coding)

*Adapted with permission from [45]

Table 6.8 Comparison between biological processes that are overrepresented in the two studies

	Biological processes overrepresented in different studies	
	Previous study[a]	Current study
RNA processing	GO:0006376—mRNA splice site selection	GO:0006376—mRNA splice site selection
	GO:0000398—nuclear mRNA splicing, via spliceosome	GO:0000398—nuclear mRNA splicing, via spliceosome
	GO:0000375—RNA splicing, via transesterification reactions	GO:0000375—RNA splicing, via transesterification reactions
	GO:0000381—regulation of alternative nuclear mRNA splicing, via spliceosome	GO:0000380—alternative nuclear mRNA splicing, via spliceosome
	GO:0006403—RNA localization	GO:0006396—RNA processing
		GO:0016070—RNA metabolic process
Other processes	GO:0007050—cell cycle arrest	GO:0007044—cell-substrate junction assembly
	GO:0016477—cell migration	GO:0007398—ectoderm development
	GO:0006613—cotranslational protein targeting to membrane	GO:0008544—epidermis development
	GO:0048523—negative regulation of cellular process	GO:0010467—gene expression
	GO:0006470—protein amino acid dephosphorylation	
	GO:0030150—protein import into mitochondrial matrix	
	GO:0006195—purine nucleotide catabolic process	

[a]Russo J, Balogh GA, Russo IH (2008) Full-term pregnancy induces a specific genomic signature in the human breast. Cancer Epidemiol Biomarkers Prev 16(1):1–16

6.4.2 Non-coding RNAs

A number of non-coding RNAs that included XIST, MALAT1 (also called NEAT2), and NEAT1 were upregulated in the parous breast. XIST, which inactivates X chromosome as an early developmental process, plays an essential role in female mammals by providing dosage equivalence between males and females. Up-regulation of XIST occurs upon differentiation, whereas failure to express XIST is often seen in malignancies and in early embryogenesis [29]. Our findings are supported by recent reports that suggest that XIST is expressed in adult well-differentiated cells in order to maintain gene repression [29–33]. Oxytocin, a neurotransmitter that acts through its specific receptor OXTR and is overexpressed during lactation, up-regulates the expression of MALAT1, a highly conserved non-coding RNA [34, 35]. Interestingly, both MALAT1 and OXTR remain overexpressed in the breast of postmenopausal parous women. NEAT1 and NEAT2 localize to the periphery and to the interior the spliceosome assembly factor SC35 domains or speckles. Our observation that in breast epithelial cells CCNL2 is highly enriched in nuclear speckles (Fig. 6.2) indicates that CCNL2 might colocalize with NEAT1 and NEAT2. The down-regulation of NEAT1, NEAT2, and XIST in the breast of nulliparous women, in whom this organ never reached a stage of complete differentiation similar to that achieved after completion of pregnancy and lactation [36], suggests that the undifferentiated breast is not actively involved in the RNA metabolism that is necessary for maintaining a state of differentiation.

6.4.3 Downstream to the Estrogen Receptor Pathway

Although in this study we did not observe differential expression in estrogen receptor between parous and nulliparous breasts, several genes that are directly or indirectly regulated by estrogen receptor were up- or downregulated in the parous breast (Chap. 7) and were found to be enriched in the breast cancer estrogen signaling gene set. Among them, GATA3, an important component of this gene set, is crucial to mammary gland morphogenesis and differentiation of progenitor cells. GATA3 has been suggested to be a tumor suppressor [36], a fact supported by the observations that induction of its expression in GATA3-negative undifferentiated carcinoma cells is sufficient to induce tumor differentiation and inhibition of tumor dissemination [37–39]. The down-regulation of RASD1 (RAS, dexamethasone-induced 1), a potential miR-375 target that negatively regulates ER alpha expression in breast cancer, further confirms that the genes involved in the estrogen receptor regulated pathways could be under permanent transcriptional modification as a manifestation of a higher degree of cell differentiation of the parous breast, in spite of the lack of transcriptomic differences in this receptor's levels between parous and nulliparous breast tissues.

6.4.4 *Cell Communication*

Cell communication, which is a key element in the process of cell and organ differentiation, is well represented in the breast of parous women. The parous breast exhibits up-regulation of desmocollin (DSC3), a calcium-dependent glycoprotein that is a member of the desmocollin subfamily of the cadherin superfamily. These members of the desmosomal family, along with the desmogleins, are found primarily in epithelial cells where they constitute the adhesive proteins of the desmosome cell–cell junction and are required for cell adhesion and desmosome formation. In addition, the up-regulation of matrix Gla proteins (MGP), laminins (LAMA3 and LAMC2), and keratin 5 (KRT5) in the parous breast is an indication that they reflect the greater differentiated state of the breast epithelial cells [40]. This concept is supported by the observation that the loss of MGP expression may be associated with tumor progression and metastasis [41].

6.4.5 *Insulin-Like Growth Factor 1*

Our findings that IGF1 is downregulated in the parous breast is consistent with published data reporting overall lower levels of IGF1 in parous than in nulliparous women [42] and support the association of IGF1 with increased breast cancer risk [43]. It is known that IGF1 stimulates mitosis and inhibits apoptosis, playing a significant role in signaling pathways involved in the pathogenesis of breast cancer. The down-regulation of IGF1 in the parous breast, in association with the significant down-regulation of SOX6, EBF1 (early B-cell factor 1), ABHD5, RASD1 (RAS, dexamethasone-induced 1), a potential miR-375 target that negatively regulates ER alpha expression in breast cancer [44], and RALGAPA2, could represent a significant driving force in the reduction of breast cancer risk conferred by pregnancy.

6.5 Concluding Remarks

In summary, using a core needle biopsy of postmenopausal breast parenchyma comprising of stroma and lobular structures, we found a specific genomic signature induced by full-term pregnancy (Table 6.7) [45]. This genomic signature suggests that the differentiation process of breast cells is centered in the mRNA processing reactome, which emerges as an important regulatory pathway induced by pregnancy. The biological importance of the differential expression of genes that control the spliceosome could be an indication of a safeguard mechanism at post-transcriptional level that maintains the fidelity of the transcriptional process. In addition, the critical regulatory pre-mRNA splicing mechanism could also regulate the expression of specific genes controlling estrogen signaling pathways, cell communication, and differentiation, as well as pathways related to chromatin remodeling, altogether resulting in control of cell differentiation and breast cancer prevention (Fig. 6.3). Future studies are needed to confirm these results, in particular studies focusing specifically on lobular epithelial cells selected using laser capture microdissection (LCM). Finally, digital transcriptome analysis such as RNA-Seq methods will help in understanding the precise differentiation paradigms in parous breast tissue.

References

1. Clarke CA, Purdie DM, Glaser SL (2006) Population attributable risk of breast cancer in white women associated with immediately modifiable risk factors. BMC Cancer 6:170
2. MacMahon B, Cole P, Lin TM, Lowe CR, Mirra AP, Ravnihar B, Salber EJ, Valaoras VG, Yuasa S (1970) Age at first birth and breast cancer risk. Bull World Health Organ 43:209–221
3. Jemal A, Siegel R, Ward E, Murray T, Xu J, Thun MJ (2007) Cancer statistics, 2007. CA Cancer J Clin 57:43–66
4. Russo J, Balogh GA, Russo IH (2008) Full-term pregnancy induces a specific genomic signature in the human breast. Cancer Epidemiol Biomarkers Prev 17:51–66
5. Russo J, Russo IH (1980) Influence of differentiation and cell kinetics on the susceptibility of the rat mammary gland to carcinogenesis. Cancer Res 40:2677–2687
6. Tay LK, Russo J (1981) Formation and removal of 7,12-dimethylbenz[a]anthracene—nucleic acid adducts in rat mammary epithelial cells with different susceptibility to carcinogenesis. Carcinogenesis 2:1327–1333
7. Russo IH, Koszalka M, Russo J (1991) Comparative study of the influence of pregnancy and hormonal treatment on mammary carcinogenesis. Br J Cancer 64:481–484
8. Thomas DB, Rosenblatt KA, Ray RM (2001) Re: Breastfeeding and reduced risk of breast cancer in an Icelandic cohort study. Am J Epidemiol 154:975–977
9. Sinha DK, Pazik JE, Dao TL (1988) Prevention of mammary carcinogenesis in rats by pregnancy: effect of full-term and interrupted pregnancy. Br J Cancer 57:390–394
10. Srivastava P, Russo J, Mgbonyebi OP, Russo IH (1998) Growth inhibition and activation of apoptotic gene expression by human chorionic gonadotropin in human breast epithelial cells. Anticancer Res 18:4003–4010
11. Russo J, Moral R, Balogh GA, Mailo D, Russo IH (2005) The protective role of pregnancy in breast cancer. Breast Cancer Res 7:131–142
12. Russo J, Russo IH (1997) Role of differentiation in the pathogenesis and prevention of breast cancer. Endocr Relat Cancer 4:7–21
13. Henry MD, Triplett AA, Oh KB, Smith GH, Wagner KU (2004) Parity-induced mammary epithelial cells facilitate tumorigenesis in MMTV-neu transgenic mice. Oncogene 23:6980–6985
14. Srivastava P, Russo J, Russo IH (1997) Chorionic gonadotropin inhibits rat mammary carcinogenesis through activation of programmed cell death. Carcinogenesis 18:1799–1808
15. Medina D (2004) Breast cancer: the protective effect of pregnancy. Clin Cancer Res 10:380S–384S
16. Ginger MR, Gonzalez-Rimbau MF, Gay JP, Rosen JM (2001) Persistent changes in gene expression induced by estrogen and progesterone in the rat mammary gland. Mol Endocrinol 15:1993–2009
17. D'Cruz CM, Moody SE, Master SR, Hartman JL, Keiper EA, Imielinski MB, Cox JD, Wang JY, Ha SI, Keister BA, Chodosh LA (2002) Persistent parity-induced changes in growth

factors, TGF-beta3, and differentiation in the rodent mammary gland. Mol Endocrinol 16:2034–2051

18. Russo J, Russo IH (2004) Endocrine control of breast development. In: Russo J, Russo IH (eds) Molecular basis of breast cancer: prevention and treatment, 1st edn. Springer, Berlin, pp 64–67
19. Subramanian A, Tamayo P, Mootha VK, Mukherjee S, Ebert BL, Gillette MA, Paulovich A, Pomeroy SL, Golub TR, Lander ES, Mesirov JP (2005) Gene set enrichment analysis: a knowledge-based approach for interpreting genome-wide expression profiles. Proc Natl Acad Sci U S A 102:15545–15550
20. de Graaf K, Hekerman P, Spelten O, Herrmann A, Packman LC, Bussow K, Muller-Newen G, Becker W (2004) Characterization of cyclin L2, a novel cyclin with an arginine/serine-rich domain: phosphorylation by DYRK1A and colocalization with splicing factors. J Biol Chem 279:4612–4624
21. Wahl MC, Will CL, Luhrmann R (2009) The spliceosome: design principles of a dynamic RNP machine. Cell 136:701–718
22. Taga Y, Miyoshi M, Okajima T, Matsuda T, Nadano D (2010) Identification of heterogeneous nuclear ribonucleoprotein A/B as a cytoplasmic mRNA-binding protein in early involution of the mouse mammary gland. Cell Biochem Funct 28:321–328
23. Huang PR, Hung SC, Wang TC (2010) Telomeric DNA-binding activities of heterogeneous nuclear ribonucleoprotein A3 in vitro and in vivo. Biochim Biophys Acta 1803:1164–1174
24. Han SP, Friend LR, Carson JH, Korza G, Barbarese E, Maggipinto M, Hatfield JT, Rothnagel JA, Smith R (2010) Differential subcellular distributions and trafficking functions of hnRNP A2/B1 spliceoforms. Traffic 11:886–898
25. Loyer P, Trembley JH, Grenet JA, Busson A, Corlu A, Zhao W, Kocak M, Kidd VJ, Lahti JM (2008) Characterization of cyclin L1 and L2 interactions with CDK11 and splicing factors: influence of cyclin L isoforms on splice site selection. J Biol Chem 283:7721–7732
26. Li HL, Wang TS, Li XY, Li N, Huang DZ, Chen Q, Ba Y (2007) Overexpression of cyclin L2 induces apoptosis and cell-cycle arrest in human lung cancer cells. Chin Med J (Engl) 120:905–909
27. Zhuo L, Gong J, Yang R, Sheng Y, Zhou L, Kong X, Cao K (2009) Inhibition of proliferation and differentiation and promotion of apoptosis by cyclin L2 in mouse embryonic carcinoma P19 cells. Biochem Biophys Res Commun 390:451–457
28. Brooks YS, Wang G, Yang Z, Smith KK, Bieberich E, Ko L (2009) Functional pre-mRNA trans-splicing of coactivator CoAA and corepressor RBM4 during stem/progenitor cell differentiation. J Biol Chem 284:18033–18046
29. Erwin JA, Lee JT (2010) Characterization of X-chromosome inactivation status in human pluripotent stem cells. Curr Protoc Stem Cell Biol Chapter 1:Unit 1B 6
30. Do JT, Han DW, Gentile L, Sobek-Klocke I, Wutz A, Scholer HR (2009) Reprogramming of Xist against the pluripotent state in fusion hybrids. J Cell Sci 122:4122–4129
31. Vincent-Salomon A, Ganem-Elbaz C, Manie E, Raynal V, Sastre-Garau X, Stoppa-Lyonnet D, Stern MH, Heard E (2007) X inactive-specific transcript RNA coating and genetic instability of the X chromosome in BRCA1 breast tumors. Cancer Res 67:5134–5140
32. Xiao C, Sharp JA, Kawahara M, Davalos AR, Difilippantonio MJ, Hu Y, Li W, Cao L, Buetow K, Ried T, Chadwick BP, Deng CX, Panning B (2007) The XIST noncoding RNA functions independently of BRCA1 in X inactivation. Cell 128:977–989
33. Silver DP, Dimitrov SD, Feunteun J, Gelman R, Drapkin R, Lu SD, Shestakova E, Velmurugan S, Denunzio N, Dragomir S, Mar J, Liu X, Rottenberg S, Jonkers J, Ganesan S, Livingston DM (2007) Further evidence for BRCA1 communication with the inactive X chromosome. Cell 128:991–1002
34. Breton C, Di Scala-Guenot D, Zingg HH (2001) Oxytocin receptor gene expression in rat mammary gland: structural characterization and regulation. J Mol Endocrinol 27:175–189
35. Koshimizu TA, Fujiwara Y, Sakai N, Shibata K, Tsuchiya H (2010) Oxytocin stimulates expression of a noncoding RNA tumor marker in a human neuroblastoma cell line. Life Sci 86:455–460

36. Wilson BJ, Giguere V (2008) Meta-analysis of human cancer microarrays reveals GATA3 is integral to the estrogen receptor alpha pathway. Mol Cancer 7:49
37. Chou J, Provot S, Werb Z (2010) GATA3 in development and cancer differentiation: cells GATA have it! J Cell Physiol 222:42–49
38. Pei XH, Bai F, Smith MD, Usary J, Fan C, Pai SY, Ho IC, Perou CM, Xiong Y (2009) CDK inhibitor p18(INK4c) is a downstream target of GATA3 and restrains mammary luminal progenitor cell proliferation and tumorigenesis. Cancer Cell 15:389–401
39. Kouros-Mehr H, Bechis SK, Slorach EM, Littlepage LE, Egeblad M, Ewald AJ, Pai SY, Ho IC, Werb Z (2008) GATA-3 links tumor differentiation and dissemination in a luminal breast cancer model. Cancer Cell 13:141–152
40. Fischer J, Klein PJ, Farrar GH, Hanisch FG, Uhlenbruck G (1984) Isolation and chemical and immunochemical characterization of the peanut-lectin-binding glycoprotein from human milk-fat-globule membranes. Biochem J 224:581–589
41. Chen L, O'Bryan JP, Smith HS, Liu E (1990) Overexpression of matrix Gla protein mRNA in malignant human breast cells: isolation by differential cDNA hybridization. Oncogene 5:1391–1395
42. Holmes MD, Pollak MN, Hankinson SE (2002) Lifestyle correlates of plasma insulin-like growth factor I and insulin-like growth factor binding protein 3 concentrations. Cancer Epidemiol Biomarkers Prev 11:862–867
43. Key TJ, Appleby PN, Reeves GK, Roddam AW (2010) Insulin-like growth factor 1 (IGF1), IGF binding protein 3 (IGFBP3), and breast cancer risk: pooled individual data analysis of 17 prospective studies. Lancet Oncol 11:530–542
44. de Souza Rocha Simonini P, Breiling A, Gupta N, Malekpour M, Youns M, Omranipour R, Malekpour F, Volinia S, Croce CM, Najmabadi H, Diederichs S, Sahin O, Mayer D, Lyko F, Hoheisel JD, Riazalhosseini Y (2010) Epigenetically deregulated microRNA-375 is involved in a positive feedback loop with estrogen receptor alpha in breast cancer cells. Cancer Res 70:9175–9184
45. Peri S, López de Cicco R, Santucci-Pereira J, Slifker M, Ross EA, Russo IH, Russo PA, Arslan AA, Belitskaya-Lévy I, Zeleniuch-Jacquotte A, Bordas P, Lenner P, Åhman J, Afanasyeva Y, Johansson R, Sheriff F, Hallmans G, Toniolo P, Russo J (2012) Defining the genomic signature of the parous breast. BMC Med Genomics (in press)

Chapter 7
Chromatin Remodeling and Pregnancy-Induced Differentiation

7.1 Introduction

Breast cancer is the most frequently diagnosed cancer in postmenopausal women and the leading cause of cancer death in females worldwide [1]. The global incidence of breast cancer has gradually increased over the last few decades [1, 2]. Although the reasons of this increase are uncertain, it is known that the breast cancer risk is reduced in women who gave birth to a child before age 24 [3] a reduction that is enhanced by breast-feeding and multiparity [4, 5]. Experimentally it has been demonstrated that the protection conferred by pregnancy is mediated by the differentiation of the breast, a physiological process driven by the complex hormonal milieu created by the placenta and the fetus [6–8]. The postulate that the degree of differentiation acquired through an early pregnancy changes the genomic signature that differentiates the lobular structures of early parous (P) women from those of nulliparous (NP) women has been demonstrated through the enriched analysis of the genomic profile of breasts of parous and nulliparous postmenopausal and premenopausal women [9, 10] and of rodent models [6–8, 11, 12]. These findings have allowed researchers to demonstrate that significant differences in the expression of genes controlling differentiation and transcription exist between groups that differ in their parity history. These data explain at molecular level the basis of the protective effect of pregnancy and establishes a functional genomic signature of breast cancer risk reduction, confirming a postulate published in 1997 [7].

We have demonstrated using a detailed histological, cytological, immunohistochemical (IHC), and transcriptomic analysis of breast samples obtained from nulliparous and parous postmenopausal women that the differentiation of the breast induced by an early pregnancy imprints a specific phenotypic and genotypic signature that can be detected in postmenopausal women.

J. Russo and I.H. Russo, *Role of the Transcriptome in Breast Cancer Prevention*, 309
DOI 10.1007/978-1-4614-4884-6_7, © Springer Science+Business Media New York 2013

7.2 The Methodological Approach

Breast tissue was collected from volunteering healthy women [13] between 50 and 69 years of age, postmenopausal, i.e., lack of menstrual periods for 12 preceding months and elevated circulating levels of follicle-stimulating hormone (FSH) (40–250 IU/L), consistent with menopausal condition. Breast core needle biopsies (CNBs) were taken from the upper outer quadrant of the right or the left breast under radiographic control. From the CNBs obtained from each donor one core was fixed in 70% ethanol for histological and IHC analysis; the two remaining cores were placed in RNAlater® (Ambion) solution for RNA extraction and subsequent transcriptomic analysis (see Chap. 5).

7.3 Architecture of Postmenopausal Women's Breast

Our previous studies have in great part clarified the role of pregnancy-induced breast differentiation in the reduction in breast cancer risk, as well as the identification of lobules type 1 (Lob 1) or the terminal ductal lobular unit (TDLU) as the site of origin of breast cancer [6, 9, 14]. The morphological, physiological, and genomic changes resulting from pregnancy and hormonally induced differentiation of the breast and their influence on breast cancer risk have been addressed in previous publications [6, 9, 14, 15]. Our observations that during the postmenopausal years the breast of both parous and nulliparous women contains preponderantly Lob 1 and the fact that nulliparous women are at higher risk of developing breast cancer than parous women indicate that Lob 1 in these two groups of women either differ biologically, or exhibit different susceptibility to carcinogenesis [15]. The breast tissues of the parous and nulliparous women contained ducts and Lob 1, which were characterized by containing 11.2 ± 6.3 ductules per lobular unit, as previously reported [7–9]. Each ductule was composed of an external layer of myoepithelial cells and a monolayer of cuboidal epithelial cells lining a lumen than contained proteinaceous material (Fig. 7.1a–d). IHC staining revealed that epithelium lining both ducts and ductules consisted of basal cells showing positive reactivity for keratin 5/6 (Fig. 7.1e) and myoepithelial cells reacting positively with smooth muscle antigen (SMA) (Fig. 7.1f); these two markers had similar reactivity in both parous and nulliparous breasts.

The proliferative activity of the epithelial cells or Ki67 index was expressed as the percentage of Ki67 positive cells from the total number of cells counted in ducts and Lob 1 of parous (Fig. 7.2a, b) and nulliparous (Fig. 7.2c, d) women's breast. The Ki67 index in the ductal epithelium of NP breasts was significantly higher ($p < 0.03$) than in the Lob 1 of the same tissues and it was also higher than in ducts and Lob 1 of the parous breast (Fig. 7.2b). In the parous breast, on the other hand, the Ki67 index did not differ between the epithelium of ducts and that of Lob 1 ($p > 0.55$) (Fig. 7.2b).

The ER-α and the PR were equally expressed in epithelial cells lining ducts and Lob 1 of both NP and P breast tissues. The percentage of cells positive for both receptors did not differ between NP and P women's breasts, as shown in the box plot of ER-α positive cells (Fig. 7.3).

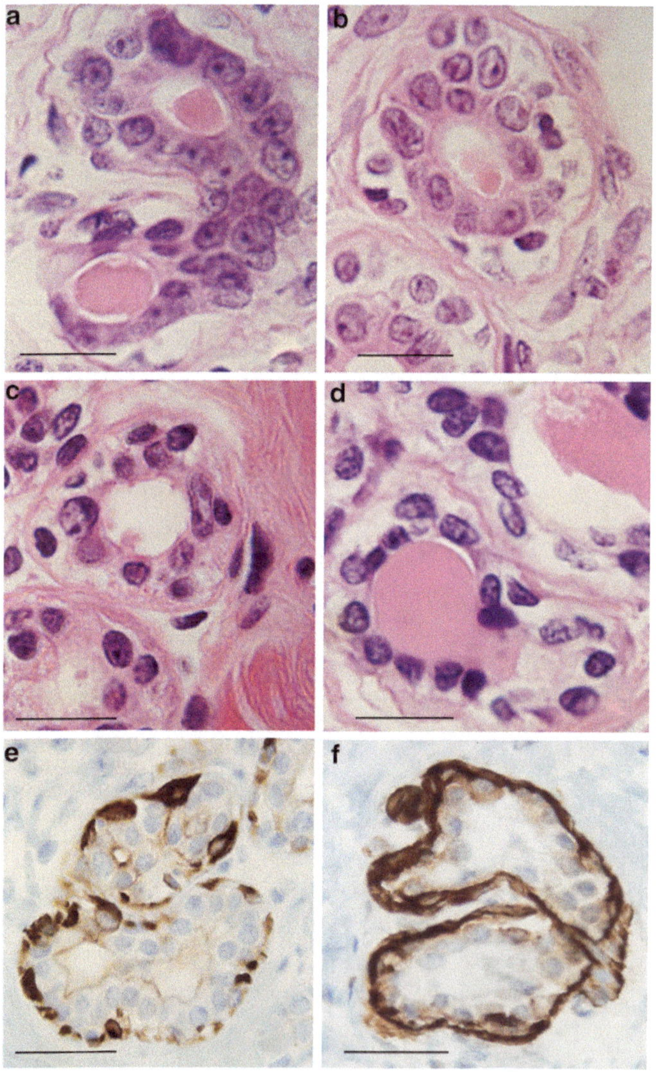

Fig. 7.1 Histological sections of HE-stained ductules in lobules type 1 (Lob 1): (**a**, **b**) from nulliparous (NP) and (**c**, **d**) from parous (P) women's breast tissues; (**e**) positive IHC stain for keratin 5/6 in basal cells; (**f**) IHC stain for SMA in myoepithelial cells. DAB with hematoxylin (H) counterstain. Magnification bar: 100 μm. All ethanol-fixed cores were processed for histopathological and IHC evaluation. All blocks of paraffin-embedded tissues were cut at a thickness of 5 μm, stained with hematoxylin and eosin (HE) and examined under an Olympus BH-2 transmitted light microscope. Each section was evaluated for the presence of mammary ducts and lobules and for determining the ratio between parenchyma and stroma. Specimens lacking epithelial components were not included in the analysis (reprinted with permission from [51])

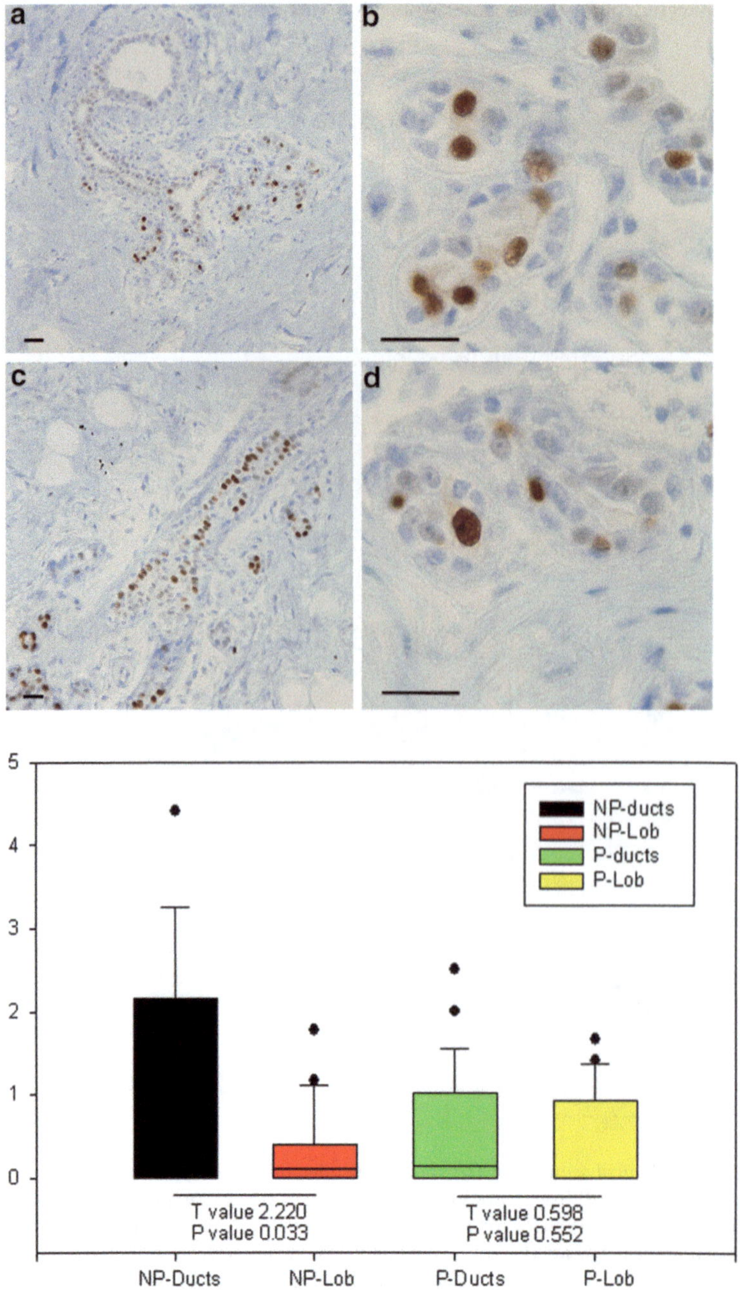

Fig. 7.2 Ki 67 immunoreactivity in the nucleus of epithelial cells in ducts (**a**) and Lob 1 (**b**) in the parous breast and in ducts (**c**) and Lob 1 (**d**) of the nulliparous breast. DAB-H counterstain; magnification bar: 100 μm. Box plot of the proliferative activity (Ki67 index) of ductal and Lob 1 epithelial cells. The Ki67 index in ductal epithelial cells of the nulliparous breast (NP-ducts) was significantly higher than in the Lob 1 (NP-Lob) of the same tissues (paired *t*-test) ($T=2.22$; $p<0.03$), but it did not differ significantly between ducts (P-ducts) and Lob 1 (P-Lob) in the parous breast. The Ki 67 index in NP-ducts was also significantly higher than in ducts and Lob 1 of the parous breast. See legend of Fig. 7.3 (reprinted with permission from [51])

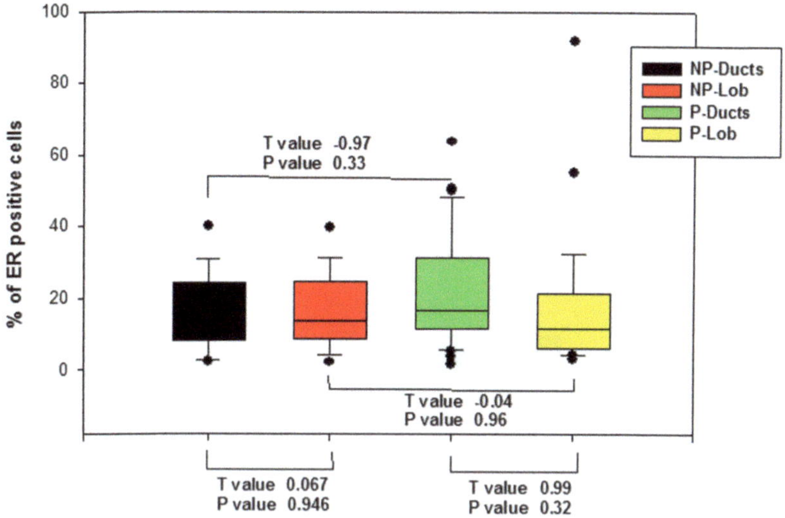

Fig. 7.3 The estrogen receptor α (ER-α) immunoreactivity in the nucleus of epithelial cells in ducts and Lob 1 is similar between parous and nulliparous breasts, as shown in the box plot. Fifty cases (21 NP and 29 P) were selected for IHC detection of the following antibodies: cytokeratin (CK) 5/6, clone D5/16 B4, ER-α clone ID5, dilution 1:50, progesterone receptor (PR) (clone PgR 636), smooth muscle antibody (SMA) clone 1A4, and Ki67, all from DakoCytomation, anti-di-methyl-histone H3 (Lys9) (H3K9me^2), tri-methyl histone H3 (Lys27) (H3K27me^3) (Cell Signaling Technology Inc.), and cyclin L2 (CCNL2) antibody (Novus Biologicals, Cambridge, UK). All assays were run with appropriate negative and positive controls; incubation and staining procedures were performed following protocols recommended by the manufacturers. Evaluation of IHC reactions was performed by a count of 1,000 cells per case and results were expressed as the percentage of positive nuclei (ER-α, PR, Ki67, H3K9me^2, H3K27me^3, and CCNL2) or cytoplasm (CK 5/6, SMA) of the total number counted and analyzed by *t*-test. Cells were evaluated according the intensity of brown staining as strongly positive (+), moderately positive (±), or negative (−) (reprinted with permission from [51])

The study of HE-stained tissues revealed that the population of luminal cells lining ducts and Lob 1 was composed of cells that were characterized by their nuclear appearance into two types: one that contained large and palely stained nuclei with prominent nucleoli (Fig. 7.1a, b) and another consisting of small hyper chromatic nuclei (Fig. 7.1c, d). The pale staining of the large former nuclei is a feature indicative of a high content of non-condensed euchromatin; these nuclei were called euchromatin-rich nuclei (EUN) (Fig. 7.1a, b). The hyperchromasia observed in the latter nuclei was indicative of chromatin condensation and high content of heterochromatin; these nuclei were identified as heterochromatin-rich nucleus (HTN) (Figs. 7.1c, d and 7.4a). The analysis of the distribution of HTN and EUN cells in histological sections of the breast core biopsies revealed that EUN were more abundant in the NP than in the P breast tissues, whereas the inverse was true for the HTN; these differences were statistically significant (Fig. 7.4b). We have confirmed the differences between the HTN and EUN depicted in Fig. 7.1a, b vs. 7.1c, d, using a quantitative image analysis system. The nuclear size (diameter, area, and perimeter) of the EUN as a whole was significantly higher ($p<0.05$) than that of the HTN in both nulliparous and parous women (Table 7.1 and Fig. 7.4b). Differences were also

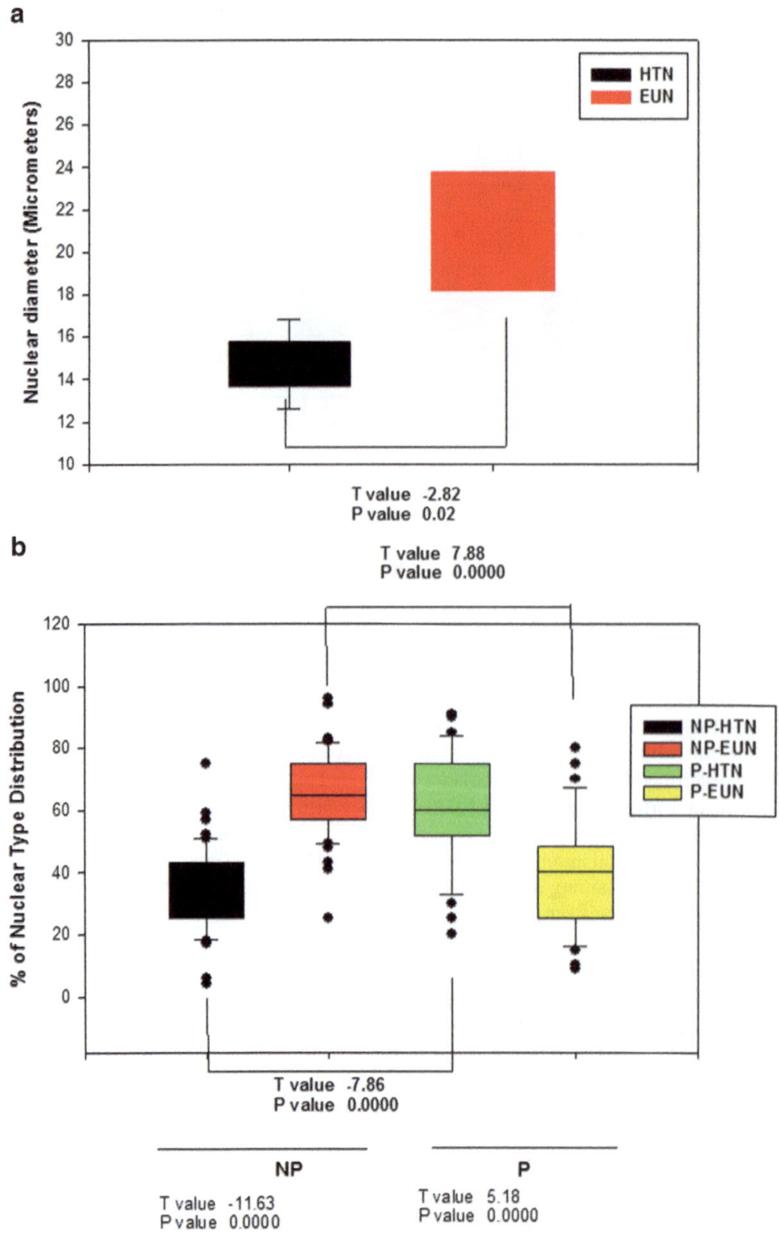

Fig. 7.4 (**a**) Box plot showing the significant difference ($T=-2.82$; $p<0.02$) in nuclear diameter between hyperchromatic heterochromatin-rich nuclei (HTN) and the palely stained euchromatin-rich nuclei (EUN) nuclei. (**b**) The box plot showing the percentage of HTN and EUN distribution in histological sections of the breast core needle biopsies of parous (P) and nulliparous (NP) women revealed that HTN were significantly more abundant in the P than in the NP breast ($T=-7.86$; $p<0.0000$), whereas EUN were prevalent in the NP vs. P breast ($T=7.88$; $p<0.0000$). The percentage of HTN in the NP breast was significantly lower than the percentage of EUN ($T=-11.63$; $p=0.0000$); in the P breast, on the other hand, HTN prevailed over EUN ($T=5.18$; $p=0.0000$) (reprinted with permission from [51])

Table 7.1 Image analysis geometric, densitometric, and textural parameters for hematoxylin-stained interphase nuclei from breast epithelial cells of postmenopausal nulliparous (NP) and parous (P) women

	Reproductive history			
Nuclear characteristics	Nulliparous (NP)		Parous (P)	
Chromatin pattern	EUN, $\overline{x} \pm SD$	HTN, $\overline{x} \pm SD$	EUN, $\overline{x} \pm SD$	HTN, $\overline{x} \pm SD$
Area (μm^2)	27.40±7.47[1]	16.37±5.08[2]	24.38±6.93[3]	15.99±4.79[4]
Perimeter (μm)	24.20±5.34[1,5]	18.42±3.72[2,6]	22.30±4.79[3,7]	16.97±3.01[4,8]
Feret ratio	0.72±0.11[1,9]	0.62±0.14[2,10]	0.72±0.11[3,11]	0.71±0.12[4,12]
Mean gray value/nucleus	198.64±11.14[1,13]	167.96±14.58[2,14]	193.85±15.90[3,15]	182.90±15.35[4,16]
Entropy	5.69±0.26[1,17]	5.85±0.32[2,18]	5.66±0.41[3,19]	5.81±0.34[4,20]
Energy	0.022±0.005[1,21]	0.019±0.004[2,22]	0.024±0.012[3,23]	0.021±0.006[4,24]

EUN euchromatin-rich nucleus; *HTN* heterochromatin-rich nucleus; $\overline{x} \pm SD$ mean ± standard deviation; ANOVA; *NS* no significant [1]EUN vs. [2]HTN ($p<0.05$); [3]EUN vs. [4]HTN ($p<0.05$); EUN[1] vs. [3]($p>0.000$); HTN[2] vs. [4](NS); EUN[5] vs. [7]($p>0.000$); HTN[6] vs. [8]($p<0.004$); EUN[9] vs. [11](NS); HTN[10] vs. [12]($p<0.000$); EUN[13] vs. [15](0.000); HTN[14] vs. [16]($p<0.000$); EUN[17] vs. [19](NS); HTN[18] vs. [20](NS); EUN[21] vs. [23]($p<0.001$); HTN[22] vs. [24](NS)

In this work we analyzed in hematoxylin-stained slides of breast tissues from four nulliparous and five parous women the nuclear texture features of interphase nuclei of epithelial cells using the Carl Zeiss/Kontron equipment. The threshold low (L) and high (H) levels were defined such that the nuclear images appeared pseudocolorized green and well separated from each other and from the background (in the present case $L=\sim 86$ and $H=\sim 200$ gray values). Quantitative information on the following geometric, densitometric, and textural parameters was obtained: nuclear area (μm^2), nuclear perimeter (μm), nuclear feret ratio (=minimum feret/maximal feret), mean gray value per nucleus, standard deviation of the total densitometric values per nucleus or absorbance variability per nucleus (SDtd), entropy, and energy [52–55] (reprinted with permission from [51]) found to be statistically significant ($p < 0.05$) regarding the nuclear shape (nuclear feret ratio) in the breast of nulliparous women, indicating that in these breasts the nuclei of the HTN had a more elongated ellipsoidal shape than the EUN (Table 7.1). The light absorbance (mean gray values/nucleus) was always greater for EUN than for HTN of both NP and P breasts, either considered as two groups or individually, an indication that under densitometric terms HTN were always more densely stained than EUN. Comparison of the EUN of nulliparous vs. parous breasts revealed significant differences in nuclear size, stainability, and densitometric energy, leading us to conclude that epithelial cell nuclei were larger, less stainable, and with smaller regions with uniform densitometric intensity in nulliparous breasts. Comparison of the HTN of nulliparous vs. parous breasts revealed significant differences in nuclear diameter (Fig. 7.4a), perimeter, shape, and stainability; cell nuclei showed larger contours and more elongated ellipsoidal shape and they were more stainable in nulliparous breasts (Table 7.1). These observations indicated that a shift of the EUN cell population to a more densely packed chromatin cell (HTN) had occurred in association with the history of pregnancy as a distinctive pattern of the postmenopausal parous breast.

Since chromatin condensation is part of the process of chromatin remodeling towards gene silencing that is highly regulated by methylation of histones, we verified this phenomenon by IHC incubating NP and P breast tissues with antibodies against histone 3 dimethylated at lysine 9 ($H3K9me^2$) (Fig. 7.5**a**-a, b) and trimethylated at lysine 27 ($H3K27me^3$) (Fig. 7.5**c**-a, b). The IHC stain revealed that methylation of H3 at both lysine 9 and 27 was increased in the heterochromatin-condensed nuclei of epithelial cells of the parous breast (Fig. 7.5**a**-b and 7.5**c**-b) when compared to the EUN of the nulliparous breast (Fig. 7.5**a**-a and 7.5**c**-a). In the nulliparous breast the reactivity in individual cells was less intense and the number of positive cells was significantly lower (Fig. 7.5**b** and 7.5**d**). These variations in chromatin reorganization were supported by the upregulation of *CBX3*, *CHD2*, *L3MBTL*, and *EZH2* genes controlling this process, as depicted in Table 7.2 and Fig. 7.6.

7.4 Transcriptomic Differences

Analysis of P and NP microarrays revealed that there were 305 differentially expressed probesets, 267 up- and 38 downregulated, corresponding to 208 distinct genes between these two groups. From these 267 genes we selected those that described biological processes that were representative of the transcriptomic differences between the parous and the nulliparous breasts. Using bioinformatics-based analysis of microarray data we found that the biological processes involving the splicing machinery and mRNA processing were prevalent in the parous breast and were represented by the following upregulated genes: *LUC7L3*, *SFRS1*, *HNRNPA2B1*, *HNRNPD*, *RBM25*, *SFRS5*, *METTL3*, *HNRNPDL*, and *SFPQ* (Table 7.2). Transcription regulation and chromatin organization were also highly

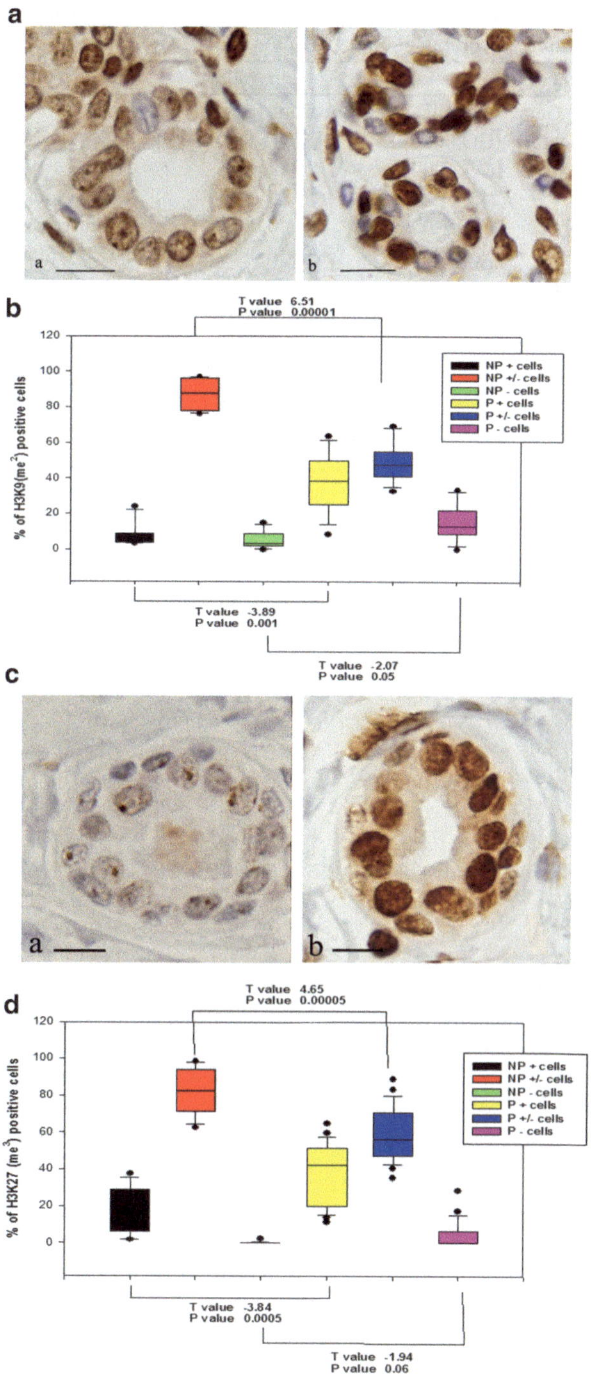

Fig. 7.5 (**a**) The H3K9(me^2) IHC staining is of higher (+) intensity in the nuclei of the P (**a,** b) breast than in NP breast (**a,** a); a moderately diffused (±) stain predominates in most of the NP breast. DAB-H counterstain. Magnification bar: 100 μm. (**b**) Box plot shows a significantly higher number of strongly positive cells (+) in P than in NP breasts ($p < 0.001$), moderately positive (±) cells predominate in the NP tissues ($p < 0.00001$), and negative cells are more numerous in the P cells ($p < 0.05$). (**c**) IHC reaction of H3K27(me^3) is of higher (+) intensity in the nuclei of the P (**c,** b) breast than in NP breast (**c,** a), in which the nuclear stain is faint and finely granular, being mostly circumscribed to the nucleoli. DAB-H counterstain. Magnification bar: 100 μm. (**d**) Box plot shows a significantly higher number of strongly positive cells (+) in P than in NP breasts ($p < 0.0005$); weakly to moderately positive (±) cells predominate in the NP tissues ($p < 0.00005$); negative cells are more numerous in the P than in the NP breast cells ($p < 0.06$) (reprinted with permission from [51])

Table 7.2 Genes displaying differential expression between parous and nulliparous breast tissues classified according to biological processes

Symbol	Log ratio	*p* Value	Gene name
(A) Genes upregulated in the parous breast			
Apoptosis (GO:0006915;GO:0006917;GO:0008624;GO:0042981)			
CASP4	0.37	0.0003	Caspase 4, apoptosis-related cysteine peptidase
RUNX3	0.36	0.0000	Runt-related transcription factor 3
LUC7L3	0.34	0.0002	LUC7-like 3 (*Saccharomyces cerevisiae*)
ELMO3	0.30	0.0003	Engulfment and cell motility 3
DNA repair (GO:0006281; GO:0006284)			
SFPQ	0.46	0.0002	Splicing factor proline/glutamine-rich
MBD4	0.36	0.0003	Methyl-CpG binding domain protein 4
RBBP8	0.32	0.0000	Retinoblastoma-binding protein 8
Cell adhesion (GO:0007155; GO:0030155)			
NRXN1	0.60	0.0001	Neurexin 1
DSC3	0.51	0.0000	Desmocollin 3
COL27A1	0.44	0.0002	Collagen, type XXVII, alpha 1
PNN	0.37	0.0001	Pinin, desmosome-associated protein
COL4A6	0.36	0.0008	Collagen, type IV, alpha 6
LAMC2	0.34	0.0008	Laminin, gamma 2
COL7A1	0.33	0.0002	Collagen, type VII, alpha 1
COL16A1	0.31	0.0000	Collagen, type XVI, alpha 1
LAMA3	0.30	0.0008	Laminin, alpha 3
Cell cycle (GO:0000075; GO:0007049; GO:0045786)			
SYCP2	0.45	0.0000	Synaptonemal complex protein 2
PNN	0.37	0.0001	Pinin, desmosome-associated protein
RUNX3	0.36	0.0000	Runt-related transcription factor 3
RBBP8	0.32	0.0000	Retinoblastoma-binding protein 8
Cell differentiation (GO:0001709; GO:0030154; GO:0030216)			
MGP	0.53	0.0003	Matrix Gla protein
KRT5	0.41	0.0002	Keratin 5
GATA3	0.35	0.0009	GATA-binding protein 3
LAMA3	0.30	0.0008	Laminin, alpha 3
Cell proliferation (GO:0008283; GO:0008284; GO:0008285; GO:0042127; GO:0050679; GO:0050680)			
PTN	0.67	0.0002	Pleiotrophin
KRT5	0.41	0.0002	Keratin 5
RUNX3	0.36	0.0000	Runt-related transcription factor 3
IL28RA	0.34	0.0003	Interleukin 28 receptor, alpha (interferon, lambda receptor)
CDCA7	0.31	0.0005	Cell division cycle associated 7
Cell motility (GO:0006928; GO:0030334)			
DNALI1	0.37	0.0001	Dynein, axonemal, light intermediate chain 1
LAMA3	0.30	0.0008	Laminin, alpha 3
G-protein coupled receptor pathway (GO:0007186)			
OXTR	0.54	0.0006	Oxytocin receptor

(continued)

Table 7.2 (continued)

Symbol	Log ratio	*p* Value	Gene name
RNA metabolic process (GO:0000398; GO:0001510; GO:0006376; GO:0006396; GO:0006397; GO:0006401; GO:0008380)			
METTL3	0.69	0.0000	Methyltransferase like 3
HNRPDL	0.65	0.0001	Heterogeneous nuclear ribonucleoprotein D-like
HNRNPD	0.59	0.0003	Heterogeneous nuclear ribonucleoprotein D (AU-rich element RNA-binding protein 1, 37 kDa)
HNRNPA2B1	0.56	0.0003	Heterogeneous nuclear ribonucleoprotein A2/B1
SFPQ	0.47	0.0006	Splicing factor proline/glutamine-rich
RBM25	0.38	0.0009	RNA-binding motif protein 25
RBMX	0.38	0.0000	RNA-binding motif protein, X-linked
LUC7L3	0.34	0.0002	LUC7-like 3 (S. cerevisiae)
SFRS1	0.30	0.0001	Splicing factor, arginine/serine-rich 1
RNA transport (GO:0050658)			
HNRNPA2B1	0.56	0.0003	Heterogeneous nuclear ribonucleoprotein A2/B1
Transcription (GO:0006350; GO:0006355; GO:0006357; GO:0006366; GO:0016481; GO:0045449; GO:0045893; GO:0045941)			
HNRPDL	0.65	0.0001	Heterogeneous nuclear ribonucleoprotein D-like
HNRNPD	0.59	0.0003	Heterogeneous nuclear ribonucleoprotein D (AU-rich element RNA-binding protein 1, 37 kDa)
CBX3	0.53	0.0003	Chromobox homolog 3 (HP1 gamma homolog, *Drosophila*)
NFKBIZ	0.48	0.0001	Nuclear factor of kappa light polypeptide gene enhancer in B-cells inhibitor, zeta
FUBP1	0.47	0.0002	Far upstream element (FUSE) binding protein 1
SFPQ	0.47	0.0006	Splicing factor proline/glutamine-rich
EZH2	0.44	0.0000	Enhancer of zeste homolog 2 (*Drosophila*)
ZNF207	0.41	0.0007	Zinc finger protein 207
ZNF711	0.41	0.0003	Zinc finger protein 711
GATA3	0.38	0.0009	GATA binding protein 3
PNN	0.37	0.0003	Pinin, desmosome-associated protein
ZNF107	0.37	0.0001	Zinc finger protein 107
RUNX3	0.36	0.0000	Runt-related transcription factor 3
CCNL1	0.35	0.0009	Cyclin L1
ZNF692	0.34	0.0000	Zinc finger protein 692
CHD2	0.33	0.0001	Chromodomain helicase DNA-binding protein 2
RBBP8	0.32	0.0000	Retinoblastoma-binding protein 8
ZNF789	0.32	0.0005	Zinc finger protein 789
CDCA7	0.31	0.0005	Cell division cycle associated 7

(continued)

Table 7.2 (continued)

Symbol	Log ratio	*p* Value	Gene name
Chromatin organization (GO:0006333; GO:0006338)			
CBX3	0.53	0.0003	Chromobox homolog 3 (HP1 gamma homolog, *Drosophila*)
CHD2	0.33	0.0001	Chromodomain helicase DNA-binding protein 2
Cell division (GO:0051301)			
SYCP2	0.45	0.0000	Synaptonemal complex protein 2
DNA metabolic process (GO:0006139; GO:0006260; GO:0006310; GO:0015074)			
METTL3	0.69	0.0000	Methyltransferase like 3
SFPQ	0.46	0.0002	Splicing factor proline/glutamine-rich
GOLGA2B	0.32	0.0001	Golgin A2 family, member B
Lactation (GO:0007595)			
OXTR	0.54	0.0006	Oxytocin receptor
(B) Downregulated genes			
Apoptosis (GO:0006917)			
SOS1	−0.23	0.0040	Son of sevenless homolog 1
Cell adhesion (GO:0007155; GO:0030155)			
PDZD2	−0.35	0.0004	PDZ domain containing 2
Cell proliferation (GO:0008283; GO:0008284; GO:0008285; GO:0042127; GO:0050679; GO:0050680)			
IGF1	−0.35	0.0002	Insulin-like growth factor 1 (somatomedin C)
Cell motility (GO:0006928; GO:0030334)			
IGF1	−0.35	0.0002	Insulin-like growth factor 1 (somatomedin C)
G-protein coupled receptor pathway (GO:0007186)			
RASD1	−0.31	0.0009	RAS, dexamethasone-induced 1
Transcription (GO:0006350; GO:0006355; GO:0006357; GO:0006366; GO:0016481; GO:0045449; GO:0045893; GO:0045941)			
SOX17	−0.28	0.0026	SRY (sex determining region Y)-box 17
EBF1	−0.33	0.0005	Early B-cell factor 1
DNA metabolic process (GO:0006139; GO:0006260; GO:0006310; GO:0015074)			
IGF1	−0.35	0.0002	Insulin-like growth factor 1 (somatomedin C)
Insulin-like growth factor receptor signaling pathway (GO:0043568)			
IGF1	−0.35	0.0002	Insulin-like growth factor 1 (somatomedin C)
(C) Overexpressed nonprotein coding (npc) regions			
Gene symbol	Probe ID	Log ratio	Gene name
CXorf50B	242292_at	0.35	Nonprotein coding RNA 246B
MALAT1	224558_s_at	0.56	Metastasis associated lung adenocarcinoma transcript 1
MALAT1	224558_s_at	0.56	Metastasis associated lung adenocarcinoma transcript 1
NCRNA00173	237591_at	0.39	Nonprotein coding RNA 173
NCRNA00201	225786_at	0.47	Nonprotein coding RNA 201
NEAT1	224565_at	0.38	Nuclear paraspeckle assembly transcript 1

(continued)

Table 7.2 (continued)

Symbol	Log ratio	*p* Value	Gene name
NEAT1	224566_at	0.50	Nuclear paraspeckle assembly transcript 1
XIST	224589_at	0.39	X (inactive)-specific transcript
XIST	221728_x_at	0.57	X (inactive)-specific transcript
XIST	214218_s_at	0.57	X (inactive)-specific transcript

All laboratory personnel were blinded to samples' parity status and other personal information. Unblinding of the parity status after completion of cDNA microarray analysis revealed that volunteer participants belonged to one of the following groups: Parous (P), 71 women that were 23.2 (±4.25) years old at the time of their first pregnancy and 24.0 (±4.6) at the time of delivery of a first full-term pregnancy (FTP); this group included women that had been pregnant once or more times (gravida ^{3}1), and delivered one or more live children (parity ^{3}1) (G^{3}1/P^{3}1); nulligravida nulliparous (NN), 30 women who never became pregnant and therefore never delivered a live child (G0/P0), and gravida-nulliparous (GN), 12 women that became pregnant one or more times, but never delivered a live child (G^{3}1/P0). Pregnancies in 11 of the women in this group were terminated between the 6th and 12th week of gestation, and one had a miscarriage at the 20th week of pregnancy. Because of the similarities in gene expression levels between NN and GN these two groups were further analyzed as a single group of nulliparous (NP) women. For microarray gene analysis total RNA was isolated from the core biopsy samples using the Qiagen Allprep RNA/DNA Mini Kit (Qiagen, Alameda, CA, USA) according to manufacturer's instructions. The GeneChip Expression 3¢-Amplification Two-Cycle cDNA Synthesis Kit (Affymetrix, Santa Clara, CA) was used for the Affymetrix microarray gene analysis. A total of 169 chips were run; from these, 113 chips, 71 from P and 42 from NP, were selected for the differential expression analysis of parous vs. nulliparous after completion of standard Affymetrix quality control measures (average background, scale factors, percent present calls) and probe-level model (PLM) analysis. Nineteen good quality chips that represented technical replicates were excluded from the P/NP comparison. Affymetrix CEL files were preprocessed using RMA [56], which incorporates background adjustment, quantile normalization of probe intensities across arrays, and summarization using the median polish algorithm. To account for between-batch variability in the arrays, the data were adjusted using ComBat, an empirical Bayes framework developed by Johnson et al. [57]. A variance filter was applied for removing all probesets with variance across all samples below the first quartile. A total of 18,694 probesets remained for further analysis after filtering. The limma package [58], which uses empirical Bayes methods to moderate standard errors of model coefficients (i.e., log2 fold-changes), was implemented in the R/Bioconductor platform [59] that was used for identifying probesets differentially expressed in the P/NP comparisons. Probesets for downstream analysis from pairwise comparisons were selected using both the *p*-value of 0.001 from the empirical Bayes moderated *t*-statistics, and a minimum log2 fold-change of 0.3 threshold as criteria of significance; unless otherwise noted. A heatmap using the RMA expression values and average linkage method to make hierarchical clustering on selected genes was built for depicting the genes that were differentially expressed between parous and nulliparous women. Data mining methods were applied for identifying statistically significant biological processes, pathways, and gene networks that were differentially expressed in the P/NP comparisons. Gene ontology (GO) functional categories enriched in differentially expressed genes were identified using conditional hypergeometric tests in the GOstats package (R/BioConductor). This analysis was carried out independently for up- and downregulated genes; a *p*-value cut off of 0.01 was used to select GO terms.
To identify pathways and associations to other knowledge datasets, Gene Set Enrichment Analysis (GSEA) was performed against the lists of differentially expressed genes. Since we were interested in finding pathways and co-regulated genes, we relaxed the *p*-value to 0.01 and did not apply any fold change filter to identify pathways from more genes. Pathways obtained from MSigDB (database of gene sets provided by GSEA) were tested for enrichment. Default parameters were chosen, except that the maximum intensity of probes was only selected while collapsing probe sets for a single gene. The gene expression profile obtained was deposited to the Gene Expression Omnibus (GEO) Series GSE26457: http://www.ncbi.nlm.nih.gov/geo/query/acc.cgi?token=zpmfjygscwaemdo&acc=GSE26457 (reprinted with permission from [51])

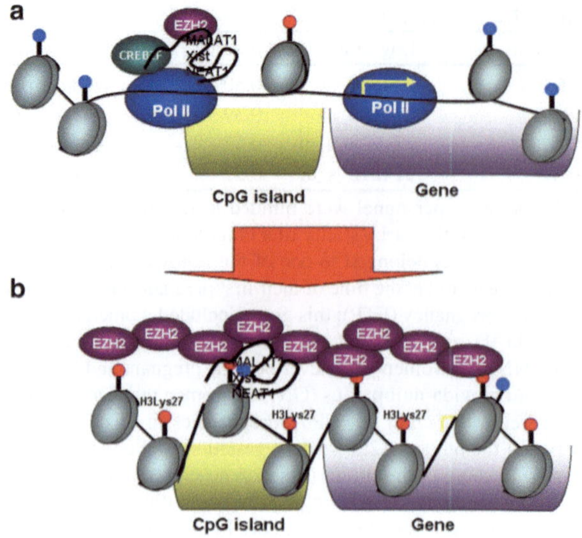

Fig. 7.6 (**a**) Transcriptionally active chromatin is predominantly expressed in the EUN of the nulliparous women's breast. (**b**) Transcriptionally inactive chromatin is more frequently found in the heterochromatin-rich nuclei (HTN) of the parous breast; its presence is associated with histone 3 methylation at lysines 9 and 27, and transcriptional silencing in heterochromatin complexes

represented in the parous breast by the upregulation of *CBX3*, *EBF1*, *GATA3*, *RBBP8*, *CCNL1*, *CCNL2*, *CDCA7*, *EZH2*, *FUBP1*, *NFKBIZ*, *RUNX3*, *ZNF107*, *ZNF207*, *ZNF692*, *ZNF711*, *ZNF789*, *CDCA7*, and *ZNF692* (Table 7.2). The parous breast also expressed upregulation of six noncoding regions that included *X inactive-specific transcript* (*XIST*), *MALAT-1* (or *NEAT2*), and *NEAT1* (Table 7.2).

Genes that were downregulated in the parous breast represented transcription regulation, encompassing *CBL*, *FHL5*, *NFATC3*, *NCR3C1*, *TCF7L2*, and a set of genes that were involved in IGF-like growth factor signaling, somatic stem cell maintenance, muscle cell differentiation and apoptosis, such as *IGF1*, *RASD1*, *EBF1*, *SOX1*, *SOX6*, *SOX17*, *RALGAPA2*, and *ABHD5* (Table 7.2). The level of expression was confirmed to be differentially expressed between nulliparous and parous breast tissues by real-time RT-PCR for the following genes: *CREBZF*, *XIST*, *MALAT1*, *NEAT1*, *CCNL2*, *GATA3*, *DDX17*, *HNRPDL*, *SOX6*, *SNHG12*, *SOX17*, and *C1orf168*. In addition to the level of expression, the localization of the alternative splicing regulator cyclin-cyclin L2 protein (*CCNL2*) [16] was verified by IHC. CCNL2 protein was expressed in the nucleus of epithelial cells in breast tissues from NP and P women, although the level of expression was significantly higher in Lob 1 in the parous breast when compared with similar structures found in the breast of nulliparous women. These observations confirmed the localization of this gene product in the splicing factor compartment (nuclear speckles) [17].

7.5 Functional Significance

We demonstrated that the changes in cell types and increases in chromatin condensation are novel markers for defining the concept of differentiation in the adult breast. These findings confirm the universality of the histone 3 methylation in lysines 9 and 27 during differentiation, since a similar phenomenon has been described to occur during embryonic stem cell (ESC) differentiation [18]. The observed chromatin changes in parous epithelial cells are complemented by the expression of genes related to increasing cell adhesion and differentiation, such as *NRXN1*, *DSC3*, *COL27A1*, *PNN*, *COL4A6*, *LAMC2*, *COL7A1*, *COL16A1*, *MGP*, *KRT5*, *GATA3*, and *LAMA3*. In contrast to the findings of Asztalos et al. [10] of downregulation of the expression of ER-α following recent (<2 years) and distant (5–10 years) pregnancies in premenopausal women, our current genomic and IHC study did not reveal differences in the level of expression of ER-α in the epithelial cells of ducts and Lob 1 between parous and nulliparous postmenopausal women. Nevertheless, numerous genes that are regulated downstream by the ER-α were found to be upregulated in the parous breast, supporting a-parity-mediated protective effect evident in younger parous women [10] but lasting until menopause. Among the ER-α downstream-regulated genes was *GATA3*, which encodes a protein that belongs to the GATA family of transcription factors that regulates T lymphocyte differentiation and maturation. *GATA3* is crucial to mammary gland morphogenesis and differentiation of progenitor cells and a putative tumor suppressor [19]. Induction of *GATA3* expression in *GATA3*-negative undifferentiated carcinoma cells is sufficient to induce tumor differentiation and inhibition of tumor dissemination [20]. Therefore, the observation that genes involved in the estrogen receptor-regulated pathways are upregulated in the parous breast in spite of the lack of transcriptomic differences in this receptor's levels between parous and nulliparous postmenopausal breast tissues suggests that they could be under permanent transcriptional modification as a manifestation of a higher degree of cell differentiation.

Studies of breast development under the influence of parity in women and in animal models are in agreement on the pregnancy-induced differentiation of the breast, a process that ultimately becomes manifested as a specific genomic signature in the mammary gland [6–12]. Although variations in gene expression among different studies and species are expected, an increase in immune activity, including overexpression of lipopolysaccharide-binding protein (*LBP*/*Lbp*) has been reported in the postpregnancy breast of premenopausal women [10] and in the mammary gland of four different strains of rats [12]. Interestingly, this response observed in both recently pregnant and in distant pregnant groups was not observed in the postmenopausal group reported in this study. These discrepancies might indicate that the upregulation of inflammation/immune response-related genes persists during postpartum involution, but wanes after menopause sets in. However, it cannot be ruled out the possibility that the cyclic hormonal changes occurring during the menstrual/estrus cycle influence the genomic profile of the breast activating pathways that greatly differ from those expressed in the postmenopausal parous women.

7.6 Evidence of a Shifting of the Stem Cell Population in the Human Breast

We found a shift in the cell population of the postmenopausal breast as a manifestation of the reprogramming of the organ after pregnancy. These observations are in agreement with what is observed in the rat mammary gland, which also contains two types of luminal epithelial cells, designated dark (DC) and intermediate (IC) cells, in addition to the myoepithelial cells [21]. The DC and IC are equivalent to the HTN and EUN cells described in the present work. DCs increase after pregnancy and lactational involution; whereas the ICs significantly outnumber the DC in ductal hyperplasias and ductal carcinomas [21, 22]. Our analysis of nuclear ultrastructural and morphometric parameters of rodent IC have allowed us to differentiate the mammary progenitor stem cell from the cancer stem cells [15, 21, 22]. Nuclear morphometric analysis of breast and ovarian carcinomas has confirmed the predictive value of nuclear grade on the progression of premalignant lesions to invasiveness [23–25]. Our present findings of a significant decrease in the number of EUN with a subsequent increase in the number of HTN cells expressing specific biomarkers identified at the chromatin and transcriptional levels support the value of morphometric analysis as an adjuvant to molecular studies (Fig. 7.5**a-d**). Our data clearly indicate that there are morphological indications of chromatin remodeling in the parous breast, such as the increase in the number of epithelial cells with condensed chromatin and increased reactivity with anti-$H3K9me^2$ and $H3K27me^3$ antibodies. Histone methylation is a major determinant for the formation of active and inactive regions of the genome and is crucial for the proper programming of the genome during development [26]. In the parous breast there is upregulation of transcription factors and chromatin remodeling genes such as *CHD2* or *chromodomain helicase DNA-binding protein 2* and the *CBX3* or *Chromobox homolog 3*, whose products are required for controlling recruitment of protein/protein or DNA/protein interactions. *CBX3* is involved in transcriptional silencing in heterochromatin-like complexes, and recognizes and binds H3 tails methylated at lysine 9, leading to epigenetic repression. Two other important genes related to the polycomb group (PcG) protein that are upregulated in the parous breast are the *L3MBTL* gene or l (3) mbt-like and the histone-lysine N-methyltransferase or *EZH2*. Members of the PcG form multimeric protein complexes that maintain the transcriptional repressive state of genes over successive cell generations. *EZH2* is an enzyme that acts mainly as a gene silencer, performing this role by the addition of three methyl groups to lysine 27 of histone 3, a modification that leads to chromatin condensation [18, 27, 28].

7.7 Role of Noncoding RNA in Chromatin Remodeling

Recent studies indicate that RNA molecules recruit PcG complexes to the locus of transcription or to sites located elsewhere in the genome. An important role has been attributed to noncoding RNAs (ncRNAs) [29]. It is possible to postulate that the increased chromatin condensation in the parous breast reported herewith could have been initiated by ncRNAs, a postulate supported by the observed upregulation of several ncRNAs that included nuclear paraspeckle assembly transcript 1 (*NEAT1*), *MALAT-1* (*NEAT2*), and *XIST* [30], all critical components of the speckles. The expression of *MALAT-1* is upregulated by the neurotransmitter oxytocin during lactation, which acts through its specific receptor OTR. It is of interest the fact that both *OTR* and *MALAT-1* remain upregulated in the breast of postmenopausal parous women even in the absence of circulating oxytocin. These observations indicate that in parous women the breast remains actively involved in the RNA metabolism that is necessary for maintaining a state of differentiation. Upregulation of *XIST* occurs upon differentiation, resulting in X chromosome inactivation. An ncRNA transcribed from a portion of the *Xist* gene locus forms hairpin structures that recruit the PRC2 complex to the X-inactivation center *X(ic)* [31]. Transcription of full-length *Xist* RNA, which forms the same hairpin structures, leads to further PRC2 recruitment and the spread of PcG-mediated repression across the inactive X chromosome. *Xist* repression, which is often seen in malignancies, also occurs in early embryogenesis and during the acquisition of pluripotency in undifferentiated ES cells by the binding of *Nanog*, *Oct4*, and *Sox2* directly to the chromatin of the *Xist* gene [31]. It is possible that in the postmenopausal nulliparous breast the upregulation of *DDX*, *Sox1*, *Sox6*, and *Sox17*, which might be equivalent to *Nanog*, *Oct4*, and *Sox2*, play a direct pivotal role in the repression of *XIST* transcription. Although this postulate needs to be functionally verified, it is possible that these genes may play a role in controlling *XIST* in the parous breast. The upregulation of *XIST* has important implications in the understanding of the differentiation pattern of the parous breast. In recent studies it has been shown that the reprogramming of X-chromosome inactivation during the acquisition of pluripotency in vivo and in vitro is accompanied by the repression of *XIST* [31–33]. Reprogramming experiments have further reinforced the concept that X-inactivation is intimately linked to differentiation and support our findings that *XIST* is expressed in adult well-differentiated cells, participating in the maintenance of gene repression [31–33]. There is a relationship between the chromatin remodeling process and posttranscriptional control maintained by the spliceosome machinery that is stored in nuclear speckles. Among the components of the spliceosome machinery that are upregulated in the parous breast are the heterogeneous nuclear ribonucleoproteins *HNRPA3*, *HNRPA2B1*, *HNRPD*, and the *HNRPU* shown in Table 7.2. The functional role of these *HNRPs* in the postmenopausal breast could be implicated in the regulation of mRNA stability, other functions like mammary gland involution [34], acting as negative regulators of telomere length maintenance [35] or regulating the trafficking of mRNA molecules [36]. Other members of the spliceosome complex are the small nuclear ribonucleoproteins (snRNPs), which function as suppressors of tumor cell growth and may have major implications as cancer therapeutic targets. Among these we have found that the transcripts regulated by the genes *SF3B1*, *SFRS2*, *SFRS7*, *SFRS8*, *SFRS14*, *SFRS16*, *SNRP70*, *SNRPB*, *SNRPA1*, *PRF3*, and *PHF5A* are overexpressed in the parous breast. Other members of the splicing factor compartment that are localized in the nuclear speckles are *CCNL1* and *CCNL2*. We have demonstrated through immunohistochemistry that CCNL2 protein is overexpressed in the nucleus of epithelial cells composing the Lob 1 of the parous breast. *CCNL1* and *CCNL2* are transcriptional regulators that participate in the pre-mRNA splicing process and the expression of critical factors leading to cell apoptosis, possibly through the Wnt signal transduction pathway [37, 38], which we found to be downregulated in the parous breast.

Another component of the spliceosome complex that regulates genes involved in the apoptotic process is the RNA-binding motif protein 5 (*RBM5*). The overexpression of *RBM5* retards ascites-associated tumor growth and enhances *p53*-mediated inhibition of cell growth and colony formation [39, 40], mechanisms that could also be operational in the parous breast. The spliceosome plays a critical role in differentiating mouse ESC, and self-renewal, pluripotency, and tissue lineage specification of human ESC [41]. Posttranscriptional modifications of RNA, including packaging into the nuclear speckles of the breast epithelial cells and recognition by RNA-binding proteins and/or microRNAs are crucial processes in differentiating breast epithelial cells. Although it is known that these regulatory mechanisms decrease the susceptibility of the cell to carcinogenesis, more studies need to be conducted for identifying the specific pathways involved in this process. Data presented here contribute to emphasize the importance of posttranscriptional regulatory mechanisms as a critical component underlying the differentiation of the breast.

7.8 Inducing Chromatin Remodeling by HCG

In our preclinical studies of chemically induced mammary tumor model [6, 42–45], we have shown that the initiation of mammary cancer is prevented when the carcinogen is administered after completion of the first pregnancy or after a 21-day treatment of virgin rats with either human urinary or recombinant hCG, u-hCG, and r- hCG, respectively (see Chap. 2). The preventive effect of both pregnancy and hCG treatments is mediated by the induction of differentiation of the mammary gland, depression of DNA synthesis, and changes in the genomic profile of this organ [42, 43, 45] (Fig. 7.7). Moreover, a short-term treatment of virgin rats with r-hCG prior to DMBA administration induces a degree of mammary gland differentiation that results in a dramatic decline in mammary cancer incidence [7, 42, 45–47]. Like full-term pregnancy, r-hCG treatment induces a permanent genomic signature in the mammary epithelial cells associated with lower cell proliferation and efficient DNA repair capacity, creating a differentiated epithelium that is more resistant to carcinogenesis [48, 49]. Based on our in vivo studies we proposed that in the breast, pregnancy or hCG are able to shift the Stem Cells 1 that are susceptible to be transformed by a carcinogen to Stem Cells 2 that are refractory [47, 48]. The Stem Cells 2 are progenitor cells originated after post-lactation involution of the breast, but they can proliferate and differentiate under the stimulus of a new pregnancy [47, 48]. This hypothesis, called *the terminal differentiation hypothesis of breast cancer prevention*, predicts that the loss of Stem Cells 1 through their differentiation to Stem Cells 2 and the general increased differentiation of the breast

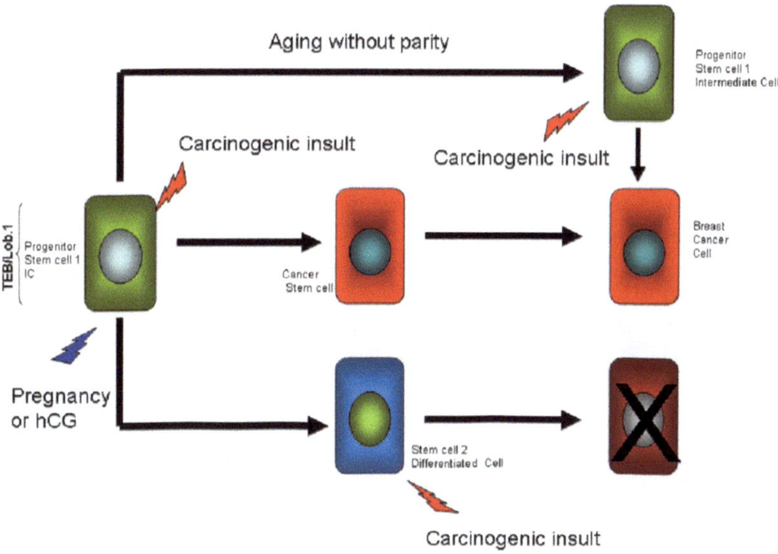

Fig. 7.7 The initially normal progenitor stem cell 1/IC that is present in the Lob 1 or TEB and gives origin to the parenchymal tree, when affected by a carcinogen becomes the cancer stem cell (CSC) that originates breast cancer. Aging in the absence of pregnancy retains the stem cell 1, which when affected by a carcinogen can become a CSC. Both early pregnancy or hCG treatment of virgin animals induce the differentiation of the progenitor stem cell 1 to the stem cell 2, which has become resistant to undergo neoplastic transformation, although it retains proliferative activity and the capability to regenerate the complete lobular system during the next pregnancy (from Russo and Russo [15])

following pregnancy or hCG treatment will result in protection from tumorigenesis [7, 46, 48] (Fig. 7.7). As it is described in Chap. 4, we demonstrated in vitro that r-hCG prevented the expression of transformation phenotypes induced in MCF-10F cells by E2 treatment and stimulated ductulogenesis by increasing the length of the ducts and producing tertiary branching of the breast epithelial cells [50].

In order to determine if some of the genes listed in Table 7.2 were also present in MCF-10F cells and to determine if hCG induces activation of chromatin remodeling genes we treated the cells with 10, 50, 100 IU/mL of r-hCG for 48 h. Cell lysates were prepared using 1XRIPA buffer at the end of treatment and 40 μg of cell lysates were resolved by 4–12% Bis-Tris gel and transferred on nitrocellulose membrane followed by incubation with primary mouse anti-human EZH2 antibody (BD). The immunoreactive protein was detected by IRDye 800CW goat. The expression of EZH2 was significantly increased by the 50 and 100 IU r-hCG treatment (Fig. 7.8A). These data were confirmed by IF using the antibody mouse anti-human EZH2 1:200 (BD) and labeling was detected with Alexa fluor488 goat anti-mouse or Alexa fluor555 goat anti-rabbit secondary antibody (Fig. 7.8B). Nuclei were counter-stained with DAPI and the fluorescent images were photographed using an Olympus

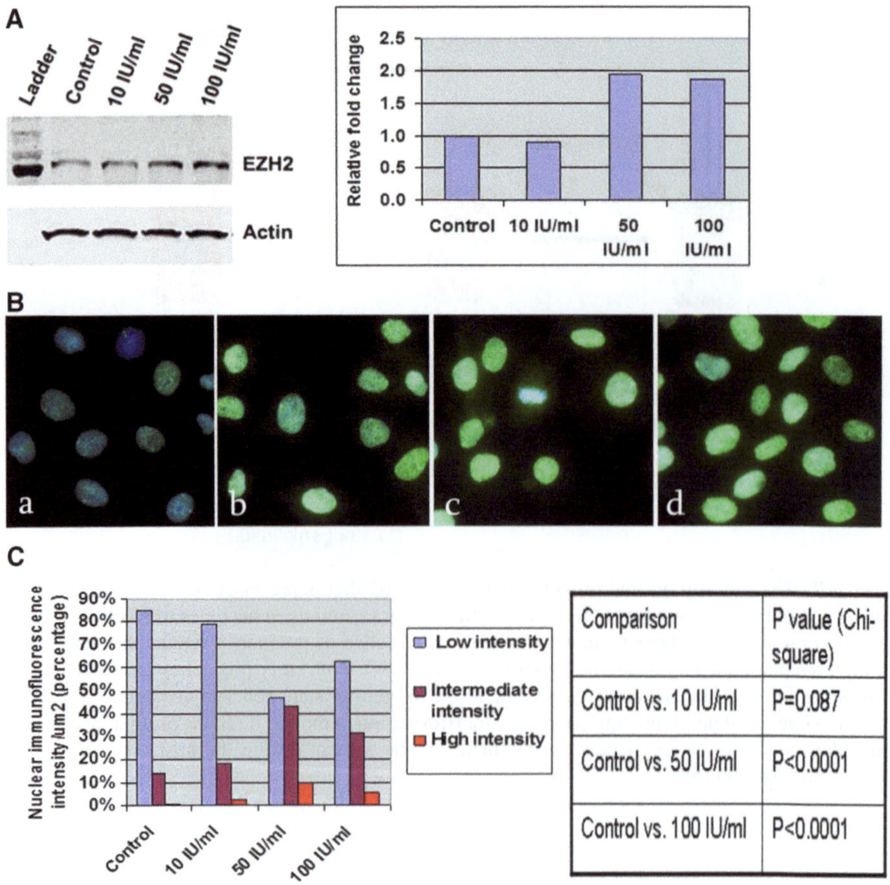

Comparison	P value (Chi-square)
Control vs. 10 IU/ml	P=0.087
Control vs. 50 IU/ml	P<0.0001
Control vs. 100 IU/ml	P<0.0001

Fig. 7.8 EZH2 determination in MCF-10F cells treated with r-hCG. (**A**) Western Blot, (**B**) immunofluorescence (IF): (**a**) 0 IU (control); (**b**) 10; (**c**) 50; and (**d**) 100 IU r-hCG, (**C**) fluorescence quantitation

Bx53 IF microscope and quantified using Metamorph software (Fig. 7.8**C**). The significant increase in the expression of the nuclear protein was confirmed by Western blot and by RT-PCR.

The level of *XIST* expression in MCF-10F cells treated with r-hCG at the doses of 0, 10, 50, and 100 IU for 48 h was evaluated by RT-PCR (*probe* Hs00300535_s1) (Fig. 7.9). A significant dose-dependent increase in *XIST* expression was detected in the MCF-10F cells treated with r-hCG. Determination of level of expression of CREBZF in MCF-10F cells treated with r-hCG for 48 h by IF using rabbit anti-human CREBZF ab (Lifespan Biosciences) at a dilution of 1:100 revealed that the treatment with r-hCG significantly increased the level of expression of CREBZF in MCF-10F cells in a dose-dependent manner. RT-PCR (probe Hs00300535_s1) was utilized for confirmation and quantitation of values (Fig. 7.10). CREB/ATF bZIP

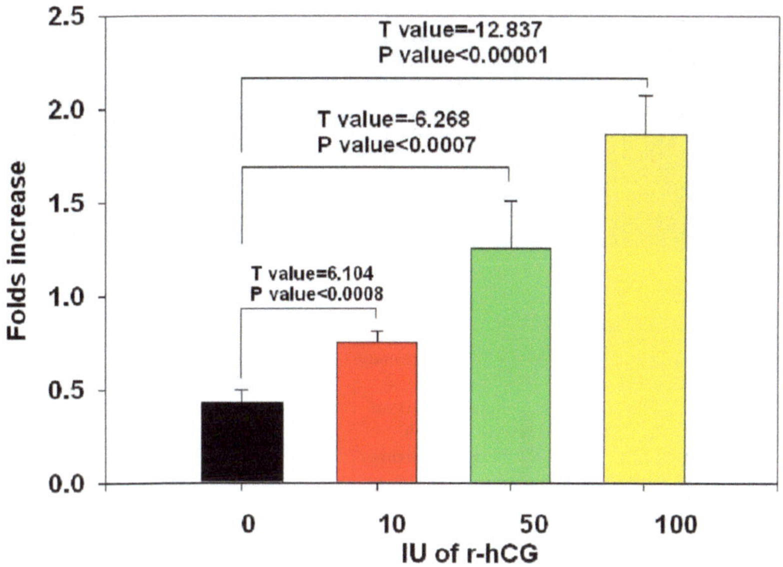

Fig. 7.9 Determination of XIST level of expression in MCF-10F cells treated with 0, 10, 50, and 100 IU r-hCG for 48 h and quantitated by RT-PCR

A

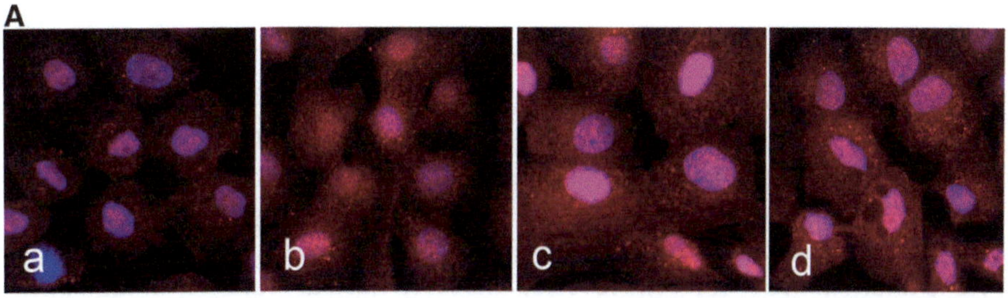

B

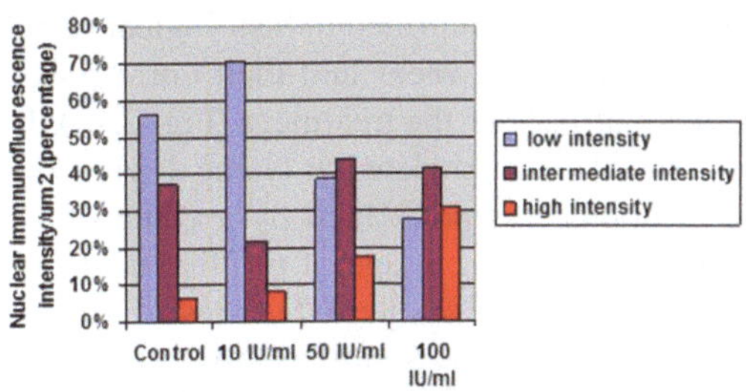

Comparison	P value (Chi-square)
Control vs. 10 IU/ml	P<0.0001
Control vs 50 IU/ml	P<0.0001
Control vs 100 IU/ml	P<0.0001

Fig. 7.10 CREBZF detection in MCF-10F cells treated with r-hCG for 48 h. (**A**) IF, (**a**) 0; (**b**) 10; (**c**) 50; and (**d**) 100 IU r-hCG. (**B**) RT-PCR quantification

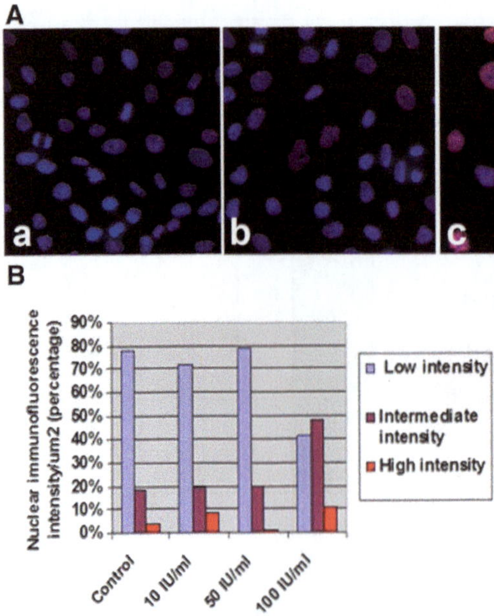

Comparison	P value (Chi-square)
Control vs. 10 IU/ml	P=0.057
Control vs. 50 IU/ml	P=0.043 (decreased in 50 IU/ml)
Control vs. 100 IU/ml	P<0.0001 (increased in 100 IU/ml)

Fig. 7.11 Expression of H3K27me^3 in MCF-10F cells treated with r-hCG for 48 h. (**A**) IF, (**a**) 0 (control); (**b**) 10; (**c**) 50; and (**d**) 100 IU r-hCG. High intensity reactivity observed in cells treated with 100 IH r-hCG. (**B**) Quantitation

transcription factor also called ZF or Zhangfei, which is also upregulated in the parous breast tissues (Table 7.1), is member of the CREB/ATF subfamily of bZIP transcription factors that are widely recognized as critical regulators of gene expression (see Chap. 6) and may play an important role in the chromatin remodeling induced by hCG. The IF analysis of histone 3 trimethylation in lysine 27 (H3K27me^3) was performed using the rabbit anti H3K27me^3 (Cell Signaling Technology Inc.) at a 1:200 dilution. MCF-10F cells revealed increased nuclear reactivity of high intensity in cells treated with 100 IU r-hCG (Fig. 7.11). Further evidence that this effect was due to the differentiating effect of r-hCG was confirmed in histological sections of MCF-10F cells treated with 50 IU r-hCG for 2 weeks and their corresponding controls, which were grown in collagen matrix after the treatment (Fig. 7.12). IHC was performed using antibody against the H3 trimethylated at lysine 4 (H3K4me^3) and H3K27me^3. Evaluation of IHC reactions was performed by a count of ~800 cells per case and results were expressed as the percentage of positive nuclei over the total number of cells counted and statistically analyzed by *t*-test. Cells were evaluated according the intensity of brown staining as strongly positive (+++), moderately positive (±), or negative (−). More than 80% of the MCF-10F control cells (Fig. 7.12a, b) were strongly positive with the H3K4me^3 antibody, consistent with the presence of an active euchromatin, whereas 60% of the r-hCG-treated cells

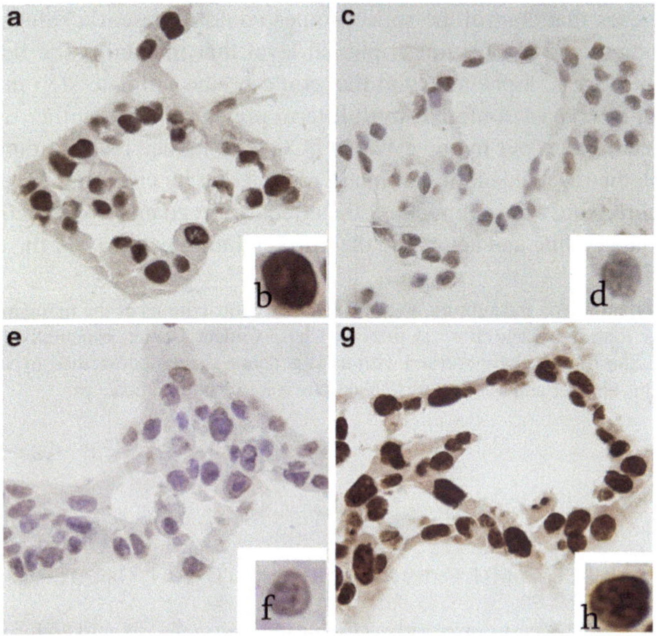

Fig. 7.12 MCF-10F cells growing in collagen after a 2-week treatment with 50 IU r-hCG. IHC reactivity with antibody against the H3K4me3 (**a**–**d**) or H3K27me3 (**e**–**h**). Untreated controls (**a**, **b**) were strongly positive with the H3K4me3 antibody, consistent with the presence of an active euchromatin, whereas r-hCG-treated cells (**c**, **d**) were predominantly negative. MCF-10F cells immunoreacted with H3K27me3 antibody showed strong nuclear reactivity in r-hCG-treated cells (**g**, **h**), whereas the untreated control cells were negative (**e**, **f**)

(Fig. 7.12c, d) were moderately positive or negative. The opposite reactivity was observed in the cells immunoreacted with the H3K27me3 antibody, which showed strong nuclear reactivity in 100% of r-hCG-treated cells (Fig. 7.12g, h), whereas greater than 80% of control cells were either weakly positive or negative (Fig. 7.12e, f).

7.9 Relevance of Chromatin Remodeling in Breast Cancer Prevention

Our work [51] clearly demonstrates that the breast of parous postmenopausal women exhibits a specific signature that has been induced by a full-term pregnancy. This signature reveals for the first time that the differentiation process is centered in chromatin remodeling and the mRNA processing reactome, which emerge as important regulatory pathways induced by pregnancy. The biological importance of the pathways identified in this specific population cannot be sufficiently emphasized due to the fact that the upregulation of the noncoding sequences that control gene repression and of the genes that control the spliceosomes could represent a safeguard mechanism at genomic and at posttranscriptional level that maintains the fidelity of the transcription process, a phenomenon that could be the ultimate step mediating the protection of the breast conferred by full-term pregnancy. Altogether our data provide rationale basis to our hypothesis that hCG may induce its differentiation effect by activating the mechanism of chromatin remodeling by changing the euchromatin to a heterochromatic state, mimicking the effect of pregnancy by selectively silencing part of the genome and activating the differentiating pathway of the cells.

Acknowledgements We, the authors, acknowledge the contributions of the many members of the Breast Cancer Research Laboratory at the Fox Chase Cancer Center, especially Drs. Y Su, R. Lopez, and F. Sheriff, who have worked with us to generate the data described in Sect. 7.8 incorporated into this chapter and allowed us to elaborate it into a unified concept.

References

1. Jemal A, Bray F, Center MM, Ferlay J, Ward E, Forman D (2011) Global cancer statistics. CA Cancer J Clin 61:69–90
2. Harford JB (2011) Breast-cancer early detection in low-income and middle-income countries: do what you can versus one size fits all. Lancet Oncol 12:306–312
3. MacMahon B, Cole P, Lin TM, Lowe CR, Mirra AP, Ravnihar B, Salber EJ, Valaoras VG, Yuasa S (1970) Age at first birth and breast cancer risk. Bull World Health Organ 43:209–221
4. Hinkula M, Pukkala E, Kyyronen P, Kauppila A (2001) Grand multiparity and the risk of breast cancer: population-based study in Finland. Cancer Causes Control 12:491–500
5. Yang XR, Chang-Claude J, Goode EL, Couch FJ, Nevanlinna H, Milne RL, Gaudet M, Schmidt MK, Broeks A, Cox A, Fasching PA, Hein R et al (2011) Associations of breast cancer risk factors with tumor subtypes: a pooled analysis from the Breast Cancer Association Consortium studies. J Natl Cancer Inst 103:250–263
6. Russo IH, Koszalka M, Russo J (1991) Comparative study of the influence of pregnancy and hormonal treatment on mammary carcinogenesis. Br J Cancer 64:481–484
7. Russo J, Russo IH (1997) Role of differentiation in the pathogenesis and prevention of breast cancer. Endocr Relat Cancer 4:7–21
8. Russo J, Russo IH (eds) (2004) Molecular basis of breast cancer: prevention and treatment. Springer, Berlin, p 447
9. Russo J, Balogh GA, Russo IH (2008) Full-term pregnancy induces a specific genomic signature in the human breast. Cancer Epidemiol Biomarkers Prev 17:51–66
10. Asztalos S, Gann PH, Hayes MK, Nonn L, Beam CA, Dai Y, Wiley EL, Tonetti DA (2010) Gene expression patterns in the human breast after pregnancy. Cancer Prev Res 3:301–311
11. Medina D (2004) Breast cancer: the protective effect of pregnancy. Clin Cancer Res 10:380S–384S
12. D'Cruz CM, Moody SE, Master SR, Hartman JL, Keiper EA, Imielinski MB, Cox JD, Wang JY, Ha SI, Keister BA, Chodosh LA (2002) Persistent parity-induced changes in growth factors, TGF-beta3, and differentiation in the rodent mammary gland. Mol Endocrinol 16:2034–2051
13. Belitskaya-Levy I, Zeleniuch-Jacquotte A, Russo J, Russo IH, Bordas P, Ahman J, Afanasyeva Y, Johansson R, Lenner P, Li X, de Cicco-Lopez RL, Peri S, Ross E, Russo PA, Santucci-Pereira J, Sheriff FS, Slifker M, Hallmans G, Toniolo P, Arslan AA (2011) Characterization of a genomic signature of pregnancy identified in the breast. Cancer Prev Res 4:1457–1464

14. Russo J, Rivera R, Russo IH (1992) Influence of age and parity on the development of the human breast. Breast Cancer Res Treat 23:211–218
15. Russo IH, Russo J (2011) Pregnancy-induced changes in breast cancer risk. J Mammary Gland Biol Neoplasia 16:221–233
16. Long JC, Caceres JF (2009) The SR protein family of splicing factors: master regulators of gene expression. Biochem J 417:15–27
17. Herrmann A, Fleischer K, Czajkowska H, Muller-Newen G, Becker W (2007) Characterization of cyclin L1 as an immobile component of the splicing factor compartment. FASEB J 21:3142–3152
18. Golob JL, Paige SL, Muskheli V, Pabon L, Murry CE (2008) Chromatin remodeling during mouse and human embryonic stem cell differentiation. Dev Dyn 237:1389–1398
19. Wilson BJ, Giguere V (2008) Meta-analysis of human cancer microarrays reveals GATA3 is integral to the estrogen receptor alpha pathway. Mol Cancer 7:49
20. Chou J, Provot S, Werb Z (2010) GATA3 in development and cancer differentiation: cells GATA have it! J Cell Physiol 222:42–49
21. Russo IH, Russo J (1996) Mammary gland neoplasia in long-term rodent studies. Environ Health Perspect 104:938–967
22. Russo J, Tait L, Russo IH (1983) Susceptibility of the mammary gland to carcinogenesis. III. The cell of origin of rat mammary carcinoma. Am J Pathol 113:50–66
23. Bussolati G, Marchio C, Gaetano L, Lupo R, Sapino A (2008) Pleomorphism of the nuclear envelope in breast cancer: a new approach to an old problem. J Cell Mol Med 12:209–218
24. Tan PH, Goh BB, Chiang G, Bay BH (2001) Correlation of nuclear morphometry with pathologic parameters in ductal carcinoma in situ of the breast. Mod Pathol 14:937–941
25. Palmer JE, Sant Cassia LJ, Irwin CJ, Morris AG, Rollason TP (2008) The prognostic value of nuclear morphometric analysis in serous ovarian carcinoma. Int J Gynecol Cancer 18:692–701
26. Cao R, Wang L, Wang H, Xia L, Erdjument-Bromage H, Tempst P, Jones RS, Zhang Y (2002) Role of histone H3 lysine 27 methylation in Polycomb-group silencing. Science 298:1039–1043
27. Kubicek S, Schotta G, Lachner M, Sengupta R, Kohlmaier A, Perez-Burgos L, Linderson Y, Martens JH, O'Sullivan RJ, Fodor BD, Yonezawa M, Peters AH, Jenuwein T (2006) The role of histone modifications in epigenetic transitions during normal and perturbed development. Ernst Schering Res Found Workshop 57:1–27
28. Lin W, Dent SY (2006) Functions of histone-modifying enzymes in development. Curr Opin Genet Dev 16:137–142
29. Guenther MG, Young RA (2010) Transcription. Repressive transcription. Science 329:150–151
30. Erwin JA, Lee JT (2010) Characterization of X-chromosome inactivation status in human pluripotent stem cells. Curr Protoc Stem Cell Biol Chapter 1:Unit 1B.6
31. Navarro P, Chambers I, Karwacki-Neisius V, Chureau C, Morey C, Rougeulle C, Avner P (2008) Molecular coupling of Xist regulation and pluripotency. Science 321:1693–1695
32. Surani MA, Hayashi K, Hajkova P (2007) Genetic and epigenetic regulators of pluripotency. Cell 128:747–762
33. Lee J (2010) Characterization of X-chromosome inactivation status in human pluripotent stem cells. Curr Protoc Stem Cell Biol Chapter 1:Unit 1B.6
34. Taga Y, Miyoshi M, Okajima T, Matsuda T, Nadano D (2010) Identification of heterogeneous nuclear ribonucleoprotein A/B as a cytoplasmic mRNA-binding protein in early involution of the mouse mammary gland. Cell Biochem Funct 28:321–328
35. Huang PR, Hung SC, Wang TC (2010) Telomeric DNA-binding activities of heterogeneous nuclear ribonucleoprotein A3 in vitro and in vivo. Biochim Biophys Acta 1803:1164–1174
36. Han SP, Friend LR, Carson JH, Korza G, Barbarese E, Maggipinto M, Hatfield JT, Rothnagel JA, Smith R (2010) Differential subcellular distributions and trafficking functions of hnRNP A2/B1 spliceoforms. Traffic 11:886–898

37. Loyer P, Trembley JH, Grenet JA, Busson A, Corlu A, Zhao W, Kocak M, Kidd VJ, Lahti JM (2008) Characterization of cyclin L1 and L2 interactions with CDK11 and splicing factors: influence of cyclin L isoforms on splice site selection. J Biol Chem 283:7721–7732
38. Yang L, Li N, Wang C, Yu Y, Yuan L, Zhang M, Cao X (2004) Cyclin L2, a novel RNA polymerase II-associated cyclin, is involved in pre-mRNA splicing and induces apoptosis of human hepatocellular carcinoma cells. J Biol Chem 279:11639–11648
39. Fushimi K, Ray P, Kar A, Wang L, Sutherland LC, Wu JY (2008) Up-regulation of the proapoptotic caspase 2 splicing isoform by a candidate tumor suppressor, RBM5. Proc Natl Acad Sci U S A 105:15708–15713
40. Kobayashi T, Ishida J, Musashi M, Ota S, Yoshida T, Shimizu Y, Chuma M, Kawakami H, Asaka M, Tanaka J, Imamura M, Kobayashi M, Itoh H, Edamatsu H, Sutherland LC, Brachmann RK (2011) p53 transactivation is involved in the antiproliferative activity of the putative tumor suppressor RBM5. Int J Cancer 128:304–318
41. Salomonis N, Schlieve CR, Pereira L, Wahlquist C, Colas A, Zambon AC, Vranizan K, Spindler MJ, Pico AR, Cline MS, Clark TA, Williams A, Blume JE, Samal E, Mercola M, Merrill BJ, Conklin BR (2010) Alternative splicing regulates mouse embryonic stem cell pluripotency and differentiation. Proc Natl Acad Sci U S A 107:10514–10519
42. Russo J, Russo IH (2000) Human chorionic gonadotropin in breast cancer prevention. In: Ethier SP (ed) Endocrine oncology. Humana Press, Totowa, NJ, pp 121–136
43. Russo J, Mailo D, Hu YF, Balogh G, Sheriff F, Russo IH (2005) Breast differentiation and its implication in cancer prevention. Clin Cancer Res 11:931s–936s
44. Russo IH, Russo J (2000) Hormonal approach to breast cancer prevention. J Cell Biochem Suppl 34:1–6
45. Russo J, Moral R, Balogh GA, Mailo D, Russo IH (2005) The protective role of pregnancy in breast cancer. Breast Cancer Res 7:131–142
46. Russo J, Balogh GA, Chen J, Fernandez SV, Fernbaugh R, Heulings R, Mailo DA, Moral R, Russo PA, Sheriff F, Vanegas JE, Wang R, Russo IH (2006) The concept of stem cell in the mammary gland and its implication in morphogenesis, cancer and prevention. Front Biosci 11:151–172
47. Russo J, Russo IH (1994) Toward a physiological approach to breast cancer prevention. Cancer Epidemiol Biomarkers Prev 3:353–364
48. Russo J, Russo IH (1987) Biological and molecular bases of mammary carcinogenesis. Lab Invest 57:112–137
49. Russo IH, Russo J (2007) Primary prevention of breast cancer by hormone-induced differentiation. Recent Results Cancer Res 174:111–130
50. Kocdor H, Kocdor MA, Russo J, Snider KE, Vanegas JE, Russo IH, Fernandez SV (2009) Human chorionic gonadotropin (hCG) prevents the transformed phenotypes induced by 17 beta-estradiol in human breast epithelial cells. Cell Biol Int 33:1135–1143
51. Russo J, Santucci-Pereira J, López de Cicco R, Sheriff F, Russo PA, Peri S, Slifker M, Ross E, Mello MLS, Vidal BC, Belitskaya-Lévy I, Arslan A, Zeleniuch-Jacquotte A, Bordas P, Lenner P, Ahman J, Afanasyeva Y, Hallmans G, Toniolo P, Russo IH (2012) Pregnancy-induced chromatin remodeling in the breast of postmenopausal women. Int J Cancer 131(5):1059–1070. doi:10.1002/ijc.27323
52. Mello ML, Vidal BC, Russo IH, Lareef MH, Russo J (2007) DNA content and chromatin texture of human breast epithelial cells transformed with 17-beta-estradiol and the estrogen antagonist ICI 182,780 as assessed by image analysis. Mutat Res 617:1–7
53. Mello ML, Russo P, Russo J, Vidal BC (2009) Entropy of Feulgen-stained 17-beta-estradiol-transformed human breast epithelial cells as assessed by restriction enzymes and image analysis. Oncol Rep 21:1483–1487
54. Doudkine A, Macaulay C, Poulin N, Palcic B (1995) Nuclear texture measurements in image cytometry. Pathologica 87:286–299
55. Isharwal S, Miller MC, Marlow C, Makarov DV, Partin AW, Veltri RW (2008) p300 (histone acetyltransferase) biomarker predicts prostate cancer biochemical recurrence and correlates with changes in epithelia nuclear size and shape. Prostate 68:1097–1104

56. Bolstad BM, Irizarry RA, Astrand M, Speed TP (2003) A comparison of normalization methods for high density oligonucleotide array data based on variance and bias. Bioinformatics 19:185–193
57. Johnson WE, Li C, Rabinovic A (2007) Adjusting batch effects in microarray expression data using empirical Bayes methods. Biostatistics 8:118–127
58. Smyth GK (2005) Limma: linear models for microarray data. In: Gentleman R, Carey V, Dudoit S, Irizarry R, Huber W (eds) Bioinformatics and computational biology solutions using R and bioconductor. Springer, New York, pp 397–420
59. Gentleman RC, Carey VJ, Bates DM, Bolstad B, Dettling M, Dudoit S, Ellis B, Gautier L, Ge Y, Gentry J, Hornik K, Hothorn T, Huber W, Iacus S, Irizarry R, Leisch F, Li C, Maechler M, Rossini AJ, Sawitzki G, Smith C, Smyth G, Tierney L, Yang JY, Zhang J (2004) Bioconductor: open software development for computational biology and bioinformatics. Genome Biol 5:R80

Chapter 8
The Role of Spliceosome in the Human Breast

8.1 Introduction

In 1977, work by the Sharp and Roberts labs revealed that genes of higher organisms are "split" or present in several distinct segments along the DNA molecule [1, 2]. The coding regions of the gene are separated by noncoding DNA that is not involved in protein expression. The split gene structure was found when adenoviral mRNAs were hybridized to endonuclease cleavage fragments of single-stranded viral DNA [1]. It was observed that the mRNAs of the mRNA-DNA hybrids contained 5′ and 3′ tails of non-hydrogen bonded regions. When larger fragments of viral DNAs were used, forked structures of looped out DNA were observed when hybridized to the viral mRNAs. It was realized that the looped out regions, the introns, are excised from the precursor mRNAs in a process Sharp named "splicing." The split gene structure was subsequently found to be common to most eukaryotic genes. Phillip Sharp and Richard J. Roberts were awarded the 1993 Nobel Prize in Physiology or Medicine for their discovery of introns and the splicing process. The advances in this field is unprecedented mainly due to the new implications in our understanding of the basic biological process and its application to the treatment and prevention of many diseases [3, 4]. In this chapter we will describe the main pathways of the splicing mechanism that help the reader to understand the new findings in the human breast and their role in breast cancer prevention.

8.2 The Splicing Mechanism

A spliceosome is a complex of specialized RNA and protein subunits that removes introns from a transcribed pre-mRNA (hnRNA) segment. This process is generally referred to as splicing. Each spliceosome is composed of five small nuclear RNA proteins, called snRNPs, and a range of non-snRNP-associated protein factors. The snRNPs that make up the nuclear spliceosome are named U1, U2, U4, U5, and U6,

J. Russo and I.H. Russo, *Role of the Transcriptome in Breast Cancer Prevention*,
DOI 10.1007/978-1-4614-4884-6_8, © Springer Science+Business Media New York 2013

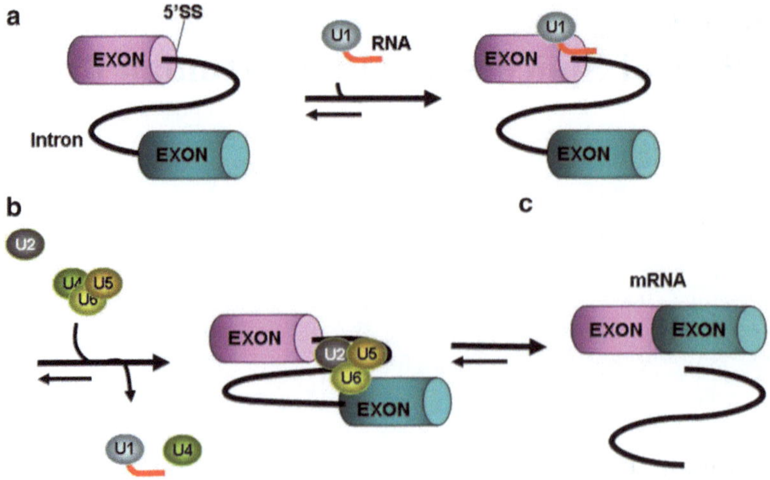

Fig. 8.1 Spliceosome assembly and RNA splicing

and participate in several RNA–RNA and RNA–protein interactions (Fig. 8.1). The canonical assembly of the spliceosome comprises the conversion of precursor messenger RNA into mature messenger RNA (mRNA). The pre-mRNA molecule undergoes three main modifications, which occur in the cell nucleus before the RNA is translated: (1) mRNA capping, (2) Processing of intron-containing pre-mRNA and (3) mRNA 3′ end processing. These three main steps are executed by a large number of proteins that are listed in Tables 8.1 and 8.2.

The capping of the pre-mRNA involves the addition of 7-methylguanosine (m7G) to the 5′ end. The cap protects the 5′ end of the primary RNA transcript from attack by ribonucleases (Fig. 8.2). The processing of intron-containing pre-mRNA is the process by which introns, regions of RNA that do not code for protein, are removed from the pre-mRNA and the remaining exons connected to re-form a single continuous molecule (Fig. 8.3). The hnRNA contains specific sequence elements that are recognized and utilized during spliceosome assembly. These include the 5′ end splice, the branch point sequence (BPS), the polypyrimidine tract (PPT), and the 3′ end splice site. The spliceosome catalyzes the removal of introns, and the ligation of the flanking exons. Introns typically have a GU nucleotide sequence at the 5′ end splice site, and an AG at the 3′ end splice site. The 3′ splice site can be further defined by a variable length of polypyrimidines, called the PPT, which serves the dual function of recruiting factors to the 3′ splice site and possibly recruiting factors to the BPS. The BPS contains the conserved Adenosine required for the first step of splicing. A group of less abundant snRNPs, U11, U12, U4atac, and U6atac, together with U5, are subunits of the so-called minor spliceosome that splices a rare class of pre-mRNA introns, denoted U12-type. These snRNPs form the U12 spliceosome and are located in the cytosol [5]. The last step in the process is the mRNA 3′ end processing that consists in the cleavage of its 3′ end and addition of adenine residues to form the poly(A) tail, which protects the 3′ end from ribonuclease digestion.

Table 8.1 Components of the splicing mechanism

mRNA capping				POLR2A RNMT SUPT5H RNGTT
Processing of intron-containing pre-mRNA	Internal methylation of mRNA			NCBP1 NCBP2 METTL3
	Formation of pre-mRNPs (heterogeneous nuclear ribonucleoproteins)			HNRPA1 HNRPA3P1 HNRPA2B1 HNRPAB HNRPC HNRPD RBMX HNRPH1 HNRPH2 HNRPK HNRPL HNRPM HNRPR HNRPU
	mRNA splicing (major pathway)	Formation of the spliceosomal E complex	U1snRNP	U1snRNA SNRP70 SNRPA SNRPB SNRPD1 SNRPD2 SNRPD3 SNRPE SNRPF SNRPG
			U2AF·	U2AF1 U2AF2 SFRS1 SFRS2 SFRS3 SFRS5 SFRS6 SFRS7 SFRS9
			RNA helicase A	FUS NSEP1 SF4 RBM5 CD2BP2 SMC1LI

(continued)

Table 8.1 (continued)

		Formation of the spliceosomal A complex	U2 snRNP	RNU2 SF3A1 SF3A2 SF3A3 SNRPA1 SNRPB2 SF3b14b PHF5A SF3B1 SF3B2 SF3B3 SF3B4 SF3B5
			SR proteins	SFRS4
			RNA helicase	DHX3B
			Additional factors	CDC40 DNAJC8 PRPF8 PTBP1
		Formation of the spliceosomal B Complex	U4:U5:U6 tri-snRNP complex	U4 snRNA SSFA1 PRPF4 RNU6 SSFA1 LSM2 U5snRNA TXNL4A WDR57 U5-116KD LSM2 PRPF8 PRPF18
mRNA 3′ end processing				NUDT21 HEAB CPSF1 CPSF2 CPSF3 CPSF4 PABPN1 PAPOLA CSTF1 CSTF2T CSTF2 CSTF3

Table 8.2 Accessory proteins for splicing

Category	Genes
SR protein kinases	CLK1, CLK2, CLK3, CLK4, PRPF4B, SRPK1, SRPK2, PSKH1
SR-protein phosphatases	PPM1G
Additional SR proteins	SFRS8, SFRS10, SFRS12, SFRS14, SFRS16, TMP21, FUSIP1, SRRM1, SRP54
Spliceosome-associated helicases	DDX1, DDX20, DHX8, DHX15, DHX16
mRNA splice site selection	BRUNOL4, CUGBP2, PTBP2
hnRNP regulators	HRMT1L2, HRMT1L1, PCBP2
Putative alternative splicing regulators	SNRPN, RNPS1
SR-repressor proteins	FUSIP1
RNAi pathway	DICER1
Miscellaneous	CUGBP1, RNPC2, NONO, XRN2, SPOP, PRPF3, FNBP3, RBM17, LSM7, SNRPN, NXF1, SFPQ

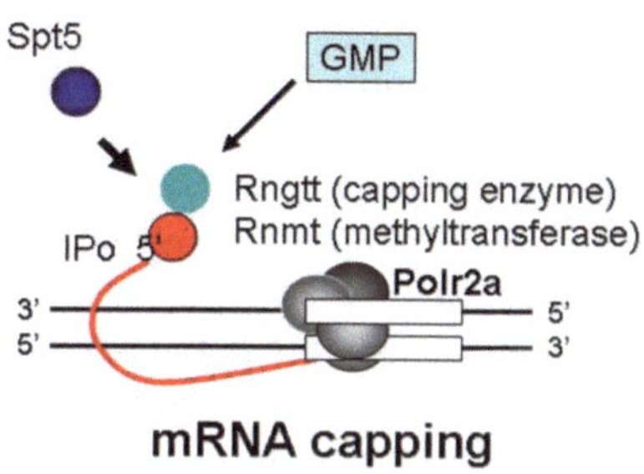

Fig. 8.2 The cap protects the 5′ end of primary RNA transcript from attack by endonucleases

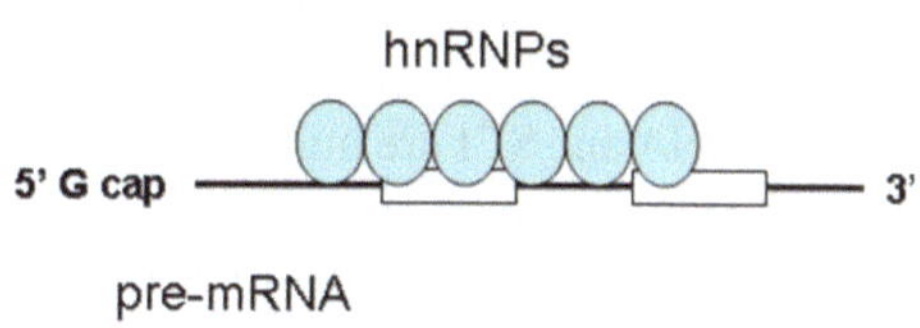

Fig. 8.3 Internal methylation of mRNA and formation of pre-mRNPs

8.3 Spliceosome Assembly

The model for formation of the spliceosome active site involves an ordered, stepwise assembly of discrete snRNP particles on the hnRNA substrate. The first recognition of hnRNAs involves U1 snRNP binding to the 5′ end splice site of the hnRNA and other non-snRNP-associated factors to form the commitment complex, or early (E) complex in mammals [6, 7] (Table 8.1 and Fig. 8.4). The commitment complex is an ATP-independent complex that commits the hnRNA to the splicing pathway [8]. U2 snRNP is recruited to the branch region through interactions with the complex component U2AF (U2 snRNP auxiliary factor) and possibly U1 snRNP (Table 8.1). In an ATP-dependent reaction, U2 snRNP becomes tightly associated with the BPS to form complex A. A duplex formed between U2 snRNA and the hnRNA branch region bulges out the branch adenosine specifying it as the nucleophile for the first transesterification [9] (Fig. 8.4). The presence of a pseudouridine residue in U2 snRNA, nearly opposite of the branch site, results in an altered conformation of the RNA-RNA duplex upon the U2 snRNP binding. Specifically, the altered structure of the duplex induced by the pseudouridine places the 2′ OH of the bulged adenosine in a favorable position for the first step of splicing [10].

The U4/U5/U6 tri-snRNP (Fig. 8.5 and Table 8.1) is recruited to the assembling spliceosome to form complex B, and following several rearrangements, complex C (the spliceosome) is activated for catalysis [11, 12]. It is unclear how the triple snRNP is recruited to complex A, but this process may be mediated through protein–protein interactions and/or base pairing interactions between U2 snRNA and U6 snRNA. The U5 snRNP interacts with sequences at the 5′ and 3′ splice sites via the invariant loop of U5 snRNA [13] and U5 protein components interact with the 3′ splice site region [14]. Upon recruitment of the triple snRNP, several RNA-RNA rearrangements precede the first catalytic step and further rearrangements occur in the catalytically active spliceosome. Several of the RNA–RNA interactions are mutually exclusive; however, it is not known what triggers these interactions, nor the order of these rearrangements. The first rearrangement is probably the displacement of U1 snRNP from the 5′ splice site and formation of a U6 snRNA interaction. It is known that U1 snRNP is only weakly associated with fully formed spliceosomes [15], and U1 snRNP is inhibitory to the formation of a U6-5′ splice site interaction on a model of substrate oligonucleotide containing a short 5′ exon and 5′ splice site [16]. Binding of U2 snRNP to the BPS is one example of an RNA–RNA interaction displacing a protein-RNA interaction. Upon recruitment of U2 snRNP, the branch binding protein SF1 in the commitment complex is displaced since the binding site of U2 snRNA and SF1 are mutually exclusive events (Table 8.1 and Fig. 8.5). Within the U2 snRNA, there are other mutually exclusive rearrangements that occur between competing conformations. For example, in the active form, stem loop IIa is favored; in the inactive form a mutually exclusive interaction between the loop and a downstream sequence predominates [12]. It is unclear how U4 is displaced from U6 snRNAm, although RNA has been implicated in spliceosome assembly, and may function to unwind U4/U6 and promote the formation of a U2/U6 snRNA

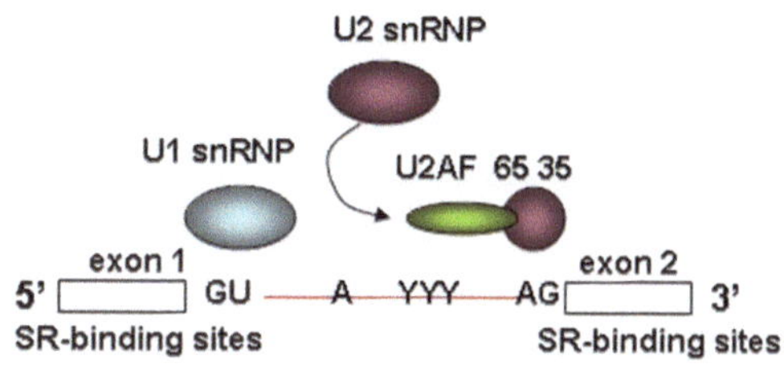

Fig. 8.4 Formation of the spliceosomal A complex

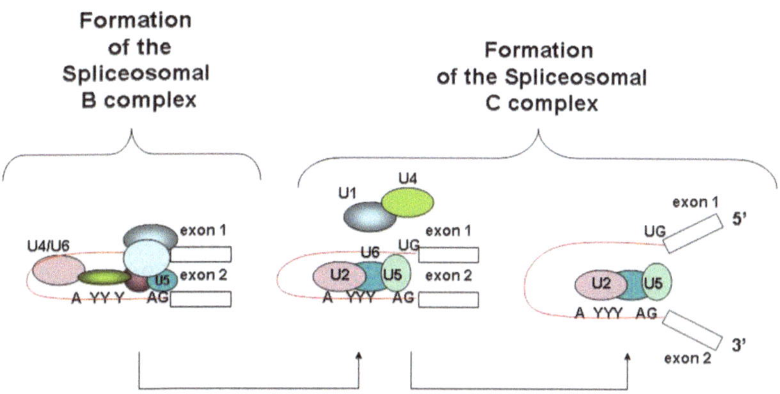

Fig. 8.5 Formation of the spliceosomal B and C complex

interaction. The interactions of U4/U6 stem loops I and II dissociate and the freed stem loop II region of U6 folds on itself to form an intramolecular stem loop and U4 is no longer required in further spliceosome assembly. The freed stem loop I region of U6 base pairs with U2 snRNA forming the U2/U6 helix I. However, the helix I structure is mutually exclusive with the 3′ half of an internal 5′ stem loop region of U2 snRNA.

8.4 The Role of Spliceosome in the Human Breast

We have reported [17, 18] that there is a group of genes that are significantly upregulated in the parous breast tissue as it is depicted in the Tables 8.3, 8.4, and 8.5 related to the mRNA processing reactome in the parous breast emerging as an important regulatory pathway induced by pregnancy. The biological importance of this pathway cannot be overemphasized enough because the pre-mRNAs contain

Table 8.3 Overrepresented GO biological processes for differentially expressed genes

GO term ID	GO term	Genes upregulated in parous samples
GO:0016071	mRNA metabolic process	CIRBP, RBMX, HNRNPA1, HNRNPA2B1, HNRNPD, LUC7L3, PNN, PRPF39, RBM25, SFPQ, SFRS1, SFRS5, SFRS7, PABPN1, PRPF4B
GO:0006397	mRNA processing	RBMX, HNRNPA1, HNRNPA2B1, LUC7L3, PNN, PRPF39, RBM25, SFPQ, SFRS1, SFRS5, SFRS7, PABPN1, PRPF4B
GO:0034059	Response to anoxia	OXTR
GO:0016070	RNA metabolic process	DDX17, CHD2,C BX3, CIRBP, ZNF785, EZH2, L3MBTL, GATA3, RBMX, ZNF789, HNRNPA1, HNRNPA2B1, HNRNPD, LUC7L3, PNN, PRPF39, ZNF83, METTL3, CREBZF, RBM25, RBBP8, RPS24, CENPK, SFPQ, SFRS1, SFRS5, SFRS7, ZNF814, ZNF207, PABPN1, RUNX3, FUBP1, PRPF4B, HNRPDL
GO:0006396	RNA processing	DDX17, RBMX, HNRNPA1, HNRNPA2B1, HNRNPD, LUC7L3, PNN, PRPF39, RBM25, RPS24, SFPQ, SFRS1, SFRS5, SFRS7, PABPN1, PRPF4B, HNRPDL
GO:0008380	RNA splicing	RBMX, HNRNPA1, HNRNPA2B1, HNRNPD, LUC7L3, PNN, PRPF39, RBM25, SFPQ, SFRS1, SFRS5, SFRS7, PABPN1, PRPF4B

Table 8.4 Overrepresented GSEA gene sets for differentially expressed genes

Pathways enriched by upregulated genes	NES	FDR q-val	Genes
mRNA processing reactome	1.626	0.093	METTL3, HNRPD, HNRPA2B1, PRPF4B, SFRS7, CLK4, SFRS5, PABPN1, CSTF3, HNRPU, RBM5, SNRP70, SFRS14, SNRPA1, CLK2, NXF1, SFRS8, SFRS2, PTBP2, FUS, SFRS6, SFRS16, SF3B1, HNRPA3, SNRPB, PRPF3, SFRS12, U2AF1, PHF5A, TXNL4A, CUGBP2

noncoding sequences (introns) that must be removed in order to accurately place the coding sequences (exons) in the correct reading frame. The upregulation of these gene products in the breast epithelia of parous women could be a clear indication of a safe guard mechanism that will maintain the fidelity of the transcription process and this could be a mechanism of protection conferred by the differentiated breast. This critical regulatory pre-mRNA splicing event is fundamental in development and cancer. Infidelity in this process can have dramatic consequences for protein production, with errors resulting in mRNA instability or the production of aberrant protein products. The spliceosome machinery involved in this process is composed

Table 8.5 Important differentially expressed genes in parous vs. nulliparous ($p<0.001$ and log 2-fold change of at least 0.3)

Gene symbol	Log ratio	Gene name
CCNL1	0.40	Cyclin L2
CCNL2	0.47	Cyclin L2
HNRNPA1	0.50	Heterogeneous nuclear ribonucleoprotein A1
HNRNPA2B1	0.56	Heterogeneous nuclear ribonucleoprotein A2/B1
HNRNPD	0.59	Heterogeneous nuclear ribonucleoprotein D (AU-rich element RNA-binding protein 1, 37 kDa)
HNRPDL	0.65	Heterogeneous nuclear ribonucleoprotein D-like
METTL3	0.69	Methyltransferase like 3
SFPQ	0.47	Splicing factor proline/glutamine-rich
SFRS1	0.30	Splicing factor, arginine/serine-rich 1
SFRS18	0.40	Splicing factor, arginine/serine-rich 18
SFRS5	0.36	Splicing factor, arginine/serine-rich 5
SFRS7	0.40	Splicing factor, arginine/serine-rich 7, 35 kDa
SNHG10	0.62	Small nucleolar RNA host gene 10 (nonprotein coding)
SNHG12	0.53	Small nucleolar RNA host gene 12 (nonprotein coding)
SNORD104	0.43	Small nucleolar RNA, C/D box 104

of RNA and proteins, which undergoes dynamic changes in RNA–RNA, RNA–protein, and protein–protein interactions during the splicing reaction. Part of this interaction is clearly shown in all the upregulated genes controlling the splicing mechanism of the parous breast tissue.

8.4.1 Internal Methylation of mRNA and the Methyltransferase Like 3

The MTTL3 or methyltransferase like 3 that is upregulated in the parous breast is involved in the posttranscriptional methylation of internal adenosine residues in eukaryotic mRNAs, forming N6-methyladenosine playing a role in the efficiency of mRNA splicing, transport or translation (Fig. 8.3). The role of this gene needs to be placed in relevance with the different mechanisms involved in the control of gene expression. The regulation of gene expression is a cellular process that controls the level and the interval of time in which genes are in a state of transcription or translation. This regulation also dictates the structure and function of the cell, and is fundamental to control differentiation, morphogenesis, and growth. By their diverse actions in eukaryotic cells, they can have a transcriptional, posttranscriptional, translational, or posttranslational effect on gene activity. Epigenetics are involved in some of these processes and can be defined as the reversible heritable changes in gene function that occur during cell division without changes in nuclear DNA sequence. They include modifications that take place on genomic DNA such as methylation of cytosine residues, and posttranscriptional modifications on the tail domains of histones by methylation, acetylation, phosphorylation, ubiquitination, or sumoylation [19–21]. DNA methylation is generally associated with transcriptional repression and is involved in genomic imprinting. This modification is active during the entire life of a cell, and it is essential for modeling and modulating the genome during gametogenesis and in the early stages of mammalian embryo development and differentiation where epigenetic events are crucial. However the cells must not only contain the appropriate epigenetic factors, but also need to accumulate mRNAs and proteins to allow the cell to perform its functions. In eukaryotic cells, pre-mRNAs have to undergo several modifications to excise the introns present prior to translation of the matured mRNA. Interestingly, this splicing process can be affected by the methylation of internal adenosine residues located within the 5′ cap and 3′ poly (A) tail [22, 23] (Fig. 8.3). The N6-methyladenosine is present at internal sites in mRNA isolated from all higher eukaryotes and prokaryotes [24]. This nucleoside modification occurs only in a sequence-specific context that appears to be conserved across diverse species and may play a role in the efficiency of mRNA splicing, transport, or translation during sporulation [23]. The high levels of *METTL3* present in the parous breast may in fact be necessary for pre-mRNA processing, because of the minor gene activation occurring in the resting breast of the parous woman and may act as a mechanism of methylation of internal adenosine residues located within the 5′ cap and 3′ poly (A) tail.

8.4.2 Formation of Pre-mRNP or Heterogeneous Nuclear Ribonucleoproteins

During the processing of intron-containing pre-mRNA the second step after the internal methylation of mRNA is the formation of pre-mRNPs (Table 8.1 and Fig. 8.3). The RNPs or heterogeneous nuclear ribonucleoproteins are main components of the spliceosome machinery and among them are the HNRPA3. HNRPA2B1, HNRPD, and the HNRPU that all of them are upregulated in the parous breast (Tables 8.3, 8.4, and 8.5). These proteins are associated with pre-mRNAs in the nucleus and appear to influence pre-mRNA processing and other aspects of mRNA metabolism and transport. While all of the hnRNPs are present in the nucleus, some seem to shuttle between the nucleus and the cytoplasm. Two other components of the hnRNP complex are FUS and U2AF1. FUS protein belongs to the FET family of RNA-binding proteins which have been implicated in cellular processes that include regulation of gene expression, maintenance of genomic integrity, and mRNA/microRNA processing [25–27] (Table 8.1). The U2AF1 or U2 small nuclear RNA auxiliary factor 1 belongs to the splicing factor SR family of genes. U2 auxiliary factor, comprising a large and a small subunit, is a non-snRNP protein required for the binding of U2 snRNP to the pre-mRNA branch site. This gene encodes the small subunit which plays a critical role in both constitutive and enhancer-dependent RNA splicing by directly mediating interactions between the large subunit and proteins bound to the enhancers. Whereas the precise functional role of the heterogeneous

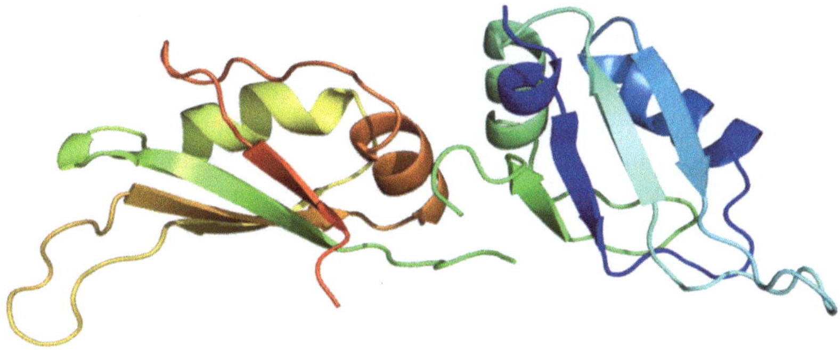

Fig. 8.6 Structure of the HNRPA1 protein. Based on PyMOL rendering of PDB 1ha1. Permission is granted to copy, distribute and/or modify this document under the terms of the GNU Free Documentation License, Version 1.2 or any later version published by the Free Software Foundation

nuclear ribonucleoproteins in the postmenopausal breast epithelia is not known they may play an important regulatory function as transcriptional regulators [28, 29]. These genes are known for coding proteins implicated in the regulation of mRNA stability as well as other function like mammary gland involution [30] or acting as negative regulator of telomere length maintenance [31], or regulating the trafficking of mRNA molecules from the nucleus to distal processes in neural cells [32].

8.4.2.1 Heterogeneous Nuclear Ribonucleoprotein A1

This protein belongs to the A/B subfamily of ubiquitously expressed hnRNPs and along with other proteins, is exported from the nucleus, probably bound to mRNA, and is immediately re-imported. Its M9 domain acts as both a nuclear localization and nuclear export signal (Fig. 8.6). The encoded protein is involved in the packaging of pre-mRNA into hnRNP particles, transport of poly A+ mRNA from the nucleus to the cytoplasm, and may modulate splice site selection. Multiple alternatively spliced transcript variants have been found for this gene but only two transcripts are fully described. These variants have multiple alternative transcription initiation sites and multiple polyA sites [32]. The parous breast shows an upregulation of the HNRNPA1 and we have interpreted that this transcript may play a role in the genomic signature of prevention detected in the breast of parous women [17, 18]. The basis for this assumption are from data in literature demonstrating that alternative pre-mRNA splicing defects can contribute to, or result from, various diseases, including cancer. Aberrant mRNAs, splicing factors and other RNA processing factors have therefore become targets for new therapeutic interventions [33]. For example the natural polyphenol resveratrol can modulate alternative splicing in a target-specific manner. For this purpose minigenes of several alternatively spliceable primary mRNAs has been transected into HEK293 cells in the presence or absence of 1, 5, 20, and 50 μM resveratrol and measured exon levels by semi-quantitative PCR after separation by agarose gel electrophoresis. Using this protocol has been found that 20 and 50 μg/mL of resveratrol affected exon inclusion of SRp20 and SMN2 pre-mRNAs, but not CD44v5 or tau pre-mRNAs. This effect was due to the ability of resveratrol to change the protein level but not the localization of several RNA processing factors. The processing factors that increased significantly were ASF/SF2, HNRNPA1 and HuR, but resveratrol did not change the levels of RBM4, PTBP1, and U2AF35. Using siRNA-mediated knockdown the cells were depleted of SIRT1, regarded as a major target of resveratrol, and showed that the effect on splicing was not dependent on SIRT1 suggesting that resveratrol might have an effect on the splicing machinery in which HNRNPA1 was upregulated [33]. Another example on how the regulation of the HNRNPA1 could be corrective of the splicing mechanisms is in the spinal muscular atrophy (SMA) that is a common autosomal recessive neuromuscular disorder that is caused by loss of the survival motor neuron gene, SMN1. SMA treatment strategies have focused on production of the survival of motor neuron (SMN) protein from the almost identical gene, SMN2. For this purpose has been used valproic acid (VPA) that is a histone deacetylase (HDAC) inhibitor that can increase SMN levels in some SMA cells or SMA patients through activation of SMN2 transcription or splicing correction of SMN2 exon 7. Of great interest is that in two fibroblast cell lines from Japanese SMA patients, more than 1 mM of VPA increased SMN2 expression at both the transcript and protein levels. VPA increased not only full-length (FL) transcript level but also exon 7-excluding (Δ7) transcript level in the cell lines and did not change the ratio of FL/Δ7, suggesting that SMN2 transcription was mainly activated. VPA modulated splicing factor expression: VPA increased the expression of splicing factor 2/alternative splicing factor (SF2/ASF) and decreased the expression of heterogeneous nuclear ribonucleoprotein A1 [34].

HNRNPA1 can also play an important role in the maintenance of genomic integrity by promoting telomere capping [35]. Telomeres are repetitive DNA elements mainly found at the ends of human chromosomes. In most normal cells, telomeres shorten with each cell division. Telomere shortening can be compensated for by a ribonucleoprotein complex, called telomerase. Telomerase, consisting of an integral RNA and catalytic protein component as well as several auxiliary factors, extends the 3′-G-rich strand of the ends of the telomeres. Telomerase bound hnRNPs in promoting telomere access by interacting with telomeres. Telomere bound hnRNPs include HNRNP A1, A2-B1, D and E and telomerase bound HNRNPs including HNRNPA1, C1/C2, and D. Maintenance of telomeres requires both DNA replication and telomere "capping" by shelterin. These two processes use two single-stranded DNA (ssDNA)-binding proteins, replication protein A (RPA), and protection of telomeres 1 (POT1). Purified POT1 and its functional partner TPP1 are unable to prevent RPA binding to telomeric ssDNA efficiently but the heterogeneous nuclear ribonucleoprotein A1 (HNRNPA1) recapitulates the RPA displacing activity. The RPA displacing activity is inhibited by the telomeric repeat-containing RNA in early S phase, but is then unleashed in late S phase when telomeric repeat-containing RNA levels decline at telomeres. Interestingly, telomeric repeat-containing RNA also promotes POT1 binding to telomeric ssDNA by removing hnRNPA1, suggesting that the re-accumulation of telomeric repeat-containing RNA after S phase helps to complete the RPA-to-POT1 switch on telomeric ssDNA. HNRPA1, TERRA, and POT1 act in concert to displace RPA from telomeric ssDNA after DNA replication, and promote telomere capping [35].

HNRNPA1 also interacts with high mobility group A protein 1a (HMGA1a) that is involved in splice site regulation of 3′ splice site 2 (A2) and 5′ splice site 3 (D3) of HIV-1 genomic RNA. HMGA1a inhibits HNRNPA1 function on exon splicing silencer of Vpr (ESSV) to activate A2 function [36]. Another type of interaction has been found between HNRNPA1 and Quaking (Qk) [37, 38]. Quaking (Qk) is required for myelin formation and has been associated with psychiatric disease. QK regulates the stability, subcellular localization, and alternative splicing of several myelin-related transcripts. QK governs these activities by enhancing HNRNPA1-RNA stability by binding a conserved 3′ UTR sequence with high affinity and specificity. A single nucleotide mutation in the binding site eliminates QK-dependent regulation, as does reduction of QK by RNAi. Analysis of exon expression across the transcriptome reveals that QK and HNRNPA1 regulate an overlapping subset of transcripts. It has been interpreted that QK regulates a large set of oligodendrocyte precursor genes indirectly by increasing the intracellular concentration of HNRNP A1 controlling of myelin gene expression [37].

HNRNPA1, hnRNPA2, and polypyrimidine tract-binding protein (PTB; also known as HNRNPI), control alternative splicing events that regulate cell proliferation and cancer and among them are the metabolic shift from oxidative phosphorylation to aerobic glycolysis that is partly achieved by a switch in the splice isoforms of the glycolytic enzyme pyruvate kinase. Although normal cells express the pyruvate kinase M1 isoform (PKM1), tumor cells predominantly express the M2 isoform (PKM2). Switching from PKM1 to PKM2 promotes aerobic glycolysis and provides a selective advantage for tumor formation. The PKM1/M2 isoforms are generated through alternative splicing of two mutually exclusive exons [39, 40]. In breast cancer a large fraction of the sequence variants of unknown significance or unclassified variants of the BRCA1 could be pathogenic by affecting mRNA splicing. These cancers exhibit a large spectrum of sequence variation but only two variants, both located in exon 18, have been shown experimentally to affect splicing regulatory elements. The effect of the variant has been tested [41, 42] by using splicing reporter hybrid minigene assays inducing a major splicing defect, with skipping of exon 23, resulting in frameshift and predicted protein termination within the second BRCT domain. Moreover, the segment c.5420–5449 of BRCA1, in the center of exon 23, exhibits splicing enhancer properties. This enhancement is abolished by the c.5434C G mutation, indicating that the nucleotide change, in this highly conserved region, affects a splicing regulatory element. Bioinformatics analyses predict that the mutation c.5434C G creates an HNRNPA1 dependent splicing silencer [41].

Although we do not know at the present time which is the precise mechanism of action of HNRNPA1 in cancer prevention it is possible to postulate that it may interact with different genes controlling apoptosis and cell proliferation. This is based on the known data from the literature that HNRNPA1 is involved with certain types of human papillomaviruses (HPVs) that are etiologically linked to cervical cancer. Their transforming capacity is encoded by a polycistronic pre-mRNA, where alternative splicing leads to the translation of functional distinct proteins such as E6, E6*, and E7. Splicing of HPV16 E6/E7 ORF cassette is regulated by the epidermal growth factor (EGF) pathway. The presence of EGF was coupled to preferential E6 expression, whereas depletion of EGF, or treatment with EGF receptor (EGFR) neutralizing antibodies or the EGFR inhibitor tyrphostin AG1478, resulted in E6 exon exclusion in favor of E6*. As a consequence, increased p53 levels and enhanced translation of E7 with a subsequent reduction of the retinoblastoma protein pRb could be discerned. E6 exon exclusion upon EGF depletion was independent from promoter usage, mRNA stability, or selective mRNA transport. Time-course experiments and incubation with cycloheximide demonstrated that E6 alternative splicing is a direct and reversible effect of EGF signal transduction, not depending on de novo protein synthesis. Within this process, Erk1/2-kinase activation was the critical event for E6 exon inclusion, mediated by the upstream MAP kinase MEK1/2. Moreover, siRNA knockdown experiments revealed an involvement of splicing factors HNRNPA1 and hnRNPA2 in E6 exon exclusion, whereas the splicing factors Brm and Sam68 were found to promote E6 exon inclusion. Because there is a natural gradient of EGF and EGFR expression in the stratified epithelium, it has been assumed that EGF modulates E6/E7 splicing during the viral life cycle and transformation [43]. In another example B23, a nucleolar protein required for rRNA processing, is localized to the cytoplasm and forms a complex with the mRNA-binding proteins HNRNPU and HNRNPA1 in a sequential manner. In addition, RNA Polymerase I, but not RNA Polymerase II inhibition, was found to account for the translocation-dependent assembly of B23/hnRNPU/HNRNPA1. Interactions among these proteins are regulated by HNRNPU-bound mRNAs such as the 3′-untranslated region (UTR) of Bcl-xL mRNA. Ectopically expressed 3′-UTR of Bcl-xL mRNA, which disrupted the interactions among B23, HNRNPU, and HNRNPA1, led to enhanced cell apoptosis induced by either actinomycin D treatment or mitotic arrest [44]. Another example is the transcription factor c-Myb which plays a key role in hematopoietic proliferation and lineage commitment and influences alternative pre-mRNA splicing. This was seen by its marked effect on the 5′-splice site selection during E1A alternative splicing, while no effect of c-Myb was observed when reporters for the 3′-splice site selection or for the constitutive splicing process were tested. Co-immunoprecipitation experiments provided evidence for interactions between c-Myb and distinct components of the splicing apparatus, such as the general splicing factor U2AF and HNRNPA1 involved in the 5′-splice site selection. The effect on 5′-splice site selection was abolished in the oncogenic variant v-Myb [45].

The protective effect of an early first full term pregnancy has been attributed to the hormonal milieu of pregnancy and its imprinting in the genomic of the postmenopausal breast [17, 18]. It is know that HNRNPA1 can be regulated by steroid hormones. Treatment of neuronal cells with estradiol results in increased expression of APP695, SC35, and HNRNPA1, and lowers the level of secreted beta-amyloid peptide (Abeta) that accumulates in senile plaques in Alzheimer's disease is formed by cleavage of the amyloid precursor protein (APP). The APP gene has several intronic Alu elements inserted in either the sense or antisense orientation. Binding of SC35 and HNRNPA1 to Alu elements on either side of exon 7 in the transcribed pre-mRNA is involved in alternative splicing of APP exons 7 and 8. Neuronal cells transfected with the full-length form of APP secrete higher levels of Abeta than cells transfected with the APP695 isoform lacking exons 7 and 8 [46]. In addition HNRNPA1 is a critical regulator of expression of the human CYP2A6 gene, a human xenobiotic-metabolizing enzyme cytochrome P450, which catalyzes the bioactivation of a number of carcinogens and drugs and is overexpressed in cases of liver diseases, such as cirrhosis, viral hepatitis, and parasitic infestation, and in certain tumor cells. Several proteins present in human hepatocytes interact specifically with the 3′-untranslated region (UTR) of CYP2A6 mRNA. Biochemical and immunological evidence show that the RNA–protein complex of highest intensity contains the heterogeneous nuclear ribonucleoprotein HNRNPA1 or a closely related protein. Mapping of the HNRNPA1 binding site within CYP2A6 3′-UTR reveals that the smallest portion of RNA supporting significant binding consists of 111 central nucleotides of the 3′-UTR. HNRNPA1 from HepG2 cancer cells exhibits modified binding characteristics to the CYP2A6 3′-UTR compared with primary hepatocytes. The level of CYP2A6 mRNA remains high in conditions of impaired transcription in primary human hepatocytes, showing that CYP2A6 expression can be affected posttranscriptionally in conditions of cellular stress. The posttranscriptional regulation involves interaction of the HNRNPA1 protein with CYP2A6 mRNA [47]. Steroid hormone resistance in New World primates occurs in the absence of abnormal expression of cognate nuclear receptors. Rather, these animals have elevated levels of heterogeneous nuclear ribonucleoproteins that act as hormone response element-binding proteins and attenuate target gene transactivation. A similar mechanism in humans via a patient with resistance to the active form of vitamin D [1,25-dihydroxyvitamin D(3) (1,25(OH)(2)D(3))] who presented with normal vitamin D receptor (VDR) expression. Initial cotransfection studies showed that the cells of the patient suppressed basal and hormone-induced transactivation by wild-type VDR. Electrophoretic mobility-shift assays and Western/Southwestern blot analyses indicated that this suppressive effect was due to overexpression of a nuclear protein that specifically interacts with a DNA response element known to bind retinoid X receptor-VDR heterodimers. Ab blocking in electrophoretic mobility-shift assays indicated that this dominant-negative acting protein was in the HNRNPA family of nucleic acid-binding proteins. Further studies have shown that several members of this family, most notably HNRNPA1, were able to suppress basal and 1,25(OH)(2)D(3)-induced luciferase activity. Vitamin D resistance in a human subject is similar to that previously described for New World primates in which abnormal expression of a hormone response element-binding protein can cause target cell resistance to 1,25(OH)(2)D(3). That this protein is a member of the HNRNP family capable of interacting with double-stranded DNA highlights a potentially important new component of the complex machinery required for steroid hormone signal transduction [48].

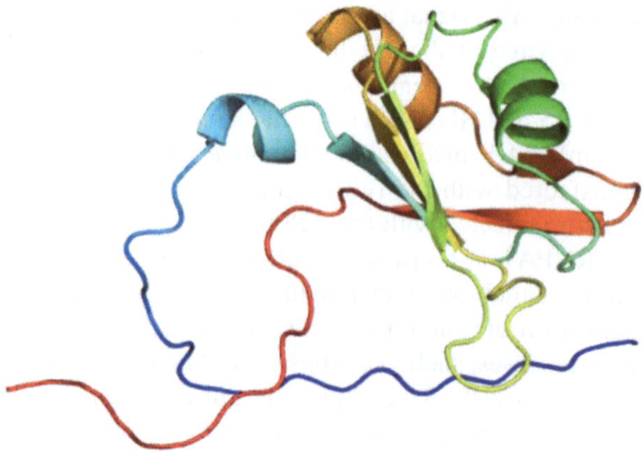

Fig. 8.7 Structure of the HNRPA2B1 protein. Based on PyMOL rendering of PDB 1x4b. Permission is granted to copy, distribute and/or modify this document under the terms of the GNU Free Documentation License, Version 1.2 or any later version published by the Free Software Foundation

8.4.2.2 Heterogeneous Nuclear Ribonucleoprotein A2/B1

The heterogeneous nuclear ribonucleoprotein A2/B1 or HNRNPA2B1 (Fig. 8.7) is upregulated in the parous breast (Tables 8.3, 8.4, and 8.5) and belongs to the A/B subfamily of ubiquitously expressed heterogeneous nuclear ribonucleoproteins (HNRNPs) [49]. The process of alternative splicing is widely misregulated in cancer, and the splicing factor HNRNP A2/B1 has been involved in cancer progression [50–52]. Knockdown of HNRNP A2/B1 in glioblastoma cells inhibited tumor formation in mice. In contrast, overexpression of HNRNPA2/B1 in immortal cells led to malignant transformation, suggesting that HNRNPA2B1 is a putative proto-oncogene [52]. However, the mechanism by which HNRNPA2B1 may be involved in cancer is not clear and it could be my modifying the splicing of other critical genes known to play a role in apoptosis. A clear example of this is the Bcl-x transcript, which has two alternatively spliced products; the anti-apoptotic Bcl-x(L) and the pro-apoptotic Bcl-x(s) [53]. Cancer cells often alter Bcl-x splicing to escape from apoptosis, which results in tumor formation, metastasis and a poor prognosis for the patient [54]. The activity of Fyn and the expression of HnRNPA2B1 were significantly increased in human metastatic pancreatic cancers. The expression and activity of Fyn were correlated with metastasis of human pancreatic cancer cells. Inhibition of Fyn activity reduced the expression of HNRNPA2B1. HnRNPA2B1 binds to endogenous Bcl-x mRNA and affects the ratio of the pro-apoptotic Bcl-x(s) mRNA to the anti-apoptotic Bcl-x (L). This study [55] provides evidence that HnRNPA2B1 is involved in apoptosis via regulation of the pro-apoptotic Bcl-x(s) mRNA. HNRNPA2B1 also regulates several tumor suppressors and oncogenes among them are c-FLIP, BIN1, and WWOX, and the proto-oncogene RON. Knockdown of RON inhibited HNRNP A2/B1 mediated transformation, which implied that RON is one of the mediators of HNRNPA2B1 oncogenic activity [52]. Another example of the role played by HNRNPA2B1 is in its association with SOX2 that is a key gene implicated in maintaining the stemness of embryonic and adult stem cells that appears to reactivate in several human cancers including glioblastoma multiforme. SOX2 was found to interact with several heterogeneous nuclear ribonucleoprotein family proteins, including HNRNPA2B1, HNRNPA3, HNRNPC, HNRNPK, HNRNPL, HNRNPM, HNRNPR, HNRNPU, as well as other ribonucleoproteins, DNA repair proteins and helicases. Gene ontology (GO) analysis revealed that the SOX2 interactome was enriched for GO terms GO:0030529 ribonucleoprotein complex and GO:0004386 helicase activity. These findings indicate that SOX2 associates with the heterogeneous nuclear ribonucleoprotein complex, suggesting a possible role for SOX2 in posttranscriptional regulation in addition to its function as a transcription factor [56]. Similar interaction has been found with the breast cancer susceptibility gene 1 (BRCA1) that plays a significant role in the development of a subset of familial breast and ovarian cancers, but increasing evidence points to a role also in sporadic tumors. BRCA1 is a multifunctional nuclear protein involved in the regulation of many nuclear cellular processes, including DNA repair, cell cycle, transcription, and chromatin remodeling. qRT-PCR analyses indicated that the HNRNPA2B1 levels increased in response to BRCA1 loss and restoration of BRCA1 expression in BRCA1 null cells reverted HNRNPA2B1 upregulation [57]. Altogether these data point towards the need to better understand the regulatory function of HNRNPA2B1 in the process of breast differentiation and prevention of breast cancer. HNRNPA2B1 is involved with pre-mRNA processing forming complexes with at least 20 other different HNRNP and heterogenous nuclear RNA in the nucleus (Tables 8.1 and 8.2) indicating that we are only understand a fraction on the role played by this gene in the normal as well as in the cancer process.

8.4.2.3 Heterogeneous Nuclear Ribonucleoprotein D (AU-Rich Element RNA-Binding Protein 1)

The HNRNPD proteins have distinct nucleic acid-binding properties [58]. The protein encoded by this gene has two repeats of quasi-RNA recognition motif (RRM) domains that bind to RNAs. It localizes to both the nucleus and the cytoplasm. This protein is implicated in the regulation of mRNA stability. The hnRNP D protein interacts with nucleic acids both in vivo and in vitro. Like many other proteins that interact with RNA, it contains RNA-binding domain (RBD) (or “RRM”) domains and arg–gly–gly (RGG) motifs (Fig. 8.8). Comparison of the predicted sequences of the hnRNP D proteins in human and mouse shows that they are 96.9% identical (98.9% similar). This very high level of conservation suggests a critical function for HNRNPD. Sequence analysis of the human HNRNPD gene shows that the protein is encoded by eight exons and that two additional exons specify sequences in the 3′ UTR. Use of two of the coding exons is determined by alternative splicing of the HNRPD mRNA. The human HNRPD gene maps to 4q21. The mouse Hnrpd gene maps to the F region of chromosome 3, which is syntenic with the human 4q21 region [59].

The HNRNPD is also upregulated in the parous breast however its precise role is not clear at the present time. However it is known that the HNRNPD transcript is

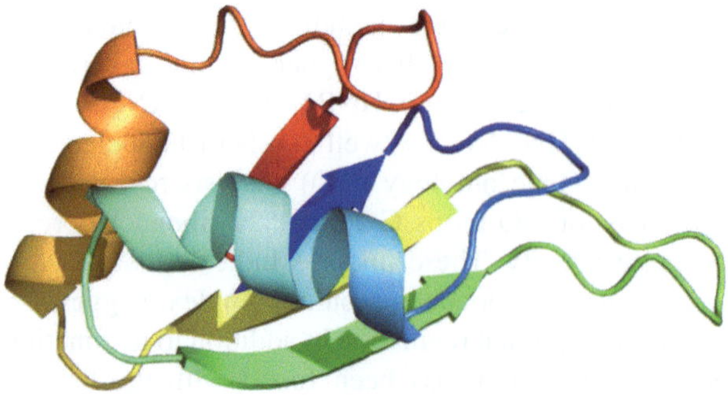

Fig. 8.8 Structure of the HNRPD protein. Based on PyMOL rendering of PDB 1hd0. Permission is granted to copy, distribute and/or modify this document under the terms of the GNU Free Documentation License, Version 1.2 or any later version published by the Free Software Foundation

alternatively spliced to produce four protein isoforms that stabilize or destabilize hundreds of mRNAs. Estradiol (E2) treatment of ovariectomized sheep increased concentrations of HNRNPD protein which stabilized estrogen receptor alpha (ER) mRNA in the uterus. Northern analysis determined that E2 treatment increased concentrations of total HNRNPD mRNAs twofold in endometrial and myometrial tissue compartments. In situ hybridization indicated that the increase was most intense in the glandular epithelium of endometrium. In a well characterized in vitro RNA stability assay, HNRNPD 3′ UTR sequences were much more stable in uterine extracts from E2-treated ewes compared to extracts from control ewes. HNRNPD mRNAs with alternative splicing of exons 2 and 7 (in the coding sequence) and exon 9 (in the 3′ UTR) were identified. The only effect of E2 treatment on alternative splicing was that it reduced the percentage of HNRNPD1 mRNAs containing exon 9-derived sequences indicating that E2 upregulates HNRNPD and ER genes coordinately by a posttranscriptional mechanism [60].

8.4.2.4 Heterogeneous Nuclear Ribonucleoproteins D Like

The HNRPDL or Heterogeneous nuclear ribonucleoproteins D like has two alternatively spliced transcript variants. One of the variants is probably not translated because the transcript is a candidate for nonsense-mediated mRNA decay. The protein encoded by this gene is similar to its family member HNRPD. The functional role of HNRPDL is promoting transcription repression by binding to double- and single-stranded DNA sequences. For example a transcription suppressor element (sequence −481 to −320) containing a G-rich motif (designated GTG) and a newly identified CAT-rich motif (designated CATR) was previously shown to modulate expression of the mouse cytochrome c oxidase Vb gene during myogenesis. The GTG element is critical for transcription activation in both undifferentiated and differentiated myocytes. Mutations of the CATR motif abolished transcription repression in myoblasts while limiting transcription activation in differentiated myotubes, suggesting contrasting functional attributes of this DNA motif at different stages of myogenesis. Results show that the activity of the transcription suppressor motif is modulated by an orchestrated interplay between ubiquitous transcription factors: ZBP-89, YY-1, and a member of the heterogeneous nuclear ribonucleoprotein D-like protein (also known as JKTBP1) family. In undifferentiated muscle cells, GTG motif-bound ZBP-89 physically and functionally interacted with CATR motif-bound YY-1 to mediate transcription repression. In differentiated myotubes, heterogeneous nuclear ribonucleoprotein D-like protein/JKTBP1 bound to the CATR motif exclusive of YY-1 and interacted with ZBP-89 in attenuating repressor activity, leading to transcription activation [61]. HNRPDL binds to the transcription suppressor CATR sequence of the COX5B promoter and also binds with high affinity to RNA molecules that contain AU-rich elements (AREs) found within the 3′-UTR of many proto-oncogenes and cytokine mRNAs. It has also been shown that HNRPDL binds both to nuclear and cytoplasmic poly(A) mRNAs an to the poly(G) and poly(A), but not to poly(U) or poly(C) RNA homopolymers [62]. These data indicate that the protein of HNRPDL contains two repeats of a putative RBD, each composed of canonical RNP-2 and RNP-1 motifs, and a glycine- and tyrosine-rich carboxyl terminus. The sequences of these two repeats are highly homologous with those of the 2× RBD-Gly rich group of HNRNPs. Northern blotting showed that two mRNAs of approximately 1.4 and 2.8 kb were present in most cultured cells examined. The recombinant protein expressed in Escherichia coli interacted with the double-stranded form of JKT41 as well as with its single-stranded form. This interaction was competitively inhibited by the same unlabeled JKT41 and to nearly the same extent by unrelated oligonucleotides. Moreover, the recombinant protein interacted with poly(G) and poly(A), but not with poly(U) or poly(C). Transient expression of the protein in SKM-1 cells repressed the expression of chloramphenicol acetyltransferase reporter genes located downstream of the intron 9 element of JKT41 or intron 7 element of FERE27 [62]. The protein of the HNRPDL shows a remarkable specificity for the (CCCTAA)*n* repeated motif, and the recombinant proteins expressed in Escherichia coli and have been shown to retain their binding specificity toward the C-block repeated sequence. In the light of the current knowledge about these proteins, their possible involvement in telomere functioning has been suggested [63].

As indicated above the transcription repression function of HNRPDL could also be a driving mechanism in the breast of parous women. Supporting data that the transcript of HNRPDL could be related to terminal differentiation has been shown by Northern blotting indicating ubiquitous but varied expressions of approximately 1.4 and 2.8 kb mRNAs in various tissues. Immunoblotting indicated that the amounts of protein of about 38 kDa were higher in the brain and testis than in other tissues. An additional protein of about 53 kDa was found in the brain and testis. Germ cell-deficient W/W(v) mutant mice and aged mice had the reduced amounts of HNRPDL in the testes. Immunohistochemical staining indicated cell type-specific expression of HNRPDL in tissues: neurons and spermatocytes displayed strong signal intensities. The signals were confined to the nucleus. The amount of 38 kDa HNRPDL was estimated to be approximately 1.3×10^7 molecules per HL-60 cell. These results indicate that HNRPDL is an abundant, highly conserved nuclear protein [29, 64].

8.4.3 Formation of the Spliceosome E Complex

8.4.3.1 RNA-Binding Motif Protein 5

A component of the spliceosome complex is RBM5 or RNA-binding motif protein 5 that regulates alternative splicing of a number of mRNAs (Table 8.1) is upregulated in the parous breast (Tables 8.3, 8.4, and 8.5). RBM5 modulates splice site pairing after recruitment of the U1 and U2 snRNPs to the 5′ and 3′ splice sites of the intron (Fig. 8.4) and both positively and negatively regulate apoptosis by regulating the alternative splicing of several genes involved in this process, including FAS and CASP2/caspase-2 [65, 66]. Overexpression of RBM5 by the regulation of alternative splicing retards ascites-associated tumor growth in immunocompromised mice, a phenomenon that may be related to an associated ability to modulate apoptosis and the cell cycle [67–69]. Overexpression of RBM5 enhanced p53-mediated inhibition of cell growth and colony formation and resulted in increased mRNA and protein levels for endogenous p53 target genes [70]. The recognition of single-stranded RNA (ssRNA) is an important aspect of gene regulation, and a number of different classes of protein domains that recognize ssRNA in a sequence-specific manner have been identified. The RNA-binding motif protein 5, also known as Luca15 or H37 [68], is a component of prespliceosomal complexes that regulates the alternative splicing of several mRNAs, such as Fas and caspase-2 [65]. The RBM5 play a role in tumor progression. In particular, down-regulation of RBM5 is involved in lung cancer and other cancers upon Ras activation, and, also, represents a molecular signature associated with metastasis in various solid tumors. On the other hand, upregulation of RBM5 occurs in breast and ovarian cancer. Moreover, RBM5 was also found to be involved in the early stage of the HIV-1 viral cycle, representing a potential target for the treatment of the HIV-1 infection. While the molecular basis for RNA recognition and ubiquitin interaction has been structurally characterized, small molecules binding this zinc finger (ZF) domain that might contribute to characterizing their activity and to the development of potential therapeutic agents have not yet been reported. Using an NMR screening of a fragment library several binders have been identified and the complex of the most promising one, compound 1, with the RBM5 ZF1 was structurally characterized in solution. Interestingly, the binding mechanism reveals that one occupies the RNA-binding pocket and is therefore able to compete with the RNA to bind RBM5 RanBP2-type ZF domain, as indicated by NMR studies [71, 72].

RBM5 is a nuclear RNA-binding protein containing two RRMs. The RBM5 gene is located at the tumor suppressor locus 3p21.3. Deletion of this locus is the most frequent genetic alteration in lung cancer, but is also found in other human cancers. RBM5 is important for the activity of the tumor suppressor protein p53. Over expression enhanced p53-mediated inhibition of cell growth and colony formation. Expression of RBM5 augmented p53 transcriptional activity in reporter gene assays and resulted in increased mRNA and protein levels for endogenous p53 target genes. In contrast, shRNA-mediated knockdown of endogenous RBM5 led to decreased p53 transcriptional activity and reduced levels of mRNA and protein for endogenous p53 target genes. RBM5 affected protein, but not mRNA, levels of endogenous p53 after DNA damage suggest that RBM5 contributes to p53 activity through post-transcriptional mechanisms [67]. RBM5 is one member of a group of structurally related genes that includes RBM6 and RBM10. RBM10 maps to Xp11.23, and one allele is inactivated as a result of X chromosome inactivation. Both RBM5 and RBM6 map to 3p21.3, a tumor suppressor region that experiences loss of heterozygosity in the majority of lung cancers. Over expression of RBM5 retards ascites-associated tumor growth in immunocompromised mice, a phenomenon that may be related to an associated ability to modulate apoptosis [66, 67, 73–75] but RBM5 seems to behave differently in breast cancer [76].

8.4.3.2 Small Nuclear Ribonucleoproteins in the Spliceosome E Complex

Differentiation of the human breast during the process of pregnancy and lactation and post lactational involution requires a unique gene expression program that insures synthesis of the appropriate proteome at each stage of maturation. Our studies using expression microarrays have provided important insight into gene expression indicating that the process of terminal differentiation is mediated by RNA processing, that alters structure and function of encoded proteins. The observation among the regulated transcripts encode RNA-binding proteins such as SNRP70, SNRPB (Fig. 8.9), SNORD104 and *the* SNRPA1 (Fig. 8.10) [77, 78], indicate significant changes in the RNA processing machinery supporting the existence of a regulated alternative pre-mRNA splicing program that is critical of the differentiated breast. Similar process has been reported during erythrocytes differentiation [79]. SNRP70 also known as U1 small nuclear ribonucleoprotein 70 kDa is a protein [80] that in humans is encoded by the *SNRNP70* gene that associates with U1 spliceosomal RNA, forming part of the spliceosome (Table 8.1). This gene has been shown to be upregulated by exposure to low-dose radiation combined with a solar particle in animals [81]. SNRP70 is linked to WW domains mediate protein–protein interactions in many intracellular processes. In pre-mRNA splicing, WW domains participate in cross-intron bridging. These WW domains are characterized by a central aromatic block of three tyrosine residues. A novel protein containing the same type of WW domain named WAC, is located in human chromosome 10p11.2-10p12.1. A *Drosophila melanogaster* WAC homolog (CG8949) was identified as a Rosetta stone protein. Domain fusion analysis of the Rosetta stone protein linked WAC to the splicing factor SNRP70 and co-localized with SC35, the marker for pre-mRNA splicing machinery [82].

The SNRPB or Small nuclear ribonucleoprotein-associated proteins B and B′ is a protein that in humans is encoded by the *SNRPB* gene and is unregulated also in the parous differentiated breast. The protein encoded by this gene is one of several nuclear proteins that are found in common among U1, U2, U4/U6, and U5 small ribonucleoprotein particles (snRNPs) (Table 8.1 and Figs. 8.4 and 8.5). These snRNPs are involved in pre-mRNA splicing, and the encoded protein may also play a role in

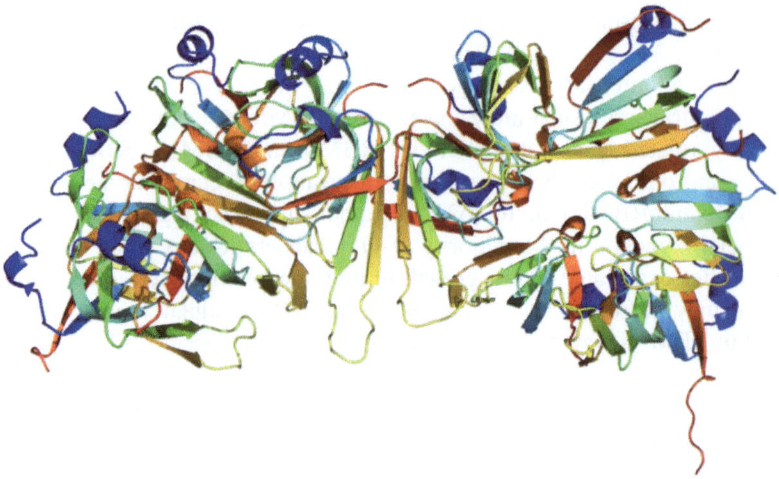

Fig. 8.9 Structure of the SNRPB protein. Based on PyMOL rendering of PDB 1d3b. Permission is granted to copy, distribute and/or modify this document under the terms of the GNU Free Documentation License, Version 1.2 or any later version published by the Free Software Foundation

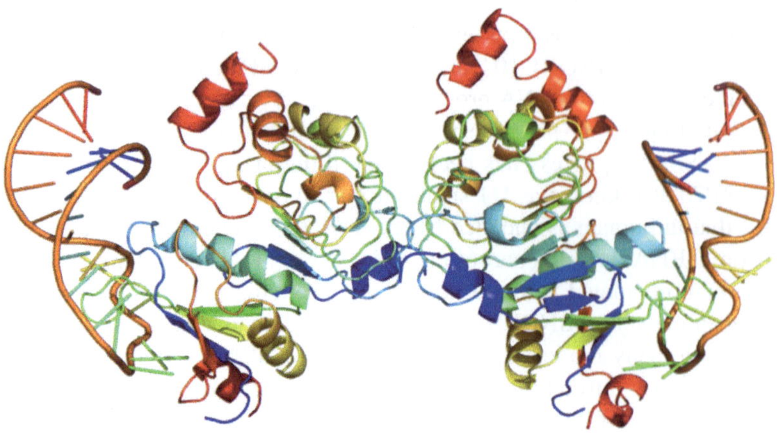

Fig. 8.10 Structure of the SNRPA1 protein. Based on PyMOL rendering of PDB 1a9n. Permission is granted to copy, distribute and/or modify this document under the terms of the GNU Free Documentation License, Version 1.2 or any later version published by the Free Software Foundation

pre-mRNA splicing or snRNP structure [83–85]. The SNRPB protein self-regulates its expression by promoting the inclusion of a highly conserved alternative exon in its own pre-mRNA that targets the spliced transcript for nonsense-mediated mRNA decay. Depletion of SNRPB protein in human cells results in reduced levels of snRNPs and a striking reduction in the inclusion levels of hundreds of additional

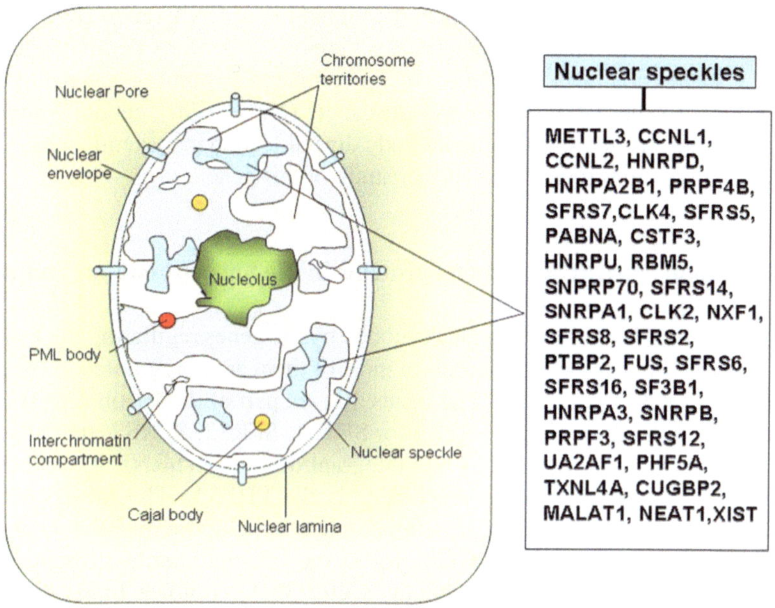

Fig. 8.11 Nuclear compartments. The nuclear speckles contain most of the transcripts related to the splicing mechanism

alternative exons, with comparatively few effects on constitutive exon splicing levels. The affected alternative exons are enriched in genes encoding RNA processing and other RNA-binding factors, and a subset of these exons also regulate gene expression by activating nonsense-mediated mRNA decay [86]. To the light of these findings the protective role of the splicing machinery in the parous breast is evident. Another important functional role of SNRPB is that single nucleotide polymorphisms (SNPs) in this gene significantly modify breast cancer risk in BRCA1 mutation carriers. The minor alleles of rs6138178 in SNRPB and rs6602595 in CAMK1D displayed the strongest associations in BRCA1 carriers (HR = 0.78, 95% CI: 0.69–0.90, P(trend) = 3.6×10^{-4} and HR = 1.25, 95% CI: 1.10–1.41, P(trend) = 4.2×10^{-4}) [87].

SNRPB protein as part in the assembly of the spliceosomal complex is located in the Cajal bodies that are subnuclear domains (Fig. 8.11). The Cajal body marker protein, coilin, interacts with SMN and Sm proteins. Therefore phosphorylation of coilin influences interaction with its target proteins and, thus, may be significant in managing the flow of snRNPs through the Cajal body [83, 88]. Interestingly coilin interacts also with Ku70 and Ku80, which are major players in the DNA repair process. Ku proteins compete with SMN and SNRPB proteins for coilin interaction sites. The binding domain on coilin for Ku proteins cannot be localized to one discrete region, and only full-length coilin is capable of inhibiting in vitro nonhomologous DNA end joining (NHEJ). Since Ku proteins do not accumulate in CBs, these findings suggest that nucleoplasmic coilin participates in the regulation of DNA repair [89]. A further functional role for SNRPB is as metastasis suppressor gene as demonstrated by is decreased expression of in the metastasizing compared to non-metastasizing tumors using the mouse allograft model of prostate cancer (NE-10) [90], genomic imprinting [91], and in the mechanisms of autoantibody diversification in systemic lupus erythematosus [92] warrants the need of further study of this gene.

8.4.3.3 Small Nuclear Ribonucleoproteins in the Spliceosome A Complex

As indicated in Table 8.1 the proteins encoded by the genes regulating the formation of complex A (Fig. 8.4) are numerous an most of them are upregulated in the parous breast (Tables 8.3, 8.4, and 8.5). The genes that are part of the B complex (Fig. 8.5) are the SFRS8, SFRS14 and the SFRS16, SF3B1, SFRS2, SFRS7, that are necessary for the splicing of pre-mRNA and integrant of the U2 snRNP. The other component of the preRNA splicing machinery is the PHF5A. This gene encodes a subunit of the splicing factor 3b protein complex. Splicing factor 3b, together with splicing factor 3a and a 12S RNA unit, forms the U2 small nuclear ribonucleoproteins complex (U2 snRNP). The splicing factor 3b/3a complex binds pre-mRNA upstream of the intron's branch site in a sequence-independent manner and may anchor the U2 snRNP to the pre-mRNA. The protein encoded by this gene contains a PHD-finger-like domain that is flanked by highly basic N- and C-termini. This protein belongs to the PHD-finger superfamily and may act as a chromatin-associated protein. This gene has several pseudogenes on different chromosomes. Acts as a transcriptional regulator by binding to the GJA1/Cx43 promoter and enhancing its upregulation by ESR1/ER-alpha. Also involved in pre-mRNA splicing. These small nuclear ribonucleoproteins are essential splicing factors and there is evidence that they function as suppressors of tumor cell growth and may have major implications as cancer therapeutics target. The pre-mRNA splicing factors are enriched in nuclear domains termed interchromatin granule clusters or nuclear speckles. During mitosis, nuclear speckles are disassembled by metaphase and reassembled in telophase in structures termed mitotic interchromatin granules. There are numerous splicing factors that we have found upregulated in the epithelia of the parous breast.

The SFRS8 or splicing factor arginine/serine-rich 8 encodes a human homolog of *Drosophila* splicing regulatory protein functioning as an alternative splicing regulator and regulate its own expression at the level of RNA processing. SFRS7 interacts with CLK4 that is a protein kinase can interact with and phosphorylate the serine- and arginine-rich (SR) proteins, which are known to play an important role in the formation of spliceosomes, and thus may be involved in the regulation of alternative splicing. The CLK2 or CDC-like kinase 2 that is also upregulated in the parous breast and may play similar function.

The SF3B1 or splicing factor 3B subunit 1 is a protein that in humans is encoded by the *SF3B1* gene. This gene encodes subunit 1 of the splicing factor 3b protein complex. Splicing factor 3b, together with splicing factor 3a and a 12S RNA unit, forms the U2 small nuclear ribonucleoproteins complex (U2 snRNP) (Table 8.1).

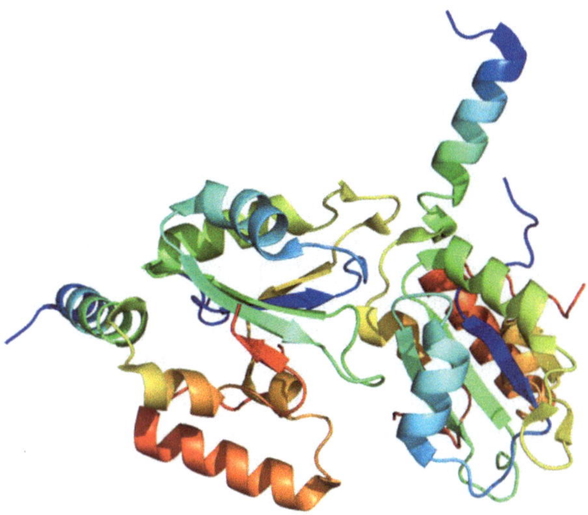

Fig. 8.12 Structure of the SF3B1 protein. Based on PyMOL rendering of PDB 2f9d. Permission is granted to copy, distribute and/or modify this document under the terms of the GNU Free Documentation License, Version 1.2 or any later version published by the Free Software Foundation

The splicing factor 3b/3a complex binds pre-mRNA upstream of the intron's branch site in a sequence-independent manner and may anchor the U2 snRNP to the pre-mRNA. Splicing factor 3b is also a component of the minor U12-type spliceosome. The carboxy-terminal two-thirds of subunit 1 have 22 nonidentical, tandem HEAT repeats that form rod-like, helical structures (Fig. 8.12). Heterozygous missense mutations in the U2AF1 and SF3B1 genes that encode spliceosome subunits. U2AF1 is frequently mutated in myeloid hematopoietic malignancies, especially in myelodysplastic syndrome (MDS), and SF3B1 is frequently mutated in both MDS [93, 94] and chronic lymphocytic leukemia (CLL). SF3B1 mutations in CLL were associated with faster disease progression and poor overall survival. The results reinforce the idea that targeting several well-known genetic pathways, including mRNA splicing, could be useful in the treatment of CLL and other malignancies [95–97].

SFRS2 or Splicing factor, arginine/serine-rich 2 also called SC35 [98, 99] is a splicing factor that is upregulated in the parous breast (Tables 8.3, 8.4, and 8.5) and may play a role in the resting stage at the postmenopause. SFRS2 has a role in blocking cell proliferation and has been shown in embryos of inbred mouse strains. In these embryos stop their cleavage at the late 2-cell stage and this phenomenon is known as the "2-cell block in vitro." Using microinjections of 5-bromouridine 5′-triphosphate (BrUTP) to examine the transcriptional status of blocked embryos and by tracing the nuclear distribution of hyperphosphorylated form of RNA polymerase II in such embryos it was found that transcriptional activity is gradually decreased when the embryos stay in block. This is accompanied by prominent increasing of the size of SFRS2 nuclear speckles (Fig. 8.11) that begin to accumulate hyperphosphorylated RNA polymerase II [100]. Another important function of

SFRS2 is in the regulation of both constitutive and alternative splicing. SFRS2 contains one RRM (domain) and a RS domain at the C-terminus which is enriched with arginine and serine residues. SFRS2 is specifically involved in major regulatory pathways for cell proliferation and cell cycle progression [101]. The SR protein SFRS2 controls cell proliferation during pituitary gland development but is completely dispensable in terminal differentiated mature cardiomyocytes in mice. SFRS2 in mouse embryonic fibroblasts induces G2/M cell cycle arrest and genomic instability, resulting at least in part from p53 hyperphosphorylation and hyperacetylation. While p53 hyperphosphorylation appears related to ATM activation, its hyperacetylation has been attributed to the increased expression of the acetyltransferase gene p300 and the aberrant splicing of the deacetylase gene SirT1. These findings reveal the involvement of SFRS2 in specific pathways in regulating cell proliferation and genomic stability during mammalian organogenesis [102]. SFRS2 affects transcriptional elongation in a gene-specific manner. SFRS2 depletion induces Pol II accumulation within the gene body and attenuated elongation, which are correlated with defective P-TEFb (a complex composed of CycT1-CDK9) recruitment and dramatically reduced CTD Ser2 phosphorylation. Recombinant SFRS2 is sufficient to rescue this defect in nuclear run-on experiments. These findings suggest a reciprocal functional relationship between the transcription and splicing machineries during gene expression [103] and support the role of the SFRS2 in the protective effect exerted by pregnancy in the postmenopausal breast.

SRSF7 or serine/arginine-rich splicing factor 7 also known as splicing factor, arginine/serine-rich 7 or splicing factor 9G8 (Table 8.1). The protein encoded by this gene is a member of the serine/arginine (SR)-rich family of pre-mRNA splicing factors that contains an RRM for binding RNA and an RS domain for binding other proteins. The RS domain is rich in serine and arginine residues and facilitates interaction between different SR splicing factors (Fig. 8.13). The SRSF7 transcript is upregulated in the parous breast (Tables 8.3, 8.4, and 8.5) however, its functional role is not clear. Literature search indicated that SRSF7 co-localizes with cyclin L2 or CCNL2, that is also upregulated in the parous breast (Tables 8.3, 8.4, and 8.5), within nuclear speckles (Fig. 8.11) and that it associates with hyperphosphorylated, but not hypophosphorylated, RNA polymerase II and cyclin-dependent kinase (CDK) p110 PITSLRE kinase via its N-terminal cyclin domains. CCNL2 it can also associate with the SRSF7 through its RS repeat region. Recombinant CCNL2 protein can stimulate in vitro mRNA splicing. Overexpression of CCNL2 suppresses the growth of human hepatocellular carcinoma SMMC 7721 cells both in vitro and in vivo, inducing cellular apoptosis. This process involves upregulation of p53 and Bax and decreased expression of Bcl-2. The data suggest that CCNL2 represents a new member of the cyclin family, which might regulate the transcription and RNA processing of certain apoptosis-related factors, resulting in tumor cell growth inhibition and apoptosis [104].

These data clearly support the concept that SRSF7 may be involve d in the resting stage of the parous breast [18]. We cannot rule out the possibility that SRSF7 might have other functional role in the parosu breast due that I also has been shown to be associated with STOX1A, a winged helix transcription factor recently

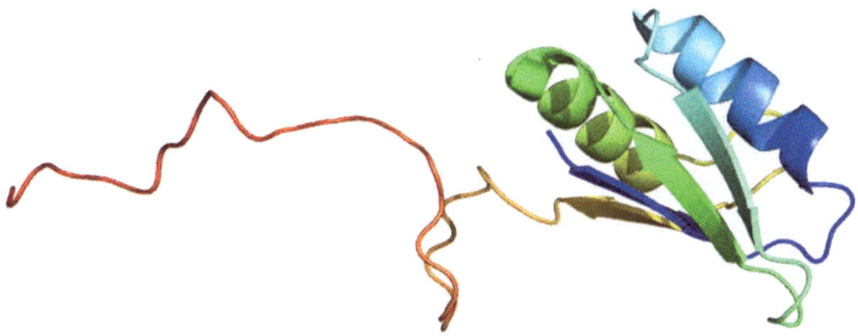

Fig. 8.13 Structure of the SFRS7 protein. Based on PyMOL rendering of PDB 2hvz. Permission is granted to copy, distribute and/or modify this document under the terms of the GNU Free Documentation License, Version 1.2 or any later version published by the Free Software Foundation

demonstrated to be involved in late onset Alzheimer's disease and affecting the amyloid processing pathway [105]. Another functional role of SRSF7 is in the cytoplasmic export of herpes simplex virus 1 [106, 107] and to function in mRNA export in conjunction with the export protein, Tap/NXF1. Tap interacts directly with the Mason-Pfizer monkey virus constitutive transport element (CTE), an element that enables export of unspliced, intron-containing mRNA [108].

SFRS8 or splicing factor suppressor of white apricot homolog (Table 8.2) encodes a human homolog of *Drosophila* splicing regulatory protein. This gene autoregulates its expression by control of splicing of its first two introns. Three SNPs in splicing factor, arginine/serine-rich 8 had an association with asthma. SFRS8 regulates the splicing of CD45, a protein which, through alternative splice variants, has an essential role in activating T cells. T cells are involved in the pathogenesis of atopic diseases such as asthma [109]. Two other genes that encode an accessory protein in the splicing mechanism is the SFS14 or putative splicing factor, arginine/serine-rich 14 [110, 111] and the SFRS16 or Splicing factor, arginine/serine-rich 16 [112, 113] (Table 8.2). They are upregulated in the parous postmenopausal breast but their functional role have not been determined.

8.4.3.4 Small Nuclear Ribonucleoproteins in the Spliceosome B Complex

A component of the spliceosome B complex that is upregulated in the parous breast are the TXNL4A that constitutes an essential component of the U5 particle, and its functions have been reported to be highly conserved throughout evolution and the PRPF3 that participates in pre-mRNA splicing and play a role in the assembly of the U4/U5/U6 tri-snRNP complex (Fig. 8.5). Another gene that is also overrepresented in the parous breast are PRPF4B or PRP4 pre-mRNA processing factor 4 homolog B that is related to the sequential transesterification steps of the pre-mRNA splicing and in signal transduction (Table 8.1) [114–116]. This protein belongs to a kinase family that includes serine/arginine-rich protein-specific kinases and CDKs. This protein is regarded as a CDK-like kinase (Clk) with homology to mitogen-activated protein kinases (MAPKs) [117]. Whereas it is not clear explanation for the upregulation of this gene in the parous breast it has been shown that PRPF4B is associated with complexes involved in the coordination of pre-mRNA processing and transcriptional regulation. PRPF4B in the *Schizosaccharomyces pombe* is enriched in SC35-containing nuclear splicing speckles. RNA interference of *Caenorhabditis elegans* PRPF4B indicates that it is essential in metazoans. In support of a role for PRPF4B in pre-mRNA splicing, is that PRP6, SWAP, and pinin are interacting proteins and demonstrated that PRPF4B is a U5 snRNP-associated kinase [118]. In addition, BRG1 and N-CoR, components of nuclear hormone coactivator and corepressor complexes, also interact with PRPF4B. PRPF4B coimmunoprecipitates with N-CoR, BRG1, pinin, and PRP6, and we present data suggesting that PRP6 and BRG1 are substrates of this kinase. Lastly, PRP4K, BRG1, and PRP6 can be purified as components of the N-CoR-2 complex. PRPF4B is an essential kinase that, in association with the both U5 snRNP and N-CoR deacetylase complexes, demonstrates a possible coordination of pre-mRNA splicing with chromatin remodeling events involved in transcriptional regulation [119]. We speculate that similar functional role is played in the parous breast mainly during the chromatin remodeling process [18]. PRPF4B can also be induced that intensive exercise triggering the cascade processes of body adaptation, including modulation of spliceosome functioning, and can lead to modification of its activity and choice of alternative exons [119]. PRPF4B has also shown to be related to the activation of resting T lymphocytes initiates differentiation into mature effector cells over 3–7 days. The chemokine CCL5 (RANTES) and its major transcriptional regulator, Krüppel-like factor 13 (KLF13), are expressed late (3–5 days) after activation in T lymphocytes. Using yeast two-hybrid screening of a human thymus cDNA library, PRPF4B was identified as a KLF13-binding protein. Specific interaction of KLF13 and PRPF4B was confirmed by reciprocal co-immunoprecipitation. Knockdown of PRPF4B by small interfering RNA markedly decreases CCL5 expression in T lymphocytes [120]. Using a yeast two-hybrid screen of a T-cell cDNA library it was found that PRPF4B protein binds to the human immunodeficiency virus type 2 (HIV-2) Gag polyprotein. Specific interaction of PRPF4B and HIV-2 Gag was confirmed in in vitro and in vivo assays. The interacting region of HIV-2 Gag is located in the conserved matrix and capsid domains, while both the RS (arginine/serine-rich) domain and the KS (kinase) domain of PRPF4B are able to bind to HIV-2 Gag. PRPF4B is not incorporated into virus particles. HIV-2 Gag is able to inhibit PRPF4B-mediated phosphorylation of the splicing factor SF2. This is also observed with Gag from simian immunodeficiency virus, a closely related virus, but not with Gag from human T-cell lymphotropic virus type 1. It is possible that Gag accumulates in the cell, down-regulation of splicing occurs through reduced phosphorylation of SF2 [121].

8.5 mRNA 3′ End Processing

This is the last step in the splicing mechanism and consists in the cleavage of its 3′ end and addition of adenine residues to form the poly(A) tail, which protects the 3′ end from ribonuclease digestion (Fig. 8.14). There are several proteins involved in this step as outlined in Table 8.1 and some of the transcripts regulating this process are upregulated in the parous breast (Tables 8.3, 8.4, and 8.5). Among them PABPN1 or poly(A) binding protein and CSTF3 (Fig. 8.15).

PABPN1 encodes an abundant nuclear protein that binds with high affinity to nascent poly(A) tails. The protein Involved in the 3′-end formation of mRNA precursors (pre-mRNA) by the addition of a poly(A) tail of 200–250 nt to the upstream cleavage product. Stimulates poly(A) polymerase (PAPOLA) conferring processivity on the poly(A) tail elongation reaction and controls also the poly(A) tail length. Increases the affinity of poly(A) polymerase for RNA. Is also present at various stages of mRNA metabolism including nucleocytoplasmic trafficking and nonsense-mediated decay (NMD) of mRNA. The type II poly(A)-binding protein PABP2/PABPN1 functions in general mRNA metabolism by promoting poly(A) tail formation in mammals and flies. It also participates in poly(A) tail shortening of specific mRNAs in flies, and snoRNA biogenesis in yeast [122]. The addition of a 3′ poly(A) tail is a prerequisite for the maturation of the majority of eukaryotic transcripts. In most eukaryotic species, RNA poly(A) tails are bound by two important poly(A)-binding proteins (PABPs) [123]: In eukaryotic cells, newly synthesized mRNAs acquire a poly(A) tail that plays several fundamental roles in export, translation and mRNA decay. Poly(A) tails of mRNAs are synthesized in the cell nucleus with a defined length, approximately 250 nucleotides in mammalian cells. The same type of length control is seen in an in vitro polyadenylation system reconstituted from three proteins: poly(A) polymerase, cleavage and polyadenylation specificity factor (CPSF), and the nuclear PABP. CPSF, binding the polyadenylation signal AAUAAA, and PABPN1, binding the growing poly(A) tail, cooperatively stimulate poly(A) polymerase such that a complete poly(A) tail is synthesized in one processive event, which terminates at a length of approximately 250 nucleotides [124]. It has been shown that PABPN1 and PABPC1 function solely in the nucleus and cytoplasm, respectively. 3′ poly(A) tails can also act as a degradation mark via the exosome complex of 3′–5′ exonucleases, involving the nuclear PABP in posttranscriptional gene regulation [125, 126]. PABPN1 is an aggregation-prone nuclear protein that could play a role in increased aggregation of misfolded proteins associated with aging. It characterizes a number of related neurodegenerative disorders caused by homopolymeric amino acid expansion mutations. However, Natural aggregation of wild-type (WT) PABPN1 is not known to be disease-associated, but alanine-expanded PABPN1 (expPABPN1) accumulates in insoluble intranuclear inclusions in muscle of patients with oculopharyngeal muscular dystrophy (OPMD) [126, 127]. OPMD caused by a polyalanine expansion mutation in the coding region of the poly-(A) binding protein nuclear 1 (PABPN1) gene. In unaffected individuals, (GCG)(6) encodes the first six alanines in a homopolymeric stretch of ten alanines.

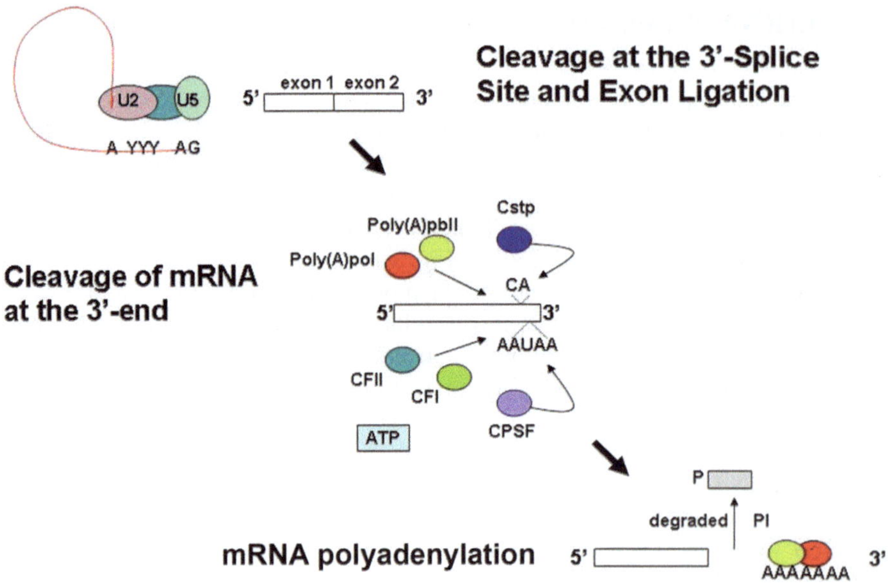

Fig. 8.14 Cleavage of the 3′ splice site and exon ligation followed by cleavage of mRNA at the 3′ end and the final step mRNA polyadenylation

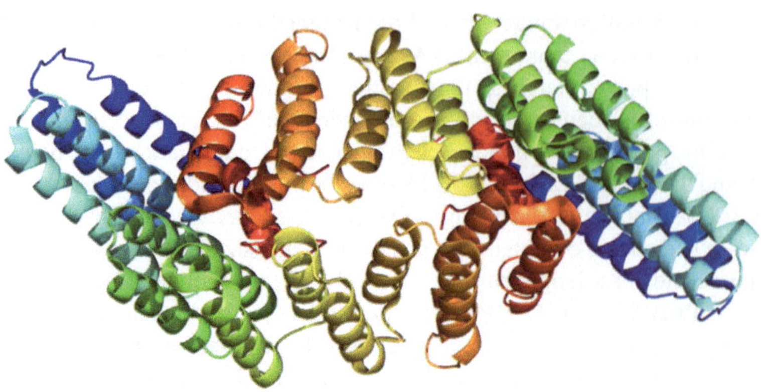

Fig. 8.15 Structure of the CSTF3 protein. Based on PyMOL rendering of PDB 2ond. Permission is granted to copy, distribute and/or modify this document under the terms of the GNU Free Documentation License, Version 1.2 or any later version published by the Free Software Foundation

In most patients, this (GCG)(6) repeat is expanded to (GCG)(8–13), leading to a stretch of 12–17 alanines in mutant PABPN1, which is thought to confer a toxic gain of function [128]. The developmental pathways of the canonical Wnt signaling can modulate muscular pathology in mutant PABPN1 nematodes, and cooperate with the Sir2-FoxO longevity pathway to confer protection against mutant PABPN1 toxicity at the cellular and behavioral levels. Mutant PABPN1 toxicity was modified by genes along the canonical Wnt pathway, several of which depend on daf-16 for activity. ss-catenin and pop-1/TCF RNAi suppressed the protection from mutant PABPN1 conferred by loss-of-function mutations in sir-2.1 and daf-16. Moreover, the aggravation of muscle cell pathology by increased sir-2.1 dosage was reversed by ss-catenin and pop-1 RNAi. The chemical inhibition of GSK-3ss, a repressor of ss-catenin activity, protected against mutant PABPN1 toxicity in a daf-16-dependent manner, which is consistent with a cross-talk between ss-catenin signaling and Sir2-FoxO signaling in protecting from mutant PABPN1 toxicity. In OPMD, a disease caused by polyalanine expansion in the nuclear protein PABPN1, the genetic inhibition of sirtuins and treatment with sirtuin inhibitors protect from mutant PABPN1 toxicity in transgenic nematodes [129].

The CSTF3 or Cleavage stimulation factor 77 kDa subunit [130, 131] is one of three (including CSTF1 and CSTF2) cleavage stimulation factors that combine to form the cleavage stimulation factor complex (CSTF). This complex is involved in the polyadenylation and 3′ end cleavage of pre-mRNAs. The encoded protein functions as a homodimer and interacts directly with both CSTF1 and CSTF2 in the CSTF complex (Fig. 8.15). Alternative splicing results in multiple transcript variants encoding different isoforms [132]. CSTF3 is upregulated in gastric cancer by 5-Fluorouracil (5-FU) an anticancer drug that is widely used in the treatment of cancer [133].

8.6 Other Accessory Proteins Related to the Splicing Mechanism

As depicted in Table 8.2 there are numerous accessory proteins that are involved in the splicing mechanism and some of them are also overrepresented in the expression profile of the parous breast (Tables 8.3, 8.4, and 8.5). Among them are the NXF1 belonging to the family of nuclear RNA export factor genes. PTBP2 that encodes a protein that binds to the intronic cluster of RNA regulatory elements and CUGBP2 that is involved in mRNA splice selection. NXF1 or Nuclear RNA export factor 1 [134, 135] is one member of a family of nuclear RNA export factor genes. Common domain features of this family are a noncanonical RNP-type RNA-binding domain (RBD), 4 leucine-rich repeats (LRRs), a nuclear transport factor 2 (NTF2)-like domain that allows heterodimerization with NTF2-related export protein-1 (NXT1), and a ubiquitin-associated domain that mediates interactions with nucleoporins. Alternative splicing results in transcript variants. The LRRs and NTF2-like domains are required for export activity. The encoded protein of this gene shuttles between the nucleus and the cytoplasm and binds in vivo to poly(A)+ RNA [136]. It is the vertebrate homologue of the yeast protein Mex67p [137]. The encoded protein overcomes the mRNA export block caused by the presence of saturating amounts of CTE RNA of type D retroviruses and other virus [138–140].

A variant allele of the homologous Nxf1 gene in mice suppresses a class of mutations caused by integration of an endogenous retrovirus (intracisternal A particle) into an intron [141].

PTBP2 or Polypyrimidine tract-binding protein 2 [142] is encoded by this gene binds to the intronic cluster of RNA regulatory elements, downstream control sequence (DCS). It is implicated in controlling the assembly of other splicing regulatory proteins. This protein is very similar to the polypyrimidine tract-binding protein PTBP1 but it is expressed primarily in the brain [143]. PTBP2 play an important role in the alternative splicing of the CaV1.2 calcium channels. This gene function in diverse cellular processes such as gene regulation, muscle contraction, and membrane excitation and are diversified in their activity through extensive. The mutually exclusive exons 8a and 8 encode alternate forms of transmembrane segment 6 (IS6) in channel domain 1. The human genetic disorder Timothy syndrome is caused by mutations in either of these two CaV1.2 exons, resulting in disrupted Ca(2+) homeostasis and severe pleiotropic disease phenotypes. The tissue-specific pattern of exon 8/8a splicing leads to differences in symptoms between patients with exon 8 or 8a mutations. The polypyrimidine tract-binding protein (PTB) mediates a switch from exon 8 to 8a splicing. PTB and its neuronal homolog, nPTB, are widely studied splicing regulators controlling large sets of alternative exons. During neuronal development, PTB expression is downregulated with a concurrent increase in nPTB expression. Exon 8a is largely repressed in embryonic mouse brain but is progressively induced during neuronal differentiation as PTB is depleted. This splicing repression is mediated by the direct binding of PTB to sequence elements upstream of exon 8a. The nPTB protein is a weaker repressor of exon 8a, resulting in a shift in exon choice when nPTB replaces PTB in cells [144]. PTBP2 interacts with the cytidine deaminase AID to switch-region DNA. Knockdown of PTBP2 mediated by short hairpin RNA in B cells led to a decrease in binding of AID to transcribed switch regions, which resulted in considerable impairment of immunoglobulin class-switch recombination [145]. How all these different function of PTBP2 are related to signature of prevention of the postmenopausal breast is not clear, however, PTBP2 is considered as “global regulators” of RNA alternative splicing, stability, and translation in non-neuronal (including ectodermal) tissues examined to date in diverse species, and REST/NRSF (RE-1 Silencing Transcription Factor/Neuron Restrictive Silencing Factor) represses >2,000 neuronal genes in all non-neuronal tissues examined. During neurogenesis these factors are replaced by what has been considered neuron-specific HuB/C/D, nPTB, and alternatively spliced REST (REST4), which work with miR-124 to activate this battery of genes, comprehensively reprogram neuronal alternative splicing, and maintain their exclusive expression in post-mitotic neurons [146]. Therefore it is possible to speculate that this genes may play an important role in the reprogramming the breast after pregnancy [17, 18]. The upregulation of PTBP2 in the parous breast provides an evidence that this gene has a regulatory function, previously considered to have a unique role in governing neurogenesis [147] can also be applied to the breast epithelia.

CUGBP2 or CUG-BP- and ETR-3-like factor 2 [148–150] is a member of the CELF/BRUNOL protein family are RNA-binding proteins and contain two N-terminal RRM domains, one C-terminal RRM domain, and a divergent segment of 160–230 aa between the second and third RRM domains. Members of this protein family regulate pre-mRNA alternative splicing and may also be involved in mRNA editing, and translation. Alternative splicing results in multiple transcript variants encoding different isoforms. CUGBP2 is upregulated in the parous breast and whereas its function in this organ is unknown this gene has an important role in alternative pre-mRNA splicing by adjusting the transcriptional output of the genome by generating related mRNAs from a single primary transcript, thereby expanding protein diversity. The CUGBP2 splicing regulator plays a key role in the brain region-specific silencing of the NI exon of the NMDA R1 receptor. In a recent study [151] has been shown that CUGBP2 to GU-rich motifs closely positioned at the boundaries of the branch sites of the NI exon, and has been demonstrated an autoregulatory role for CUGBP2 as indicated by its direct interaction with functionally significant RNA motifs surrounding the branch sites upstream of exon 6 of the CUGBP2 transcript itself. The perimeter-binding model explains how CUGBP2 can effectively embrace the branch site region to achieve the specificity needed for the selection of exon targets and the fine-tuning of alternative splicing patterns [151]. CUGBP2, acting as translation inhibitor, induces colon cancer cells to undergo apoptosis [152, 153].

8.7 Other Transcripts That Could Play a Role in RNA Splicing in the Human Breast

As it is depicted in Tables 8.3, 8.4, and 8.5, there are other genes that could play a role in the splicing of RNA in the human breast at menopause. The DEAD box RNA helicases p68 (DDX5) and p72 (DDX17) play important roles in multiple cellular processes that are commonly dysregulated in cancers, including transcription, pre-mRNA processing/alternative splicing, and miRNA processing [154]. DDX17 can unwind double-stranded RNA and also contribute to the remodeling of ribonucleoprotein complexes. These activities of p68/p72 are required for efficient RNA splicing and microRNA processing. In addition, p68/p72 perform functions that are independent of their enzymatic activity. This is especially common to their role in gene regulation, where p68/p72 coactivate various transcription factors, including the tumor suppressor p53, estrogen receptor alpha, and beta-catenin. P68/p72 are posttranslationally modified by SUMO attachment and phosphorylation that regulate their coactivation potential [155], binding to known interactants or protein stability. Knock-out mouse models revealed that both DDX5 and DDX17 are essential genes during development. Furthermore, together with their ability to stimulate cell proliferation and prevent apoptosis, the reported overexpression of p68/p72 in three of the major human cancers (colon, breast, prostate) strongly suggests that p68/p72 promote tumorigenesis and might even represent proto-oncoproteins [156]. DDX5 and DDX17, are substrates for the acetyltransferase p300 in vitro and in vivo. Mutation of acetylation sites affected the binding of p68/p72 to HDACs, but not to p300 or estrogen receptor. Acetylation additionally increased the stability of p68 and p72 RNA helicase and stimulated their ability to coactivate the estrogen receptor [157, 158], thereby potentially contributing to its aberrant activation in breast tumors. Also, acetylation of p72, but not of p68 RNA helicase, enhanced p53-dependent activation of the MDM2 promoter, pointing at another mechanism of how p72 acetylation may facilitate carcinogenesis by boosting the negative p53-MDM2 feedback loop. Furthermore, blocking p72 acetylation caused cell cycle arrest and apoptosis, revealing an essential role for p72 acetylation [159]. The muscleblind 1 (MBNL1) is an splice regulator in the development of RNA splice defects in myotonic dystrophy I (DM1). The variant of MBNL1(CUG) bind ten proteins involved in remodeling ribonucleoprotein complexes including hnRNP H, H2, H3, F, A2/B1, K, L, DDX5, DDX17, and DHX9. The expression of expanded CUG repeats alters the stoichiometry of MBNL1 (CUG) complexes to allow both the reinforcement and expansion of RNA processing defects [160]. Intensive exercise triggers the cascade processes of body adaptation, including modulation of spliceosome functioning, and can lead to modification of its activity and choice of alternative exons. We studied the effect of exercise of the maximum aerobic power on activation of transcription of genes involved in the splicing process. Short-term exercise resulted in a significant increase of mRNA expression of genes encoding proteins involved in the formation of precatalytic spliceosome: DDX17, DDX46, HNRNPR, PRPF4B, and SRPK2. The role of the detected regulators in initiation of spliceosome assembly under conditions of maximally intensive exercise is discussed [119].

LUC7L3 or LUC7-like 3 (*S. cerevisiae*) encodes a protein with an N-terminal half that contains cysteine/histidine motifs and leucine zipper-like repeats, and the C-terminal half is rich in arginine and glutamate residues (RE domain) and arginine and serine residues (RS domain). This protein localizes with a speckled pattern in the nucleus, and has been shown to be involved in the formation of spliceosome via the RE and RS domains. This genes has been shown to be upregulated in heart failure tissues demonstrated that 17 splicing factors, associated with all major spliceosome components, were upregulated. Two of these splicing factors, RBM25 and LUC7L3 were elevated in human heart failure tissue and mediated truncation of SCN5A mRNA in both Jurkat cells and human embryonic stem cell-derived cardiomyocytes [161]. The cardiac voltage-gated Na+ channel current (encoded by SCN5A), and the changes have been implicated in the increased risk of sudden death in heart failure.

PNN or pinin a desmosome-associated protein is a transcriptional activator binding to the E-box 1 core sequence of the E-cadherin promoter gene; the core-binding sequence is 5′CAGGTG-3′. Capable of reversing CTBP1-mediated transcription repression. Component of a splicing-dependent multiprotein exon junction complex (EJC) deposited at splice junction on mRNAs. The EJC is a dynamic structure consisting of a few core proteins and several more peripheral nuclear and cytoplasmic-associated factors that join the complex only transiently either during EJC assembly or during subsequent mRNA metabolism. PNN participates in the regulation of alternative pre-mRNA splicing. Associates to spliced mRNA within 60 nt upstream of the 5′-splice sites [162]. Pinin (Pnn), a nuclear speckle-associated protein, zones of accumulation of transcriptional and mRNA splicing factors, where Pnn is involved in mRNA processing [162]. PNN has been shown to function in maintenance of epithelial integrity through altering expression of several key adhesion molecules [163]. Pnn plays a crucial role in small intestinal development by influencing expression of an intestinal homeobox gene, Cdx2. Conditional inactivation of Pnn within intestinal epithelia resulted in significant down-regulation of a caudal type homeobox gene, Cdx2, leading to obvious villus dysmorphogenesis and severely disrupted epithelial differentiation. Additionally, in Pnn-deficient small intestine, we observed upregulated Tcf/Lef reporter activity, as well as misregulated expression/distribution of beta-catenin and Tcf4. Since regulation of Cdx gene expression has been closely linked to Wnt/beta-catenin signaling activity, we explored the possibility of Pnn's interaction with beta-catenin, a major effector of the canonical Wnt signaling pathway. Co-immunoprecipitation assays revealed that Pnn, together with its interaction partner CtBP2, a transcriptional co-repressor, was in a complex with beta-catenin [164]. Moreover, both of these proteins were found to be recruited to the proximal promoter area of Cdx2. Pnn is essential for tight regulation of Wnt signaling and Cdx2 expression during small intestinal development [165]. PNN and other SR proteins including SC35 are differentially expressed in the adult mouse CNS, displaying cell type-specific distribution patterns [166]. Depletion of Pnn expression, a SR-related protein with functions involved in pre-mRNA splicing and mRNA export, induces reduced expression of a subset of cellular proteins, especially that of SR family proteins, including SC35, SRm300, SRp55, and SRp40, but not that of other nuclear proteins, such as p53, Mdm2, and ki67. Knocking down Pnn expression was achieved in vitro by siRNA transfection. Expression levels of SR and SR-related proteins in Pnn-depleted cells as compared to those in control cells were evaluated by immunofluorescent staining and Western blot with specific antibodies. In addition, we also demonstrate that loss of Pnn expression could modulate splice site selection of model reporter gene in vivo. Pnn may play a general role in the control of the cellular amount of family SR proteins through down-regulation of its own expression, thereby providing us with a better understanding of the cellular mechanism by which Pnn fulfills its biological function [167].

During mouse embryo development, PNN transcripts display two isoforms due to differential utilization of a polyadenylation site and exhibit tissue variable expression with thymus expressing the highest level of transcript. Analysis of pnn expression in mouse embryos revealed N-pnn expression starts from the two-cell fertilized egg stage and is ubiquitous at all stages of mouse embryo development. ISH and immunofluorescent staining of embryo cryosections showed that during mouse organogenesis N-pnn is highly expressed in the central nervous system. In addition, N-pnn was found to be highly expressed in the cortex region of thymus of E16.5 mouse fetus, while in the hepatic primordium the strongest signals were noted at E13.5 to E14.5 rather than at later developmental stages. The subcellular location of N-pnn in photoreceptors of developing retinas was determine by nuclear fractionation and Western blot, because N-pnn displayed a staining pattern reminiscent of cytoplasmic proteins at the microscopic level in developing mouse photoreceptors [168].

PRPF4 or pre-mRNA processing factor 4 homolog (yeast) is involved in pre-mRNA splicing. Human splicing factors Hprp3p and Hprp4p are associated with the U4/U6 small nuclear ribonucleoprotein particle, which is essential for the assembly of an active spliceosomes [169–172]. Silencing of PRPF4, a splicing factor hitherto unrelated to Retinitis pigmentosa, evoked the same defects in vision, photoreceptor morphology, and retinal gene expression. RP can be elicited by mutations that affect the tri-snRNP subunit of the pre-mRNA splicing machinery. In zebrafish by silencing the RP-associated splicing factor PRPF4 and observed detrimental effects on visual function and photoreceptor morphology. Despite reducing the level of a constitutive splicing factor, no general defects in gene expression were found. Instead, retinal genes were selectively affected, providing the first in vivo link between mutations in splicing factors and the RP phenotype [173]. High oxygen consumption and cyclical changes related to dark-adaptation are characteristic of the outer retina. Oxygenation changes may contribute to the selective vulnerability of the retina in retinitis pigmentosa (RP) patients, especially for those forms involving genes with global cellular functions. Genes coding for components of the U4/U6.U5 tri small nuclear ribonucleoprotein (tri-snRNP) complex of the spliceosome stand out, because mutations in four genes cause RP, i.e., RP9 (PAP1), RP11 (PRPF31), RP13 (PRPF8), and RP18 (PRPF3), while there is no degeneration outside the retina despite global expression of these genes. With the assumption that variable oxygenation plays a role in RP forms related to pre-mRNA splicing and the retina and brain are similar, we searched a data collection of ischemia-hypoxia regulated genes of the brain for oxygen regulated genes of the U4/U6.U5 tri-snRNP complex [174].

RBM25 or RNA-binding motif protein 25 acts as a regulator of alternative pre-mRNA splicing. Involved in apoptotic cell death through the regulation of the apoptotic factor BCL2L1 isoform expression. Modulates the ratio of pro-apoptotic BCL2L1 isoform S to anti-apoptotic BCL2L1 isoform L mRNA expression. When overexpressed, stimulates pro-apoptotic BCL2L1 isoform S 5′-splice site (5′-ss) selection, whereas its depletion caused the accumulation of anti-apoptotic BCL2L1 isoform L. Promotes BCL2L1 isoform S 5′-ss usage through the 5′-CGGGCA-3′ RNA sequence. Its association with LUC7L3 promotes U1 snRNP binding to a weak 5′ ss in a 5′-CGGGCA-3′-dependent manner. Binds to the exonic splicing enhancer 5′-CGGGCA-3′ RNA sequence located within exon 2 of the BCL2L1 pre-mRNA [175].

RBMX or RNA-binding motif protein, X-linked belongs to the RBMY gene family which includes candidate Y chromosome spermatogenesis genes and function as RNA-binding protein which may be involved in pre-mRNA splicing [176–179].

SFPQ or splicing factor proline/glutamine-rich is a DNA- and RNA-binding protein, involved in several nuclear processes. Essential pre-mRNA splicing factor required early in spliceosome formation and for splicing catalytic step II, probably as an heteromer with NONO. SFPQ binds to pre-mRNA in spliceosome C complex, and specifically binds to intronic PPTs. Interacts with U5 snRNA, probably by binding to a purine-rich sequence located on the 3′ side of U5 snRNA stem 1b. It may be involved in a pre-mRNA coupled splicing and polyadenylation process as component of a snRNP-free complex with SNRPA/U1A. The SFPQ-NONO heteromer associated with MATR3 may play a role in nuclear retention of defective RNAs. SFPQ may be involved in homologous DNA pairing; in vitro, promotes the invasion of ssDNA between a duplex DNA and produces a D-loop formation. The SFPQ-NONO heteromer may be involved in DNA unwinding by modulating the function of topoisomerase I/TOP1; in vitro, stimulates dissociation of TOP1 from DNA after cleavage and enhances its jumping between separate DNA helices. The SFPQ-NONO heteromer may be involved in DNA nonhomologous end joining (NHEJ) required for double-strand break repair and V(D)J recombination and may stabilize paired DNA ends; in vitro, the complex strongly stimulates DNA end joining, binds directly to the DNA substrates and cooperates with the Ku70/G22P1-Ku80/XRCC5 (Ku) dimer to establish a functional preligation complex. SFPQ is involved in transcriptional regulation. Transcriptional repression is probably mediated by an interaction of SFPQ with SIN3A and subsequent recruitment of HDACs. The SFPQ-NONO/SF-1 complex binds to the CYP17 promoter and regulates basal and cAMP-dependent transcriptional activity. SFPQ isoform Long binds to the DNA binding domains (DBD) of nuclear hormone receptors, like RXRA and probably THRA, and acts as transcriptional co-repressor in absence of hormone ligands. Binds the DNA sequence 5′-CTGAGTC-3′ in the insulin-like growth factor response element (IGFRE) and inhibits IGF-I-stimulated transcriptional regulation [180–186]. PSF or SFPQ stimulate double-strand break repair in cell free systems, most likely via direct interaction with the repair substrate. Prior in vitro studies are, however, insufficient to demonstrate whether PSF contributes to DNA repair in living cells. miRNA-mediated PSF knockdown in human (HeLa) cells. Mutational analysis suggests that sequences required for viability and radioresistance are partially separable, and that the latter requires a unique N-terminal PSF domain. As an independent means to investigate PSF sequences involved in DNA repair, was established using an assay based on real-time relocalization of PSF-containing complexes to sites of dense, laser-induced DNA damage in living cells. The relocalization is driven by sequences in PSF, rather than its dimerization partner, p54(nrb)/NONO, and that sequences required for relocalization reside in the same N-terminal domain that contributes to radioresistance. Further evidence for the importance of PSF sequences in mediating relocalization is provided by observations that PSF promotes relocalization of a third protein, PSPC1, under conditions where p54(nrb) is limiting. Together, these observations support the model derived from prior biochemical studies that PSF influences repair via direct, local, interaction with the DNA substrate [184, 186].

Lipids can influence pre-mRNA processing by regulating the phosphorylation status of specific regulatory factors, which is mediated by protein phosphatase activity. Ceramides are lipid-signaling molecules composed of sphingosine and a fatty acid. C6 pyridinium ceramide (PyrCer) binds to the PP1 catalytic subunit and inhibits the dephosphorylation of several splicing regulatory proteins containing the evolutionarily conserved RVxF PP1-binding motif (including PSF/SFPQ, Tra2-beta1, and SF2/ASF) [180].

CCNL1 and CCNL2 or cyclin L1 and cyclin L2 are two closely related members of the cyclin family that contain C-terminal arginine- and serine-rich (RS) domains and are localized in the splicing factor compartment (nuclear speckles) [187–189] are significantly upregulated in the parous breast.. They are transcriptional regulators which participates in regulating the pre-mRNA splicing process [190, 191]. Also modulates the expression of critical apoptotic factor, leading to cell apoptosis possibly through the Wnt signal transduction pathway [104, 192]. Cyclin L1 and cyclin L2 are two closely related members of the cyclin family that contain C-terminal arginine- and serine-rich (RS) domains and are localized in the splicing factor compartment (nuclear speckles). Using photobleaching techniques was show that a green fluorescent protein (GFP) fusion protein of cyclin L1, in contrast to cyclin L2, was not mobile within the nucleus of living COS7 cells. Transcriptional arrest by actinomycin D caused accumulation of GFP-cyclin L2 in rounded and enlarged nuclear speckles but did not affect the subnuclear pattern of distribution of GFP-cyclin L1. Although immobile in most phases of the cell cycle, GFP-cyclin L1 was diffusely distributed and highly mobile in the cytoplasm of metaphase cells. By analysis of a series of chimeras, deletion constructs, and a point mutant, a segment within the RS domain of cyclin L1 was identified to be necessary for the immobility of the protein in nuclear speckles [187]. Whereas the CCNL1 has an inhibitory effect on growth of MDA-MB-231 cells it seems that interact with the tissue inhibitor of matrix metalloproteinase-1 (TIMP1) [193]. CCNL1 and TIMP1 expression was significantly elevated in breast cancer tissues compared with that in peri-breast cancer tissues of patients by cDNA microarray and these results were further confirmed by real-time RT-PCR and western blotting. Co-expression or co-repression of these two genes did not affect cell growth. Overexpression of CCNL1 and TIMP1 individually induced overexpression of each other [193]. Previous studies using the yeast two-hybrid assay (Y2H) have identified cyclin L1 (CCNL1) and Ewing sarcoma breakpoint region 1 protein (EWSR1) as being interacting partners of tuftelin-interacting protein 11 (TFIP11). All three proteins are functionally related to the spliceosome and involved in pre-mRNA splicing activities. The spliceosome is a dynamic ribonucleoprotein complex responsible for pre-mRNA splicing of intronic regions, and is composed of five small nuclear RNAs (snRNAs) and µ140 proteins. TFIP11 appears to play a role in spliceosome disassembly allowing for the release of the bound lariat-intron. The roles of CCNL1 and EWSR1 in the spliceosome are poorly understood. Using fluorescently-tagged proteins and confocal microscopy TFIP11, CCNL1, and EWSR1 frequently co-localize to speckled nuclear domains. These data would suggest that all three proteins participate in a common cellular activity related to RNA splicing events [194]. Cyclin L1 and L2 genes generate 14 mRNA variants encoding six cyclin L proteins, one of which has not been described previously. Using cyclin L gene-specific antibodies, have demonstrated expression of multiple endogenous cyclin L proteins in human cell lines and mouse tissues. Interactions between CDK11(p110), mitosis-specific CDK11(p58), and apoptosis-specific CDK11(p46) with both cyclin L-alpha and -beta proteins and the co-elution of these proteins following size exclusion chromatography. CDK11(p110) and associated cyclin L-alpha/beta proteins localize to splicing factor compartments and nucleoplasm and interact with serine/arginine-rich proteins. Importantly, we also determine the effect of CDK11-cyclin L complexes on pre-mRNA splicing. Preincubation of nuclear extracts with purified cyclin L-alpha and -beta isoforms depletes the extract of in vitro splicing activity. Ectopic expression of cyclin L1alpha, L1beta, L2alpha, or L2beta or active CDK11(p110) individually enhances intracellular intron splicing activity, whereas expression of CDK11(p58/p46) or kinase-dead CDK11(p110) represses splicing activity. Expression of cyclins L-alpha and -beta and CDK11(p110) strongly and differentially affects alternative splicing in vivo. Together, these data establish that CDK11(p110) interacts physically and functionally with cyclin L-alpha and -beta isoforms and SR proteins to regulate splicing [190].

The expression and amplification of cyclin L1 (CCNL1) gene, a potential oncogene localized in the commonly amplified 3q25-28 region, in human head and neck squamous cell carcinomas (HNSCCs) with no relationships to the clinico-pathological parameters is located in the nuclear speckles in tumor cells compatible with a role for CCNL1 in RNA splicing [195].

CrkRS is a Cdc2-related protein kinase that contains an arginine- and serine-rich (SR) domain, a characteristic of the SR protein family of splicing factors. CrkRS interacts with cyclin L1 and cyclin L2, and thus rename it as the long form of cyclin-dependent kinase 12 (CDK12(L)). A shorter isoform of CDK12, CDK12(S), that differs from CDK12(L) only at the carboxyl end, was also identified. Both isoforms associate with cyclin L1 through interactions mediated by the kinase domain and the cyclin domain, suggesting a bona fide CDK/cyclin partnership. Furthermore, CDK12 isoforms alter the splicing pattern of an E1a minigene, and the effect is potentiated by the cyclin domain of cyclin L1. When expression of CDK12 isoforms is perturbed by small interfering RNAs, a reversal of the splicing choices is observed. The activity of CDK12 on splicing is counteracted by SF2/ASF and SC35, but not by SRp40, SRp55, and SRp75. Together, our findings indicate that CDK12 and cyclin L1/L2 are CDK and cyclin partners and regulate alternative splicing [196]. Cyclin L (ania-6a), is commonly overexpressed in primary tumors compared with corresponding normal tissues. This cyclin was previously pinpointed as a candidate for a role in promoting cell cycle entry. Thus, we propose cyclin L as a candidate oncogene in head and neck cancer [197].

Cyclin L2, as a substrate of the nuclear protein kinase DYRK1A contains an N-terminal cyclin domain and a C-terminal arginine/serine-rich domain (RS domain), which is a hallmark of many proteins involved in pre-mRNA processing. The gene for cyclin L2 encodes the full-length cyclin L2, which is predominantly expressed in testis, as well as a truncated splicing variant (cyclin L2S) that lacks the RS domain and is ubiquitously expressed in human tissues. Full-length cyclin L2, but not cyclin L2S, was associated with the CDK PITSLRE. Cyclin L2 interacted with splicing factor 2 in vitro and was co-localized with the splicing factor SC35 in the nuclear speckle compartment. Photobleaching experiments showed that a fusion protein of GFP and cyclin L2 in nuclear speckles rapidly exchanged with unbleached molecules in the nucleus, similar to other RS domain-containing proteins. In striking contrast, the closely related GFP-cyclin L1 was immobile in the speckle compartment. DYRK1A interacted with cyclin L2 in pull-down assays, and overexpression of DYRK1A stimulated phosphorylation of cyclin L2 in COS-7 cells. These data characterize cyclin L2 as a highly mobile component of nuclear speckles and suggest that DYRK1A may regulate splicing by phosphorylation of cyclin L2. Human cyclin L2 shares significant homology to cyclin L1, K, T1, T2, and C, which are involved in transcriptional regulation via phosphorylation of the C-terminal domain of RNA polymerase II. The cyclin L2 protein contains an N-terminal "cyclin box" and C-terminal dipeptide repeats of alternating arginines and serines, a hallmark of the SR family of splicing factors. A new isoform and the mouse homologue of human cyclin L2 have also been cloned in this study. Recombinant cyclin L2 protein can stimulate in vitro mRNA splicing. Overexpression of human cyclin L2 suppresses the growth of human hepatocellular carcinoma SMMC 7721 cells both in vitro and in vivo, inducing cellular apoptosis. This process involves upregulation of p53 and Bax and decreased expression of Bcl-2. The data suggest that cyclin L2 represents a new member of the cyclin family, which might regulate the transcription and RNA processing of certain apoptosis-related factors, resulting in tumor cell growth inhibition and apoptosis [104]. Stable CCNL2-overexpressing P19 cells were less differentiated after treatment with 1% DMSO and that expression of myocardial cell differentiation-related genes (such as cardiac actin, GATA4, Mef2C, Nkx2.5, and BNP) were reduced compared to vector-only transfected P19. Moreover, P19 cells overexpressing the CCNL2 gene had a reduced growth rate and a remarkably decreased S phase and these cells underwent apoptosis, as detected by two different apoptosis assays. The anti-apoptotic Bcl-2 protein was also downregulated in these cells. Expression of Wnt and beta-catenin was suppressed and GSK3beta was induced in the CCNL2-overexpressing P19 cells. Overexpression of CCNL2 inhibited proliferation and differentiation of mouse embryonic carcinoma P19 cells and induced them to undergo apoptosis, possibly through the Wnt signal transduction pathway [192]. Overexpression of cyclin L2 inhibited the growth of human lung adenocarcinoma cells (A549 cell). Cell cycle analysis in cells transfected with pCCNL2 revealed an increment in proportion in G0/G1 phase ($68.07\% \pm 4.2\%$) in contrast to $60.39\% \pm 2.82\%$ of the cells transfected with mock vector. Apoptosis occurred in $7.25\% \pm 0.98\%$ cells transfected with pCCNL2, as compared with $1.25\% \pm 0.21\%$ of the mock vector control group. Cyclin L2-induced-G0/G1 arrest and apoptosis involved upregulation of caspase-3 and down-regulation of Bcl-2 and survivin. The results indicate that overexpression of cyclin L2 protein may promote efficient growth inhibition of human lung adenocarcinoma cells by inducing G0/G1 cell cycle arrest and apoptosis [191]. This function is in agreement with our data in which the CCDL2 is highly expressed in the parous breast and localized in the nuclear compartment (Figs. 8.16 and 8.17).

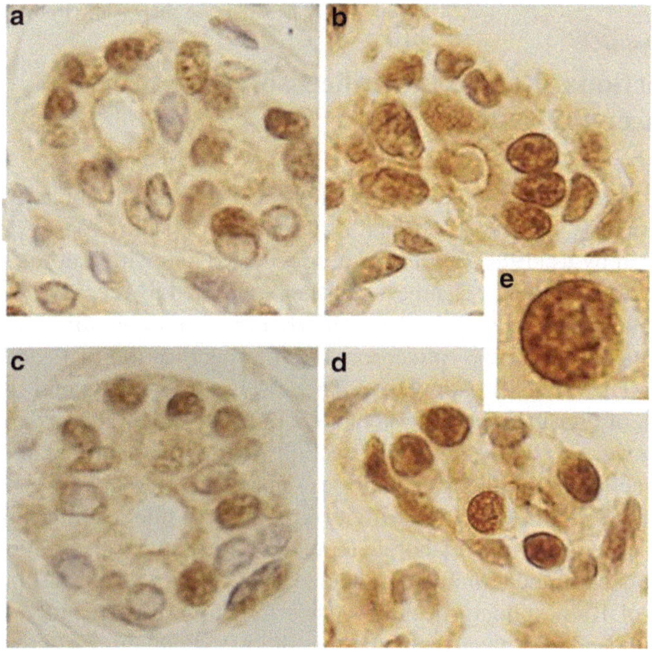

Fig. 8.16 Immunohistochemistry of cyclin-cyclin L2 protein (CCNL2) performed in paraffin embedded tissues of nulliparous and parous samples. CCNL2 protein was overexpressed in the nucleus of epithelial cells of lobules type 1 in parous breast (**b, d** and **e**) when compared to nulliparous women (**a** and **c**)

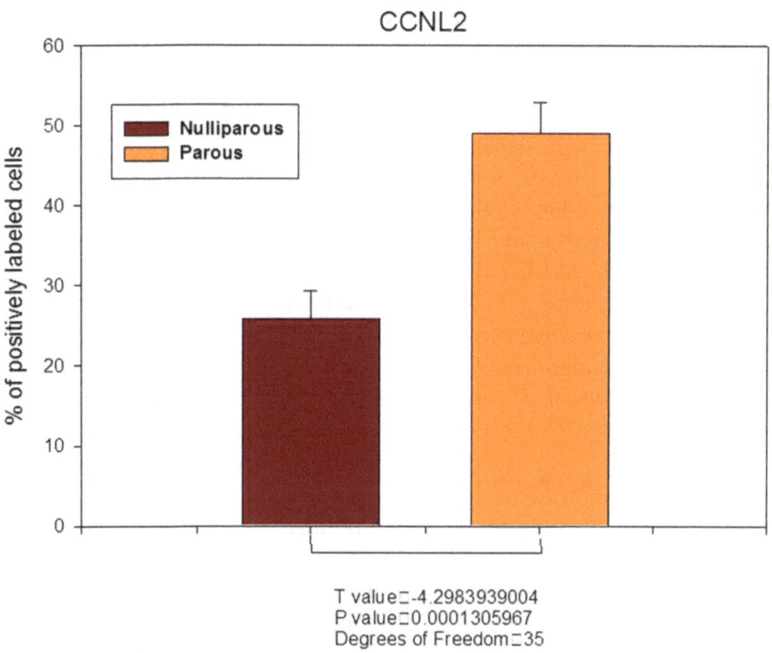

Fig. 8.17 Histogram showing quantization of CCNL2. There is a significant difference in the percentage of positive cells for CCNL2 in the parous vs. the nulliparous breast

8.8 Functional Role of the Spliceosomes in Breast Cancer Prevention

How these data explain the protective effect of parity against breast cancer? The concept that parity induces a terminal differentiation of the breast epithelial cells was postulated by us [198–206], the finding reported herewith that the spliceosome is mainly the target of these changes is further supported by recent work [207] indicating the role of alternative splicing in differentiating mouse embryonic stem (ES) point the critical role for the spliceosome in the specification of ES cells with differentiation. The same also apply to self-renewal, pluripotency, and tissue lineage specification of human embryonic stem cells [208–211]. Another example is in the *D. melanogaster* on how sex-specific functions is not a single regulatory event that governs the activities of all downstream sex determination regulatory genes-turning on Sex lethal (Sxl) RNA splicing activity in females while leaving it turned off in males-there are, in addition, elaborate temporal and spatial transcriptional controls on the expression of the terminal regulatory genes, dsx and fru [212] indicating the importance of RNA splicing in the sex determination at each individual somatic cell. Retinoic acid treatment regulates the alternative splicing mechanism during neural differentiation [213]. Or in the role of spliced interleukin (IL)-7 in distinct anatomic areas in the adult, in developing human brains and in normal human neuronal progenitor cells [214]. Splicing, nuclear transport, and extramatrix proteins may be involved in sex determination. The male sex determination pathway switches on the expression of genes driving Sertoli cell differentiation. Sertoli cells orchestrate testicular differentiation. In the absence of Sry, the predomination of the female pathway results in the realization of a robust genetic program that drives ovarian differentiation [215]. Alternative splicing is also regulating the preferentially metabolization of glucose by aerobic glycolysis, characterized by increased lactate production in cancer cells. The aerobic glycolysis process is controlled by hnRNP A1 and A2, as well as the polypyrimidine tract-binding protein PTB [216]. Alternative splicing occurs during complex disease and may govern for example experimental autoimmune encephalomyelitis [217], the differentiation of erythroid cells and megakaryocytes by GATA1 [218].

Whereas more studies need to be conducted to understand the specific pathway/s of the genes involved in this process. Our data [17, 18, 219] *emphasize the importance of posttranscriptional regulatory mechanisms as a critical component underlying the differentiation of the breast. From the moment a gene is transcribed, it undergoes a series of posttranscriptional regulatory modifications in the nucleus and cytoplasm until its final deployment as a functional protein. Initially, a message is subjected to extensive structural regulation through alternative splicing, which is capable of greatly expanding the protein repertoire by generating, in some cases, thousands of functionally distinct isoforms from a single gene locus. Then, RNA packaging into the nucleus of the breast epithelial cells and recognition by RNA-binding proteins and/or microRNAs is capable of restricting protein synthesis to selective locations and under specific input conditions. This ability of the posttran-*

scriptional apparatus to expand the informational content of the breast cells and control the lower susceptibility of the cell to carcinogenesis susceptibility is determined by the signature induced y a full term pregnancy.

References

1. Berget SM, Moore C, Sharp PA (1977) Spliced segments at 5′ terminus of adenovirus 2 late messenger-RNA. Proc Natl Acad Sci U S A 74:3171–3175
2. Chow LT, Roberts JM, Lewis JB, Broker TR (1977) A map of cytoplasmic RNA transcripts from lytic adenovirus type 2, determined by electron microscopy of RNA:DNA hybrids. Cell 11:819–836
3. Query CC (2009) Spliceosome subunit revealed. Nature 458:418–419
4. Will CL, Lührmann R (2011) Spliceosome structure and function. Cold Spring Harb Perspect Biol 3:a003707
5. König H, Matter N, Bader R, Thiele W, Müller F (2007) Splicing segregation: the minor spliceosome acts outside the nucleus and controls cell proliferation. Cell 131:718–729
6. Jamison SF, Crow A, Garcia-Blanco MA (1992) The spliceosome assembly pathway in mammalian extracts. Mol Cell Biol 12:4279–4287
7. Seraphin B, Rosbash M (1989) Identification of functional U1 snRNA pre-messenger RNA complexes committed to spliceosome assembly and splicing. Cell 59:349–358
8. Legrain P, Seraphin B, Rosbash M (1988) Early commitment of yeast pre-mRNA to the spliceosome pathway. Mol Cell Biol 8:3755–3760
9. Query CC, Moore MJ, Sharp P (1994) Branch nucleophile selection in pre-mRNA splicing: evidence for the bulged duplex model. Genes Dev 8:587–597
10. Newby MI, Greenbaum NL (2002) Sculpting of the spliceosomal branch site recognition motif by a conserved pseudouridine. Nat Struct Biol 9:958–965
11. Burge CB et al (1999) Splicing precursors to mRNAs by the spliceosomes. In: Gesteland RF, Cech TR, Atkins JF (eds) The RNA world. Cold Spring Harbor Laboratory Press, Cold Spring Harbor, pp 525–560
12. Staley JP, Guthrie C (1998) Mechanical devices of the spliceosome: motors, clocks, springs, and things. Cell 92:315–326
13. Newman AJ, Teigelkamp S, Beggs JD (1995) snRNA interactions at 5′ and 3′ splice sites monitored by photoactivated crosslinking in yeast spliceosomes. RNA 1:968–980
14. Chiara MD, Palandjian L, Feld Kramer R, Reed R (1997) Evidence that U5 snRNP recognizes the 3′ splice site for catalytic step II in mammals. EMBO J 16:4746–4759
15. Moore MJ, Sharp PA (1993) Evidence for two active sites in the spliceosome provided by stereochemistry of pre-mRNA splicing. Nature 365:364–368
16. Konforti BB, Koziolkiewicz MJ, Konarska MM (1993) Disruption of base pairing between the 5′ splice site and the 5′ end of U1 snRNA is required for spliceosome assembly. Cell 75:863–873
17. Belitskaya-Levy I, Zeleniuch-Jacquotte A, Russo J, Russo IH, Bordas P, Ahman J, Afanasyeva Y, Johansson R, Lenner P, Li X, de Cicco-Lopez RL, Peri S, Ross E, Russo PA, Santucci-Pereira J, Sheriff FS, Slifker M, Hallmans G, Toniolo P, Arslan AA (2011) Characterization of a genomic signature of pregnancy identified in the breast. Cancer Prev Res 4:1457–1464
18. Russo J, Santucci-Pereira J, de Cicco RL, Sheriff F, Russo PA, Peri S, Slifker M, Ross E, Mello ML, Vidal BC, Belitskaya-Levy I, Arslan A, Zeleniuch-Jacquotte A, Bordas P, Lenner P, Ahman J, Afanasyeva Y, Hallmans G, Toniolo P, Russo IH (2012) Pregnancy-induced chromatin remodeling in the breast of postmenopausal women. Int J Cancer 131(5):1059–1070
19. Jenuwein T, Allis CD (2001) Translating the histone code. Science 293:1074–1080

20. Gill G (2004) SUMO and ubiquitin in the nucleus: different functions, similar mechanisms? Genes Dev 18:2046–2059
21. Morgan HD, Santos F, Green K, Dean W, Reik W (2005) Epigenetic reprogramming in mammals. Hum Mol Genet 14:R47–R58
22. Rottman FM, Bokar JA, Narayan P, Shambaugh ME, Ludwiczak R (1994) N6-adenosine methylation in mRNA: substrate specificity and enzyme complexity. Biochimie 76:1109–1114
23. Clancy MJ, Shambaugh ME, Timpte CS, Bokar JA (2002) Induction of sporulation in Saccharomyces cerevisiae leads to the formation of N6-methyladenosine in mRNA: a potential mechanism for the activity of the IME4 gene. Nucleic Acids Res 30:4509–4518
24. Bujnicki JM, Feder M, Radlinska M, Blumenthal RM (2002) Structure prediction and phylogenetic analysis of a functionally diverse family of proteins homologous to the MT-A70 subunit of the human mRNA:m(6)A methyltransferase. J Mol Evol 55:431–444
25. Sugawara T, Oguro H, Negishi M, Morita Y, Ichikawa H, Iseki T, Yokosuka O, Nakauchi H, Iwama A (2010) FET family proto-oncogene Fus contributes to self-renewal of hematopoietic stem cells. Hematology 38:696–706
26. Andersson MK, Ståhlberg A, Arvidsson Y, Olofsson A, Semb H, Stenman G, Nilsson O, Aman P (2008) The multifunctional FUS, EWS and TAF15 proto-oncoproteins show cell type-specific expression patterns and involvement in cell spreading and stress response. BMC Cell Biol 9:37
27. Baechtold H, Kuroda M, Sok J, Ron D, Lopez BS, Akhmedov AT (1999) Human 75-kDa DNA-pairing protein is identical to the pro-oncoprotein TLS/FUS and is able to promote D-loop formation. J Biol Chem 274:34337–34342
28. Reboll MR, Oumard A, Gazdag AC, Renger I, Ritter B, Schwarzer M, Hauser H, Wood M, Yamada M, Resch K, Nourbakhsh M (2007) NRF IRES activity is mediated by RNA binding protein JKTBP1 and a 14-nt RNA element. RNA 13:1328–1340
29. Akagi T, Kamei D, Tsuchiya N, Nishina Y, Horiguchi H, Matsui M, Kamma H, Yamada M (2000) Molecular characterization of a mouse heterogeneous nuclear ribonucleoprotein D-like protein JKTBP and its tissue-specific expression. Gene 245:267–273
30. Taga Y, Miyoshi M, Okajima T, Matsuda T, Nadano D (2010) Identification of heterogeneous nuclear ribonucleoprotein A/B as a cytoplasmic mRNA-binding protein in early involution of the mouse mammary gland. Cell Biochem Funct 28:321–328
31. Huang PR, Hung SC, Wang TC (2010) Telomeric DNA-binding activities of heterogeneous nuclear ribonucleoprotein A3 in vitro and in vivo. Biochim Biophys Acta 1803:1164–1174
32. Han SP, Friend LR, Carson JH, Korza G, Barbarese E, Maggipinto M, Hatfield JT, Rothnagel JA, Smith R (2010) Differential subcellular distributions and trafficking functions of hnRNP A2/B1 spliceoforms. Traffic 11:886–898
33. Markus MA, Marques FZ, Morris BJ (2011) Resveratrol, by modulating RNA processing factor levels, can influence the alternative splicing of pre-mRNAs. PLoS One 6:e28926
34. Harahap IS, Saito T, San LP, Sasaki N, Gunadi, Nurputra DK, Yusoff S, Yamamoto T, Morikawa S, Nishimura N, Lee MJ, Takeshima Y, Matsuo M, Nishio H (2012) Valproic acid increases SMN2 expression and modulates SF2/ASF and hnRNPA1 expression in SMA fibroblast cell lines. Brain Dev 34(3):213–222
35. Flynn RL, Centore RC, O'Sullivan RJ, Rai R, Tse A, Songyang Z, Chang S, Karlseder J, Zou L (2011) TERRA and hnRNPA1 orchestrate an RPA-to-POT1 switch on telomeric single-stranded DNA. Nature 471:532–536
36. Tsuruno C, Ohe K, Kuramitsu M, Kohma T, Takahama Y, Hamaguchi Y, Hamaguchi I, Okuma K (2011) HMGA1a is involved in specific splice site regulation of human immunodeficiency virus type 1. Biochem Biophys Res Commun 406:512–517
37. Zearfoss NR, Clingman CC, Farley BM, McCoig LM, Ryder SP (2011) SourceQuaking regulates Hnrnpa1 expression through its 3′ UTR in oligodendrocyte precursor cells. PLoS Genet 7:e1001269
38. Zhao L, Mandler MD, Yi H, Feng Y (2010) Quaking I controls a unique cytoplasmic pathway that regulates alternative splicing of myelin-associated glycoprotein. Proc Natl Acad Sci U S A 107:19061–19066

39. Chen M, Zhang J, Manley JL (2010) Turning on a fuel switch of cancer: hnRNP proteins regulate alternative splicing of pyruvate kinase mRNA. Cancer Res 70:8977–8980
40. David CJ, Chen M, Assanah M, Canoll P, Manley JL (2010) HnRNP proteins controlled by c-Myc deregulate pyruvate kinase mRNA splicing in cancer. Nature 463:364–368
41. Gaildrat P, Krieger S, Théry JC, Killian A, Rousselin A, Berthet P, Frébourg T, Hardouin A, Martins A, Tosi M (2010) The BRCA1 c.5434C->G (p.Pro1812Ala) variant induces a deleterious exon 23 skipping by affecting exonic splicing regulatory elements. J Med Genet 47:398–403
42. Goina E, Skoko N, Pagani F (2008) Binding of DAZAP1 and hnRNPA1/A2 to an exonic splicing silencer in a natural BRCA1 exon 18 mutant. Mol Cell Biol 28:3850–3860
43. Rosenberger S, De-Castro Arce J, Langbein L, Steenbergen RD, Rösl F (2010) Alternative splicing of human papillomavirus type-16 E6/E6* early mRNA is coupled to EGF signaling via Erk1/2 activation. Proc Natl Acad Sci U S A 107:7006–7011
44. Yao Z, Duan S, Hou D, Wang W, Wang G, Liu Y, Wen L, Wu M (2010) B23 acts as a nucleolar stress sensor and promotes cell survival through its dynamic interaction with hnRNPU and hnRNPA1. Oncogene 29:1821–1834
45. Orvain C, Matre V, Gabrielsen OS (2008) The transcription factor c-Myb affects pre-mRNA splicing. Biochem Biophys Res Commun 372:309–313
46. Donev R, Newall A, Thome J, Sheer D (2007) A role for SC35 and hnRNPA1 in the determination of amyloid precursor protein isoforms. Mol Psychiatry 12:681–690
47. Christian K, Lang M, Maurel P, Raffalli-Mathieu F (2004) Interaction of heterogeneous nuclear ribonucleoprotein A1 with cytochrome P450 2A6 mRNA: implications for post-transcriptional regulation of the CYP2A6 gene. Mol Pharmacol 65:1405–1414
48. Chen H, Hewison M, Hu B, Adams JS (2003) Heterogeneous nuclear ribonucleoprotein (hnRNP) binding to hormone response elements: a cause of vitamin D resistance. Proc Natl Acad Sci U S A 100:6109–6114
49. He Y, Brown MA, Rothnagel JA, Saunders NA, Smith R (2005) Roles of heterogeneous nuclear ribonucleoproteins A and B in cell proliferation. J Cell Sci 118:3173–3183
50. Yan-Sanders Y, Hammons GJ, Lyn-Cook BD (2002) Increased expression of heterogeneous nuclear ribonucleoprotein A2/B1 (hnRNP) in pancreatic tissue from smokers and pancreatic tumor cells. Cancer Lett 183:215–220
51. Tockman MS, Mulshine JL, Piantadosi S, Erozan YS, Gupta PK, Ruckdeschel JC, Taylor PR, Zhukov T, Zhou WH, Qiao YL, Yao SX (1997) Prospective detection of preclinical lung cancer: results from two studies of heterogeneous nuclear ribonucleoprotein A2/B1 overexpression. Clin Cancer Res 3:2237–2246
52. Golan-Gerstl R, Cohen M, Shilo A, Suh SS, Bakàcs A, Coppola L, Karni R (2011) Splicing factor hnRNP A2/B1 regulates tumor suppressor gene splicing and is an oncogenic driver in glioblastoma. Cancer Res 71:4464–4472
53. Boise LH, Gonzalez-Garcia M, Postema CE, Ding L, Lindsten T, Turka LA, Mao X, Nunez G, Thompson CB (1993) bcl-x, a bcl-2-related gene that functions as a dominant regulator of apoptotic cell death. Cell 74:597–608
54. Olopade OI, Adeyanju MO, Safa AR, Hagos F, Mick R, Thompson CB, Recant WM (1997) Overexpression of BCL-x protein in primary breast cancer is associated with high tumor grade and nodal metastases. Cancer J Sci Am 3:230–237
55. Chen ZY, Cai L, Zhu J, Chen M, Chen J, Li ZH, Liu XD, Wang SG, Bie P, Jiang P, Dong JH, Li XW (2011) Fyn requires HnRNPA2B1 and Sam68 to synergistically regulate apoptosis in pancreatic cancer. Carcinogenesis 32:1419–1426
56. Fang X, Yoon JG, Li L, Tsai YS, Zheng S, Hood L, Goodlett DR, Foltz G, Lin B (2011) Landscape of the SOX2 protein-protein interactome. Proteomics 11:921–934
57. Santarosa M, Del Col L, Viel A, Bivi N, D'Ambrosio C, Scaloni A, Tell G, Maestro R (2010) BRCA1 modulates the expression of hnRNPA2B1 and KHSRP. Cell Cycle 9:4666–4673
58. Elliott DJ, Venables JP, Newton CS, Lawson D, Boyle S, Eperon IC, Cooke HJ (2000) An evolutionarily conserved germ cell-specific hnRNP is encoded by a retrotransposed gene. Hum Mol Genet 9:2117–2124

59. Dempsey LA, Li MJ, DePace A, Bray-Ward P, Maizels N (1998) The human HNRPD locus maps to 4q21 and encodes a highly conserved protein. Genomics 49:378–384
60. Ing NH (2010) Estradiol up-regulates expression of the A+U-rich binding factor 1 (AUF1) gene in the sheep uterus. J Steroid Biochem Mol Biol 122:172–179
61. Boopathi E, Lenka N, Prabu SK, Fang JK, Wilkinson F, Atchison M, Giallongo A, Avadhani NG (2004) Regulation of murine cytochrome c oxidase Vb gene expression during myogenesis: YY-1 and heterogeneous nuclear ribonucleoprotein D-like protein (JKTBP1) reciprocally regulate transcription activity by physical interaction with the BERF-1/ZBP-89 factor. J Biol Chem 279:35242–35254
62. Tsuchiya N, Kamei D, Takano A, Matsui T, Yamada M (1998) Cloning and characterization of a cDNA encoding a novel heterogeneous nuclear ribonucleoprotein-like protein and its expression in myeloid leukemia cells. J Biochem 123:499–507
63. Bandiera A, Tell G, Marsich E, Scaloni A, Pocsfalvi G, Akintunde Akindahunsi A, Cesaratto L, Manzini G (2003) Cytosine-block telomeric type DNA-binding activity of hnRNP proteins from human cell lines. Arch Biochem Biophys 409:305–314
64. Kamei D, Tsuchiya N, Yamazaki M, Meguro H, Yamada M (1999) Two forms of expression and genomic structure of the human heterogeneous nuclear ribonucleoprotein D-like JKTBP gene (HNRPDL). Gene 228:13–22
65. Kotlajich MV, Hertel KJ (2008) Death by splicing: tumor suppressor RBM5 freezes splice-site pairing. Mol Cell 32:162–164
66. Fushimi K, Ray P, Kar A, Wang L, Sutherland LC, Wu JY (2008) Up-regulation of the proapoptotic caspase 2 splicing isoform by a candidate tumor suppressor, RBM5. Proc Natl Acad Sci U S A 105:15708–15713
67. Sutherland LC, Wang K, Robinson AG (2010) RBM5 as a putative tumor suppressor gene for lung cancer. J Thorac Oncol 5:294–298
68. Rintala-Maki ND, Sutherland LC (2009) Identification and characterisation of a novel antisense non-coding RNA from the RBM5 gene locus. Gene 445:7–16
69. Shu Y, Rintala-Maki ND, Wall VE, Wang K, Goard CA, Langdon CE, Sutherland LC (2007) The apoptosis modulator and tumour suppressor protein RBM5 is a phosphoprotein. Cell Biochem Funct 25:643–653
70. Kobayashi T, Ishida J, Musashi M, Ota S, Yoshida T, Shimizu Y, Chuma M, Kawakami H, Asaka M, Tanaka J, Imamura M, Kobayashi M, Itoh H, Edamatsu H, Sutherland LC, Brachmann RK (2011) p53 transactivation is involved in the antiproliferative activity of the putative tumor suppressor RBM5. Int J Cancer 128:304–318
71. Farina B, Fattorusso R, Pellecchia M (2011) Targeting zinc finger domains with small molecules: solution structure and binding studies of the RanBP2-type zinc finger of RBM5. Chembiochem 12:2837–2845
72. Nguyen CD, Mansfield RE, Leung W, Vaz PM, Loughlin FE, Grant RP, Mackay JP (2011) Characterization of a family of RanBP2-type zinc fingers that can recognize single-stranded RNA. J Mol Biol 407:273–283
73. Oh JJ, Boctor BN, Jimenez CA, Lopez R, Koegel AK, Taschereau EO, Phan DT, Jacobsen SE, Slamon DJ (2008) Promoter methylation study of the H37/RBM5 tumor suppressor gene from the 3p21.3 human lung cancer tumor suppressor locus. Hum Genet 123:55–64
74. Wang K, Ubriaco G, Sutherland LC (2007) RBM6-RBM5 transcription-induced chimeras are differentially expressed in tumours. BMC Genomics 8:348
75. Oh JJ, Koegel AK, Phan DT, Razfar A, Slamon DJ (2007) The two single nucleotide polymorphisms in the H37/RBM5 tumour suppressor gene at 3p21.3 correlated with different subtypes of non-small cell lung cancers. Lung Cancer 58:7–14
76. Rintala-Maki ND, Goard CA, Langdon CE, Wall VE, Traulsen KE, Morin CD, Bonin M, Sutherland LC (2007) Expression of RBM5-related factors in primary breast tissue. J Cell Biochem 100:1440–1458
77. Sillekens PT, Beijer RP, Habets WJ, van Verooij WJ (1989) Molecular cloning of the cDNA for the human U2 snRNA-specific A′ protein. Nucleic Acids Res 17:1893–1906

78. Entrez gene: SNRPA1 small nuclear ribonucleoprotein polypeptide A′. http://www.ncbi.nlm.nih.gov/sites/entrez?Db=gene&Cmd=ShowDetailView&TermToSearch=6627
79. Yamamoto ML, Clark TA, Gee SL, Kang JA, Schweitzer AC, Wickrema A, Conboy JG (2009) Alternative pre-mRNA splicing switches modulate gene expression in late erythropoiesis. Blood 113:3363–3370
80. Spritz RA, Strunk K, Surowy CS, Hoch SO, Barton DE, Francke U (1987) The human U1-70K snRNP protein: cDNA cloning, chromosomal localization, expression, alternative splicing and RNA-binding. Nucleic Acids Res 15:10373–10391
81. Gridley DS, Coutrakon GB, Rizvi A, Bayeta EJ, Luo-Owen X, Makinde AY, Baqai F, Koss P, Slater JM, Pecaut MJ (2008) Low-dose photons modify liver response to simulated solar particle event protons. Radiat Res 169:280–287
82. Xu GM, Arnaout MA (2002) WAC, a novel WW domain-containing adapter with a coiled-coil region, is colocalized with splicing factor SC35. Genomics 79:87–94
83. Sleeman JE, Ajuh P, Lamond AI (2001) snRNP protein expression enhances the formation of Cajal bodies containing p80-coilin and SMN. J Cell Sci 114(pt 24):4407–4419
84. Gubitz AK, Mourelatos Z, Abel L, Rappsilber J, Mann M, Dreyfuss G (2002) Gemin5, a novel WD repeat protein component of the SMN complex that binds Sm proteins. J Biol Chem 277:5631–5636
85. Kaufman KM, Kirby MY, McClain MT, Harley JB, James JA (2001) Lupus autoantibodies recognize the product of an alternative open reading frame of SmB/B′. Biochem Biophys Res Commun 285:1206–1212
86. Saltzman AL, Pan Q, Blencowe BJ (2011) Regulation of alternative splicing by the core spliceosomal machinery. Genes Dev 25:373–384
87. Wang X, Pankratz VS, Fredericksen Z, Tarrell R, Karaus M, McGuffog L, Pharaoh PD, Ponder BA, Dunning AM, Peock S, Cook M, Oliver C, Frost D et al (2010) Common variants associated with breast cancer in genome-wide association studies are modifiers of breast cancer risk in BRCA1 and BRCA2 mutation carriers. Hum Mol Genet 19:2886–2897
88. Toyota CG, Davis MD, Cosman AM, Hebert MD (2010) Coilin phosphorylation mediates interaction with SMN and SmB′. Chromosoma 119:205–215
89. Velma V, Carrero ZI, Cosman AM, Hebert MD (2010) Coilin interacts with Ku proteins and inhibits in vitro non-homologous DNA end joining. FEBS Lett 584:4735–4759
90. Yi Y, Nandana S, Case T, Nelson C, Radmilovic T, Matusik RJ, Tsuchiya KD (2009) Candidate metastasis suppressor genes uncovered by array comparative genomic hybridization in a mouse allograft model of prostate cancer. Mol Cytogenet 2:18
91. Rapkins RW, Hore T, Smithwick M, Ager E, Pask AJ, Renfree MB, Kohn M, Hameister H, Nicholls RD, Deakin JE, Graves JA (2006) Recent assembly of an imprinted domain from non-imprinted components. PLoS Genet 2:e182
92. Deshmukh US, Kannapell CC, Fu SM (2002) Immune responses to small nuclear ribonucleoproteins: antigen-dependent distinct B cell epitope spreading patterns in mice immunized with recombinant polypeptides of small nuclear ribonucleoproteins. J Immunol 168(10):5326–5332
93. Patnaik MM, Lasho TL, Hodnefield JM, Knudson RA, Ketterling RP, Garcia-Manero G, Steensma DP, Pardanani A, Hanson CA, Tefferi A (2012) SF3B1 mutations are prevalent in myelodysplastic syndromes with ring sideroblasts but do not hold independent prognostic value. Blood 119:569–572
94. Yoshida K, Sanada M, Shiraishi Y, Nowak D, Nagata Y, Yamamoto R, Sato Y, Sato-Otsubo A, Kon A, Nagasaki M, Chalkidis G, Suzuki Y, Shiosaka M, Kawahata R, Yamaguchi T, Otsu M, Obara N, Sakata-Yanagimoto M, Ishiyama K, Mori H, Nolte F, Hofmann WK, Miyawaki S, Sugano S, Haferlach C, Koeffler HP, Shih LY, Haferlach T, Chiba S, Nakauchi H, Miyano S, Ogawa S (2011) Frequent pathway mutations of splicing machinery in myelodysplasia. Nature 478:64–69
95. Quesada V, Conde L, Villamor N, Ordóñez GR, Jares P, Bassaganyas L, Ramsay AJ, Beà S, Pinyol M, Martínez-Trillos A, López-Guerra M, Colomer D, Navarro A, Baumann T,

Aymerich M, Rozman M, Delgado J, Giné E, Hernández JM, González-Díaz M, Puente DA, Velasco G, Freije JM, Tubío JM, Royo R, Gelpí JL, Orozco M, Pisano DG, Zamora J, Vázquez M, Valencia A, Himmelbauer H, Bayés M, Heath S, Gut M, Gut I, Estivill X, López-Guillermo A, Puente XS, Campo E, López-Otín C (2011) Exome sequencing identifies recurrent mutations of the splicing factor SF3B1 gene in chronic lymphocytic leukemia. Nat Genet 44:47–52
96. Wang L, Lawrence MS, Wan Y, Stojanov P, Sougnez C, Stevenson K, Werner L, Sivachenko A, DeLuca DS, Zhang L, Zhang W, Vartanov AR, Fernandes SM, Goldstein NR, Folco EG, Cibulskis K, Tesar B, Sievers QL, Shefler E, Gabriel S, Hacohen N, Reed R, Meyerson M, Golub TR, Lander ES, Neuberg D, Brown JR, Getz G, Wu CJ (2011) SF3B1 and other novel cancer genes in chronic lymphocytic leukemia. N Engl J Med 365:2497–2506
97. Rossi D, Bruscaggin A, Spina V, Rasi S, Khiabanian H, Messina M, Fangazio M, Vaisitti T, Monti S, Chiaretti S, Guarini A, Del Giudice I, Cerri M, Cresta S, Deambrogi C, Gargiulo E, Gattei V, Forconi F, Bertoni F, Deaglio S, Rabadan R, Pasqualucci L, Foà R, Dalla-Favera R, Gaidano G (2011) Mutations of the SF3B1 splicing factor in chronic lymphocytic leukemia: association with progression and fludarabine-refractoriness. Blood 118:6904–6908
98. Bermingham JR Jr, Arden KC, Naumova AK, Sapienza C, Viars CS, Fu XD, Khotz J, Manley JL, Rosenfeld MG (1996) Chromosomal localization of mouse and human genes encoding the splicing factors ASF/SF2 (SFRS1) and SC-35 (SFRS2). Genomics 29:70–79
99. Fu XD, Maniatis T (1992) Isolation of a complementary DNA that encodes the mammalian splicing factor SC35. Science 256:535–538
100. Bogolyubova IO (2011) Transcriptional activity of nuclei in 2-cell blocked mouse embryos. Tissue Cell 43:262–265
101. Clayton JC, Phelan M, Goult BT, Hautbergue GM, Wilson SA, Lian LY (2011) The 1H, 13C and 15N backbone and side-chain assignment of the RRM domain of SC35, a regulator of pre-mRNA splicing. Biomol NMR Assign 5:7–10
102. Xiao R, Sun Y, Ding JH, Lin S, Rose DW, Rosenfeld MG, Fu XD, Li X (2007) Splicing regulator SC35 is essential for genomic stability and cell proliferation during mammalian organogenesis. Mol Cell Biol 27:5393–5402
103. Lin S, Coutinho-Mansfield G, Wang D, Pandit S, Fu XD (2008) The splicing factor SC35 has an active role in transcriptional elongation. Nat Struct Mol Biol 15:819–826
104. Yang L, Li N, Wang C, Yu Y, Yuan L, Zhang M, Cao X (2004) Cyclin L2, a novel RNA polymerase II-associated cyclin, is involved in pre-mRNA splicing and induces apoptosis of human hepatocellular carcinoma cells. J Biol Chem 279:11639–11648
105. van Abel D, Hölzel DR, Jain S, Lun FM, Zheng YW, Chen EZ, Sun H, Chiu RW, Lo YM, van Dijk M, Oudejans CB (2011) SFRS7-mediated splicing of tau exon 10 is directly regulated by STOX1A in glial cells. PLoS One 6:e21994
106. Escudero-Paunetto L, Li L, Hernandez FP, Sandri-Goldin RM (2010) SR proteins SRp20 and 9G8 contribute to efficient export of herpes simplex virus 1 mRNAs. Virology 401:155–164
107. Valente ST, Gilmartin GM, Venkatarama K, Arriagada G, Goff SP (2009) HIV-1 mRNA 3′ end processing is distinctively regulated by eIF3f, CDK11, and splice factor 9G8. Mol Cell 36:279–289
108. Swartz JE, Bor YC, Misawa Y, Rekosh D, Hammarskjold ML (2007) The shuttling SR protein 9G8 plays a role in translation of unspliced mRNA containing a constitutive transport element. J Biol Chem 282:19844–19853
109. Brasch-Andersen C, Tan Q, Børglum AD, Haagerup A, Larsen TR, Vestbo J, Kruse TA (2006) Significant linkage to chromosome 12q24.32-q24.33 and identification of SFRS8 as a possible asthma susceptibility gene. Thorax 61:874–879
110. Sampson ND, Hewitt JE (2003) SF4 and SFRS14, two related putative splicing factors on human chromosome 19p13.11. Gene 305:91–100
111. Entrez gene: SFRS14 splicing factor, arginine/serine-rich 14. http://www.ncbi.nlm.nih.gov/sites/entrez?Db=gene&Cmd=ShowDetailView&TermToSearch=10147

112. Katsu R, Onogi H, Wada K, Kawaguchi Y, Hagiwara M (2002) Novel SR-rich-related protein clasp specifically interacts with inactivated Clk4 and induces the exon EB inclusion of Clk. J Biol Chem 277:44220–44228
113. Entrez gene: SFRS16 splicing factor, arginine/serine-rich 16. http://www.ncbi.nlm.nih.gov/sites/entrez?Db=gene&Cmd=ShowDetailView&TermToSearch=11129
114. Nagase T, Ishikawa K, Miyajima N, Tanaka A, Kotani H, Nomura N, Ohara O (1998) Prediction of the coding sequences of unidentified human genes. IX. The complete sequences of 100 new cDNA clones from brain which can code for large proteins in vitro. DNA Res 5:31–39
115. Kojima T, Zama T, Wada K, Onogi H, Hagiwara M (2001) Cloning of human PRP4 reveals interaction with Clk1. J Biol Chem 276:32247–32256
116. Huang Y, Deng T, Winston BW (2000) Characterization of hPRP4 kinase activation: potential role in signaling. Biochem Biophys Res Commun 271:456–463
117. Entrez gene: PRPF4B PRP4 pre-mRNA processing factor 4 homolog B (yeast). http://www.ncbi.nlm.nih.gov/sites/entrez?Db=gene&Cmd=ShowDetailView&TermToSearch=8899
118. Dellaire G, Makarov EM, Cowger JJ, Longman D, Sutherland HG, Lührmann R, Torchia J, Bickmore WA (2002) Mammalian PRP4 kinase copurifies and interacts with components of both the U5 snRNP and the N-CoR deacetylase complexes. Mol Cell Biol 22:5141–5156
119. Tonevitsky EA, Trushkin EV, Shkurnikov MU, Akimov EB, Sakharov DA (2009) Changed profile of splicing regulator genes expression in response to exercise. Bull Exp Biol Med 147:733–736
120. Huang B, Ahn YT, McPherson L, Clayberger C, Krensky AM (2007) Interaction of PRP4 with Kruppel-like factor 13 regulates CCL5 transcription. J Immunol 178:7081–7087
121. Bennett EM, Lever AM, Allen JF (2004) Human immunodeficiency virus type 2 Gag interacts specifically with PRP4, a serine-threonine kinase, and inhibits phosphorylation of splicing factor SF2. J Virol 78:11303–11312
122. Hurschler BA, Harris DT, Grosshans H (2011) The type II poly(A)-binding protein PABP-2 genetically interacts with the let-7 miRNA and elicits heterochronic phenotypes in Caenorhabditis elegans. Nucleic Acids Res 39:5647–5657
123. Lemay JF, D'Amours A, Lemieux C, Lackner DH, St-Sauveur VG, Bähler J, Bachand F (2010) The nuclear poly(A)-binding protein interacts with the exosome to promote synthesis of noncoding small nucleolar RNAs. Mol Cell 37:34–45
124. Kühn U, Gündel M, Knoth A, Kerwitz Y, Rüdel S, Wahle E (2009) Poly(A) tail length is controlled by the nuclear poly(A)-binding protein regulating the interaction between poly(A) polymerase and the cleavage and polyadenylation specificity factor. J Biol Chem 284:22803–22814
125. Lemay JF, Lemieux C, St-André O, Bachand F (2010) Crossing the borders: poly(A)-binding proteins working on both sides of the fence. RNA Biol 7:291–295
126. Raz V, Abraham T, van Zwet EW, Dirks RW, Tanke HJ, van der Maarel SM (2011) Reversible aggregation of PABPN1 pre-inclusion structures. Nucleus 2:208–218
127. Raz V, Routledge S, Venema A, Buijze H, van der Wal E, Anvar S, Straasheijm KR, Klooster R, Antoniou M, van der Maarel SM (2011) Modeling oculopharyngeal muscular dystrophy in myotube cultures reveals reduced accumulation of soluble mutant PABPN1 protein. Am J Pathol 179:1988–2000
128. Davies JE, Rubinsztein DC (2011) Over-expression of BCL2 rescues muscle weakness in a mouse model of oculopharyngeal muscular dystrophy. Hum Mol Genet 20:1154–1163
129. Pasco MY, Rotili D, Altucci L, Farina F, Rouleau GA, Mai A, Neri C (2010) Characterization of sirtuin inhibitors in nematodes expressing a muscular dystrophy protein reveals muscle cell and behavioral protection by specific sirtinol analogues. J Med Chem 53:1407–1411
130. Takagaki Y, Manley JL (1994) A polyadenylation factor subunit is the human homologue of the Drosophila suppressor of forked protein. Nature 372:471–474
131. Entrez gene: CSTF3 cleavage stimulation factor, 3′ pre-RNA, subunit 3, 77kDa. http://www.ncbi.nlm.nih.gov/sites/entrez?Db=gene&Cmd=ShowDetailView&TermToSearch=1479

132. Takagaki Y, Manley JL (2000) Complex protein interactions within the human polyadenylation machinery identify a novel component. Mol Cell Biol 20:1515–1525
133. Park JS, Young Yoon S, Kim JM, Yeom YI, Kim YS, Kim NS (2004) Identification of novel genes associated with the response to 5-FU treatment in gastric cancer cell lines using a cDNA microarray. Cancer Lett 214:19–33
134. Yoon DW, Lee H, Seol W, DeMaria M, Rosenzweig M, Jung JU (1997) Tap: a novel cellular protein that interacts with tip of herpesvirus saimiri and induces lymphocyte aggregation. Immunity 6:571–582
135. Gruter P, Tabernero C, von Kobbe C, Schmitt C, Saavedra C, Bachi A, Wilm M, Felber BK, Izaurralde E (1998) TAP, the human homolog of Mex67p, mediates CTE-dependent RNA export from the nucleus. Mol Cell 1:649–659
136. Atsapkina AA, Golubkova EV, Kasatkina VV, Avanesian EO, Ivankova NA, Mamon LA (2010) Spermatogenesis in Drosophila melanogaster: the role of the basic transport receptor of the mRNA (Dm NXF1). Tsitologiia 52:574–579
137. Katahira J, Strässer K, Podtelejnikov A, Mann M, Jung JU, Hurt E (1999) The Mex67p-mediated nuclear mRNA export pathway is conserved from yeast to human. EMBO J 18:2593–2609
138. Teplova M, Wohlbold L, Khin NW, Izaurralde E, Patel DJ (2011) Structure-function studies of nucleocytoplasmic transport of retroviral genomic RNA by mRNA export factor TAP. Nat Struct Mol Biol 18:990–998
139. Coyle JH, Bor YC, Rekosh D, Hammarskjold ML (2011) The Tpr protein regulates export of mRNAs with retained introns that traffic through the Nxf1 pathway. RNA 17:1344–1356
140. Hernandez FP, Sandri-Goldin RM (2010) Head-to-tail intramolecular interaction of herpes simplex virus type 1 regulatory protein ICP27 is important for its interaction with cellular mRNA export receptor TAP/NXF1. MBio 1(5):e00268–10
141. Floyd JA, Gold DA, Concepcion D, Poon TH, Wang X, Keithley E, Chen D, Ward EJ, Chinn SB, Friedman RA, Yu HT, Moriwaki K, Shiroishi T, Hamilton BA (2003) A natural allele of Nxf1 suppresses retrovirus insertional mutations. Nat Genet 35:221–228
142. Markovtsov V, Nikolic JM, Goldman JA, Turck CW, Chou MY, Black DL (2000) Cooperative assembly of an hnRNP complex induced by a tissue-specific homolog of polypyrimidine tract binding protein. Mol Cell Biol 20:7463–7479
143. Entrez gene: PTBP2 polypyrimidine tract binding protein 2. http://www.ncbi.nlm.nih.gov/sites/entrez?Db=gene&Cmd=ShowDetailView&TermToSearch=58155
144. Tang ZZ, Sharma S, Zheng S, Chawla G, Nikolic J, Black DL (2011) Regulation of the mutually exclusive exons 8a and 8 in the CaV1.2 calcium channel transcript by polypyrimidine tract-binding protein. J Biol Chem 286:10007–10016
145. Nowak U, Matthews AJ, Zheng S, Chaudhuri J (2011) The splicing regulator PTBP2 interacts with the cytidine deaminase AID and promotes binding of AID to switch-region DNA. Nat Immunol 12:160–166
146. Bitel CL, Perrone-Bizzozero NI, Frederikse PH (2010) HuB/C/D, nPTB, REST4, and miR-124 regulators of neuronal cell identity are also utilized in the lens. Mol Vis 16:2301–2316
147. Boutz PL, Stoilov P, Li Q, Lin CH, Chawla G, Ostrow K, Shiue L, Ares M Jr, Black DL (2007) A post-transcriptional regulatory switch in polypyrimidine tract-binding proteins reprograms alternative splicing in developing neurons. Genes Dev 21:1636–1652
148. Lu X, Timchenko NA, Timchenko LT (1999) Cardiac elav-type RNA-binding protein (ETR-3) binds to RNA CUG repeats expanded in myotonic dystrophy. Hum Mol Genet 8:53–60
149. Entrez gene: CUGBP2 CUG triplet repeat, RNA binding protein 2. http://www.ncbi.nlm.nih.gov/sites/entrez?Db=gene&Cmd=ShowDetailView&TermToSearch=10659
150. Anant S, Henderson JO, Mukhopadhyay D, Navaratnam N, Kennedy S, Min J, Davidson NO (2001) Novel role for RNA-binding protein CUGBP2 in mammalian RNA editing. CUGBP2 modulates C to U editing of apolipoprotein B mRNA by interacting with apobec-1 and ACF, the apobec-1 complementation factor. J Biol Chem 276:47338–47351
151. Dembowski JA, Grabowski PJ (2009) The CUGBP2 splicing factor regulates an ensemble of branchpoints from perimeter binding sites with implications for autoregulation. PLoS Genet 5:e1000595

152. Subramaniam D, Natarajan G, Ramalingam S, Ramachandran I, May R, Queimado L, Houchen CW, Anant S (2008) Translation inhibition during cell cycle arrest and apoptosis: Mcl-1 is a novel target for RNA binding protein CUGBP2. Am J Physiol Gastrointest Liver Physiol 294:G1025–G1032
153. Ramalingam S, Natarajan G, Schafer C, Subramaniam D, May R, Ramachandran I, Queimado L, Houchen CW, Anant S (2008) Novel intestinal splice variants of RNA-binding protein CUGBP2: isoform-specific effects on mitotic catastrophe. Am J Physiol Gastrointest Liver Physiol 294:G971–G9781
154. Fuller-Pace FV, Moore HC (2011) RNA helicases p68 and p72: multifunctional proteins with important implications for cancer development. Future Oncol 7:239–251
155. Mooney SM, Grande JP, Salisbury JL, Janknecht R (2010) Sumoylation of p68 and p72 RNA helicases affects protein stability and transactivation potential. Biochemistry 49(1):1–10
156. Janknecht R (2010) Multi-talented DEAD-box proteins and potential tumor promoters: p68 RNA helicase (DDX5) and its paralog, p72 RNA helicase (DDX17). Am J Transl Res 2:223–234
157. Dutertre M, Gratadou L, Dardenne E, Germann S, Samaan S, Lidereau R, Driouch K, de la Grange P, Auboeuf D (2010) Estrogen regulation and physiopathologic significance of alternative promoters in breast cancer. Cancer Res 70:3760–3770
158. Fuller-Pace FV, Ali S (2008) The DEAD box RNA helicases p68 (Ddx5) and p72 (Ddx17): novel transcriptional co-regulators. Biochem Soc Trans 36:609–612
159. Mooney SM, Goel A, D'Assoro AB, Salisbury JL, Janknecht R (2010) Pleiotropic effects of p300-mediated acetylation on p68 and p72 RNA helicase. J Biol Chem 285:30443–30452
160. Paul S, Dansithong W, Jog SP, Holt I, Mittal S, Brook JD, Morris GE, Comai L, Reddy S (2011) Expanded CUG repeats dysregulate RNA splicing by altering the stoichiometry of the muscleblind 1 complex. J Biol Chem 286:38427–38438
161. Gao G, Xie A, Huang SC, Zhou A, Zhang J, Herman AM, Ghassemzadeh S, Jeong EM, Kasturirangan S, Raicu M, Sobieski MA II, Bhat G, Tatooles A, Benz EJ Jr, Kamp TJ, Dudley SC Jr (2011) Role of RBM25/LUC7L3 in abnormal cardiac sodium channel splicing regulation in human heart failure. Circulation 124:1124–1131
162. Alpatov R, Munguba GC, Caton P, Joo JH, Shi Y, Shi Y, Hunt ME, Sugrue SP (2004) Nuclear speckle-associated protein Pnn/DRS binds to the transcriptional corepressor CtBP and relieves CtBP-mediated repression of the E-cadherin gene. Mol Cell Biol 24:10223–10235
163. Jeronimo C, Forget D, Bouchard A, Li Q, Chua G, Poitras C, Thérien C, Bergeron D, Bourassa S, Greenblatt J, Chabot B, Poirier GG, Hughes TR, Blanchette M, Price DH, Coulombe B (2007) Systematic analysis of the protein interaction network for the human transcription machinery reveals the identity of the 7SK capping enzyme. Mol Cell 27:262–274
164. Alpatov R, Shi Y, Munguba GC, Moghimi B, Joo JH, Bungert J, Sugrue SP (2008) Corepressor CtBP and nuclear speckle protein Pnn/DRS differentially modulate transcription and splicing of the E-cadherin gene. Mol Cell Biol 28:1584–1595
165. Joo JH, Taxter TJ, Munguba GC, Kim YH, Dhaduvai K, Dunn NW, Degan WJ, Oh SP, Sugrue SP (2010) Pinin modulates expression of an intestinal homeobox gene, Cdx2, and plays an essential role for small intestinal morphogenesis. Dev Biol 345:191–203
166. Hsu SY, Chen YJ, Ouyang P (2011) Pnn and SR family proteins are differentially expressed in mouse central nervous system. Histochem Cell Biol 135:361–373
167. Chiu Y, Ouyang P (2006) Loss of Pnn expression attenuates expression levels of SR family splicing factors and modulates alternative pre-mRNA splicing in vivo. Biochem Biophys Res Commun 341:663–671
168. Leu S, Ouyang P (2006) Spatial and temporal expression profile of pinin during mouse development. Gene Expr Patterns 6:620–631
169. Gonzalez-Santos JM, Wang A, Jones J, Ushida C, Liu J, Hu J (2002) Central region of the human splicing factor Hprp3p interacts with Hprp4p. J Biol Chem 277:23764–23772
170. Heng HH, Wang A, Hu J (1998) Mapping of the human HPRP3 and HPRP4 genes encoding U4/U6-associated splicing factors to chromosomes 1q21.1 and 9q31-q33. Genomics 48:273–275

171. Ayadi L, Callebaut I, Saguez C, Villa T, Mornon JP, Banroques J (1998) Functional and structural characterization of the prp3 binding domain of the yeast prp4 splicing factor. J Mol Biol 284:673–687
172. Lauber J, Plessel G, Prehn S, Will CL, Fabrizio P, Gröning K, Lane WS, Lührmann R (1997) The human U4/U6 snRNP contains 60 and 90kD proteins that are structurally homologous to the yeast splicing factors Prp4p and Prp3p. RNA 3:926–941
173. Linder B, Dill H, Hirmer A, Brocher J, Lee GP, Mathavan S, Bolz HJ, Winkler C, Laggerbauer B, Fischer U (2011) Systemic splicing factor deficiency causes tissue-specific defects: a zebrafish model for retinitis pigmentosa. Hum Mol Genet 20:368–377
174. Schmidt-Kastner R, Yamamoto H, Hamasaki D, Yamamoto H, Parel JM, Schmitz C, Dorey CK, Blanks JC, Preising MN (2008) Hypoxia-regulated components of the U4/U6.U5 tri-small nuclear riboprotein complex: possible role in autosomal dominant retinitis pigmentosa. Mol Vis 14:125–135
175. Zhou A, Ou AC, Cho A, Benz EJ Jr, Huang SC (2008) Novel splicing factor RBM25 modulates Bcl-x pre-mRNA 5′ splice site selection. Mol Cell Biol 28:5924–5936
176. Kanhoush R, Beenders B, Perrin C, Moreau J, Bellini M, Penrad-Mobayed M (2010) Novel domains in the hnRNP G/RBMX protein with distinct roles in RNA binding and targeting nascent transcripts. Nucleus 1:109–122
177. Kanhoush R, Praseuth D, Perrin C, Chardard D, Vinh J, Penrad-Mobayed M (2011) Differential RNA-binding activity of the hnRNP G protein correlated with the sex genotype in the amphibian oocyte. Nucleic Acids Res 39:4109–4121
178. Adamik B, Islam A, Rouhani FN, Hawari FI, Zhang J, Levine SJ (2008) An association between RBMX, a heterogeneous nuclear ribonucleoprotein, and ARTS-1 regulates extracellular TNFR1 release. Biochem Biophys Res Commun 371:505–509
179. Elliott DJ (2004) The role of potential splicing factors including RBMY, RBMX, hnRNPG-T and STAR proteins in spermatogenesis. Int J Androl 27:328–334
180. Sumanasekera C, Kelemen O, Beullens M, Aubol BE, Adams JA, Sunkara M, Morris A, Bollen M, Andreadis A, Stamm S (2012) C6 pyridinium ceramide influences alternative pre-mRNA splicing by inhibiting protein phosphatase-1. Nucleic Acids Res 40:4025–4039
181. Landeras-Bueno S, Jorba N, Pérez-Cidoncha M, Ortín J (2011) The splicing factor proline-glutamine rich (SFPQ/PSF) is involved in influenza virus transcription. PLoS Pathog 7:e1002397
182. Kunde SA, Musante L, Grimme A, Fischer U, Müller E, Wanker EE, Kalscheuer VM (2011) The X-chromosome-linked intellectual disability protein PQBP1 is a component of neuronal RNA granules and regulates the appearance of stress granules. Hum Mol Genet 20:4916–4931
183. Cristobo I, Larriba MJ, Ríos Vde L, García F, Muñoz A, Casal JI (2011) Proteomic analysis of 1α,25-dihydroxyvitamin D(3) action on human colon cancer cells reveals a link to splicing regulation. J Proteomics 75:384–397
184. Ha K, Takeda Y, Dynan WS (2011) Sequences in PSF/SFPQ mediate radioresistance and recruitment of PSF/SFPQ-containing complexes to DNA damage sites in human cells. DNA Repair 10(3):252–259
185. Rajesh C, Baker DK, Pierce AJ, Pittman DL (2011) The splicing-factor related protein SFPQ/PSF interacts with RAD51D and is necessary for homology-directed repair and sister chromatid cohesion. Nucleic Acids Res 3:132–145
186. Salton M, Lerenthal Y, Wang SY, Chen DJ, Shiloh Y (2010) Involvement of Matrin 3 and SFPQ/NONO in the DNA damage response. Cell Cycle 9:1568–1576
187. Herrmann A, Fleischer K, Czajkowska H, Müller-Newen G, Becker W (2007) Characterization of cyclin L1 as an immobile component of the splicing factor compartment. FASEB J 21:3142–3152
188. de Graaf K, Hekerman P, Spelten O, Herrmann A, Packman LC, Büssow K, Müller-Newen G, Becker W (2004) Characterization of cyclin L2, a novel cyclin with an arginine/serine-rich domain: phosphorylation by DYRK1A and colocalization with splicing factors. J Biol Chem 279:4612–4624

189. Bond CS, Fox AH (2009) Paraspeckles: nuclear bodies built on long noncoding RNA. J Cell Biol 186:637–644
190. Loyer P, Trembley JH, Grenet JA, Busson A, Corlu A, Zhao W, Kocak M, Kidd VJ, Lahti JM (2008) Characterization of cyclin L1 and L2 interactions with CDK11 and splicing factors: influence of cyclin L isoforms on splice site selection. J Biol Chem 283:7721–7732
191. Li HL, Wang TS, Li XY, Li N, Huang DZ, Chen Q, Ba Y (2007) Overexpression of cyclin L2 induces apoptosis and cell-cycle arrest in human lung cancer cells. Chin Med J (Engl) 120:905–909
192. Zhuo L, Gong J, Yang R, Sheng Y, Zhou L, Kong X, Cao K (2009) Inhibition of proliferation and differentiation and promotion of apoptosis by cyclin L2 in mouse embryonic carcinoma P19 cells. Biochem Biophys Res Commun 390:451–457
193. Peng L, Yanjiao M, Ai-guo W, Pengtao G, Jianhua L, Ju Y, Hongsheng O, Xichen Z (2011) A fine balance between CCNL1 and TIMP1 contributes to the development of breast cancer cells. Biochem Biophys Res Commun 409:344–349
194. Tannukit S, Wen X, Wang H, Paine ML (2008) TFIP11, CCNL1 and EWSR1 protein-protein interactions, and their nuclear localization. Int J Mol Sci 9:1504–1514
195. Muller D, Millon R, Théobald S, Hussenet T, Wasylyk B, du Manoir S, Abecassis J (2006) Cyclin L1 (CCNL1) gene alterations in human head and neck squamous cell carcinoma. Br J Cancer 94:1041–1044
196. Chen HH, Wang YC, Fann MJ (2006) Identification and characterization of the CDK12/cyclin L1 complex involved in alternative splicing regulation. Mol Cell Biol 26:2736–2745
197. Redon R, Hussenet T, Bour G, Caulee K, Jost B, Muller D, Abecassis J, du Manoir S (2002) Amplicon mapping and transcriptional analysis pinpoint cyclin L as a candidate oncogene in head and neck cancer. Cancer Res 62:6211–6217
198. Russo J, Tay LK, Russo IH (1982) Differentiation of the mammary gland and susceptibility to carcinogenesis. Breast Cancer Res Treat 2:5–73
199. Russo J, Balogh GA, Chen J, Fernandez SV, Fernbaugh R, Heulings R, Mailo DA, Moral R, Russo PA, Sheriff F, Vanegas JE, Wang R, Russo IH (2006) The concept of stem cell in the mammary gland and its implication in morphogenesis, cancer and prevention. Front Biosci 11:151–172
200. Russo J, Tait L, Russo IH (1983) Susceptibility of the mammary gland to carcinogenesis. III. The cell of origin of rat mammary carcinoma. Am J Pathol 113:50–66
201. Russo IH, Russo J (1978) Developmental stage of the rat mammary gland as determinant of its susceptibility to 7,12-dimethylbenz[a]anthracene. J Natl Cancer Inst 61:1439–1449
202. Russo IH, Koszalka M, Russo J (1991) Comparative study of the influence of pregnancy and hormonal treatment on mammary carcinogenesis. Br J Cancer 64:481–484
203. Russo J, Russo IH (1998) Differentiation and breast cancer development. In: Heppner G (ed) Advances in oncobiology. JAI Press, Greenwich, CN, pp 1–10
204. Russo J, Russo IH (1997) Toward a unified concept of mammary carcinogenesis. Prog Clin Biol Res 396:1–16
205. Russo J, Ao X, Grill C, Russo IH (1999) Pattern of distribution of cells positive for estrogen receptor alpha and progesterone receptor in relation to proliferating cells in the mammary gland. Breast Cancer Res Treat 53:217–227
206. Russo J, Mailo D, Hu YF, Balogh G, Sheriff F, Russo IH (2005) Breast differentiation and its implication in cancer prevention. Clin Cancer Res 11:931s–936s
207. Salomonis N, Schlieve CR, Pereira L, Wahlquist C, Colas A, Zambon AC, Vranizan K, Spindler MJ, Pico AR, Cline MS, Clark TA, Williams A, Blume JE, Samal E, Mercola M, Merrill BJ, Conklin BR (2010) Alternative splicing regulates mouse embryonic stem cell pluripotency and differentiation. Proc Natl Acad Sci U S A 107:10514–10519
208. Salomonis N, Nelson B, Vranizan K, Pico AR, Hanspers K, Kuchinsky A, Ta L, Mercola M, Conklin BR (2009) Alternative splicing in the differentiation of human embryonic stem cells into cardiac precursors. PLoS Comput Biol 5:e1000553
209. Brooks YS, Wang G, Yang Z, Smith KK, Bieberich E, Ko L (2009) Functional pre-mRNA trans-splicing of coactivator CoAA and corepressor RBM4 during stem/progenitor cell differentiation. J Biol Chem 284:18033–18046

210. Yeo GW, Coufal NG, Liang TY, Peng GE, Fu XD, Gage FH (2009) An RNA code for the FOX2 splicing regulator revealed by mapping RNA-protein interactions in stem cells. Nat Struct Mol Biol 16:130–137
211. Bunaciu RP, Tang T, Mao CD (2008) Differential expression of Wnt13 isoforms during leukemic cell differentiation. Oncol Rep 20:195–201
212. Robinett CC, Vaughan AG, Knapp JM, Baker BS (2010) Sex and the single cell. II. There is a time and place for sex. PLoS Biol 8:e1000365
213. Alam AH, Suzuki H, Tsukahara T (2010) Retinoic acid treatment and cell aggregation independently regulate alternative splicing in P19 cells during neural differentiation. Cell Biol Int 34:631–643
214. Moors M, Vudattu NK, Abel J, Krämer U, Rane L, Ulfig N, Ceccatelli S, Seyfert-Margolies V, Fritsche E, Maeurer MJ (2010) Interleukin-7 (IL-7) and IL-7 splice variants affect differentiation of human neural progenitor cells. Genes Immun 11:11–20
215. Piprek RP (2009) Genetic mechanisms underlying male sex determination in mammals. J Appl Genet 50:347–360
216. Clower CV, Chatterjee D, Wang Z, Cantley LC, Vander Heiden MG, Krainer AR (2010) The alternative splicing repressors hnRNP A1/A2 and PTB influence pyruvate kinase isoform expression and cell metabolism. Proc Natl Acad Sci U S A 107:1894–1899
217. Gillett A, Maratou K, Fewings C, Harris RA, Jagodic M, Aitman T, Olsson T (2009) Alternative splicing and transcriptome profiling of experimental autoimmune encephalomyelitis using genome-wide exon arrays. PLoS One 4:e7773
218. Kobayashi E, Shimizu R, Kikuchi Y, Takahashi S, Yamamoto M (2010) Loss of the Gata1 gene IE exon leads to variant transcript expression and the production of a GATA1 protein lacking the N-terminal domain. J Biol Chem 285:773–783
219. Peri P, López de Cicco R, Santucci-Pereira J, Slifker M, Ross EA, Russo IH, Russo PA, Arslan AA, Belitskaya-Lévy I, Zeleniuch-Jacquotte A, Bordas P, Lenner P, Åhman J, Afanasyeva Y, Johansson R, Sheriff F, Hallmans G, Toniolo P, Russo J (2012) Defining the genomic signature of the parous breast. BMC Med Genomic

Chapter 9
Noncoding RNAs and Breast Cancer Prevention

9.1 Introduction

The development of the breast is a lifelong process of organogenesis that starts as an appendage of the skin in the 5-week-old embryo [1]; however, the commitment of the organ to develop as a female breast becomes established at the time of fertilization of the oocyte through the inheritance of a paternal X chromosome [2–4]. Subsequent cell divisions will generate 2-, 4-, and 8-cells, which will progress to the morula stage (human pre-embryo) and the blastocyst, within which the inner cell mass (ICM) cells continue to proliferate and constitute the ultimate totipotent cells from which the embryonic stem (ES) cells are harvested [2–4]. The ICM cells represent the ultimate undifferentiated cell type, as it gives rise to all cell types and live offspring [5]. Totipotency persists for the very first cell doublings, from the single cell and zygote to at least the 4-cell pre-embryo. Initiation of transcription in the newly formed embryonic genome reportedly occurs at the 4- and 8-cell stage, followed by decreases in abundance of individual mRNAs [6]. The XX female needs to equalize their gene dosage relative to XY males by inactivating one of their X chromosomes. An inactive chromosome X (Xi) becomes present in each cell through the X chromosome inactivation center (XCI) that contains several genetic elements essential for the transcription initiation of long noncoding RNAs (lncRNAs) [7]. Initiation of XCI requires the *cis* accumulation of a nontranslated human X inactive-specific transcript (XIST) RNA that coats the X chromosome and is followed by various epigenetic changes on the future Xi that contribute to chromosome silencing [8], which is detected as early as the 4-cell stage of mouse embryos. Defects in dosage compensation prior to implantation lead to abnormal development in a majority of the embryos and early lethality. Thus, the presence and function of an lncRNA determines the lifetime ability of the breast to develop normal growth and differentiation, which require a synchronized sequence of cellular processes that involve commitment to specific cell types and its ultimate function, milk production [9–13]. Any derangements affecting the integrated framework of signaling networks that control breast development

J. Russo and I.H. Russo, *Role of the Transcriptome in Breast Cancer Prevention*,
DOI 10.1007/978-1-4614-4884-6_9, © Springer Science+Business Media New York 2013

during puberty, pregnancy, lactation, or post lactation involution, such as inheritance [14] or exposure to genetic and environmental factors that cause accumulation of germline [3, 4, 14] or epigenetic [15, 16] mutations might lead to the neoplastic transformation of mammary tissues [17, 18]. Loss of Xi has been reported in both BRCA1 defective and in wild breast cancer cells [19]. XIST is the key player of the X chromosome silencing; the inactive X (Xi) acquires typical features of heterochromatin, such as late replication, hypoacetylation of histones H3 and H4, methylation of histone H3 at lysines 9 and 27, lack of methylation of H3 at lysine 4, and methylation of DNA CpG islands, epigenetic modifications that appear to act synergistically and stably maintain the inactive state through subsequent cell divisions [20]. Studies of human embryonic stem cells (hESCs) have demonstrated that lncRNAs are important regulators of pluripotency and neurogenesis, playing an important role in human brain development [21]. Similarly, the role played by lncRNAs, and more specifically XIST, in normal development and differentiation of the breast has been confirmed by our studies of the genomic and epigenetic characteristics of the differentiated breast of early parous women that had reached menopause free of breast cancer [22]. The reduction in breast cancer risk conferred by the first pregnancy has been attributed to the induction of complete differentiation of the virginal breast, which in nulliparous women remains undifferentiated and susceptible to carcinogenic insults [9, 10, 22]. Genome-wide studies comparing the gene expression profiles of breast biopsy specimens of these two populations revealed that the differentiated breast of parous women expressed upregulation of the lncRNA *XIST*. In addition, the nucleus of epithelial cells had condensed chromatin and increased reactivity with anti-H3K9me^2 and H3K27me^3 antibodies [11]. These observations led us to postulate that chromatin remodeling is the driving force of the observed differences between the parous and nulliparous breast that had been initiated by lncRNAs that are key players in developmental processes, maintaining pluripotency or differentiation during embryogenesis [2, 21] and maintain these roles during adult growth and differentiation [11, 22].

9.2 Nuclear Organelles and ncRNAs

The cell nucleus is a highly compartmentalized organelle harboring a variety of dynamic subnuclear bodies. Its interior is not uniform and the bodies that it contains are not membrane-bound [23]. The best-known of these existing subnuclear compartments is the nucleolus, which is mainly involved in the assembly of ribosomes for their exportation to the cytoplasm [24]. Besides the nucleolus, other subnuclear compartments are made up of unique proteins, RNA molecules, and particular parts of mitochondria. These include Cajal bodies or coiled bodies (CBs) [25], gems (dissociated Sm proteins of the survival of motor neurons [SMN] complex) [26]; PIKA (polymorphic interphase karyosomal association [27], PML (promyelocytic leukemia) bodies [28], paraspeckles, and splicing speckles [29, 30]. Increasing knowledge has accumulated since the 1900s on a number of these domains, findings that have confirmed that the nucleoplasm is not a uniform mixture, but rather an organized and compartmentalized functional structure [23–30]. Cajal bodies were discovered by Ramon y Cajal in silver stained neurons, and rediscovered by electron microscopists, who renamed them coiled bodies (CBs) [25]; CBs in fetal tissues are in proximity of gems, thus their twin appearance generated the name gemini to this duo [26]. However, the phenomenon is not observed in adult tissues in which the two structures appear fused [25]. A nucleus typically contains between 1 and 10 compact Cajal bodies that measure between 0.2 and 2.0 μm in diameter, depending upon the cell type and species [25]. When seen under an electron microscope, CBs resemble balls of tangled threads [23] and are dense foci of distribution for the protein coiling [24, 27, 29, 30]. CBs are involved in a number of different roles relating to RNA processing, specifically small nucleolar RNA (snoRNA) and small nuclear RNA (snRNA) maturation, and histone mRNA modification [30]. Gems are similar in size and shape to CBs, and in fact are virtually indistinguishable under the microscope [24]. Unlike CBs, gems do not contain small nuclear ribonucleoproteins (snRNPs), but do contain an SMN, whose function relates to snRNP biogenesis, therefore they are believed to assist CBs in snRNP biogenesis [27], though it has also been suggested from microscopic evidence that CBs and gems are different manifestations of the same structure.

The presence of speckles in the nucleus was first reported by Cajal as translucent clumps in 1910 and identified with the electron microscope as interchromatin particles by Swift in 1959, although the term "speckles" was first coined by Beck in 1961 [31, 32]. Speckles are subnuclear structures that are enriched in pre-messenger RNA splicing factors and are located in the interchromatin regions of the nucleoplasm of mammalian cells. Fluorescent microscopy shows them as irregular, punctuate structures that vary in size and shape, and the electron microscope confirms them as clusters of interchromatin granules. Speckles are dynamic structures, and both their protein and RNA-protein components can cycle continuously between speckles and other nuclear locations, including active transcription sites. Studies on the composition, structure, and behavior of speckles have provided a model for understanding the functional compartmentalization of the nucleus and the organization of the gene-expression machinery [33]. Sometimes referred to as interchromatin granule clusters or as splicing-factor compartments, speckles are rich in splicing snRNPs [31, 34] and other splicing proteins necessary for pre-mRNA processing [35]. Because of a cell's changing requirements, the composition and location of these bodies changes according to mRNA transcription and regulation via phosphorylation of specific proteins [36]. The compartmentalization allows the cell to prevent translation of unspliced mRNA [37]. Eukaryotic mRNA contains introns that must be removed before being translated to produce functional proteins. The splicing is done inside the nucleus before the mRNA can be accessed by ribosomes for translation. Without the nucleus, ribosomes would translate newly transcribed (unprocessed) mRNA, resulting in malformed and nonfunctional proteins. Paraspeckles, which were discovered by Fox et al. in 2002, are irregularly shaped compartments in the nucleus' interchromatic space [29]. First documented in HeLa cells, in which there are generally 10–30 per nucleus [31], paraspeckles are now known to also exist in all human primary cells, transformed cell lines, and tissue sections [33]. Their name is derived from their distribution in the nucleus; the "para" is short for parallel and the "speckles" refers to the splicing speckles to which they are always in close proximity [29, 31, 33, 34].

Nuclear speckles or their ultrastructural equivalent, the interchromatin granule clusters, are enriched in components of the pre-mRNA splicing machinery, particularly spliceosomal snRNP particles and other non-snRNP protein splicing factors such as SC35 and U2AF. They also contain several kinases, the PP1 phosphatase, 3′-end processing factors, some transcription factors involved in gene expression driven by the RNA polymerase II, and a population of poly(A) RNA and noncoding RNAs (ncRNAs). LncRNAs are in general considered as nonprotein coding transcripts longer than 200 nucleotides, distinguishing them from small regulatory RNAs such as microRNAs (miRNAs), short interfering RNAs (siRNAs), Piwi-interacting RNAs (piRNAs), snoRNAs, etc. The findings that only one-fifth of transcription across the human genome is associated with protein-coding genes [38, 39], whereas lncRNA sequences are fourfold more frequent indicate the need of performing large-scale complementary DNA (cDNA) sequencing projects such as FANTOM (Functional Annotation of Mammalian cDNA) for revealing the complexity of this transcription [40]. The FANTOM3 project identified ~35,000 noncoding transcripts from ~10,000 distinct loci that bear many signatures of mRNAs, including 5′ capping, splicing, and poly-adenylation, but have little or no open reading frame (ORF). Guttman et al. [41] sought to undertake systematic loss-of-function experiments on all large intergenic ncRNAs (lincRNAs) known to be expressed in mouse embryonic stem cells (ESCs). ESCs are pluripotent cells that can self-renew in culture and can give rise to cells of any of the three primary germ layers including the germline in which the signaling, transcriptional, and chromatin regulatory networks controlling pluripotency have been well characterized. The knockdown of the vast majority of ESC-expressed lincRNAs has a strong effect on gene expression patterns of comparable magnitude to that seen for the well-known ESC regulatory proteins. Loss-of-function has allowed identifying dozens of lincRNAs that exit from the pluripotent state and similarly, additional lincRNAs that, while not essential for the maintenance of pluripotency, act to repress lineage-specific gene expression programs in ESCs [41]. These studies demonstrated that most lincRNAs are directly regulated by critical pluripotency-associated transcription factors and that ~30 % of lincRNAs physically interact with specific chromatin regulatory proteins to affect gene expression, and many physically interact with chromatin proteins, affect gene expression programs, and maintain the ESC state.

9.3 Defining the RNAs

Mammalian genomes produce a wide variety of RNA transcripts [41–43]. In addition to the classical RNAs that serve as templates for protein synthesis and translation, that include the complementary RNA (cRNA), a viral RNA that is transcribed from negative-sense RNA; messenger RNA (mRNA), made up of 400–10,000 bases long molecules; ribosomal RNA (rRNA) that together with proteins forms the ribosomes and play a structural role and ribosomal binding of mRNA and transfer RNA (tRNA).

9.4 Noncoding RNAs

9.4.1 Noncoding RNA Classes

NcRNAs have been grouped into two major classes based on transcript size; small ncRNAs that are represented by a broad range of known and newly discovered RNA species, with many being associated with 5′ or 3′ regions of protein-coding genes. This class includes the well-documented miRNAs, siRNAs, piRNAs, etc. Extensive research on the molecular biology and its application to cancer research and therapy that is ongoing is beyond the scope of this chapter and is available in existing reviews in this field [44].

9.4.2 Long Noncoding RNAs

LncRNAs are a numerous class of newly discovered genes in the human genome that are defined as transcripts >200 nucleotides with little or no protein-coding potential [21]. The end product of the DNA sequence from which an ncRNA is transcribed is often called an RNA gene or ncRNA gene. They have been proposed to be key regulators of biological processes, including stem cell pluripotency and neurogenesis [21]. Several lncRNAs have been biologically characterized (including XIST, TSIX, HOTAIR, and AIR) [45], but shotgun cDNA sequencing and microarray hybridization have suggested that the vast majority of the mammalian genome can produce RNA transcripts under some circumstances [42]. The mammalian transcriptome also encodes many thousands of large noncoding transcripts that include a class of ~3,500 lincRNAs, which have been identified using a chromatin signature of actively transcribed genes [7, 41, 46]. These lincRNA genes have been shown to express clear evolutionary conservation patterns that correlate with various cellular processes and binding of key transcription factors to their promoters and the lincRNAs themselves physically associate with chromatin regulatory proteins [47]. Although it remains unclear whether the RNA transcripts themselves have biological functions, studies in ESCs and induced pluripotent stem cells (iPSCs) indicate that lncRNAs are integral members of the ESC self-renewal regulatory circuit. In addition, Loewer et al. [48] showed that lincRNA-RoR enhanced the reprogramming of fibroblasts into iPSCs. LncRNAs such as MALAT1, Evf-2, and Nkx2.2AS have also been reported to specify neural cell fate and function. LncRNAs are also dynamically expressed during neuronal–glia fate specification, and they appear to regulate the expression of protein-coding genes within the same genomic locus, suggesting lncRNA function. Additional evidence suggesting functional roles of lncRNAs in the brain includes a computational analysis of in situ hybridization data from the Allen Brain Atlas, which identified 849 lncRNAs showing specific expression in the mouse brain [49]. Furthermore, neural lncRNAs have been shown to be regulated by transcription factors and epigenetic processes. So far, most efforts aimed at understanding lncRNA functions in pluripotency and neural differentiation have been focused on the mouse as a model system [47, 49]. To date, the roles of lncRNAs in human embryonic and neural developmental gene networks are just beginning to be investigated. Interesting enough, findings on lncRNA functions in pluripotency and neural differentiation in mouse and human ESC are similar to our findings on the differentiation of the breast induced by an early pregnancy in the breast of postmenopausal women [11, 22].

NcRNAs are generated in eukaryotes by the spliceosomes that perform the splicing reactions essential for removing intron sequences, this process is required for the formation of mature mRNA (see Chap. 8). Another group of introns can catalyze their own removal from host transcripts, these are called self-splicing RNAs. There are two main groups of self-splicing RNAs, these are the group I catalytic intron and group II catalytic intron. These ncRNAs catalyze their own excision from mRNA, tRNA, and rRNA precursors in a wide range of organisms. These ncRNA are involved in critical regulatory processes that define biological processes and roles of a cell. The expression of these molecules have been shown to be a systematic transcriptional and regulatory event involving recruitment of spliceosomes machinery and nuclear export. Majority of these ncRNAs are expressed during various stages of development and are highly tissue specific. It is understood that these molecules exert a higher tier of regulation over critical structural and regulatory proteins and are critical to epigenetic processes and directing cell fate. It has been recently shown that in rats, an ncRNA, PINC (pregnancy-induced ncRNA) is induced by both pregnancy and hormonal stimulation. PINC is alternatively spliced, polyadenylated and is expressed in parous rat mammary gland. Functional studies have shown that it plays significant role in modulating cell fate in mammary epithelial cells and imparts "functional memory" of parity [50]. Although this is the only ncRNA that has been shown to be directly involved in epigenetic imprinting, no genome-wide screening for such molecules has been done. The results from the initial transcriptomic analysis in the normal breast of parous and nulliparous women reveals that genes such as nuclear paraspeckle assembly transcript 1 (*NEAT1*), *MALAT-1* (*NEAT2*), and *XIST* are upregulated in the parous breast [11, 51]. The role of these genes in epithelial cell differentiation and maturation needs to be explored. More importantly, we must assess the role of ncRNA and the genes involved in epithelial cell maturation and fate in both parous and nulliparous women. Furthermore the expression levels of these molecules can be combined with expression measurements of coding RNA to identify the systematic regulatory networks that are involved in parous and nulliparous breasts and could provide novel and significant information in the role of ncRNA in breast cancer prevention.

9.5 Noncoding RNA in the Parous Breast and its Implications in Cancer Prevention

Recent studies indicate that RNA molecules recruit PcG complexes to the locus of transcription or to sites located elsewhere in the genome. An important role has been attributed to ncRNAs [52]. It is possible to postulate that the increased chromatin condensation in the parous breast reported by us [11] could have been initiated by ncRNAs, a postulate supported by the observed upregulation of several ncRNAs that included nuclear paraspeckle assembly transcript 1 (NEAT1), MALAT-1 (NEAT2), and XIST [11, 53] (Table 9.1), all critical components of the speckles. The expression of MALAT-1 is upregulated by the neurotransmitter oxytocin during lactation, which acts through its specific receptor OTR. It is of interest the fact that both OTR and MALAT-1 remain upregulated in the breast of postmenopausal parous women even in the absence of circulating oxytocin. These observations indicate that in parous women the breast remains actively involved in the RNA metabolism that is necessary for maintaining a state of differentiation. Upregulation of XIST occurs upon differentiation, resulting in XCI. A ncRNA transcribed from a portion of the Xist gene locus forms hairpin structures that recruit the PRC2 complex to the X-inactivation center X(ic) [54]. Transcription of full-length Xist RNA, which forms the same hairpin structures, leads to further PRC2 recruitment and the spread of PcG-mediated repression across the inactive X chromosome. Xist repression, which is often seen in malignancies, also occurs in early embryogenesis and during the acquisition of pluripotency in undifferentiated ES cells by the binding of Nanog, Oct4, and Sox2 directly to the chromatin of the Xist gene [54]. It is possible that in the postmenopausal nulliparous breast the upregulation of DDX, Sox1, Sox6, and Sox17, which might be equivalent to Nanog, Oct4, and Sox2, plays a direct pivotal role in the repression of XIST transcription. Although this postulate needs to be functionally verified, it is possible that these genes may play a role in controlling XIST in the parous breast. The upregulation of XIST has important implications in the understanding of the differentiation pattern of the parous breast. In recent studies it has been shown that the reprogramming of XCI during the acquisition of pluripotency in vivo and in vitro is accompanied by the repression of XIST [54–56]. Reprogramming experiments have further reinforced the concept that X-inactivation is intimately linked to differentiation and support our findings that the upregulation in the expression of XIST in adult well-differentiated cells is an indication of its participation in the maintenance of gene repression [54–56]. Continuous search for additional ncRNA in the parous breast is pivotal for furthering our understanding of the role of these noncoding regions in gene regulation and differentiation.

Table 9.1 Over expressed nonprotein coding (NPC) regions

Gene symbol	Probe ID	Log ratio	*P* value	Gene name
CXorf50B	242292_at	0.35	0.0001	Nonprotein coding RNA 246B
MALAT1	224558_s_at	0.56	0.0000	Metastasis-associated lung adenocarcinoma transcript 1
MALAT1	224558_s_at	0.56	0.0000	Metastasis-associated lung adenocarcinoma transcript 1
NCRNA00173	237591_at	0.39	0.0002	Nonprotein coding RNA 173
NCRNA00201	225786_at	0.47	0.0004	Nonprotein coding RNA 201
NEAT1	224565_at	0.38	0.0012	Nuclear paraspeckle assembly transcript 1
NEAT1	224566_at	0.50	0.0014	Nuclear paraspeckle assembly transcript 1
XIST	224589_at	0.39	0.0000	X (inactive)-specific transcript
XIST	221728_x_at	0.57	0.0000	X (inactive)-specific transcript
XIST	214218_s_at	0.57	0.0000	X (inactive)-specific transcript

9.6 The Functional Role of XIST

X inactivation is an early developmental process in mammalian females that transcriptionally silences one of the pairs of X chromosomes, thus providing dosage equivalence between males and females (see Sect. 9.1). The process is regulated by several factors, including a region of chromosome X called the X-inactivation center. The XIST gene is expressed exclusively from the XIC of the inactive X chromosome. The transcript is spliced but apparently does not encode a protein. The transcript remains in the nucleus where it coats the inactive X chromosome. Alternatively spliced transcript variants have been identified, but their full length sequences have not been determined. Xist triggers the X-inactivation process in mice even in the absence of this gene. hESCs fall into three classes of XCI states: upregulation of XIST upon differentiation, always expressing XIST in the undifferentiated and differentiated states, and never expressing XIST in the undifferentiated and differentiated states. Failure to express XIST represents an especially concerning state in hESC, as this state does not occur in healthy female cells but it is often seen in malignancies [53]. Normally X inactivation is initiated in early embryogenesis, but recent reports identified instances where Xist is expressed and can initiate gene repression [57]. It has been demonstrated that Xist is functional in tumor cells, where SATB1 was identified as the first silencing factor for Xist-mediated chromosome silencing [58]. Xist is a unique gene in that it is reprogrammed to the state of somatic cells in fusion-induced pluripotent hybrids. In hybrids formed from the cell fusion of embryonal carcinoma cells (ECCs) with male neural stem cells (mNSCs), the Xist gene was found to be reprogrammed to the somatic cell state, whereas the pluripotency-related and tissue-specific marker genes were reprogrammed to the pluripotent cell state. Specifically, Xist is not expressed in hybrids, because the memory of the somatic cell has been retained (i.e., mNSCs do not exhibit Xist expression) and that of the pluripotent cell erased (i.e., inactivation of the partially active Xist gene of ECCs, complete methylation of the Xist region). The latter phenomenon is induced by male, but not by female, NSCs [59]. A role of XCI process in the development of breast cancer have been suggested. In particular, the relationship between the breast cancer predisposing gene BRCA1 and XIST, the main mediator of XCI, has been intensely investigated, but still remains controversial. The behavior of XIST has been investigated in different groups of breast carcinomas and in a panel of breast cancer cell lines both BRCA1 mutant and wild type, and also evaluated the occurrence of broader defects of heterochromatin in relation to BRCA1 status in breast cancer cells. In breast cancer cells BRCA1 is involved in XIST regulation on the active X chromosome, but not in its localization as previously suggested, and that XIST can be unusually expressed by an active X and can decorate it. This indicates that the detection of XIST cloud in cancer cell is not synonymous of the presence of an inactive X chromosome. Moreover, global heterochromatin defects observed in breast tumor cells are independent of BRCA1 status. These observations shed light on a possible previously uncharacterized mechanism of breast carcinogenesis mediated by XIST misbehavior, particularly in BRCA1-related cancers. Moreover, the significantly higher levels of XIST-RNA detected in BRCA1-associated respect to sporadic basal-like cancers open the possibility to use XIST expression as a marker to discriminate between the two groups of tumors [20, 60]. In particular, it has been proposed that the loss of BRCA1 function can lead to loss of XIST RNA association with the Xi. The X-chromosome status was evaluated using single-cell (RNA and DNA fluorescence in situ hybridization) and global genomic (array-comparative genomic hybridization and allelotyping) approaches on a series of 11 well-defined BRCA1 tumors. Many or most of the tumor cells contained one or more XIST RNA domains, although the number of these domains varied considerably between cells, even within a single tumor. Frequent X-chromosome allelic and copy number aberrations have been found in agreement with aberrant XIST RNA domain numbers. In summary, by combining multiple approaches to assess the genetics and epigenetics of a large series of BRCA1 primary tumors, it has been concluded that BRCA1 is not required for XIST RNA coating of the X chromosome. The intratumoral and intertumoral variability in XIST RNA domain number in BRCA1 tumors correlates with chromosomal genetic abnormalities, including gains, losses, reduplications, and rearrangements of the X-chromosome [61, 62]. The increased risk of several types of cancer in Klinefelter syndrome (47XXY), including that of the breast, suggests that the extra X chromosome may be involved in the tumorigenesis associated with this syndrome [63]. Cancer cells (PSK-1) derived from a patient with Klinefelter syndrome (47XXY) showing loss of an inactive X chromosome subsequently gained active X chromosomes. This abnormal X chromosome composition in PSK-1 is caused by a loss of an inactive X chromosome followed by multiplication of identical active X chromosomes, not by reactivation of an inactive X chromosome. In a series of 22 female-derived cancer cell lines (eight breast cancer cell lines, seven ovarian cancer cell lines, and seven cervical cancer cell lines) demonstrated that loss-of-inactive X in the female-derived cancer cells is mainly achieved by loss of an inactive X chromosome followed by multiplication of an identical active X chromosome. However, distinctive pathways, including reactivation of an inactive X chromosome, are also involved in the mechanisms for loss-of-inactive X and gain-of-active X in female-derived cancer cells [63].

9.7 The Functional Role of NEAT1

The use of high-throughput analyses of mammalian transcriptomes have revealed that more than half of the transcripts produced by RNA polymerase II are nonprotein-coding. One class of these noncoding transcripts is the lncRNAs, which are more than 200 nucleotides in length and are molecularly indistinguishable from other protein-coding mRNAs. Although the molecular functions of these lncRNAs have long remained unknown, emerging evidence implicates the functional involvement of lncRNAs in the regulation of gene expression through the modification of chromatin, maintenance of subnuclear structures, transport of specific mRNAs, and control of pre-mRNA splicing; examples of these lncRNAs are NEAT1/MENε/β/VINC, MALAT1/NEAT2, and Gomafu/RNCR2/MIAT, which accumulate abundantly within the nucleus as RNA components of specific nuclear bodies [64].

In our work [11] using the Affymetrix expression arrays to identify polyadenylated RNA transcripts displaying nuclear enrichment we have identified two noncoding nuclear-enriched abundant transcripts (NEAT). RNAs strikingly located less than 70 kb apart on human chromosome 11, NEAT1, at the locus encoding for TncRNA, and NEAT2, also known as MALAT-1. Although the two NEAT transcripts share no significant homology with each other, each is conserved within the mammalian lineage, suggesting significant function for these ncRNAs. Human cells as the murine homologs of these ncRNAs are also nuclear enriched. RNA FISH analyses suggest that these ncRNAs function in mRNA metabolism as they demonstrate an intimate association of these RNA species with SC35 nuclear speckles in both human and mouse cells. One of these transcripts, NEAT1 localizes to the periphery of such domains, whereas the neighboring transcript, NEAT2, is part of the long-sought polyadenylated component of nuclear speckles [65].

NEAT1 RNA, a highly abundant 4 kb ncRNA, is retained in nuclei in approximately 10–20 large foci that we have shown that completely coincide with paraspeckles, nuclear domains implicated in mRNA nuclear retention. Paraspeckles are dynamic structures that are altered in response to changes in cellular metabolic activity. They are transcription dependent [30] and in the absence of RNA Pol II transcription, the paraspeckle disappears and all of its associated protein components (PSP1, p54nrb, PSP2, CFI(m)68, and PSF) form a crescent-shaped perinucleolar cap in the nucleolus. This phenomenon has been demonstrated during the cell cycle, in which paraspeckles are present during interphase and all the phases of mitosis, except in telophase. During telophase, when the two daughter nuclei are formed, there is no RNA Pol II transcription so the protein components instead form a perinucleolar cap [33]. Depletion of NEAT1 RNA via RNAi eradicates paraspeckles, suggesting that it controls sequestration of the paraspeckle proteins PSP1 and p54, factors linked to A-I editing. Unlike overexpression of PSP1, NEAT1 overexpression increases paraspeckle number, and paraspeckles emanate exclusively from the NEAT1 transcription site. The PSP-1 RNA binding domain is required for its colocalization with NEAT1 RNA in paraspeckles, and biochemical analyses support that NEAT1 RNA binds with paraspeckle proteins. Unlike other nuclear-retained RNAs, NEAT1 RNA is not A-I edited, consistent with a structural role in paraspeckles. NEAT1 functions as an essential structural determinant of paraspeckles, providing a precedent for a ncRNA as the foundation of a nuclear domain [66]. Nuclear retention correlates with adenosine-to-inosine editing and is in paraspeckle-associated complexes containing the proteins p54(nrb), PSF, and PSP1 alpha. The core paraspeckle proteins (PSF/SFPQ, P54NRB/NONO, and PSPC1 [paraspeckle protein 1]) are members of the DBHS (*Drosophila melanogaster* behavior, human splicing) family. These proteins, together with the long nonprotein-coding RNA NEAT1 (MEN-epsilon/beta), associate to form paraspeckles and maintain their integrity [67]. In hESCs, were a robust editing activity is found, there is no nuclear retention, whereas p54(nrb), PSF, and PSP1 alpha are all expressed in hESCs, but paraspeckles are absent and only appear upon differentiation. Paraspeckle assembly and function depend on expression of a long nuclear-retained ncRNA, NEAT1. This RNA is not detectable in hESCs but is induced upon differentiation. This is in agreement what we find in the parous breast in which NEAT1 is upregulated. Knockdown of NEAT1 in HeLa cells results both in loss of paraspeckles and in enhanced nucleocytoplasmic export of mRNAs containing inverted Alu repeats. This large noncoding nuclear RNA has a biological function in the regulation of mRNA export [68]. These long nonprotein-coding RNAs are emerging as important regulators of cellular differentiation and support the concept that their presence in the parous breast is a marker of differentiation. Many long ncRNAs exhibit dynamic expression patterns during neuronal and oligodendrocyte (OL) lineage specification, neuronal-glial fate transitions, and progressive stages of OL lineage elaboration including myelination. Consideration of the genomic context of these dynamically regulated ncRNAs showed they were part of complex transcriptional loci that encompass key neural developmental protein-coding genes, with which they exhibit concordant expression profiles as indicated by both microarray and in situ hybridization analyses. These included ncRNAs associated with differentiation-specific nuclear subdomains such as Gomafu and Neat1, and ncRNAs associated with developmental enhancers and genes encoding important transcription factors and homeotic proteins. Changes in ncRNA expression profiles have been observed in response to treatment with trichostatin A, a histone deacetylase inhibitor that prevents the progression of OL progenitors into post-mitotic OLs by altering lineage-specific gene expression programs. LncRNA is expressed in neuronal and glial cell differentiation and in the modulation of ncRNA expression by modification of chromatin architecture. These observations explicitly link ncRNA dynamics to neural stem cell fate decisions, specification and epigenetic reprogramming [48], event that is also observed in the involution of the postmenopausal breast leading to terminal differentiation [11].

NEAT1 is virus inducible ncRNA in the brain of mice infected with Japanese encephalitis virus and rabies virus. NEAT1 interacts with the paraspeckle protein, P54nrb through three different protein interaction regions (PIRs) one of which (PIR-1) is localized near the 5′ end while the other two (PIR-2, PIR-3) are localized near the 3′ region of NEAT1 [69]. Through this mechanism paraspeckles and their components may ultimately have a role in controlling gene expression during many cellular processes including differentiation, viral infection, and stress responses [29, 70]. The use of a live-cell imaging system for the inducible transcription of Men ε/β (also known as Neat1 ncRNAs) allows the direct visualization of the recruitment of paraspeckle proteins. Men ε/β ncRNAs are essential to initiate the de novo assembly of paraspeckles. These newly formed structures effectively harbor nuclear-retained mRNAs confirming that they are bona fide functional paraspeckles. By three independent approaches it has been shown that Men ε/β transcription, but not ncRNAs alone, regulates paraspeckle maintenance. Finally, fluorescence recovery after photobleaching (FRAP) analyses supported a critical structural role for Men ε/β ncRNAs in paraspeckle organization [71]. It has also been proposed that paraspeckles are nonessential, subpopulation-specific nuclear bodies formed secondary to particular environmental triggers [72, 73]. However there is evidence that NEAT1 bind the RNA binding protein p54(nrb) that is involved in many nuclear processes including transcription, RNA processing, and retention of hyperedited RNAs [74]. LncRNAs are dysregulated in Huntington's disease brains while the brain-specific tumor-suppressor MEG3 is downregulated. Many LncRNAs that are dysregulated gene expression through formation of epigenetic ribonucleic complexes, including TUG1 and MEG3 [75]. Therefore, elucidating lncRNA network changes will be important in understanding and treating this and other neurodegenerative processes.

9.8 The Functional Role of NEAT2

NEAT2 (also known as MALAT-1) is also upregulated in the normal parous breast. This gene is extraordinarily well conserved for a ncRNA, more so than even XIST [65]. MALAT1 is known to be misregulated in many human cancers. Reports in the literature have shown that in the endometrial stromal sarcoma (ESS) of the uterus the metastasis-associated lung adenocarcinoma transcript 1 (MALAT-1) gene is one of the major genes upregulated, whereas the full-length placental cDNA clone (CS0DI066YJ10) is one of the major genes downregulated. Samples of normal stroma in the secretory phase and menopausal state included some that were negative or weakly positive for MALAT-1. In contrast, all ESS and 12 of 13 cases of stromal cells in the proliferative phase were negative for the full-length placental cDNA clone but 10 of 13 cases of endometrial stromal cells in the secretory phase were positive for transcripts of the gene ($P<0.05$). These results indicated that endometrial stromal cells have different phenotypic characteristics between proliferative and secretory phases and the tumor cells of ESS have the phenotypic character of endometrial stromal cells in the proliferative phase [76]. The highly conserved small RNA of 61 nucleotides originating from the MALAT1 locus that is broadly expressed in human tissues is found exclusively in the cytoplasm. RNase P cleaves the nascent MALAT1 transcript downstream of a genomically encoded poly(A)-rich tract to simultaneously generate the 3′ end of the mature MALAT1 transcript and the 5′ end of the small RNA. Enzymes involved in tRNA biogenesis then further process the small RNA, consistent with its adoption of a tRNA-like structure. These findings reveal a 3′ end processing mechanism by which a single gene locus can yield both a stable nuclear-retained ncRNA with a short poly(A) tail-like moiety and a small tRNA-like cytoplasmic RNA [77], this could be related to the neoplastic process. MALAT-1 gene was over expressed in trophoblast cell invasion. Targeting of MALAT-1 mRNA expression with siRNA in trophoblast-like BeWo, JAR, and JEG-3 choriocarcinoma cells suppressed the invasion ability of these cells [78]. MALAT1 was involved in cervical cancer cell growth, cell cycle progression, and invasion through the regulation of gene expression, such as caspase-3, -8, Bax, Bcl-2, and BclxL [79]. MALAT1 is upregulated in many cancers [80] and in neuroblastoma has been found to bind to the cyclic AMP-responsive element binding (CREB) transcription was observed using chromatin immunoprecipitation (ChIP) followed by tiling array analysis, and the results were confirmed using ChIP-qPCR. The posterior pituitary hormone oxytocin increased the levels of MALAT1 and immediate early gene transcripts as early as 15 min after stimulation. Although the expression of immediate early genes returned to basal levels after 3 h, MALAT1 transcript levels peaked 6–24 h after stimulation. Indicating a shorter transcriptional initiation site and found that CREB binds to the defined proximal promoter of the MALAT1 gene [81]. An important function of MALAT1 is its interaction with the serine/arginine splicing factors that regulate tissue- or cell-type-specific alternative splicing of pre-mRNA in a concentration- and phosphorylation-dependent manner highlighting the role of this genes in the regulation of gene expression [82]. Altogether, the role of ncRNAs in the mechanism of breast cancer prevention still is unknown and deserves a significant research effort.

References

1. Russo J, Russo IH (eds) (2004) Molecular basis of breast cancer: prevention and treatment. Springer, Berlin, 11p
2. Assou S, Boumela I, Haouzi D, Anahory T, Hervé Dechaud H, De Vos J, Hamamah S (2010) Dynamic changes in gene expression during human early embryo development: from fundamental aspects to clinical applications. Hum Reprod Update 17(2):272–290
3. van den Berg IM, Laven JS, Stevens M, Jonkers I, Galjaard RJ, Gribnau J, van Doorninck JH (2009) X chromosome inactivation is initiated in human preimplantation embryos. Am J Hum Genet 84(6):771–779
4. van den Berg IM, Galjaard RJ, Laven JS, vanDoorninck JH (2011) XCI in preimplantation mouse and human embryos: first there is remodelling…. Hum Genet 130(2):203–215
5. Reubinoff BE, Pera MF, Fong CY, Trounson A, Bongso A (2000) Embryonic stem cell lines from human blastocysts: somatic differentiation in vitro. Nat Biotechnol 18:399–404

6. Taylor DM, Handyside AH, Ray PF, Dibb NJ, Winston RM, Ao A (2001) Quantitative measurement of transcript levels throughout human preimplantation development: analysis of hypoxanthine phosphoribosyl transferase. Mol Hum Reprod 7:147–154
7. Khalil AM, Guttman M, Huarte M, Garber M, Raj A, Rivea Morales D, Thomas K, Presser A, Bernstein BE, van Oudenaarden A, Regev A, Lander ES, Rinn JL (2009) Many human large intergenic noncoding RNAs associate with chromatin-modifying complexes and affect gene expression. Proc Natl Acad Sci U S A 106(28):11667–11672
8. Shen Y, Matsuno Y, Fouse SD, Rao N, Root S, Xu R, Matteo Pellegrini M, Riggs AD, Guoping Fan G (2008) X-inactivation in female human embryonic stem cells is in a nonrandom pattern and prone to epigenetic alterations. Proc Natl Acad Sci U S A 105(12):4709–4714
9. Russo J, Balogh GA, Chen J, Fernandez SV, Fernbaugh R, Heulings R, Mailo DA, Moral R, Russo PA, Sheriff F, Vanegas JE, Wang R, Russo IH (2006) The concept of stem cell in the mammary gland and its implication in morphogenesis, cancer and prevention. Front Biosci 11:151–172
10. Russo J, Balogh GA, Russo IH (2008) Full-term pregnancy induces a specific genomic signature in the human breast. Cancer Epidemiol Biomarkers Prev 17:51–66
11. Russo J, Santucci-Pereira J, de Cicco RL, Sheriff F, Russo PA, Peri S, Slifker M, Ross E, Mello ML, Vidal BC, Belitskaya-Lévy I, Arslan A, Zeleniuch-Jacquotte A, Bordas P, Lenner P, Ahman J, Afanasyeva Y, Hallmans G, Toniolo P, Russo IH (2012) Pregnancy-induced chromatin remodeling in the breast of postmenopausal women. Int J Cancer 131(5):1059–1070. doi:10.1002/ijc.27323
12. Hennighausen L, Robinson GW (2005) Information networks in the mammary gland. Nat Rev Mol Cell Biol 6:715–725
13. Koutcherov Y, Mai JK, Paxinos G (2003) Hypothalamus of the human fetus. J Chem Neuroanat 26:253–270
14. Kristiansen M, Knudsen GP, Maguire P, Margolin S, Pedersen J, Lindblom A, Ørstavik KH (2005) High incidence of skewed X chromosome inactivation in young patients with familial non-BRCA1/BRCA2 breast cancer. J Med Genet 42(11):877–880
15. Hon GC, Hawkins RD, Caballero OL, Lo C, Lister R, Pelizzola M, Valsesia A, Ye Z, Kua S, Edsall LE, Camargo AA, Stevenson BJ, Ecker JR, Bafna V, Strausberg RL, Simpson AJ, Ren B (2012) Global DNA hypomethylation coupled to repressive chromatin domain formation and gene silencing in breast cancer. Genome Res 22(2):246–258
16. Takeshima H, Yamashita S, Shimazu T, Ushijima T (2011) Effects of genome architecture and epigenetic factors on susceptibility of promoter CpG islands to aberrant DNA methylation induction. Genomics 98(3):182–188
17. Russo J, Tait L, Russo IH (1983) Susceptibility of the mammary gland to carcinogenesis: III. The cell of origin of rat mammary carcinoma. Am J Pathol 113:50–66
18. Russo J, Reina D, Frederick J, Russo IH (1988) Expression of phenotypical changes by human breast epithelial cells treated with carcinogens in vitro. Cancer Res 48:2837–2857
19. Sirchia SM, Ramoscelli L, Grati FR, Barbera F, Coradini D, Rossella F, Porta G, Lesma E, Ruggeri A, Radice P, Simoni G, Miozzo M (2005) Loss of the inactive X chromosome and replication of the active X in BRCA1-defective and wild-type breast cancer cells. Cancer Res 65(6):2139–2146
20. Sirchia SM, Tabano S, Monti L, Recalcati MP, Gariboldi M, Grati FR, Porta G, Finelli P, Radice P, Miozzo M (2009) Misbehaviour of XIST RNA in breast cancer cells. PLoS One 4(5):e5559
21. Ng S-Y, Johnson R, Stanton LW (2011) Human long non-coding RNAs promote pluripotency and neuronal differentiation by association with chromatin modifiers and transcription factors. EMBO J 31(3):522–533
22. Russo J, Russo IH (2012) Molecular basis of pregnancy-induced breast cancer prevention. Horm Mol Biol Clin Invest 9(1):3–10
23. Dundr M, Misteli T (2001) Functional architecture in the cell nucleus. Biochem J 356:297–310
24. Saunders WS, Cooke CA, Earnshaw WC (1991) Compartmentalization within the nucleus: discovery of a novel subnuclear region. J Cell Biol 115:919–931

25. Cioce M, Lamond A (2005) Cajal bodies: a long history of discovery. Annu Rev Cell Dev Biol 21:105–131
26. Matera AG, Frey MA (1998) Coiled bodies and gems: janus or gemini? Am J Hum Genet 63:317–321
27. Pombo A, Cuello P, Schul W, Yoon J, Roeder R, Cook P, Murphy S (1998) Regional and temporal specialization in the nucleus: a transcriptionally active nuclear domain rich in PTF, Oct1 and PIKA antigens associates with specific chromosomes. EMBO J 17:1768–1778
28. Seeler JS, Dejean A (1999) The PML nuclear bodies: actors or extras? Curr Opin Genet Dev 9:362–367
29. Fox AH, Lamond AI (2010) Paraspeckles. Cold Spring Harb Perspect Biol 2:a000687
30. Fox AH, Bond CS, Lamond AI (2005) P54nrb forms a heterodimer with PSP1 that localizes to paraspeckles in an RNA-dependent manner. Mol Biol Cell 16:5304–5315
31. Lamond AI, Spector DL (2003) Nuclear speckles: a model for nuclear organelles. Nat Rev Mol Cell Biol 4:605–612
32. Spector DL, Lamond AI (2011) Nuclear speckles. Cold Spring Harb Perspect Biol 3:a000646
33. Tripathi K, Parnaik VK (2008) Differential dynamics of splicing factor SC35 during the cell cycle. J Biosci 33:345–354
34. Handwerger KE, Gall JG (2006) Subnuclear organelles: new insights into form and function. Trends Cell Biol 16:19–26
35. Lehninger AL, Nelson DL, Cox MM (2000) Lehninger principles of biochemistry, 3rd edn. Worth Publishers, New York
36. Moreno F, Ahuatzi D, Riera A, Palomino CA, Herrero P (2005) Glucose sensing through the Hxk2-dependent signalling pathway. Biochem Soc Trans 33:265–268
37. Görlich D, Kutay U (1999) Transport between the cell nucleus and the cytoplasm. Annu Rev Cell Dev Biol 15:607–660
38. Lee TI, Young RA (2000) Transcription of eukaryotic protein-coding genes. Annu Rev Genet 34:77–137
39. Kapranov P, St Laurent G, Raz T, Ozsolak F, Reynolds CP, Sorensen PH, Reaman G, Milos P, Arceci RJ, Thompson JF, Triche TJ (2010) The majority of total nuclear-encoded non-ribosomal RNA in a human cell is 'dark matter' un-annotated RNA. BMC Biol 8:149
40. Carninci P et al (2005) The transcriptional landscape of the mammalian genome. Science 309:1559–1563
41. Guttman M, Amit I, Garber M, French C, Lin MF, Feldser D, Huarte M, Zuk O, Carey BW, Cassady JP, Cabili MN, Jaenisch R, Mikkelsen TS, Jacks T, Hacohen N, Bernstein BE, Kellis M, Regev A, Rinn JL, Lander ES (2009) Chromatin signature reveals over a thousand highly conserved large non-coding RNAs in mammals. Nature 458:223–227
42. ENCODE Project Consortium; Birney E, Stamatoyannopoulos JA, Dutta A, Guigó R, Gingeras TR, Margulies EH, Weng Z et al (2007) Identification and analysis of functional elements in 1% of the human genome by the ENCODE pilot project. Nature 447:799–816
43. Mattick JS (2009) The genetic signatures of noncoding RNAs. PLoS Genet 5:e1000459
44. Sana J, Faltejskova P, Svoboda M, Slaby O (2012) Novel classes of non-coding RNAs and cancer. J Transl Med 10:103
45. Washietl S, Pedersen JS, Korbel JO, Stocsits C, Gruber AR, Hackermüller J, Hertel J, Lindemeyer M, Reiche K, Tanzer A, Ucla C, Wyss C, Antonarakis SE, Denoeud F, Lagarde J, Drenkow J, Kapranov P, Gingeras TR, Guigó R, Snyder M, Gerstein MB, Reymond A, Hofacker IL, Stadler PF (2007) Structured RNAs in the ENCODE selected regions of the human genome. Genome Res 17:852–864
46. Guttman M et al (2010) Ab initio reconstruction of cell type-specific transcriptomes in mouse reveals the conserved multi-exonic structure of lincRNAs. Nat Biotechnol 28:503–510
47. Guttman M, Donaghey J, Carey BW, Garber M, Grenier JK, Munson G, Young G, Lucas AB, Ach R, Bruhn L, Yang X, Amit I, Meissner A, Regev A, Rinn JL, Root DE, Lander ES (2011) lincRNAs act in the circuitry controlling pluripotency and differentiation. Nature 477:295–300. doi:10.1038/nature10398

48. Loewer S, Cabili MN, Guttman M, Loh YH, Thomas K, Park IH, Garber M, Curran M, Onder T, Agarwal S, Manos PD, Datta S, Lander ES, Schlaeger TM, Daley GQ, Rinn JL (2010) Large intergenic non-coding RNA-RoR modulates reprogramming of human induced pluripotent stem cells. Nat Genet 42:1113–1117
49. Mercer TR, Qureshi IA, Gokhan S, Dinger ME, Li G, Mattick JS, Mehler MF (2010) Long noncoding RNAs in neuronal-glial fate specification and oligodendrocyte lineage maturation. BMC Neurosci 11:14
50. Ginger MR, Shore AN, Contreras A, Rijnkels M, Miller J, Gonzalez-Rimbau MF, Rosen JM (2006) A noncoding RNA is a potential marker of cell fate during mammary gland development. Proc Natl Acad Sci U S A 103:5781–5786
51. Belitskaya-Lévy I, Zeleniuch-Jacquotte A, Russo J, Russo IH et al (2011) Characterization of a genomic signature of pregnancy identified in the breast. Cancer Prev Res 4:1457–1464
52. Matthew GG, Young RA (2010) Repressive transcription. Science 329:150–151
53. Erwin JA, Lee JT (2010) Characterization of X-chromosome inactivation status in human pluripotent stem cells. Curr Protoc Stem Cell Biol Chapter 1:Unit 1B.6
54. Navarro P, Chambers I, Karwacki-Neisius V, Chureau C, Morey C, Rougeulle C, Avner P (2008) Molecular coupling of Xist regulation and pluripotency. Science 321:1693–1695
55. Surani MA, Hayashi K, Hajkova P (2007) Genetic and epigenetic regulators of pluripotency. Cell 128:747–762
56. Lee JT (2010) Characterization of X-chromosome inactivation status in human pluripotent stem cells. Curr Protoc Stem Cell Biol Chapter 1:Unit 1B.6
57. Agrelo R, Wutz A (2010) ConteXt of change—X inactivation and disease. EMBO Mol Med 2(1):6–15
58. Agrelo R, Wutz A (2009) Cancer progenitors and epigenetic contexts: an Xisting connection. Epigenetics 4:568–570
59. Do JT, Han DW, Gentile L, Sobek-Klocke I, Wutz A, Schöler HR (2009) Reprogramming of Xist against the pluripotent state in fusion hybrids. J Cell Sci 122:4122–4129
60. Perez DS, Hoage TR, Pritchett JR, Ducharme-Smith AL, Halling ML, Ganapathiraju SC, Streng PS, Smith DI (2007) Long, abundantly expressed non-coding transcripts are altered in cancer. Hum Mol Genet 17:642–655
61. Vincent-Salomon A, Ganem-Elbaz C, Manié E, Raynal V, Sastre-Garau X, Stoppa-Lyonnet D, Stern MH, Heard E (2007) X inactive-specific transcript RNA coating and genetic instability of the X chromosome in BRCA1 breast tumors. Cancer Res 67:5134–5140
62. Silver DP, Dimitrov SD, Feunteun J, Gelman R, Drapkin R, Lu SD, Shestakova E, Velmurugan S, Denunzio N, Dragomir S, Mar J, Liu X, Rottenberg S, Jonkers J, Ganesan S, Livingston DM (2007) Further evidence for BRCA1 communication with the inactive X chromosome. Cell 128:991–1002
63. Kawakami T, Zhang C, Taniguchi T, Kim CJ, Okada Y, Sugihara H, Hattori T, Reeve AE, Ogawa O, Okamoto K (2004) Characterization of loss-of-inactive X in Klinefelter syndrome and female-derived cancer cells. Oncogene 23:6163–6169
64. Ip JY, Nakagawa S (2011) Long non-coding RNAs in nuclear bodies. Dev Growth Differ 54(1):44–54. doi:10.1111/j.1440-169X.2011.01303.x
65. Hutchinson JN, Ensminger AW, Clemson CM, Lynch CR, Lawrence JB, Chess A (2007) A screen for nuclear transcripts identifies two linked noncoding RNAs associated with SC35 splicing domains. BMC Genomics 8:39
66. Clemson CM, Hutchinson JN, Sara SA, Ensminger AW, Fox AH, Chess A, Lawrence JB (2009) An architectural role for a nuclear noncoding RNA: NEAT1 RNA is essential for the structure of paraspeckles. Mol Cell 33:717–726
67. Bond CS, Fox AH (2009) Paraspeckles: nuclear bodies built on long noncoding RNA. J Cell Biol 186:637–644
68. Chen LL, Carmichael GG (2009) Altered nuclear retention of mRNAs containing inverted repeats in human embryonic stem cells: functional role of a nuclear noncoding RNA. Mol Cell 35:467–478

69. Murthy UM, Rangarajan PN (2010) Identification of protein interaction regions of VINC/NEAT1/Men epsilon RNA. FEBS Lett 584:1531–1535
70. Meehan M, Burke FM, Macken S, Owen P (2010) Characterization of the haem-uptake system of the equine pathogen Streptococcus equi subsp. equi. Microbiology 156:1824–1835
71. Mao YS, Sunwoo H, Zhang B, Spector DL (2011) Direct visualization of the co-transcriptional assembly of a nuclear body by noncoding RNAs. Nat Cell Biol 13:95–101
72. Nakagawa S, Naganuma T, Shioi G, Hirose T (2011) Paraspeckles are subpopulation-specific nuclear bodies that are not essential in mice. J Cell Biol 193:31–39
73. Honsa ES, Fabian M, Cardenas AM, Olson JS, Maresso AW (2011) The five near-iron transporter (NEAT) domain anthrax hemophore, IsdX2, scavenges heme from hemoglobin and transfers heme to the surface protein IsdC. J Biol Chem 286:33652–33660
74. Bruelle C, Bédard M, Blier S, Gauthier M, Traish AM, Vincent M (2011) The mitotic phosphorylation of p54(nrb) modulates its RNA binding activity. Biochem Cell Biol 89:423–433
75. Johnson R (2012) Long non-coding RNAs in Huntington's disease neurodegeneration. Neurobiol Dis 46(2):245–254
76. Yamada K, Kano J, Tsunoda H, Yoshikawa H, Okubo C, Ishiyama T, Noguchi M (2006) Phenotypic characterization of endometrial stromal sarcoma of the uterus. Cancer Sci 97:106–112
77. Wilusz JE, Freier SM, Spector DL (2008) 3′ end processing of a long nuclear-retained noncoding RNA yields a tRNA-like cytoplasmic RNA. Cell 135:919–932
78. Tseng JJ, Hsieh YT, Hsu SL, Chou MM (2009) Metastasis associated lung adenocarcinoma transcript 1 is up-regulated in placenta previa increta/percreta and strongly associated with trophoblast-like cell invasion in vitro. Mol Hum Reprod 15:725–731
79. Guo F, Li Y, Liu Y, Wang J, Li Y, Li G (2010) Inhibition of metastasis-associated lung adenocarcinoma transcript 1 in CaSki human cervical cancer cells suppresses cell proliferation and invasion. Acta Biochim Biophys Sin (Shanghai) 42:224–229
80. Diederichs S (2010) Non-coding RNA in malignant tumors. A new world of tumor biomarkers and target structures in cancer cells. Pathologe suppl 2:258–262
81. Koshimizu TA, Fujiwara Y, Sakai N, Shibata K, Tsuchiya H (2010) Oxytocin stimulates expression of a noncoding RNA tumor marker in a human neuroblastoma cell line. Life Sci 86:455–460
82. Tripathi V, Ellis JD, Shen Z, Song DY, Pan Q, Watt AT, Freier SM, Bennett CF, Sharma A, Bubulya PA, Blencowe BJ, Prasanth SG, Prasanth KV (2010) The nuclear-retained noncoding RNA MALAT1 regulates alternative splicing by modulating SR splicing factor phosphorylation. Mol Cell 39:925–938

Chapter 10
The Role of Stem Cell in Breast Cancer Prevention

10.1 Evidence for a Stem Cell in the Mammary Gland

Stem cells in adult structures have been defined by their ability for self-renewal and for generating a differentiated progeny. In the mammary gland, Deome et al. [1] demonstrated that fragments of different parenchymal portions were able to generate fully functional mammary outgrowths in mice, forming ductal and lobuloalveolar structures composed by epithelial and myoepithelial cells. This concept was further developed by Kordon and Smith [2] who demonstrated that the progeny from a single cell might comprise the epithelial population of a fully developed lactating mammary outgrowth in mice. Thus, the development of the complete mammary tree from a small portion of a duct or from single cells attests of their multifaceted potential. However, it was not known whether these progenitor/stem cells would be capable of initiating cancer when exposed to a carcinogenic agent. This issue was addressed by Russo and coworkers [3–5], who demonstrated that cancer started in terminal end buds (TEBs) present in the mammary gland of young virgin rats. The analysis of these structures by electron microscopy allowed them to characterize their cellular composition based upon cell and nuclear size, nuclear-cytoplasmic ratio, amount of chromatin condensation, electron density of the cytoplasm, number and distribution of organelles, and the presence or absence of Mg^{2+} and $Na^{+}K^{+}$-dependent ATPases. Based upon these criteria, in addition to myoepithelial cells, three types of epithelial cells were identified: Light, intermediate, and dark cells [4, 5]. Dark cells were found to be the predominant type in TEBs; intermediate and myoepithelial cells were present in significantly lower percentages and light cells were only occasionally seen; therefore, their percentage was combined with that of intermediate cells. The analysis of the DNA labeling index revealed that all the cell types proliferated, although at different rates, depending upon the type of cells and of their location within the mammary gland tree. Cell proliferation was maximal in intermediate cells located in TEBs, being significantly lower in dark and myoepithelial cells found in the same location. High cell proliferation was associated with greater incorporation of H^3-DMBA, and a progressive dominance of

J. Russo and I.H. Russo, *Role of the Transcriptome in Breast Cancer Prevention*,
DOI 10.1007/978-1-4614-4884-6_10,

intermediate cells in DMBA-induced intraductal proliferations (IDPs) and in ductal carcinomas [5, 6]. These results indicated that intermediate cells were not only the targets of the carcinogen but also the stem cells of mammary carcinomas. Further work by Bennett et al. [7] demonstrated that intermediate cells isolated from DMBA-induced mammary tumors originated two cell types in culture, the dark cell, representing a terminally differentiated cell or a class in transition to differentiation, and intermediate cells, which could represent an undifferentiated, or stem cell, a progenitor of dark and myoepithelial cells. Rudland et al. [8] isolated and characterized from the normal rat mammary gland and from DMBA-induced mammary adenocarcinomas epithelial cells that were cuboidal and gave rise to a mixture of cuboidal and spindle-shaped cells resembling fibroblasts. In confluent cultures, cuboidal cells acquired the morphology of a third type of cells, which were dark, polygonal, and with many small vacuoles, resembling the dark cells ultrastructurally described by Russo et al. [5]. Chepko and Smith [9] differentiated three division-competent cell populations in the murine mammary epithelium, a subset of "large light cells" structurally and functionally compatible with early stages of secretory differentiation, "small light cells" that were the least differentiated, suggesting that the large light cells were a direct precursor to terminally differentiated cells, both secretory and myoepithelial. These results confirmed the Russo's work [5].

10.2 Cell Markers for Identifying the Stem Cell in the Mammary Gland

A shift from the pioneering work done for characterizing by morphology and by in vitro behavior the progenitor/stem cells started with the search for immunocytochemical and genomic markers was done by Smith et al. [10] utilizing the expression of keratins 6 and 14 in mouse mammary epithelium for defining subsets of morphologically distinct luminal mammary epithelial cells with kinetic properties expected for latent mammogenic stem cells. Keratin 6 was confined to a small number of mammary epithelial cells found in the growing end buds and among the luminal epithelium, whereas keratin 14 was expressed in basally located fusiform cells as the myoepithelial cells. These authors emphasized the usefulness of these markers for identifying mammary epithelium-specific primordial cells. Stingl et al. [11, 12] utilized new molecular markers for selecting subpopulations of cells with distinct differentiation potential. They described bipotent human mammary epithelial progenitor cells based on the expression of epithelial-specific antigen (ESA), sialomucin 1 (MUC1), common acute lymphoblast antigen (CALLA/CD10), and alpha-integrin, in combination with exclusion of rhodamine dye. Hebbard et al. [13] observed that CD44, a member of the family of cell surface proteins that is expressed in breast carcinomas, is also expressed in the normal mammary gland. In rodents, CD44 expression is first detected at puberty, and thereafter it is regulated by the estrous cycle; it disappears during lactation, reappearing during involution, suggesting that the expression of this protein is a marker of a stem cell. Novel studies in mice mammary gland [14] have identified stem cells in TEBs and ducts by pulse labeling HC-11 primary mammary epithelial cells with fluorescent TRITC-cell linker membrane label and BrdU, the cells were then transplanted into cleared juvenile syngenic mammary fat pads, in which they were identified as long-lived, label-retaining mammary epithelial cells (LRCs) in mammary ducts that were actively growing or static. This study demonstrated that LRCs are stem cells and their progeny (transitional cells) are arranged as transitional units (TUs) and that both express Zonula Occludens-1 and alpha-catenin proteins, data that suggest that TUs retain stem cells.

The study of markers for other stem cells has been useful in the identification of mammary stem/progenitor cells. Sca1 (stem cell antigen 1) was first described in mice as a hematopoietic stem cell antigen [15]. Welm et al. [16] detected in the luminal epithelium of mice an Sca1+ cell population that is enriched for functional stem/progenitor cells. These cells are BrdU label retaining, lack expression of differentiation markers, and are progesterone receptor negative. The Sca1+ population also shows "side population" (SP) properties, a characteristic first defined in bone marrow cells [15], as cells with Hoechst dye-effluxing properties that have phenotypic markers of multipotential hematopoietic stem cells. It has been proposed that the protein responsible for that phenotype is breast cancer resistance protein 1 (BCRP1), suggesting that the expression of this protein could serve as a marker for stem cells from various sources [17]. Mammary epithelial cells with SP properties were also identified in human mammary gland. Alvi et al. [18] showed that 0.2–0.45% of both human and mouse epithelia were formed by distinct SP cells. These cells generated ductal and lobuloalveolar structures when transplanted into murine cleared mammary fat pads. The SP cells had a high expression of BCRP1, sca1, telomerase catalytic subunit, and low levels of differentiated markers for luminal (epithelial membrane antigen and cytokeratin 19) and myoepithelial cell types (cytokeratin 14). These cells were detected in all human breast samples studied, but their presence was not correlated with age, parity, contraceptive use, or day of menstrual cycle. Further investigations identified new markers which may be specific for the human stem/progenitor cells. Gudjonsson et al. [19] isolated a cell line derived from human mammary cells expressing ESA and lacking sialomucin (MUC) expression that could give rise to both luminal epithelial and myoepithelial cells in culture. One single ESA+/MUC− cell had the ability of generating a terminal ductal-lobular unit-like structure in basement membrane gel, similar to that formed when the cell line was implanted in mice. In contrast, an ESA+/MUC+ subpopulation was differentiated, luminal epithelial-restricted without stem cell properties. Dontu et al. [20] developed a system to enrich the population of human mammary progenitor/stem cells by culturing them in suspension where they formed "nonadherent mammospheres." These structures were able to differentiate along all three mammary epithelial lineages and to clonally generate complex functional structures in 3D culture systems. Cytological and immunocytochemical analysis of secondary mammospheres revealed that these structures contained cells positive for alpha-6 integrin, cytokeratin 5, which was widely expressed, and CD10; ESA-positive and cytokeratin 14-positive cells were less frequently found. Muc 1, alpha-smooth muscle antigen (ASMA), and cytokeratin 18 were not detected. In addition to cells, mammospheres contained extracellular material (ECM). However, immunostains for fibronectin and collagen IV, the classical components of adult gland ECM material were negative, although ~20% of the mammospheres stained positive for laminin. In contrast, abundant expression of the embryonic ECM components, tenascin and decorin, were detected in mammospheres (see ref. [20]). Moreover, the comparison of the genomic profile of undifferentiated cells from mammospheres to that of differentiated cells cultured on collagen identified genes candidates for stem/progenitor cell markers. Some of these genes have been already described as involved in stem/progenitor cell-specific functions or regulation of self-renewal, whereas abnormal expression of some of them has been correlated with breast cancer development such as proliferation, cell survival, and invasion. Recently, new studies showed that the null mutation of the peroxisome proliferator-activated receptor-binding protein (PBP) resulted in defective mammary gland development and in the inability of the mammary epithelial cells to form mammospheres, suggesting a role of PBP in the survival of mammary stem cells or in the mammosphere formation process [21].

10.3 Estrogen Receptor as a Marker of Stem Cells in the Mammary Gland

The identification of the stem cell and of its role in the development and differentiation of the mammary gland from birth to senesce requires an understanding of the effect of estrogen and its cognate ligand receptor alpha (ERalpha) in these processes. The importance of the role played by the ERalpha in mammary gland development has been highlighted by the development of the ERalpha KO mouse [22]. At birth, the mammary gland of intact animals consists of a rudimentary ductal tree that develops and fills the stroma of the gland in response to increased ovarian estrogen at puberty. The mammary gland of ERalpha KO females does not grow beyond the rudimentary ducts, illustrating the role of estrogens in ductal elongation. The importance of active ductal growth driven by estrogen has been further emphasized by the higher susceptibility of the breast to be transformed during a "high risk" window in the lifespan of a female encompassed between menarche and a first full term pregnancy [6]. This period is characterized by rapid ductal growth and active proliferative activity of the mammary epithelium of Lob 1. These structures are composed of a rapidly proliferating epithelium that has a high content of ERalpha and progesterone receptor (PR)-positive cells. With the progressive maturation of Lob 1 to Lob 2, Lob 3, and Lob 4 there is a progressive decrease in the percentage of proliferating cells, a reduction in the percentage of cells positive for steroid hormone receptors, and a reduction in the susceptibility of the cells to be transformed by chemical carcinogens [23]. These data indicate that the stem cells that originate the mammary tree as well as cancerous lesions are located in a specific compartment of the mammary parenchyma, namely the Lob 1 or TDLU; these are the cells that have been called Stem cell 1 by Russo and Russo [24]. Supporting studies by

Petersen et al. [25] have shown that a subset of suprabasal breast luminal epithelial cells that are able to generate themselves as well as differentiated luminal epithelial and myoepithelial cells, and to form terminal ductal lobular unit (TDLU)-like structures are distinguished by cytokeratin 19. The suprabasal population of breast stem cells consists of undifferentiated "intermediate" cells with Hoechst dye-effluxing "side population" (SP) properties. These cells lack expression of myoepithelial and luminal apical membrane markers such as CALLA and MUC1. They are rich for ERalpha-positive cells and express several fold higher levels of the ERalpha, p21 (CIP1), and Msi1 genes than non-SP cells. They also form branching structures in matrigel which included cells of both luminal and myoepithelial lineages. These data suggest a model where scattered steroid receptor-positive cells are stem cells that self-renew through asymmetric cell division and generate patches of transit amplifying and differentiated cells [26, 27]. ERalpha/PR+ breast cancers exhibit loss of the two key regulators of asymmetric cell division, Musashi-1 and Notch-1, and thus they may arise from symmetric division of the ERalpha/PR+ stem cell [26]. These data are supported by the observations of Russo et al. [23] that epithelial cells of the Lob 1 co-express ERalpha, PR and the proliferation marker Ki67, suggesting that these cells could originate ERalpha-positive tumors. However, these cells represent less than 1% of the total cell population, whereas the majority of ERalpha/PR+ cells do not express the proliferation marker, an indication that the cells that contain the receptors are not capable of proliferating. The findings that proliferating cells are different from those that are ERalpha/PR-positive support data that indicate that estrogen controls cell proliferation by an indirect mechanism. Further support is the finding that when Lob 1 of normal breast tissue are placed in culture, they lose the ERalpha-positive cells, indicating that only proliferating cells that are also ERalpha-negative can survive, representing a type of stem cell that may originate ER-negative tumors [23]. The fact that the majority of proliferating breast epithelial cells do not express ERalpha and PR receptors could explain Clayton et al. [28] data that cells characterized as human mammary stem cells, present ESA expression, Hoechst dye exclusion, low levels of MUC-1 and CALLA, and lack detectable expression of ER alpha and beta. Cells expressing that phenotype had high cloning efficiency in culture from a single cell, generating mixed colonies containing luminal and myoepithelial cells.

10.3.1 Estrogen Receptor Beta and the Breast Stem Cells

Estrogens and ERs are required for the proliferation of stem cells. For example, it was observed that the human breast carcinoma cells PMC42, which have stem cell characteristics, did not proliferate in serum-free medium unless 17β-estradiol (E_2) or progesterone were added, though their ER content was lower than that described for MCF-7 and T47D. The addition of both hormones induced a more than additive increase in proliferation whereas the addition of tamoxifen significantly decreased cell numbers and inhibited the stimulatory effects of E_2 [29]. Estrogens also have profound effects on function and plasticity of rat neural stem cells. Both embryonic and adult rat neural stem cells express ERalpha and ERbeta. E_2 treatment increased the proliferation of embryonic neural stem cells and these effects were inhibited by the ER antagonist, ICI-182780, showing an involvement of ERs [30]. It has also been shown that estrogens have significant effects on spermatogonial stem cells of the Japanese eel (*Anguilla japonica*) and these effects are mediated via ERs [31]. Together, these observations indicate that estrogens and ERalpha/ERbeta are required for the proliferation of stem cells. However the data regarding the role of the second ER isoforms ERbeta in regulation of cell proliferation are controversial [22, 23, 25–34]. ERbeta has been assigned two different and opposed actions as an inhibitor or a stimulator of E_2-induced proliferation in human breast cells. For example, there are several reports indicating that over-expression of ERbeta and its variants in breast cancer cell lines and breast cancer cells inhibited ERalpha-mediated cell proliferation [35–37]. In ERbeta-knock out mice, the presence of ERalpha but not ERbeta was necessary for the development of mouse mammary gland [38, 39]. Thus, it was hypothesized that ERbeta is acting as antagonist for the actions of ERalpha, as an inhibitor of cell proliferation [35–37, 40–42]. However, this hypothesis is challenged by the following data: (a) There are proliferating cells in breast which express ERbeta [43], but the ERalpha-expressing cells in breast cancer do not express proliferation markers [44, 45]; (b) The expression of ERbeta in breast cancer cells correlated with the enhanced expression of cell proliferating markers (e.g., Ki67 and cyclin A) [43–46]; (c) ERbeta is by far the more abundant of the two ERs in human breast cells [47] and rat mammary gland [48, 49] and its expression is higher in normal breast cells than in breast cancer cells [50–54]; (d) both wild-type and ERbeta variants are expressed in higher grade human breast tumors [45–55] and the expression of ERbeta correlated with accepted prognostic indicators including lymph node status and tumor grades [56]; (e) high percentage ERalpha-negative tumors were positive for ERbeta. The presence of ERbeta was associated with an increase in survival rates in women treated with tamoxifen [57]; and (f) in addition, it has been found an inverse relationship between the methylation rate of the ERbeta gene and tamoxifen resistance. The tamoxifen-resistant tumors showed denser methylation of the ERbeta gene than control tumors [58].

There are several lines of evidence suggesting that ERbeta is involved in the control of stem cell proliferation. Proliferation of pluripotent, bone marrow stem cells, which develop to lymphoid and myeloid progenitors, is negatively regulated by estrogens. In estrogen deficiency and in ERbeta KO mice, there is significant alteration in bone marrow hematopoiesis. Shim et al. [59] observed that 1.5-year-old ERbeta KO mice developed pronounced splenomegaly that is much more severe in females than in males. Further characterization of these mice revealed myelogenous hyperplasia in bone marrow, an increase in the number of granulocytes and B lymphocytes in blood, lymphadenopathy, and infiltration of leukocytes in the liver and lung. Analysis by flow cytometry of the bone marrow cells revealed that the percentage and total number of Gr-1hi/Mac-1hi-positive granulocytes were increased. The number of B cells in the bone marrow and spleen were significantly higher in ERbeta$^{-/-}$ mice than in WT littermates. Some of the ERbetaKO mice also had a severe lymphoproliferative phenotype. Thus the absence of ERbeta results in a myeloproliferative disease resembling human chronic myeloid leukemia with lymphoid blast crisis. These results indicate a role for ERbeta in regulating the differentiation of pluripotent hematopoietic progenitor cells [59]. In the prostate, there are high levels of ERbeta but no ERalpha, suggesting a direct estrogenic influence on prostatic epithelium mediated by ERbeta. Imamov et al. [60] reported that loss of ERbeta results in epithelial hypercellularity in the ventral prostate. In ERbeta$^{-/-}$ mouse prostates, there is over-expression of the androgen receptor and of the anti-apoptotic factor Bcl-2 in the prostate. It is normally expressed only in the basal cells in the prostate. This apparent expansion of the "stem cell-like population" in the ERbeta$^{-/-}$ mouse prostate has been further examined. They found a higher expression of cytokeratin 5 in ERbeta$^{-/-}$ mouse prostates so that the ratio of cytokeratin 5 to that of 19 is much higher in ERbeta$^{-/-}$ than in wild-type littermates. In addition, labeling of DNA with BrdU showed a 3.5-fold higher proliferation rate in ERbeta$^{-/-}$ mouse prostate. Despite these clear differences, the piling up of epithelial cells never progressed to high-grade prostatic intraepithelial neoplasia (PIN)-like lesions. Hyperplastic foci in ERbeta$^{-/-}$ mice show accumulation of cells without signs of atypia, resembling low-grade PIN in humans. The reason for this appeared to be a high rate of cellular detachment and subsequent fall off into the lumen in ERbeta$^{-/-}$ mice. The fall off phenomenon is possibly related to the finding that the expression of the cell adhesion molecule E-cadherin was reduced. It is concluded that in ERbeta$^{-/-}$ mouse prostates, the epithelial cell population contains more epithelial cells in the intermediate stage of differentiation, possessing both the ability to proliferate as the basal cells and the ability to secrete as the highly differentiated luminal epithelium.

Estrogen exposure has been linked to a risk for the development of testicular germ cell cancers. Pais et al. [61] compared the localization and expression levels of ER alpha and beta subtypes in testicular germ cell cancers with normal testis. These authors observed that ERalpha was not expressed in the human normal testis and was also absent in all the testicular germ cell cancers studied. In contrast, ERbeta was strongly expressed in various germ cells of the normal testis, suggesting that only ERbeta mediates the action of estrogen in the human male gonad [61]. Palmieri et al. [62] evaluated the expression of ERalpha and ERbeta by immunochemistry in normal breast tissue samples, and in purified human breast fibroblasts by Western blotting, RT-PCR analysis, and ligand-binding sucrose gradient assay. They observed that ERbeta variants, including ERbeta1, ERbeta2, ERbeta5, and ERbeta delta but not ERalpha, were expressed in human adult mammary fibroblasts. These results are supported by the findings that an ERbeta-selective ligand, BAG, but not the ERalpha high-affinity ligand E_2, can induce fibroblast growth factor-7 release and activate transcription from an estrogen-responsive element promoter in these adult human mammary fibroblasts. Together, these observations revealed that, in the adult breast and in breast cancer, the proliferative signals derived from the stroma of adult mammary glands in response to estrogen are not mediated by ERalpha and provide new insights into the nature of stromal-epithelial interactions in the adult mammary gland. In addition, the expression of these ERbeta variants in cells where there is no ERalpha suggested that these ERbeta splice forms may have functions other than that of modulating ERalpha activity [62].

MCF-10F cells are immortalized human breast epithelial cells (HBEC) negative for ERalpha but positive for ERbeta. Earlier passages of these cells have low levels of ERbeta mRNA expression but when they were transformed either by a chemical carcinogen, or estrogen or its metabolites [63, 64], the levels of ERbeta expression were enhanced [65]. E_2, 2-OH E_2, and 4-OH E_2 are capable of enhancing cell proliferation, and of transforming HBECs, inducing phenotypes that were not abrogated by the antiestrogen ICI182780 [64–68]. Although these observations suggest that ERbeta may play a role in E_2-mediated cell proliferation and transformation, the definitive role of this receptor remains elusive.

10.3.2 Influence of the Stroma in the Genomic Profile of the MCF-10F Cell that Behaves as a Stem Cell In Vitro

Considering that the HBEC MCF-10F could behave like a stem cell we aimed to determine the role of the stroma in the growth pattern of these cells in vitro. We have found that MCF-10F cells growing in collagen matrix form ductular structures mimicking the breast epithelia in vivo (Fig. 10.1). We performed cDNA microarray in order to determine the differential gene expression profile between the cells growing in monolayer and those growing in a tridimensional matrix and determining the role of the stroma in the ductulogenic process. We found 161 genes differentially expressed and up-modulated (log mean of difference >2.0, with $P<0.05$) in the ductular structures in comparison to the MCF-10F cells in monolayer [63]. Those genes are related to several biological functions such as gene transcription or regulation of transcription, such as Myeloid cell nuclear differentiation antigen (MNDA) [59–75], protein biosynthesis (such as Stromal cell-derived factor 2) [76], amino acid transport, and membrane trafficking (collagen, type IV, alpha 5 and RAB4, a member of the RAS oncogene family), DNA repair system (such as ADP-ribosyltransferase (NAD+, poly(ADP ribose) polymerase)-like 2) [77–87] and genes related to regulation of cell transformation such as transforming growth factor beta receptor III. Two of the genes that are highly relevant are the MNDA and the ADP-ribosyltransferase (NAD+, poly(ADP ribose) polymerase)-like 2 or PARP. The MNDA is expressed in a lineage-specific manner in myeloid cells [72–74]. MNDA may have an important role in myelomonocytic cell differentiation by exerting an antiproliferative effect on myeloid cell growth. In our specific model the MCF-10F cells express it under the stroma like effect of the collagen matrix and if could be involved in the expression of the organization of the ductal structures. MNDA may be related to the stem cell differentiation process in the HBECs.

ADP-ribosyltransferase (NAD+, poly (ADP ribose) polymerase)-like 2 is also upregulated in the ductular structures and is thought to participate in chromatin condensation, maintenance of genomic stability, and the repair of oxidative DNA

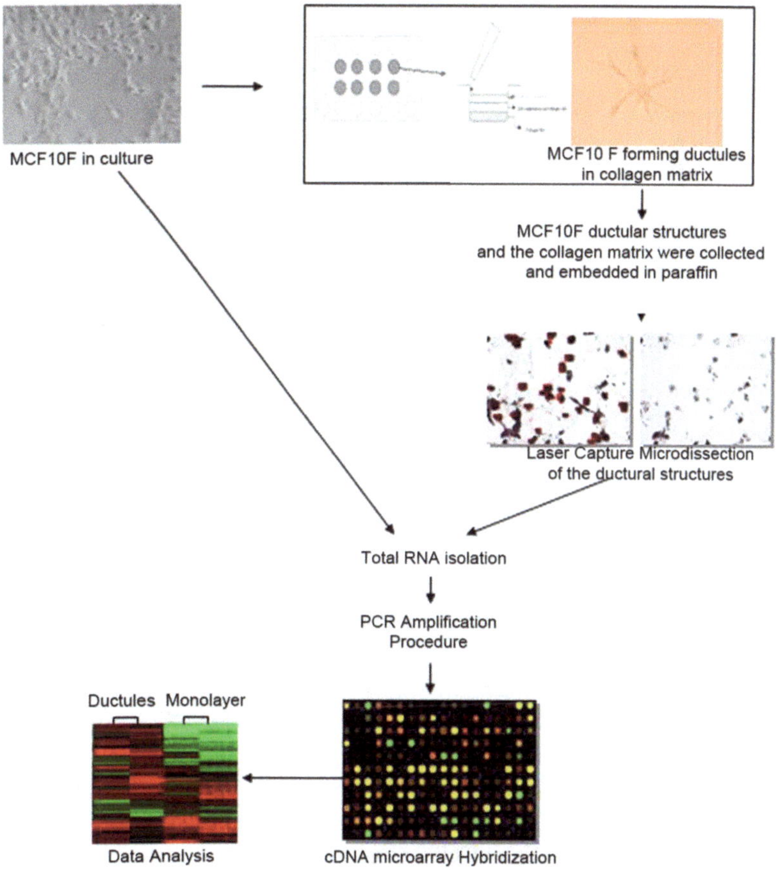

Fig. 10.1 Schematic representation of the steps to determine the differential gene expression profile between MCF-10F cells growing in monolayer and those forming ductular-like structures in collagen matrix after 21 days (modified from Russo et al. [63])

damage [77]. PARP binds to double and single DNA strand breaks, generated by reactive oxygen species and the DNA-bound repair enzymes during the repair process. Upon binding to strand breaks sites via two zinc fingers in its N-terminal region, PARP's catalytic activity increases 500-fold [78, 79]. PARP catalyzes the transfer of the ADP-ribose moiety of NAD+ onto a host of acceptor proteins such as histones, DNA topoisomerases, p53, DNA-dependent protein kinase, and other DNA binding proteins, including itself, thus forming long branched polymers of ADP-ribose [80–83]. The high negative charge associated with poly ADP-ribosylation electrostatically repels the modified proteins from DNA and this is thought to clear the damaged site of chromatin and other extraneous proteins and facilitate repair [84, 85]. Although PARP is necessary for the repair of damaged DNA that allows continued cell

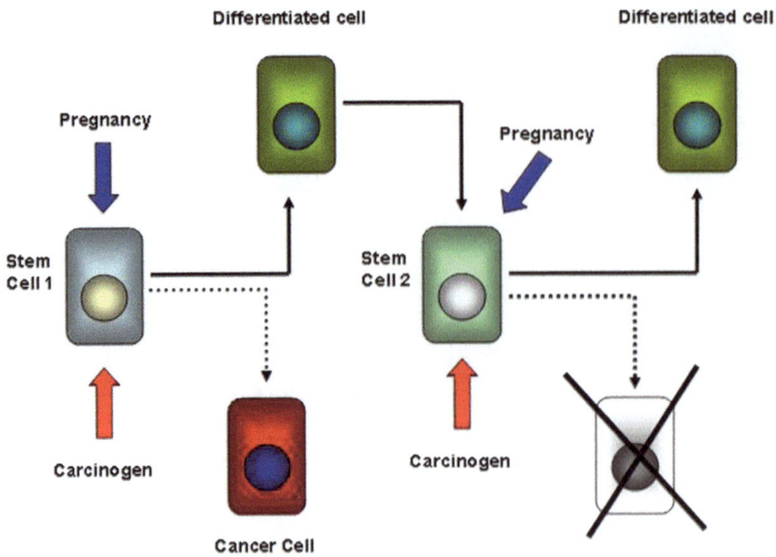

Fig. 10.2 The terminal differentiation hypothesis of breast cancer prevention (modified from Russo, J. and Russo, I.H. Role of differentiation in the pathogenesis and prevention of breast cancer. Endocrine Related Cancer 4:7–21, 1997)

survival, it is widely recognized that in the face of extensive DNA strand breaks, PARP activation can lead to depletion of NAD+, decreases in intracellular ATP levels, and cell death [86, 87], all properties that are part of the genomic make up of a differentiated cell like the Stem Cell 2 (Fig. 10.2).

10.3.3 The MCF-10F Cell as the Stem Cell in Estrogen-Induced Carcinogenesis

There is substantial amount of epidemiological, clinical and experimental evidence pointing to estrogens, e.g., 17β-estradiol (E_2), as being one of the most important etiological factors for the development and progression of breast cancer [64]. To test the transforming ability of estrogens on MCF-10F cells that are ERalpha negative, ERbeta positive and progesterone receptor negative, they were treated twice a week during 2 weeks with 70 nM 17β-E_2 [64]. These cells expressed transformation phenotypes such as the formation of colonies in agar methocel, and the loss of the ductulogenic capacity when they grew in a collagen matrix. In order to identify the more aggressive transformed cells capable of forming tumors after E_2 treatment, we have selected the highly invasive populations of MCF-10F cells treated with E_2

in their ninth passage by seeding them in Boyden chambers (see Chap. 3). Those cells crossing the membrane were collected, expanded, and designated B2, B3, B4, B5, C2, C3, C4 and C5. Four of them, B2, C3, C4 and C5 cells were injected to severe combined immune depressed (SCID) mice. Only C3 and C5 cells were tumorigenic in 2/12 and 9/10 animals injected, respectively. The tumors were poorly differentiated adenocarcinomas, ERalpha, and PR negative, and expressed basic keratin of high molecular weight, E-Cadherin, CAM5.2, and vimentin. The genomic profile of C3 and C5 cells analyzed by cDNA microarray, revealed that C5 cells overexpressed more than fivefold tankyrase (chr 8p23.1), claudin 1 (chr 3q28), homeobox C10 (HOX-C10; chr 12q13.3), and Notch homolog 3 (chr 19p13.12). It also exhibited downregulation of telomeric repeat binding factor 1 (chr 8q21.11) and tumor metastasis suppressor LASS2 (chr 1q21.3) genes. Four tumoral cell lines were obtained from four of the nine tumors derived from C5: C5-A1-T1, C5-A4-T4, C5-A6-T6, and C5-A8-T8 and all of them produced tumors when they were injected to SCID mice. Comparative genomic hybridization (CGH) analysis was performed to identify gains and losses of genetic material in the different cell lines during the tumorigenic process. CGH analyses showed that the E_2-transformed cells (trMCF) (see Fig. 4.12) had no differences when compared with untreated MCF-10F cells, except for a loss in 9p11-13. The four tumors (An1, An4, An6, and An8) showed identical pattern of genomic imbalances. CGH analyses showed similar genomic patterns between the four tumors (A1, A4, A6, and A8) and the four cell lines derived from them (C5-A1-T1, C5-A4-T4, C5-A6-T6, and C5-A8-T8); and there were no additional chromosomal alterations after in vitro cell culture. All the tumors and derived cell lines showed gains of 1p, 5q15-qter, and 8q24.1-qter and losses of chromosome 4, 3p12.3-13, 8p11.1-21, 9p21-pter, and 18q24.1. The parental cell line C5 showed a tendency for gain of 1p and 5q15-qter and loss of chromosome 4 and it is likely that in the tumors derived from C5, a sub-clone with these changes had a selective advantage in vivo and became more distinct. Losses of 3p12.3-13, 8p11.1-21, 9p21-pter, and 18q appear to be new changes in the tumor. Interestingly, C5 and the cells treated with E_2 had loss of 9p11-13 while in the tumors the 9p21-pter was lost. The chromosomal alterations that we found in vitro are similar to those reported in primary breast cancer. Altogether our data show that 17β-estradiol is able to transform an HBEC and that the MCF-10F cell line has all the properties of a stem cell that is able to generate a tumor when challenged with a carcinogen agent.

10.4 The Evidence for the Shifting of Stem Cell 1 to Stem Cell 2 in the Mammary Gland Post-Pregnancy

Epidemiological studies in humans and experimental carcinogenesis models have provided wide evidence of the protective effect of pregnancy from breast cancer development [88–97]. Russo and coworkers [95, 98, 99] have postulated that the mechanism of pregnancy-induced protection is mediated by the induction of mammary gland differentiation driven by the hormonal milieu of pregnancy, which creates a specific genomic signature in the mammary gland that makes this organ permanently refractory to carcinogenesis [100, 101]. Alternative explanations attributed the protective effect of pregnancy to changes in the environmental milieu [102] and/or alterations in the immunological profile of the host [92]. A further refinement of the hypothesis of how pregnancy could be affecting cancer susceptibility through induction of differentiation of the mammary gland was first proposed by Russo and Russo [24], who postulated that the Lob 1 and the TEB found in the breast of nulliparous women or of young virgin rats, respectively, had not completed their differentiation into Lob 2, Lob 3, and Lob 4, retaining a high concentration of stem cells called Stem cell 1, which are susceptible to undergo neoplastic transformation when exposed to a carcinogenic agent (see previous section, Fig. 10.2) [24]. After the postmenopausal involution of the mammary gland, the architecture of the parous breast is similar to that of the nulliparous breast, containing predominantly Lob 1 composed of Stem cell 2, an epithelial cell population that is refractory to transformation. It was further postulated that the degree of differentiation acquired through early pregnancy permanently changes the "genomic signature" that differentiate the Lob 1 from early parous women from that of nulliparous women, shifting the Stem cell 1 to Stem cell 2 that is refractory to carcinogenesis. These cells were called Stem cell 2 because after post-lactational involution, the mammary epithelium remains capable of responding with proliferation and differentiation to the stimulus of a new pregnancy; however, these cells are refractory to carcinogenesis, even though they are stimulated to proliferate and to regenerate the whole mammary gland (Fig. 10.2). The Stem cell 2 is characterized by having a genomic signature that has been induced by the first cycle of differentiation. During the last 8 years, supporting evidence to this hypothesis has been generated by Russo and coworkers as well as by other researchers. Studies by Smith and coworkers [103–105] using transgenic WAP-driven Cre and Rosa 26-fl-stop-fl-LacZ mice provided evidence of a new mammary epithelial cell population that originates from differentiated cells during pregnancy; 5–10% of this parity-induced epithelium survives post-lactational involution after the first pregnancy. With successive pregnancies, their percentage increases, reaching 60% of the total epithelium in multiparous females. The parity-induced mammary epithelial cells (PI-MEC) is equivalent to the Stem cell 2 postulated by Russo and Russo [24], since these cells show capacity for self-renewal and contribute to mammary outgrowth in transplantation studies. PI-MEC can function as alveolar progenitors in subsequent pregnancies, and it is thought that they would be related to differences in response to hormonal stimulation and carcinogenic agents observed between nulliparous and parous females [103–105].

The crucial role of the number of mammary stem cells in breast cancer risk has also been postulated by Trichopoulos et al. [106], number that would be reduced through the process of terminal differentiation after the first full-term pregnancy that in certain way is the same idea of shifting the number of Stem cell 1 to another more differentiated cells or Stem cell 2 postulated earlier by Russo and Russo [24]. Several authors have focused in finding molecular changes as a mechanism of the pregnancy-induced protection [107–114]. Russo and coworkers have found that the post-pregnancy involuted rat mammary gland exhibits a genomic signature characterized by elevated expression of genes involved in the apoptotic pathways, such as testosterone repressed prostate message 2 (TRPM2), interleukin 1 beta-converting enzyme (ICE), bcl-XL, bcl-XS, p53, p21, and c-myc, which can be from 3- to 5-fold upregulated [107, 108, 115]. The activation of programmed cell death genes occurs through a p53-dependent process, modulated by c-myc and with partial dependence on the bcl2-family-related genes. In addition, inhibin A and B, heterodimeric nonsteroidal secreted glycoproteins with tumor suppressor activity are also upregulated [107, 108, 115, 116]. Genes whose level of expression progressively increases with time of pregnancy reaching their highest levels between 21 and 42 days postpartum are those coding for a fragment of glycogen phosphorylase, AMP-activated kinase, bone morphogenetic protein 4, and vesicle-associated protein 1. G/T mismatch-specific thymine DNA glycosylase gene is also increased by fivefold in this model. These data indicate that the activation of genes involved in the DNA repair process is part of the signature induced in the mammary gland by pregnancy. These observations confirm previous findings that in vivo the ability of the cells to repair carcinogen-induced damage by unscheduled DNA synthesis and adduct removal is more efficient in the parous animal mammary gland [98]. In concordance with the studies of Srivastava et al. [107], Sivaraman et al. [111] observed that p53 can be implicated in the protective effect of parity, which can be mimicked by treatment of virgin rats with estrogen and progesterone. Studies by Medina et al. [109, 110] in the same hormonal model reported that the function of p53 is required for the hormone-mediated protection of DMBA-induced mammary tumorigenesis in mice. Genomic analysis of the mammary gland of virgin rats treated with estrogen and progesterone at doses that have been reported to mimic pregnancy, showed down-regulation of certain growth-promoting molecules, whereas markers involved in cell cycle control or the modulation of transforming growth factor beta (TGF-beta) signaling pathway were upregulated in the posttreatment involuted mammary gland [112]. In this study, an unknown noncoding RNA (designated G.B7) and RbAp46, which has been implicated in a number of complexes involving chromatin remodeling, were found to be persistently upregulated in the lobules of the regressed glands. Using gene profile analysis, D'Cruz et al. [114] also observed down regulation of growth factors potentially involved in epithelial proliferation as well as persistent upregulation of TGF-beta3 and several of its transcripts targets in the involuted gland of parous rats and mice. The proposed model of parity-induced specific changes [24] has been further confirmed by Ginger and Rosen [113], who reported that pregnancy induces multiple changes in the mammary epithelial cells, including nuclear accumulation of p53 and induction of whey acidic protein (WAP). During involution, a large component of the epithelium is eliminated through apoptosis, and a specific subpopulation of epithelial cells survives this process. The involuted mammary gland has persistent changes in gene expression, nuclear localization of p53, and an altered proliferative capacity in response to a carcinogen. Pregnancy would induce epigenetic changes, such as chromatin remodeling, DNA methylation/demethylation, and histone modifications, affecting cell fate in the parous mammary gland. As it has been previously published [63] all the genes that have been related to the Stem cell 2 seem to work in a different functional pathways than those described for the Stem cell 1.

Collectively, the data described above present evidence that pregnancy, through the process of cell differentiation, shifts the Stem cell 1 to Stem cell 2 (Fig. 10.2), cells that exhibit a specific genomic signature that could be responsible for the refractoriness of the mammary gland to carcinogenesis.

10.5 Isolation of the Stem Cells from the Rat Mammary Gland

10.5.1 Isolation of Stem Cells

In order to propagate sufficient rat mammary stem cells we adapted the methodology employed for the propagation of mouse mammary stem cells utilizing StemCell Technologies (Fig. 10.3). Right and left mammary abdominal glands were obtained from anesthetized 50–99-day-old virgin female Sprague Dawley rats. Dissections were performed in a sterile laminar flow hood. The tissue was then placed in 1× gentle collagenase/hyaluronidase solution and incubated 15 h at 37°C with gentle shaking. After dissociation, cell pellets were resuspended with a 1:4 mixture of ammonium chloride (NH_4Cl) and cold Hanks' Balanced Salt Solution supplemented with 2% FBS and centrifuged at 350×*g* for 5 min. The resultant organoids were sequentially resuspended in 0.25% Trypsin-EDTA for 2 min, 5 mg/mL Dispase I plus 0.1 mg/mL DNase I for 2 min, and followed by filtration through a 40 μm cell strainer to obtain single cell suspensions. For the enrichment of mammary epithelial cells a single cell suspension at a concentration of 1×10^8 cells/mL was prepared in Hanks' Balanced Salt Solution supplemented with 2% FBS (HF), followed by 15 min incubation of EasySep Negative Selection Mouse Mammary Epithelial Cell Enrichment Cocktail and another 15 min incubation of EasySep Biotin Selection Cocktail. Magnet Nanoparticles were then added in and $CD45^+$/$Ter119^+$, and $CD31^+$ cells were removed by magnet selection. Cells were ready for culturing after the viability was checked by trypan blue staining. After selection of cells with EasySep mouse mammary stem cell enrichment kit, the cells were resuspended in HF and stained with a 1:50 dilution of CD24-PE and CD49f-FITC for 30 min on ice followed by 2 μg/mL propidium iodide. Analysis of CD24-PE- or CD49f-FITC-positive cells was done by FACS Vantage SE Becton Dickinson BD Flow Cytometer (Fig. 10.4).

10.5.2 Mammosphere Culture Conditions

Mammary epithelial cells enriched single cells were grown in 6-well ultra-low attachment plate at a density of 25,000 or 50,000 cells/mL in complete EpiCult-B medium (#06100, StemCell technology) containing 10 ng/mL EGF, 10 ng/mL basic

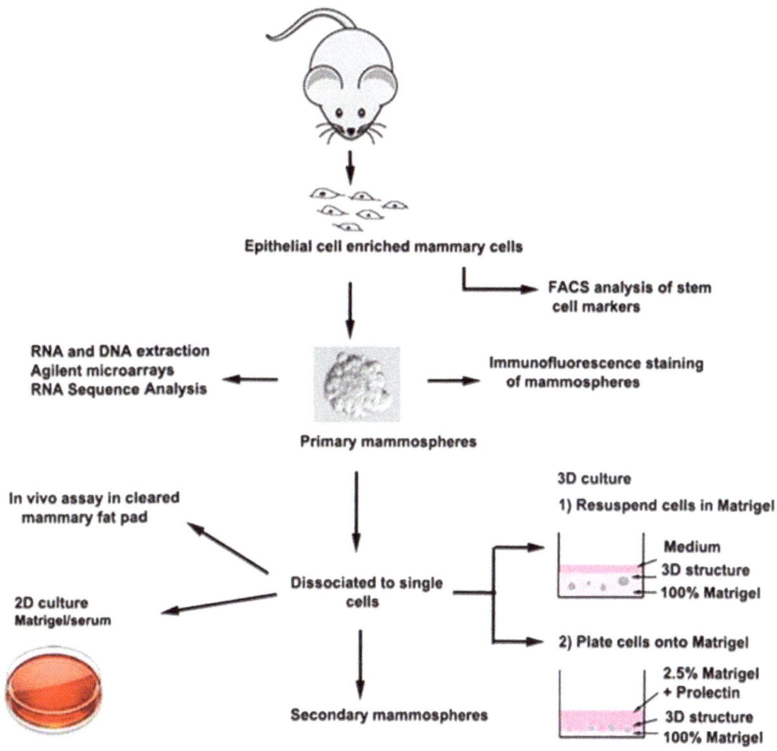

Fig. 10.3 Different steps involved in the preparation and analysis of mammospheres

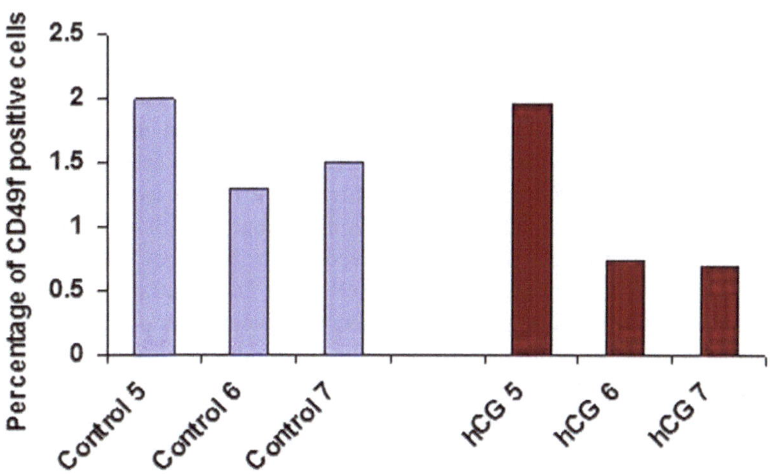

Fig. 10.4 FACS analysis of stem cell markers. CD49f: alpha 6 integrin that is associated with bipotent progenitor cells and myoepithelial cells

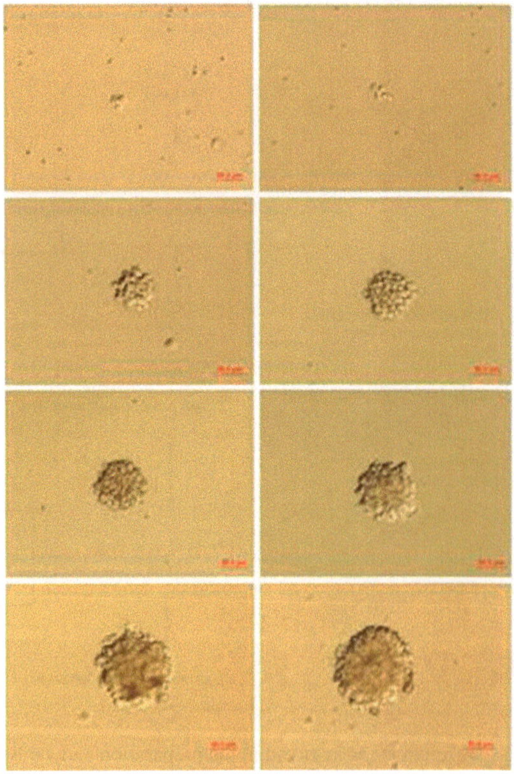

Fig. 10.5 Freshly isolated rat mammary gland cells form mammospheres. Epithelial cells enriched rat mammary cells were plated on ultra-low attachment 6-well plate at a density of 25,000 cells/mL in complete EpiCult-B medium

fibroblast growth factor (bFGF), 4 μg/mL Heparin, and 1× Pen/Strep/Fungizone. The formation of mammospheres was daily monitored by examination under an inverted microscope and photographed every other day (Fig. 10.5). After 7–8 days in culture, mammospheres were counted and then collected using a 40 μm cell strainer and dissociated with 0.05% Trypsin-EDTA for 2 min at 37°C for obtaining single cell suspensions. Primary mammosphere-derived cells were plated at a density of 25,000 cells/mL for the culture of secondary mammospheres. Primary mammosphere-derived single cells were mixed with Matrigel at a density of 600 cells/400 μL Matrigel per well in 24-well plate. Differentiation assay medium was added onto the Matrigel after it solidified. One week after plating, the medium was changed with differentiation assay medium containing 1 μg/mL prolactin and refreshed every week. Cells were fixed with 10% formalin for 30 min at room temperature and followed with immunofluorescence staining after 25 days of culture. We were able to culture mammospheres from single rat mammary epithelial cells in a suspension culture in low-attachment dishes. We were successful in culturing and passing these to produce mammospheres demonstrating their self-renewal capability, results similar to reports of mammosphere formation from human mammary

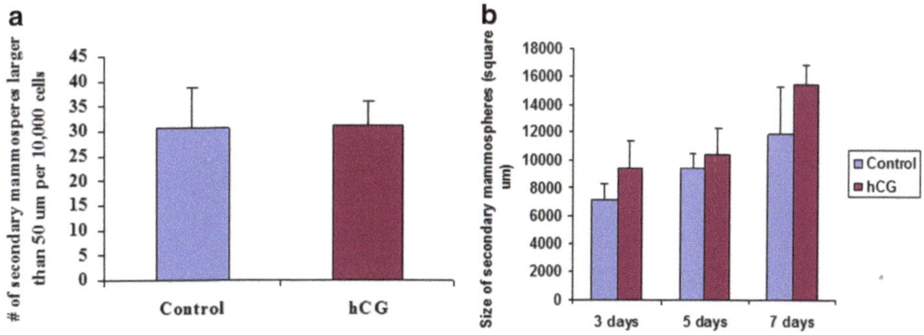

Fig. 10.6 There are no significant differences in the number and size of secondary mammospheres

cells [20]. The frequencies of primary mammospheres formed from epithelial cells enriched rat mammary cells are 2–6 spheres/1,000 cells, which are similar to other reports on human (~7 spheres/1,000 cells) [20] and mouse; (~2 spheres/1,000 cells) [117] mammary cells. Twenty five to fifty percent of dissociated cells from rat mammary epithelial mammospheres were recovered and regenerated new mammospheres. The frequency of secondary mammospheres formed from primary mammosphere-derived cells were 2–4 spheres/1,000 cells, which is similar to previous report in humans [20].

10.5.3 *Effect of hCG the Mimicking Hormone of Pregnancy in Mammospheres Formation*

We have isolated the stem cells of the mammary gland of rats treated with hCG for 21 days and allowed to rest another additional 21 days (see Chap. 2) and compared if there was a difference in the formation of mammospheres between the control and hCG-treated cells. We have found that the mammary epithelial cells from rats treated with hCG formed significantly less primary mammospheres supporting the concept in reduction of stem cells; however, the size of the mammospheres was not significantly different. There were also no differences in the number and size of the secondary mammospheres (Fig. 10.6a, b) or tertiary mammospheres (Fig. 10.7a, b).

10.5.4 *Characterization of Cells from Mammospheres*

For immunofluorescence staining the mammospheres were centrifuged on glass slides and fixed with acetone-methanol (1:1) for 10 min at −20°C. The staining of

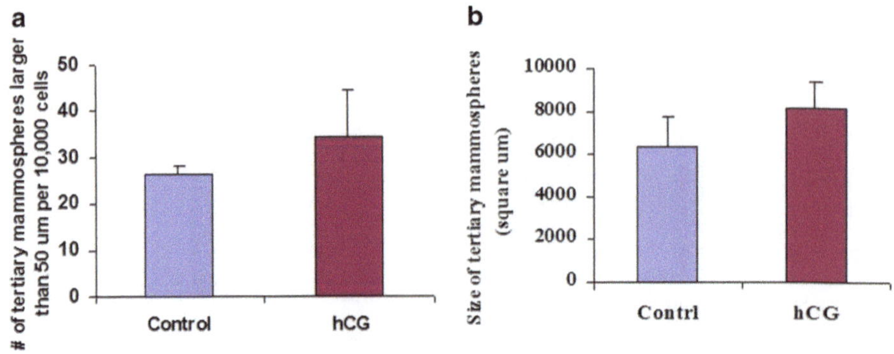

Fig. 10.7 There are no significant differences in the number and size of tertiary mammospheres

2D differentiation assay was performed in 3 cm dishes. The following primary antibodies were used: ESA, CK14, CK18, and β-casein. Alexa fluor 555 donkey anti-rabbit, alexa fluor 488 donkey anti-mouse, and alexa fluor 647 donkey anti-goat secondary antibodies were used to detect the staining. As it is depicted in Fig. 10.8, primary mammospheres reacted with ESA (EpCAM) that is a marker of bipotent progenitor cells and differentiated luminal cells and also reacted with CK14 that is attributed to differentiated myoepithelial cells or to putative progenitor cells. Of interest is that the primary mammospheres are positive for CD24 that is significantly reduced in the mammary gland of hCG-treated animals (Fig. 10.9). Immunostaining with CK14 showed that this antibody was expressed in some of the cells in primary mammospheres obtained from hCG-treated rats, whereas it was rarely observed in the spheres from control animals (Fig. 10.10).

Primary mammosphere-derived cells are capable of differentiation into different types of colonies under differentiating conditions (Fig. 10.11). Using ESA, CK14, and beta casein as markers of cell differentiation we found that there are more colonies with three lineages differentiation after hCG treatment (Fig. 10.12). Of interest is the finding that hCG induces the formation of more colonies containing myoepithelial cells (Fig. 10.13).

We have compared the transcriptomic profile of the stems cells of the mammary gland from the control and hCG-treated animals (Table 10.1) and we demonstrated by both microarray and real-time RT-PCR that CD24 is significantly reduced in the mammospheres from hCG-treated rats (Fig. 10.14 and Table 10.2). MME (CD10) is significantly reduced in mammospheres from hCG-treated rats based on the real-time RT-PCR result, whereas it did not appear significantly changed by microarray analysis (FDR 0.138). The myoepithelial markers Krt (CK14) and ASMA showed upregulation in the mammospheres from hCG-treated rats by both microarray and real-time RT-PCR analysis, but none of them reached statistical significance (P=0.086, FDR 0.269 and P=0.032, FDR 0.164, respectively)) (Table 10.2 and Fig. 10.14). Genes reported in the literature to be highly specific for myoepithelial

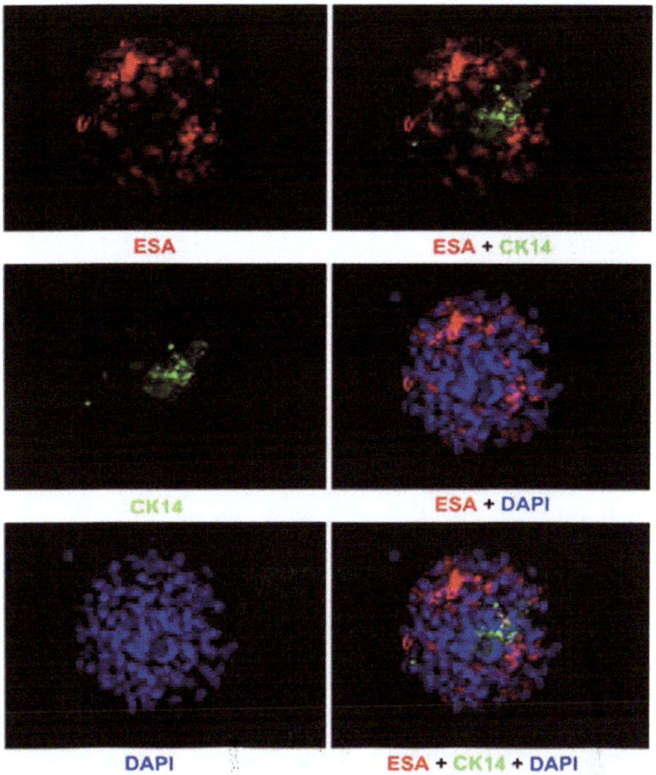

Fig. 10.8 Cellular composition of primary mammospheres from rat mammary gland. ESA (EpCAM) is a bipotent progenitor cells and differentiated luminal cells. CK14: differentiated myoepithelial cells and attributed to putative progenitor cells. Seven-day-old primary mammospheres were centrifuged on slides and fixed with acetone-methanol (1:1). The cellular composition was checked by the antibodies ESA and CK14 staining indicated under pictures

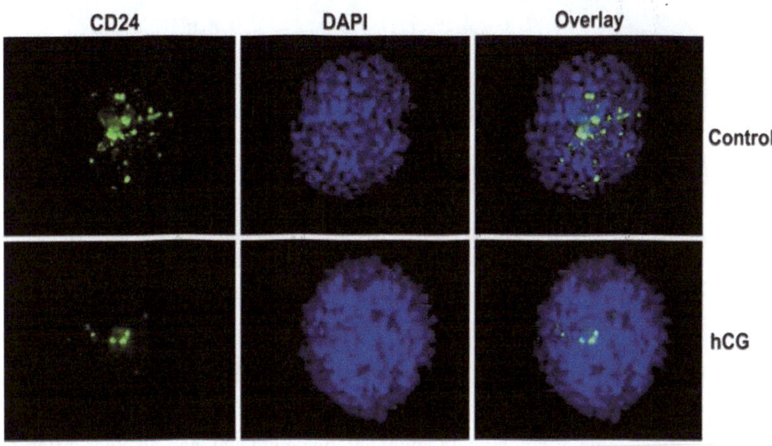

Fig. 10.9 CD24-positive cells are reduced in the primary mammospheres from rats of 21 days post hCG treatment. Staining on cytospin slides (mammospheres)

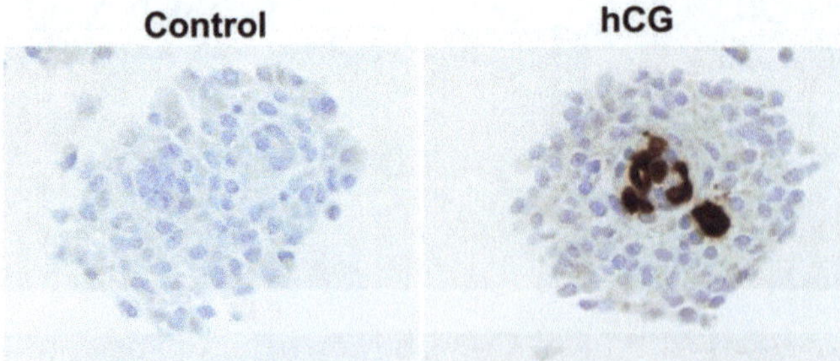

Fig. 10.10 Immunostaining with CK14 showed CK14 is expressed in some of the cells in primary mammospheres from hCG-treated rats, whereas is hard to observed in the spheres from control

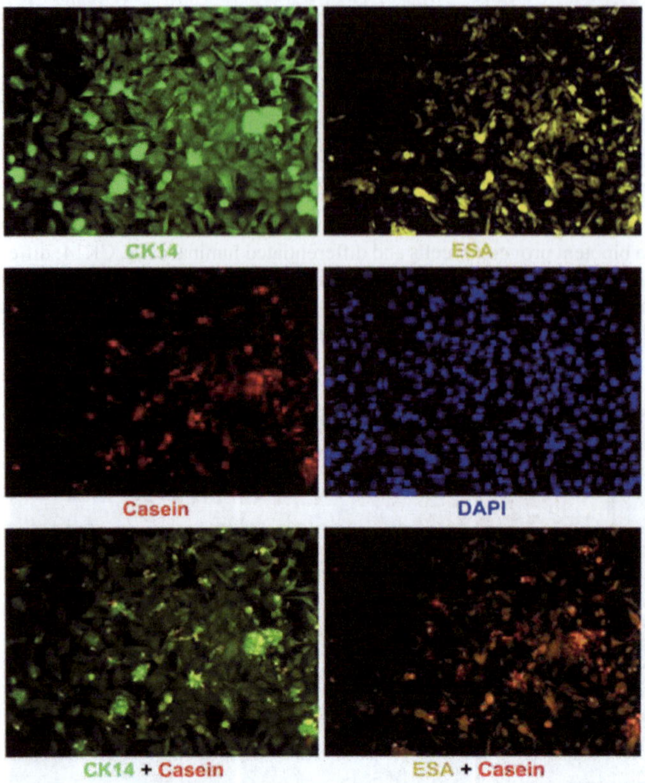

Fig. 10.11 ICC/IF staining of colony with epithelial, myoepithelial, and alveolar differentiation. Images are taken by monochrome camera, the color showing is pseudocolor

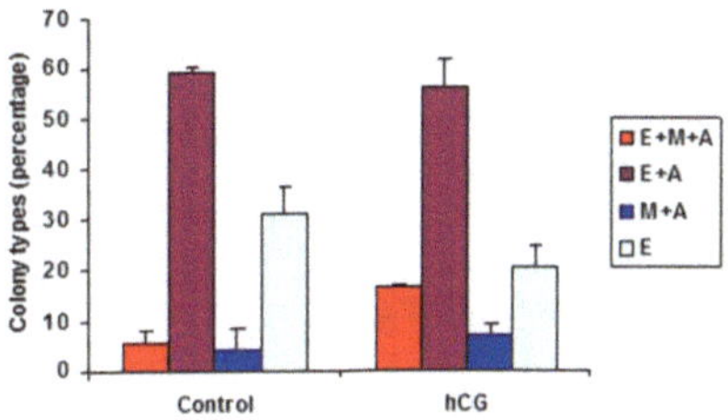

E: epithelial differentiation by ESA staining
M: myoepitheilal differentiation by CK14 staining
A: aveolar differentiation by Beta-casein staining

Percentage	E+M+A	E+A	M+A	E
Control	5.4±2.5	59.4±1.0	4.1±4.2	31.0±2.6
hCG	16.5±0.4	56.1±5.4	6.8±2.3	20.6±4.5

Fig. 10.12 There are more colonies with three lineages differentiation after hCG treatment

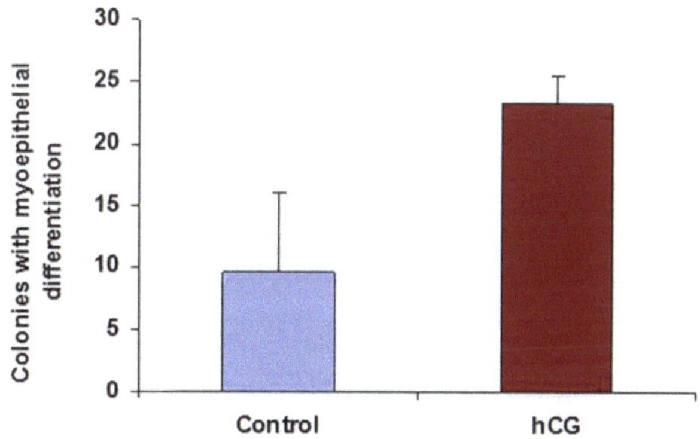

Fig. 10.13 There are more colonies with myoepithelial differentiation after hCG treatment (2D differentiation assay). Test: $P = 0.026$

Table 10.1 Level of Expression of Transcripts detected in the Mammary Gland of Rats treated with hCG vs. Control

Markers used to characterize mammospheres in the literature			Microarray data			
Marker	Symbol	Gene name	Log FC	Fold change	*P*-value	FDR
ASMA	Acta2	Smooth muscle alpha-actin	0.38	1.31	0.032	0.164
Cd24	Cd24	CD24 molecule	−1.42	0.37	0.000	0.033
ESA	Epcam	Epithelial cell adhesion molecule	−0.27	0.83	0.503	0.702
Alpha 6 integrin (CD49f)	Itga6	Integrin, alpha 6	−0.05	0.97	0.728	0.855
CK14	Krt14	Keratin 14	0.92	1.89	0.086	0.269
CK18	Krt18	Keratin 18	−0.19	0.88	0.674	0.820
CK5	Krt5	Keratin 5	0.69	1.61	0.162	0.378
CD10	MME	Membrane metallo-endopeptidase	−0.78	0.58	0.021	0.138
Muc1	Muc1	Mucin 1, cell surface associated	Not found in the arrays			

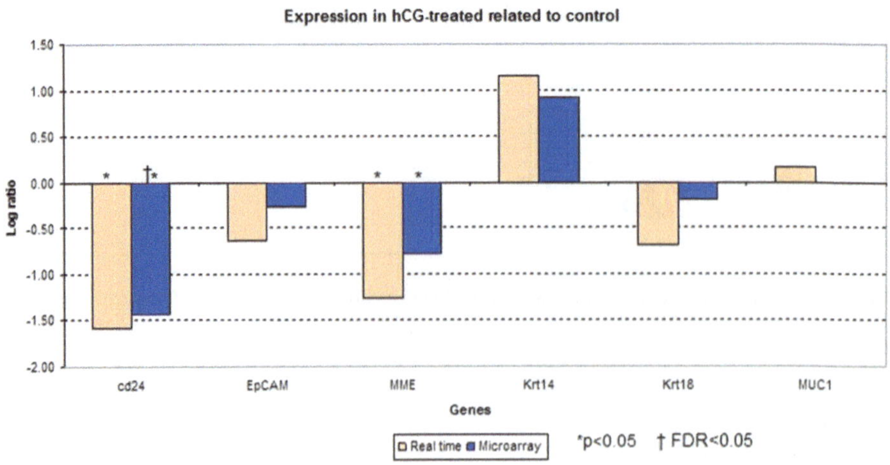

Fig. 10.14 Comparison of microarray data to qPCR results

Table 10.2 Comparison of the transcriptomic profile of the mammary gland of control and hCG-treated rats evaluated by real time RT-PCR and microarray

	Real-time RT-PCR			Microarray			
Detector	Log FC	Fold change	*P* value	Log FC	Fold change	*P* value	FDR
CD24	−1.58	0.33	0.000	−1.42	0.37	0.000	0.033
EpCAM (ESA)	−0.64	0.64	0.216	−0.27	0.83	0.503	0.702
MME (CD10)	−1.26	0.42	0.008	−0.78	0.58	0.021	0.138
Krt14 (CK14)	1.15	2.22	0.138	0.92	1.89	0.086	0.269
Krt18 (CK18)	−0.69	0.62	0.383	−0.19	0.88	0.674	0.820
Muc1	0.16	1.12	0.725	Not found in the array			

Table 10.3 Level of Expression of Myoepithelial Cell Markers detected in the Mammary Gland of Rats treated with hCG vs. Control

Symbol	Gene name	Log FC	Fold change	*P* value	FDR
Adamts1	ADAM metallopeptidase with thrombospondin type 1 motif, 1	0.68	1.61	0.001	0.047
Cyr61	Cystein-rich, angiogenic inducer, 61	0.78	1.72	0.000	0.033
Igfbp3	Insulin-like growth factor binding protein 3	0.78	1.71	0.001	0.042
Tpm1	Tropomyosin 1	1.05	2.06	0.001	0.042

cells, such as Adamts1, Cyr61, Igfbp3, and Tpm1, are significantly upregulated in the primary mammospheres from hCG-treated rats (Table 10.3). The adamalysin-thrombospondin (ADAMTS) proteinases have been implicated in various cellular events, including cleavage of proteoglycans, extracellular matrix degradation, inhibition of angiogenesis, gonadal development, and organogenesis. The expression of ADAMTS1 in breast tissues is higher in stromal fibroblasts and myoepithelial cells, but it is poorly expressed in luminal epithelial cells. ADAMTS1 is significantly downregulated in invasive breast carcinoma compared to non-neoplastic mammary tissue [118]. ADAMTS1 is cancer-specific hypermethylated in colorectal tumors [119], and its expression is decreased in prostate cancer, and might be involved in the early steps of prostate cancer development [120].

Although IGFBP-3 has no direct inhibitory effect on breast cancer cells Hs578T, it could accentuate apoptosis induced by the physiological trigger ceramide in an IGF-independent manner [121], whereas the expression of IGFBP-3 in MCF-7 cells leads to the induction of apoptosis through the activation of caspases involved in a death receptor-mediated pathway, an indication that IGFBP-3 functions as a negative regulator of breast cancer cell growth, independent of the IGF-IGF receptor axis [122]. Another gene that is upregulated in myoepithelial cells is Tropomyosin-1 that functions as a suppressor of transformation [123] and has been shown can resensitize breast cancer cells to anoikis [124].

Canonical pathway analyses of microarray data obtained from mammospheres of the mammary gland of rats treated with hCG have shown that pathways involved in the immune system are downregulated after hCG treatment, which is consistent with our previous microarray data from rat mammary gland tissues of in vivo experiment discussed in Chap. 3.

10.6 The Importance of the Mammary Gland Stem Cell and Pregnancy in the Prevention of Breast Cancer

Our comparative studies of human and rodent mammary development in relation to age and parity [99, 125–129] have revealed that the development of the mammary gland is a progressive process of growth initiated at childhood [130, 131]. Epidemiological studies in humans and experimental carcinogenesis models have provided wide evidence of the protective effect of pregnancy from breast cancer development [83–89, 132–134]. Russo and coworkers [98, 99, 135] have postulated that the mechanism of pregnancy-induced protection is mediated by the induction of mammary gland differentiation driven by the hormonal milieu of pregnancy, which creates a specific genomic signature in the mammary gland that makes this organ permanently refractory to carcinogenesis. A further refinement of the hypothesis of how pregnancy could be affecting cancer susceptibility through induction of differentiation of the mammary gland was first proposed by Russo and Russo [24], who postulated that the Lob 1 and the TEB found in the breast of nulliparous women or of young virgin rats, respectively, had not completed their differentiation into Lob 2, Lob 3, and Lob 4, retaining a high concentration of S/PC or Stem cell 1, which is susceptible to undergo neoplastic transformation when exposed to a carcinogenic agent [24] (Fig. 10.2). Although after the postmenopausal involution of the mammary gland, the architecture of the breast in parous women is similar to that of the nulliparous women, both containing predominantly Lob 1, in parous women the Lob 1 is composed of Stem cell 2, an epithelial cell population that through the completion of differentiation induced by pregnancy has permanently changed its "genomic signature" and becomes refractory to transformation [100, 101]. Nevertheless, the Stem cell 2 remains capable of responding with proliferation and differentiation to the stimulus of a new pregnancy. The Stem cell 2 is characterized by a genomic signature that has been induced by the first cycle of differentiation. The crucial role of the number of mammary stem cells in breast cancer risk has been postulated by Trichopoulos et al. [106] but the concept that their number would be reduced through the process of terminal differentiation after the first full-term pregnancy has been indicated previously [24]. *However, an important concept in our study is that in the process of differentiation is not only the number of stem cells but the shifting of stem cell 1 to stem cell 2 by changing the genomic and epigenomic profile of these cells, as it has been recently reported to be the case in the breast of postmenopausal parous women* [100, 101]. Several authors have focused in finding molecular changes as a mechanism of the pregnancy-induced protection. Russo and coworkers have found that the post-pregnancy involuted mammary gland exhibits a specific genomic signature as well as epigenetic changes, such as chromatin remodeling, DNA methylation/demethylation, and histone modifications that affect cell fate in the breast of parous women [100, 101]. *Collectively, the data described above present evidence that pregnancy, through the process of cell differentiation, shifts the Stem cell 1 to Stem cell 2. These cells exhibit a specific genomic signature that could be responsible for the refractoriness of the mammary gland to carcinogenesis* [100, 101].

Acknowledgments We, the authors, acknowledge the contributions of the many members of the Breast Cancer Research Laboratory, and more specifically Yanrong Su, Ph.D.; Julia Pereira, Ph.D.; Ricardo Lopez de Cicco, Ph.D.; Fathima Sheriff, M.D.; Mr. Thomas Pogash; and Ms. Theresa Nguyen who have worked with us to generate the data incorporated in Sect. 10.5 in this chapter and allowed us to elaborate it into a unified concept.

References

1. Deome KB, Faulkin LJ Jr, Bern HA, Blair PB (1959) Development of mammary tumors from hyperplastic alveolar nodules transplanted into gland-free mammary fat pads of female C3H mice. Cancer Res 19:515–520
2. Kordon EC, Smith GH (1998) An entire functional mammary gland may comprise the progeny from a single cell. Development 125:1921–1930
3. Russo J, Saby J, Isenberg WM, Russo IH (1977) Pathogenesis of mammary carcinomas induced in rats by 7,12-dimethylbenz(a)anthracene. J Natl Cancer Inst 59:436–445
4. Russo J, Isenberg W, Ireland M, Russo I (1976) Ultrastructural changes in the mammary epithelial cell population during neoplastic development induced by a chemical carcinogen. Proceedings Electron Microscopy Society of America (G.W. Bailey, ed.), Claitors' Publishing Division, Baton Rouge, Louisiana, 34:250–251

5. Russo J, Tait L, Russo IH (1983) Susceptibility of the mammary gland to carcinogenesis. III. The cell of origin of rat mammary carcinoma. Am J Pathol 113:50–66
6. Russo J, Tay LK, Russo IH (1982) Differentiation of the mammary gland and susceptibility to carcinogenesis. Breast Cancer Res Treat 2:5–73
7. Bennett DC, Peachey LA, Durbin H, Rudland PS (1978) A possible mammary stem cell line. Cell 15:283–298
8. Rudland PS, Bennett DC, Warburton MJ (1980) Isolation and characterization of epithelial stem-cell cell lines from the rat mammary gland. Br J Cancer 41:666–668
9. Chepko G, Smith GH (1997) Three division-competent, structurally-distinct cell populations contribute to murine mammary epithelial renewal. Tissue Cell 29:239–253
10. Smith GH, Mehrel T, Roop DR (1990) Differential keratin gene expression in developing, differentiating, preneoplastic, and neoplastic mouse mammary epithelium. Cell Growth Differ 1:161–170
11. Stingl J, Eaves CJ, Kuusk U, Emerman JT (1998) Phenotypic and functional characterization in vitro of a multipotent epithelial cell present in the normal adult human breast. Differentiation 63:201–213
12. Stingl J, Eaves CJ, Zandieh I, Emerman JT (2001) Characterization of bipotent mammary epithelial progenitor cells in normal adult human breast tissue. Breast Cancer Res Treat 67:93–109
13. Hebbard L, Steffen A, Zawadzki V, Fieber C, Howells N, Moll J, Ponta H, Hofmann M, Sleeman J (2000) CD44 expression and regulation during mammary gland development and function. J Cell Sci 113(pt 14):2619–2630
14. Kenney NJ, Smith GH, Lawrence E, Barrett JC, Salomon DS (2001) Identification of stem cell units in the terminal end bud and duct of the mouse mammary gland. J Biomed Biotechnol 1:133–143
15. Spangrude GJ, Aihara Y, Weissman IL, Klein J (1988) The stem cell antigens Sca-1 and Sca-2 subdivide thymic and peripheral T lymphocytes into unique subsets. J Immunol 141:3697–3707
16. Welm BE, Tepera SB, Venezia T, Graubert TA, Rosen JM, Goodell MA (2002) Sca-1(pos) cells in the mouse mammary gland represent an enriched progenitor cell population. Dev Biol 245:42–56
17. Zhou S, Schuetz JD, Bunting KD, Colapietro AM, Sampath J, Morris JJ, Lagutina I, Grosveld GC, Osawa M, Nakauchi H, Sorrentino BP (2001) The ABC transporter Bcrp1/ABCG2 is expressed in a wide variety of stem cells and is a molecular determinant of the side-population phenotype. Nat Med 7:1028–1034
18. Alvi AJ, Clayton H, Joshi C, Enver T, Ashworth A, Vivanco MM, Dale TC, Smalley MJ (2003) Functional and molecular characterisation of mammary side population cells. Breast Cancer Res 5:R1–R8
19. Gudjonsson T, Villadsen R, Nielsen HL, Ronnov-Jessen L, Bissell MJ, Petersen OW (2002) Isolation, immortalization, and characterization of a human breast epithelial cell line with stem cell properties. Genes Dev 16:693–706
20. Dontu G, Abdallah WM, Foley JM, Jackson KW, Clarke MF, Kawamura MJ, Wicha MS (2003) In vitro propagation and transcriptional profiling of human mammary stem/progenitor cells. Genes Dev 17:1253–1270
21. Jia Y, Qi C, Zhang Z, Zhu YT, Rao SM, Zhu YJ (2005) Peroxisome proliferator-activated receptor-binding protein null mutation results in defective mammary gland development. J Biol Chem 280:10766–10773
22. Couse JF, Korach KS (1999) Estrogen receptor null mice: what have we learned and where will they lead us? Endocr Rev 20:358–417
23. Russo J, Ao X, Grill C, Russo IH (1999) Pattern of distribution of cells positive for estrogen receptor alpha and progesterone receptor in relation to proliferating cells in the mammary gland. Breast Cancer Res Treat 53:217–227
24. Russo J, Russo IH (1997) Role of differentiation in the pathogenesis and prevention of breast cancer. Endocr Relat Cancer 4:7–21

25. Petersen OW, Gudjonsson T, Villadsen R, Bissell MJ, Ronnov-Jessen L (2003) Epithelial progenitor cell lines as models of normal breast morphogenesis and neoplasia. Cell Prolif 36(suppl 1):33–44
26. Clarke RB, Anderson E, Howell A, Potten CS (2003) Regulation of human breast epithelial stem cells. Cell Prolif 36(suppl 1):45–58
27. Clarke RB, Spence K, Anderson E, Howell A, Okano H, Potten CS (2005) A putative human breast stem cell population is enriched for steroid receptor-positive cells. Dev Biol 277:443–456
28. Clayton H, Titley I, Vivanco M (2004) Growth and differentiation of progenitor/stem cells derived from the human mammary gland. Exp Cell Res 297:444–460
29. Whitehead RH, Quirk SJ, Vitali AA, Funder JW, Sutherland RL, Murphy LC (1984) A new human breast carcinoma cell line (PMC42) with stem cell characteristics. III. Hormone receptor status and responsiveness. J Natl Cancer Inst 73:643–648
30. Brannvall K, Korhonen L, Lindholm D (2002) Estrogen-receptor-dependent regulation of neural stem cell proliferation and differentiation. Mol Cell Neurosci 21:512–520
31. Miura T, Miura C, Ohta T, Nader MR, Todo T, Yamauchi K (1999) Estradiol-17beta stimulates the renewal of spermatogonial stem cells in males. Biochem Biophys Res Commun 264:230–234
32. Kuiper GG, Enmark E, Pelto-Huikko M, Nilsson S, Gustafsson JA (1996) Cloning of a novel receptor expressed in rat prostate and ovary. Proc Natl Acad Sci U S A 93:5925–5930
33. Ogawa S, Inoue S, Watanabe T, Hiroi H, Orimo A, Hosoi T, Ouchi Y, Muramatsu M (1998) The complete primary structure of human estrogen receptor beta (hER beta) and its heterodimerization with ER alpha in vivo and in vitro. Biochem Biophys Res Commun 243:122–126
34. Balfe PJ, McCann AH, Welch HM, Kerin MJ (2004) Estrogen receptor beta and breast cancer. Eur J Surg Oncol 30:1043–1050
35. Skliris GP, Munot K, Bell SM, Carder PJ, Lane S, Horgan K, Lansdown MR, Parkes AT, Hanby AM, Markham AF, Speirs V (2003) Reduced expression of oestrogen receptor beta in invasive breast cancer and its re-expression using DNA methyl transferase inhibitors in a cell line model. J Pathol 201:213–220
36. Paruthiyil S, Parmar H, Kerekatte V, Cunha GR, Firestone GL, Leitman DC (2004) Estrogen receptor beta inhibits human breast cancer cell proliferation and tumor formation by causing a G2 cell cycle arrest. Cancer Res 64:423–428
37. Shaaban AM, O'Neill PA, Davies MP, Sibson R, West CR, Smith PH, Foster CS (2003) Declining estrogen receptor-beta expression defines malignant progression of human breast neoplasia. Am J Surg Pathol 27:1502–1512
38. Krege JH, Hodgin JB, Couse JF, Enmark E, Warner M, Mahler JF, Sar M, Korach KS, Gustafsson JA, Smithies O (1998) Generation and reproductive phenotypes of mice lacking estrogen receptor beta. Proc Natl Acad Sci U S A 95:15677–15682
39. Korach KS, Couse JF, Curtis SW, Washburn TF, Lindzey J, Kimbro KS, Eddy EM, Migliaccio S, Snedeker SM, Lubahn DB, Schomberg DW, Smith EP (1996) Estrogen receptor gene disruption: molecular characterization and experimental and clinical phenotypes. Recent Prog Horm Res 51:159–186; discussion 158–186
40. Weihua Z, Makela S, Andersson LC, Salmi S, Saji S, Webster JI, Jensen EV, Nilsson S, Warner M, Gustafsson JA (2001) A role for estrogen receptor beta in the regulation of growth of the ventral prostate. Proc Natl Acad Sci U S A 98:6330–6335
41. Weihua Z, Saji S, Makinen S, Cheng G, Jensen EV, Warner M, Gustafsson JA (2000) Estrogen receptor (ER) beta, a modulator of ERalpha in the uterus. Proc Natl Acad Sci USA 97:5936–5941
42. Weihua Z, Warner M, Gustafsson JA (2002) Estrogen receptor beta in the prostate. Mol Cell Endocrinol 193:1–5
43. Jensen EV, Cheng G, Palmieri C, Saji S, Makela S, Van Noorden S, Wahlstrom T, Warner M, Coombes RC, Gustafsson JA (2001) Estrogen receptors and proliferation markers in primary and recurrent breast cancer. Proc Natl Acad Sci U S A 98:15197–15202

44. Clarke RB, Howell A, Anderson E (1997) Estrogen sensitivity of normal human breast tissue in vivo and implanted into athymic nude mice: analysis of the relationship between estrogen-induced proliferation and progesterone receptor expression. Breast Cancer Res Treat 45:121–133
45. Clarke RB, Howell A, Potten CS, Anderson E (1997) Dissociation between steroid receptor expression and cell proliferation in the human breast. Cancer Res 57:4987–4991
46. Tonetti DA, Rubenstein R, DeLeon M, Zhao H, Pappas SG, Bentrem DJ, Chen B, Constantinou A, Craig Jordan V (2003) Stable transfection of an estrogen receptor beta cDNA isoform into MDA-MB-231 breast cancer cells. J Steroid Biochem Mol Biol 87:47–55
47. Gustafsson JA, Warner M (2000) Estrogen receptor beta in the breast: role in estrogen responsiveness and development of breast cancer. J Steroid Biochem Mol Biol 74:245–248
48. Saji S, Jensen EV, Nilsson S, Rylander T, Warner M, Gustafsson JA (2000) Estrogen receptors alpha and beta in the rodent mammary gland. Proc Natl Acad Sci USA 97:337–342
49. Saji S, Sakaguchi H, Andersson S, Warner M, Gustafsson J (2001) Quantitative analysis of estrogen receptor proteins in rat mammary gland. Endocrinology 142:3177–3186
50. Foley EF, Jazaeri AA, Shupnik MA, Jazaeri O, Rice LW (2000) Selective loss of estrogen receptor beta in malignant human colon. Cancer Res 60:245–248
51. Iwao K, Miyoshi Y, Egawa C, Ikeda N, Noguchi S (2000) Quantitative analysis of estrogen receptor-beta mRNA and its variants in human breast cancers. Int J Cancer 88:733–736
52. Roger P, Sahla ME, Makela S, Gustafsson JA, Baldet P, Rochefort H (2001) Decreased expression of estrogen receptor beta protein in proliferative preinvasive mammary tumors. Cancer Res 61:2537–2541
53. Rutherford T, Brown WD, Sapi E, Aschkenazi S, Munoz A, Mor G (2000) Absence of estrogen receptor-beta expression in metastatic ovarian cancer. Obstet Gynecol 96:417–421
54. Speirs V, Malone C, Walton DS, Kerin MJ, Atkin SL (1999) Increased expression of estrogen receptor beta mRNA in tamoxifen-resistant breast cancer patients. Cancer Res 59:5421–5424
55. Speirs V, Adams IP, Walton DS, Atkin SL (2000) Identification of wild-type and exon 5 deletion variants of estrogen receptor beta in normal human mammary gland. J Clin Endocrinol Metab 85:1601–1605
56. Speirs V, Kerin MJ (2000) Prognostic significance of oestrogen receptor beta in breast cancer. Br J Surg 87:405–409
57. Swain SM (2001) Tamoxifen for patients with estrogen receptor-negative breast cancer. J Clin Oncol 19:93S–97S
58. Chang HG, Kim SJ, Chung KW, Noh DY, Kwon Y, Lee ES, Kang HS (2005) Tamoxifen-resistant breast cancers show less frequent methylation of the estrogen receptor beta but not the estrogen receptor alpha gene. J Mol Med 83:132–139
59. Shim GJ, Wang L, Andersson S, Nagy N, Kis LL, Zhang Q, Makela S, Warner M, Gustafsson JA (2003) Disruption of the estrogen receptor beta gene in mice causes myeloproliferative disease resembling chronic myeloid leukemia with lymphoid blast crisis. Proc Natl Acad Sci U S A 100:6694–6699
60. Imamov O, Morani A, Shim GJ, Omoto Y, Thulin-Andersson C, Warner M, Gustafsson JA (2004) Estrogen receptor beta regulates epithelial cellular differentiation in the mouse ventral prostate. Proc Natl Acad Sci U S A 101:9375–9380
61. Pais V, Leav I, Lau KM, Jiang Z, Ho SM (2003) Estrogen receptor-beta expression in human testicular germ cell tumors. Clin Cancer Res 9:4475–4482
62. Palmieri C, Saji S, Sakaguchi H, Cheng G, Sunters A, O'Hare MJ, Warner M, Gustafsson JA, Coombes RC, Lam EW (2004) The expression of oestrogen receptor (ER)-beta and its variants, but not ERalpha, in adult human mammary fibroblasts. J Mol Endocrinol 33:35–50
63. Russo J, Balogh GA, Chen J, Fernandez SV, Fernbaugh R, Heulings R, Mailo DA, Moral R, Russo PA, Sheriff F, Vanegas JE, Wang R, Russo IH (2006) The concept of stem cell in the mammary gland and its implication in morphogenesis, cancer and prevention. Front Biosci 11:151–172

64. Russo J, Hasan Lareef M, Balogh G, Guo S, Russo IH (2003) Estrogen and its metabolites are carcinogenic agents in human breast epithelial cells. J Steroid Biochem Mol Biol 87:1–25
65. Hu YF, Lau KM, Ho SM, Russo J (1998) Increased expression of estrogen receptor beta in chemically transformed human breast epithelial cells. Int J Oncol 12:1225–1228
66. Russo J, Lareef MH, Tahin Q, Hu YF, Slater C, Ao X, Russo IH (2002) 17Beta-estradiol is carcinogenic in human breast epithelial cells. J Steroid Biochem Mol Biol 80:149–162
67. Lareef MH, Garber J, Russo PA, Russo IH, Heulings R, Russo J (2005) The estrogen antagonist ICI-182-780 does not inhibit the transformation phenotypes induced by 17-beta-estradiol and 4-OH estradiol in human breast epithelial cells. Int J Oncol 26:423–429
68. Fernandez SV, Russo IH, Lareef M, Balsara B, Russo J (2005) Comparative genomic hybridization of human breast epithelial cells transformed by estrogen and its metabolites. Int J Oncol 26:691–695
69. Kehrl JH (1995) Hematopoietic lineage commitment: role of transcription factors. Stem Cells 13:223–241
70. Shivdasani RA, Orkin SH (1995) Erythropoiesis and globin gene expression in mice lacking the transcription factor NF-E2. Proc Natl Acad Sci U S A 92:8690–8694
71. Tsai S, Bartelmez S, Sitnicka E, Collins S (1994) Lymphohematopoietic progenitors immortalized by a retroviral vector harboring a dominant-negative retinoic acid receptor can recapitulate lymphoid, myeloid, and erythroid development. Genes Dev 8:2831–2841
72. Briggs JA, Burrus GR, Stickney BD, Briggs RC (1992) Cloning and expression of the human myeloid cell nuclear differentiation antigen: regulation by interferon alpha. J Cell Biochem 49:82–92
73. Briggs R, Dworkin L, Briggs J, Dessypris E, Stein J, Stein G, Lian J (1994) Interferon alpha selectively affects expression of the human myeloid cell nuclear differentiation antigen in late stage cells in the monocytic but not the granulocytic lineage. J Cell Biochem 54:198–206
74. Briggs RC, Briggs JA, Ozer J, Sealy L, Dworkin LL, Kingsmore SF, Seldin MF, Kaur GP, Athwal RS, Dessypris EN (1994) The human myeloid cell nuclear differentiation antigen gene is one of at least two related interferon-inducible genes located on chromosome 1q that are expressed specifically in hematopoietic cells. Blood 83:2153–2162
75. Briggs RC, Kao WY, Dworkin LL, Briggs JA, Dessypris EN, Clark J (1994) Regulation and specificity of MNDA expression in monocytes, macrophages, and leukemia/B lymphoma cell lines. J Cell Biochem 56:559–567
76. Hamada T, Tashiro K, Tada H, Inazawa J, Shirozu M, Shibahara K, Nakamura T, Martina N, Nakano T, Honjo T (1996) Isolation and characterization of a novel secretory protein, stromal cell-derived factor-2 (SDF-2) using the signal sequence trap method. Gene 176:211–214
77. Lindahl T, Satoh MS, Poirier GG, Klungland A (1995) Post-translational modification of poly(ADP-ribose) polymerase induced by DNA strand breaks. Trends Biochem Sci 20:405–411
78. Menissier-de Murcia J, Molinete M, Gradwohl G, Simonin F, de Murcia G (1989) Zinc-binding domain of poly(ADP-ribose)polymerase participates in the recognition of single strand breaks on DNA. J Mol Biol 210:229–233
79. Boulikas T (1991) Relation between carcinogenesis, chromatin structure and poly(ADP-ribosylation) (review). Anticancer Res 11:489–527
80. Althaus FR, Hofferer L, Kleczkowska HE, Malanga M, Naegeli H, Panzeter PL, Realini CA (1994) Histone shuttling by poly ADP-ribosylation. Mol Cell Biochem 138:53–59
81. Malanga M, Pleschke JM, Kleczkowska HE, Althaus FR (1998) Poly(ADP-ribose) binds to specific domains of p53 and alters its DNA binding functions. J Biol Chem 273:11839–11843
82. Pleschke JM, Kleczkowska HE, Strohm M, Althaus FR (2000) Poly(ADP-ribose) binds to specific domains in DNA damage checkpoint proteins. J Biol Chem 275:40974–40980
83. Zahradka P, Ebisuzaki K (1982) A shuttle mechanism for DNA-protein interactions. The regulation of poly(ADP-ribose) polymerase. Eur J Biochem 127:579–585

84. Le Rhun Y, Kirkland JB, Shah GM (1998) Cellular responses to DNA damage in the absence of Poly(ADP-ribose) polymerase. Biochem Biophys Res Commun 245:1–10
85. Cosi C, Marien M (1999) Implication of poly (ADP-ribose) polymerase (PARP) in neurodegeneration and brain energy metabolism. Decreases in mouse brain NAD+ and ATP caused by MPTP are prevented by the PARP inhibitor benzamide. Ann N Y Acad Sci 890:227–239
86. Ha HC, Snyder SH (2000) Poly(ADP-ribose) polymerase-1 in the nervous system. Neurobiol Dis 7:225–239
87. Pieper AA, Verma A, Zhang J, Snyder SH (1999) Poly (ADP-ribose) polymerase, nitric oxide and cell death. Trends Pharmacol Sci 20:171–181
88. MacMahon B, Cole P, Lin TM, Lowe CR, Mirra AP, Ravnihar B, Salber EJ, Valaoras VG, Yuasa S (1970) Age at first birth and breast cancer risk. Bull World Health Organ 43:209–221
89. Lambe M, Hsieh CC, Chan HW, Ekbom A, Trichopoulos D, Adami HO (1996) Parity, age at first and last birth, and risk of breast cancer: a population-based study in Sweden. Breast Cancer Res Treat 38:305–311
90. Kelsey JL, Gammon MD, John EM (1993) Reproductive factors and breast cancer. Epidemiol Rev 15:36–47
91. Moon RC (1981) Influence of pregnancy and lactation on experimental mammary carcinogenesis. In: Pike MC, Siiteri PK, Welsch CW (eds) Banbury report 8 hormones and breast cancer. Cold Spring Harbor Laboratory Press, Cold Spring Harbor, NY, pp 353–394
92. Sinha DK, Pazik JE, Dao TL (1988) Prevention of mammary carcinogenesis in rats by pregnancy: effect of full-term and interrupted pregnancy. Br J Cancer 57:390–394
93. Yang J, Yoshizawa K, Nandi S, Tsubura A (1999) Protective effects of pregnancy and lactation against N-methyl-N-nitrosourea-induced mammary carcinomas in female Lewis rats. Carcinogenesis 20:623–628
94. Welsch CW (1985) Host factors affecting the growth of carcinogen-induced rat mammary carcinomas: a review and tribute to Charles Brenton Huggins. Cancer Res 45:3415–3443
95. Russo J, Russo IH (1980) Influence of differentiation and cell kinetics on the susceptibility of the rat mammary gland to carcinogenesis. Cancer Res 40:2677–2687
96. Swanson SM, Whitaker LM, Stockard CR, Myers RB, Oelschlager D, Grizzle WE, Juliana MM, Grubbs CJ (1997) Hormone levels and mammary epithelial cell proliferation in rats treated with a regimen of estradiol and progesterone that mimics the preventive effect of pregnancy against mammary cancer. Anticancer Res 17:4639–4645
97. Rajkumar L, Guzman RC, Yang J, Thordarson G, Talamantes F, Nandi S (2001) Short-term exposure to pregnancy levels of estrogen prevents mammary carcinogenesis. Proc Natl Acad Sci U S A 98:11755–11759
98. Tay LK, Russo J (1981) Formation and removal of 7,12-dimethylbenz[a]anthracene—nucleic acid adducts in rat mammary epithelial cells with different susceptibility to carcinogenesis. Carcinogenesis 2:1327–1333
99. Russo IH, Koszalka M, Russo J (1991) Comparative study of the influence of pregnancy and hormonal treatment on mammary carcinogenesis. Br J Cancer 64:481–484
100. Russo J, Santucci-Pereira J, de Cicco RL, Sheriff F, Russo PA, Peri S, Slifker M, Ross E, Mello ML, Vidal BC, Belitskaya-Levy I, Arslan A, Zeleniuch-Jacquotte A, Bordas P, Lenner P, Ahman J, Afanasyeva Y, Hallmans G, Toniolo P, Russo IH (2012) Pregnancy-induced chromatin remodeling in the breast of postmenopausal women. Int J Cancer 31(5):1059–1070. doi:10.1002/ijc.27323
101. Belitskaya-Levy I, Zeleniuch-Jacquotte A, Russo J, Russo IH, Bordas P, Ahman J, Afanasyeva Y, Johansson R, Lenner P, Li X, de Cicco-Lopez RL, Peri S, Ross E, Russo PA, Santucci-Pereira J, Sheriff FS, Slifker M, Hallmans G, Toniolo P, Arslan AA (2011) Characterization of a genomic signature of pregnancy identified in the breast. Cancer Prev Res 4:1457–1464
102. Thordarson G, Jin E, Guzman RC, Swanson SM, Nandi S, Talamantes F (1995) Refractoriness to mammary tumorigenesis in parous rats: is it caused by persistent changes in the hormonal environment or permanent biochemical alterations in the mammary epithelia? Carcinogenesis 16:2847–2853

103. Wagner KU, Boulanger CA, Henry MD, Sgagias M, Hennighausen L, Smith GH (2002) An adjunct mammary epithelial cell population in parous females: its role in functional adaptation and tissue renewal. Development 129:1377–1386
104. Henry MD, Triplett AA, Oh KB, Smith GH, Wagner KU (2004) Parity-induced mammary epithelial cells facilitate tumorigenesis in MMTV-neu transgenic mice. Oncogene 23:6980–6985
105. Boulanger CA, Wagner KU, Smith GH (2005) Parity-induced mouse mammary epithelial cells are pluripotent, self-renewing and sensitive to TGF-beta1 expression. Oncogene 24:552–560
106. Trichopoulos D, Lagiou P, Adami HO (2005) Towards an integrated model for breast cancer etiology: the crucial role of the number of mammary tissue-specific stem cells. Breast Cancer Res 7:13–17
107. Srivastava P, Russo J, Russo IH (1997) Chorionic gonadotropin inhibits rat mammary carcinogenesis through activation of programmed cell death. Carcinogenesis 18:1799–1808
108. Srivastava P, Russo J, Russo IH (1999) Inhibition of rat mammary tumorigenesis by human chorionic gonadotropin associated with increased expression of inhibin. Mol Carcinog 26:10–19
109. Medina D, Kittrell FS (2003) p53 function is required for hormone-mediated protection of mouse mammary tumorigenesis. Cancer Res 63:6140–6143
110. Medina D (2004) Breast cancer: the protective effect of pregnancy. Clin Cancer Res 10:380S–384S
111. Sivaraman L, Conneely OM, Medina D, O'Malley BW (2001) p53 is a potential mediator of pregnancy and hormone-induced resistance to mammary carcinogenesis. Proc Natl Acad Sci U S A 98:12379–12384
112. Ginger MR, Gonzalez-Rimbau MF, Gay JP, Rosen JM (2001) Persistent changes in gene expression induced by estrogen and progesterone in the rat mammary gland. Mol Endocrinol 15:1993–2009
113. Ginger MR, Rosen JM (2003) Pregnancy-induced changes in cell-fate in the mammary gland. Breast Cancer Res 5:192–197
114. D'Cruz CM, Moody SE, Master SR, Hartman JL, Keiper EA, Imielinski MB, Cox JD, Wang JY, Ha SI, Keister BA, Chodosh LA (2002) Persistent parity-induced changes in growth factors, TGF-beta3, and differentiation in the rodent mammary gland. Mol Endocrinol 16:2034–2051
115. Russo J, Russo IH (2004) Endocrine control of breast development. In: Russo J, Russo IH (eds) Molecular basis of breast cancer: prevention and treatment, 1st edn. Springer, Berlin, pp 64–67
116. Russo J, Russo IH (1997) Role of hCG and inhibin in breast cancer. Int J Cancer 4:297–306
117. Liao MJ, Zhang CC, Zhou B, Zimonjic DB, Mani SA, Kaba M, Gifford A, Reinhardt F, Popescu NC, Guo W, Eaton EN, Lodish HF, Weinberg RA (2007) Enrichment of a population of mammary gland cells that form mammospheres and have in vivo repopulating activity. Cancer Res 67:8131–8138
118. Porter S, Scott SD, Sassoon EM, Williams MR, Jones JL, Girling AC, Ball RY, Edwards DR (2004) Dysregulated expression of adamalysin-thrombospondin genes in human breast carcinoma. Clin Cancer Res 10:2429–2440
119. Lind GE, Kleivi K, Meling GI, Teixeira MR, Thiis-Evensen E, Rognum TO, Lothe RA (2006) ADAMTS1, CRABP1, and NR3C1 identified as epigenetically deregulated genes in colorectal tumorigenesis. Cell Oncol 28:259–272
120. Gustavsson H, Wang W, Jennbacken K, Welen K, Damber JE (2009) ADAMTS1, a putative anti-angiogenic factor, is decreased in human prostate cancer. BJU Int 104:1786–1790
121. Gill ZP, Perks CM, Newcomb PV, Holly JM (1997) Insulin-like growth factor-binding protein (IGFBP-3) predisposes breast cancer cells to programmed cell death in a non-IGF-dependent manner. J Biol Chem 272:25602–25607
122. Kim HS, Ingermann AR, Tsubaki J, Twigg SM, Walker GE, Oh Y (2004) Insulin-like growth factor-binding protein 3 induces caspase-dependent apoptosis through a death receptor-mediated pathway in MCF-7 human breast cancer cells. Cancer Res 64:2229–2237

123. Mahadev K, Raval G, Bharadwaj S, Willingham MC, Lange EM, Vonderhaar B, Salomon D, Prasad GL (2002) Suppression of the transformed phenotype of breast cancer by tropomyosin-1. Exp Cell Res 279:40–51
124. Bharadwaj S, Thanawala R, Bon G, Falcioni R, Prasad GL (2005) Resensitization of breast cancer cells to anoikis by tropomyosin-1: role of Rho kinase-dependent cytoskeleton and adhesion. Oncogene 24:8291–8303
125. Russo J, Russo IH (1978) DNA labeling index and structure of the rat mammary gland as determinants of its susceptibility to carcinogenesis. J Natl Cancer Inst 61:1451–1459
126. Russo IH, Russo J (1978) Developmental stage of the rat mammary gland as determinant of its susceptibility to 7,12-dimethylbenz[a]anthracene. J Natl Cancer Inst 61:1439–1449
127. Russo J, Gusterson BA, Rogers AE, Russo IH, Wellings SR, van Zwieten MJ (1990) Comparative study of human and rat mammary tumorigenesis. Lab Invest 62:244–278
128. Russo J (1983) Basis of cellular autonomy in the susceptibility to carcinogenesis. Toxicol Pathol 11:149–166
129. Russo J, Russo IH (1998) Role of pregnancy and chorionic gonadotropin in breast cancer prevention. In: Birkhauser MH, Rozenbaum H (eds) Proc IV European congress on menopause. ESKA, Paris, pp 133–142
130. Russo J, Russo IH (2004) Biological and molecular basis of breast cancer. Springer, Heidelberg
131. Russo J, Rivera R, Russo IH (1992) Influence of age and parity on the development of the human breast. Breast Cancer Res Treat 23:211–218
132. Vessey MP, McPherson K, Roberts MM, Neil A, Jones L (1985) Fertility in relation to the risk of breast cancer. Br J Cancer 52:625–628
133. Kelsey JL, Horn-Ross PL (1993) Breast cancer: magnitude of the problem and descriptive epidemiology. Epidemiol Rev 15:7–16
134. Russo I, Russo J (1994) Role of hCG and inhibin in breast-cancer (review). Int J Oncol 4:297–306
135. Russo J, Balogh GA, Russo IH (2008) Full-term pregnancy induces a specific genomic signature in the human breast. Cancer Epidemiol Biomarkers Prev 17:51–66

Index

J. Russo and I.H. Russo, *Role of the Transcriptome in Breast Cancer Prevention*,
DOI 10.1007/978-1-4614-4884-6, © Springer Science+Business Media New York 2013

C

D

S

MIX
Papier aus verantwortungsvollen Quellen
Paper from responsible sources
FSC® C105338

If you have any concerns about our products,
you can contact us on
ProductSafety@springernature.com

In case Publisher is established outside the EU,
the EU authorized representative is:
Springer Nature Customer Service Center GmbH
Europaplatz 3, 69115 Heidelberg, Germany

Printed by Libri Plureos GmbH
in Hamburg, Germany